Pediatric Primary Care Case Studies

Edited by

Catherine E. Burns, PhD, RN, CPNP-PC, FAAN
Professor Emeritus
School of Nursing
Oregon Health & Science University
Portland, Oregon

Beth Richardson, DNS, RN, CPNP, FAANP
Associate Professor
Coordinator of the Pediatric Nurse Practitioner Program
School of Nursing
Indiana University
Indianapolis, Indiana

Margaret A. Brady, PhD, RN, CPNP-PC
Co-Director of the Pediatric Nurse Practitioner Program
Azusa Pacific University
Azusa, California
Professor
School of Nursing
California State University, Long Beach
Long Beach, California

JONES AND BARTLETT PUBLISHERS
Sudbury, Massachusetts
BOSTON   TORONTO   LONDON   SINGAPORE

World Headquarters

Jones and Bartlett Publishers
40 Tall Pine Drive
Sudbury, MA 01776
978-443-5000
info@jbpub.com
www.jbpub.com

Jones and Bartlett Publishers
Canada
6339 Ormindale Way
Mississauga, Ontario L5V 1J2
Canada

Jones and Bartlett Publishers
International
Barb House, Barb Mews
London W6 7PA
United Kingdom

Jones and Bartlett's books and products are available through most bookstores and online booksellers. To contact Jones and Bartlett Publishers directly, call 800-832-0034, fax 978-443-8000, or visit our website, www.jbpub.com.

Substantial discounts on bulk quantities of Jones and Bartlett's publications are available to corporations, professional associations, and other qualified organizations. For details and specific discount information, contact the special sales department at Jones and Bartlett via the above contact information or send an email to specialsales@jbpub.com.

The authors, editor, and publisher have made every effort to provide accurate information. However, they are not responsible for errors, omissions, or for any outcomes related to the use of the contents of this book and take no responsibility for the use of the products and procedures described. Treatments and side effects described in this book may not be applicable to all people; likewise, some people may require a dose or experience a side effect that is not described herein. Drugs and medical devices are discussed that may have limited availability controlled by the Food and Drug Administration (FDA) for use only in a research study or clinical trial. Research, clinical practice, and government regulations often change the accepted standard in this field. When consideration is being given to use of any drug in the clinical setting, the health care provider or reader is responsible for determining FDA status of the drug, reading the package insert, and reviewing prescribing information for the most up-to-date recommendations on dose, precautions, and contraindications, and determining the appropriate usage for the product. This is especially important in the case of drugs that are new or seldom used.

Production Credits
Publisher: Kevin Sullivan
Acquisitions Editor: Emily Ekle
Acquisitions Editor: Amy Sibley
Associate Editor: Patricia Donnelly
Editorial Assistant: Rachel Shuster
Associate Production Editor: Lisa Cerrone
Marketing Manager: Rebecca Wasley
V.P., Manufacturing and Inventory Control: Therese Connell
Composition: Paw Print Media
Cover Design: Kristin E. Parker
Cover Images: *Background*—Crayon Image: © Anikasalsera/Dreamstime.com; Handprint Image: © Lori Martin/Dreamstime.com. *Photos, clockwise from top*—© Vadim Ponomarenko/Dreamstime.com; Courtesy of Catherine E. Burns; © Anette Romanenko/Dreamstime.com; Courtesy of Catherine E. Burns.
Printing and Binding: Malloy, Inc.
Cover Printing: Malloy, Inc.

Library of Congress Cataloging-in-Publication Data
Pediatric primary care case studies / [edited by] Catherine E. Burns, Beth Richardson, Margaret A. Brady.
    p. ; cm.
  Includes bibliographical references and index.
  ISBN 978-0-7637-6136-3 (pbk.)
  1. Pediatrics—Case studies. I. Burns, Catherine E. II. Richardson, Beth, CPNP. III. Brady, Margaret A.
  [DNLM: 1. Pediatrics—Problems and Exercises. 2. Primary Health Care—Problems and Exercises.
WS 18.2 P37015 2010]
  RJ58.P45 2010
  618.92—dc22
                                         2009011613

6048

Printed in the United States of America
13 12 11 10 09   10 9 8 7 6 5 4 3 2 1

Contents

Preface   ix

Contributors   xi

Chapter 1

**Diagnostic Reasoning:
A Complex Issue for Pediatric Primary Care   1**
Catherine E. Burns

UNIT 1   Developmental Problems

Chapter 2

An Infant with Gross Motor Delays   11
Elissa Jones-Hua

Chapter 3

A Toddler with Language and Social Delays   27
Brian T. Maurer

Chapter 4

A School-Age Child with School Failure Problems   43
Ann Marie McCarthy
Sharon Yearous

Chapter 5

An Adolescent with Fatigue   59
Dawn Lee Garzon

UNIT 11   Functional Health and Mental Health Problems

Chapter 6

The Well Infant   75
Anna Marie Hefner

Chapter 7

The Overweight Preschooler   85
Margaret A. Brady

Chapter 8

The Breastfed Infant Who Is Not Gaining   103
Pamela J. Hellings

Chapter 9

The Constipated 8-Year-Old   115
Tamra D. Kehoe

Chapter 10

The Teen Needing a Sports Physical   133
Catherine G. Blosser

Chapter 11

The Infant Not Sleeping Through the Night   163
Lynne Henry

Chapter 12

The Child Who Is Very Busy and Doesn't Listen   175
Larry W. Lynn

Chapter 13

The Boy Who Draws a Picture Suggesting an Abuse Situation   193

Beth Moore

Margaret A. Brady

Chapter 14

The 14-Year-Old Who Looks Depressed   207

Ann M. Guthery

Chapter 15

The Teen Who Thinks She Might Be Gay   221

Sheran M. Simo

UNIT 111   Diseases

Chapter 16

The Child with a Fever for Six Days   231

Ritamarie John

Chapter 17

The Wheezing Child   251

Deborah A. Bohan

Chapter 18

The Overweight Child with High Blood Sugar   267

Arlene Smaldone

Chapter 19

Migrant Farmworker's Toddler with Anemia   291

Veronica Kane

Chapter 20

The Child with a Headache   321
Ritamarie John

Chapter 21

The Preschooler with a Red Eye   335
Michele Saysana

Chapter 22

The Toddler with Recurrent Ear Infections   347
Kathleen M. Boyd

Chapter 23

The Athlete Who Experienced Syncope   359
Patrick E. Killeen

Chapter 24

The Child Presenting with Cough   377
Jennifer Newcombe

Chapter 25

The Child with Vomiting and Diarrhea   387
Ardys M. Dunn
Victoria Winter

Chapter 26

Three Cases of Oral Trauma   405
Prashant Gagneja
John Peterson

Chapter 27

The Preschooler with Urinary Urgency and Urinary Incontinence   417
Shelly J. King

Chapter 28

The 15-Year-Old Girl Who Wants Birth Control   427

Deborah Stiffler

Chapter 29

The 16-Year-Old Girl with a Vaginal Discharge   441

Teral Gerlt

Chapter 30

The Child with an Itchy Rash   455

Donald W. Kennerley

Chapter 31

The Teen Boy with Acne   467

Catherine E. Burns
Danielle J. Poulin

Chapter 32

The Limping Child   481

Jan Bazner-Chandler

Chapter 33

The Late-Preterm Baby Beginning Well-Child Care   493

Lori J. Silao

Chapter 34

A Child with Short Stature   507

George Anadiotis

Index   519

|Preface

Pediatric Primary Care Case Studies was written by nurse practitioner, physician, and physician assistant clinicians and educators who believe that health care for children in primary care settings should be excellent, whatever the discipline of the provider. This book is designed to exemplify the critical thinking process and diagnostic reasoning skills that clinicians should use to assess and manage treatment of the infants, young children, and adolescents who present with common signs and symptoms of childhood illnesses or behavioral problems in providers' practice settings.

These cases were developed to reflect common pediatric healthcare problems such as depression, obesity, autism, attention-deficit hyperactivity disorder, and environmental health concerns among many others. The chapter authors address key elements in the reasoning process that should be employed as the provider gathers data about a case from the initial presentation through the diagnostic decision and highlight the standards of treatment for the selected diagnosis. Additionally, the cases discuss concerns surrounding children from a variety of socioeconomic, cultural, familial, and developmental backgrounds.

We hope this book helps fill in gaps in the clinical knowledge of students who have completed didactic courses and guides their preparation for clinical work by taking an organized approach to symptom-driven presentations.

Organization of the Book

This book is divided into three sections, which follow an introductory chapter reviewing essential features of the diagnostic approach to pediatric primary care. Unit I covers developmental problems in children from infancy through adolescence—motor delays, language delays, learning problems in school, and sleeping too much. The cases in Unit II involve functional health problems, beginning with a case study illustrating principles of health maintenance. Subsequent cases include an obese child with unhealthy nutritional practices, a breastfeeding infant who is not gaining weight, a constipated child, a child needing a preparticipation sports examination, an infant not sleeping through the night, a child with attention and hyperactivity issues, a child who is abused, a child with possible depression, and a teen who thinks she might be gay. Finally, Unit III surveys common medical symptoms and related conditions which the provider will see and should not miss—wheezing, type 2 diabetes, anemia, headache, a red eye, recurrent ear infections, a heart murmur, cough, vomiting and diarrhea, dental trauma, urinary tract infection, a birth control request, sexually transmitted infection, an itchy rash, acne, a limp, preterm infant care, and a possible genetic syndrome.

This book was designed to demonstrate how a healthcare provider should incorporate the concepts of critical thinking into a practical model of diagnostic reasoning that he or she would use daily. Scenarios are presented with information emerging chronologically. The author for each case becomes the expert guiding the reader in the decision-making process, thinking through the case as it progresses. Additional elements such as familial, developmental, and cultural issues are intertwined in the case presentations to illustrate how they are factored into the assessment and decision-making process.

Generally, as in real practice, the child and family member(s) present with a "chief complaint." From there the experts begin to reason their way through the assessment process, considering some diagnoses and reflecting as they go along on the data they have collected and what they know about the etiology and pathophysiology associated with various symptoms. A Making the Diagnosis section follows some discussion of various diagnoses already considered and discarded during the assessment process. The Management section sometimes involves several visits, with additional information coming in at each visit related to confirmation of the diagnosis, initial management, long-term management, and confirmation of problem resolution. The references used reflect the "best practice" information the expert is using for decision-making, but are by no means an exhaustive review of the literature. Tables are sometimes used to display information in an easily viewed style.

Cases are initially described in terms of the symptom because that is where the clinician must begin. A symptom analysis occurs early in the presentation of each case. From there, various diagnoses are considered and either supported or refuted with further data. Of course, some diagnoses, such as acne, are predominantly self-evident whereas others, such as a syncope episode, require greater analysis before a diagnosis can be determined.

About the Authors and Contributors

The contributors for this text were selected for their expertise and experience in caring for infants, children, and adolescents. They represent a variety of specialties and are from all parts of the United States and Canada. Each of the lead authors has more than 20 years of experience practicing and teaching pediatric primary care to a variety of students in nurse practitioner and medical fields. Dr. Richardson has authored a text on pediatric physical assessment that is widely used, as well as a book of pediatric practice guidelines. The idea for this book is hers and she should be credited with its creation. Drs. Burns and Brady are coauthors on the widely used *Pediatric Primary Care* text (Elsevier, 2009), which is now in its fourth edition and used by many pediatric and family nurse practitioner programs.

We hope this book will meet a current educational need of all pediatric primary care provider students and their educators and preceptors as well as less experienced clinicians in practice.

Contributors

George Anadiotis, DO
Pediatric Development &
    Rehabilitation Services
Legacy Emanuel Hospital for
    Children
Portland, Oregon

Jan Bazner-Chandler, MSN, CNS,
    CPNP
Assistant Professor
Azusa Pacific University
Azusa, California

Catherine G. Blosser, MPA-HA,
    PNP-BC, RN
Pediatric Nurse Practitioner (Retired)
Multnomah County Health
    Department
Oak Grove, Oregon

Deborah A. Bohan, MEd, PA-C
Physician Assistant
Department of Pediatrics
Allegheny General Hospital
Pittsburgh, Pennsylvania

Kathleen M. Boyd, MD
Assistant Professor of Pediatrics
Indiana University School of
    Medicine
Indianapolis, Indiana

Ardys M. Dunn, PhD, PNP, RN
Associate Professor Emeritus
School of Nursing
University of Portland
Portland, Oregon
Professor (Retired)
Samuel Merritt College School of
    Nursing
Oakland, California

Prashant Gagneja, DDS, MS
Chairman, Pediatric Dentistry
School of Dentistry
Oregon Health & Science University
Portland, Oregon

Dawn Lee Garzon, PhD, CPNP
Assistant Professor
University of Missouri–St. Louis
St. Louis, Missouri

Teral Gerlt, MS, PNP, RN-C, WHCNP
Instructor
School of Nursing
Oregon Health and Sciences
    University
Portland, Oregon

Ann M. Guthery, PhD(c), PMHNP, RN
Clinical Assistant Professor
College of Nursing
Arizona State University
Phoenix, Arizona

Anna Marie Hefner, MSN, MAEd,
    RN, CPNP
Associate Professor
School of Nursing
Azusa Pacific University
Azusa, California

Pamela J. Hellings, PhD, RN, CPNP-R
Professor Emeritus
Oregon Health and Science
    University
Portland, Oregon

Lynne Henry, MSN, RN, CPNP
St. Vincent Health Network
North Vernon, Indiana

Ritamarie John, DNP, CPNP-PC
Program Director
Assistant Professor of Pediatrics
Columbia University
School of Nursing
New York, New York

Elissa Jones-Hua, MSN, RN, CPNP
Nurse Practitioner
Developmental Pediatrics
Riley Hospital for Children
Indiana University
Indianapolis, Indiana

Veronica Kane, PhD, CPNP
Pediatric Specialty Coordinator
Clinical Assistant Professor
MGH Institute of Health Professions
Boston, Massachusetts

Tamra D. Kehoe, MSN, RN, CPNP
Pediatric Nurse Practitioner
Multnomah County Health
    Department
Portland, Oregon

Donald W. Kennerly, MD, CCFP
Belleville General Hospital
Belleville, Ontario, Canada

Patrick E. Killeen, MS, PA-C
Department of Pediatrics
Danbury Hospital
Danbury, Connecticut

Shelly J. King, MSN, RN, CPNP
Director Children's Continence Center
Pediatric Urology, Riley Hospital for
    Children
Indiana University
Indianapolis, Indiana

Larry W. Lynn, MD
Assistant Professor
Physician Assistant Program
Butler University
Indianapolis, Indiana

Brian T. Maurer, MS, PA-C
Pediatric Physician Assistant
Enfield Pediatric Associates
Enfield, Connecticut

**Ann Marie McCarthy, PhD, RN,
    FAAN**
College of Nursing
University of Iowa
Iowa City, Iowa

Beth Moore, MSN, RN
Long Beach Memorial Medical Center
Miller Children's Hospital
Long Beach, California

**Jennifer Newcombe, MSN, CNS,
    CPNP**
Loma Linda Children's Hospital
Loma Linda, California

John Peterson, DDS
Professor (Part time)
Pediatric Dentistry
School of Dentistry
Oregon Health and Science
    University
Portland, Oregon

Danielle J. Poulin, MSN, PNP, RNC
Pediatric Nurse Practitioner
Western Medical Center–Santa Ana
Santa Ana, California

Michele Saysana, MD, FAAP
Clinical Assistant Professor of
    Pediatrics
Indiana University School of
    Medicine
Indianapolis, Indiana

Lori J. Silao, MN, RN, CNNP
Adjunct Faculty
Azusa Pacific University
Azusa, California

Sheran M. Simo, MSN, FNP-BC
Nurse Practitioner
St. Vincent Primary Care Network
Indianapolis, Indiana

Arlene Smaldone, DNSc, CPNP, CDE
Assistant Professor
Columbia University
School of Nursing
New York, New York

Deborah Stiffler, PhD, RN, CNM
Assistant Professor
Coordinator, Women's Health Nurse
    Practitioner Major
Indiana University
School of Nursing
Indianapolis, Indiana

Victoria Winter, MSN, PNP, RN
Adjunct Professor
Azusa Pacific University
Pediatric Nurse Practitioner Program
Azusa, California
Cardiothoracic Intensive Care
Children's Hospital Los Angeles
Los Angeles, California

Sharon Yearous, PhD, RN, CPNP, NCSN
Executive Director
Iowa School Nurse Association
Cedar Rapids, Iowa

Chapter 1

Diagnostic Reasoning: A Complex Issue for Pediatric Primary Care

Catherine E. Burns

Pediatric primary care providers use a critical thinking skill set to help them arrive at a diagnosis and to provide efficient, cost-effective care to their patients. Evidence-based practice has become a guiding principle that is consistent with the diagnostic reasoning process: using the best information available as one thinks through the pros and cons of various pathways that emerge along the road from diagnosis to management and problem resolution.

The clinician is typically taught to move from assessment to diagnosis to intervention and, finally, to evaluation in a linear fashion; however, in reality, the practicing clinician considers various diagnoses while conducting the assessment so that data will confirm or refute various possible diagnoses. Sometimes, management strategies also have diagnostic elements—if the plan doesn't work, then perhaps the diagnosis was wrong. For example, if iron supplementation does not result in raising a low hemoglobin level and further tests were not done initially, then perhaps the problem was not iron-deficiency anemia. Therefore, additional tests must be done to identify another diagnosis. Thus, the use of iron supplementation had diagnostic elements. The problem-solving or diagnostic reasoning process may be linear (i.e., diagnosis generally comes before intervention), but during a given episode the process generally is more convoluted than linear. The clinician also must think on his or her feet with only minimal time for reflection. Delivering primary care to pediatric patients often presents unique diagnostic challenges for healthcare providers.

Evidence-based care is the standard; however, using the best evidence available when assessing and managing patients is not always easy because new information is forever emerging, sometimes validating and sometimes refuting previous "best evidence." There is also an issue of selecting the best evidence for a particular case. Will the healthcare provider have to generalize data from adults studies to children? Are data from a study of children in another country or involving a different population appropriate to use? Is using a particular diagnostic test essential or optional? Should one consider a new therapy, a drug for example, before best evidence results are available?

Which variables, such as race, gender, culture, educational level, age, or family constellation, might make a difference in selecting the best management plan? Will a nationally recognized clinical practice guideline work to the benefit of the patient, given the setting, clinical resources, financial status, and other factors of the client at hand? Has new information emerged that the clinician isn't yet aware of? Many factors affect the assessment process, conclusions reached, and plans made. Pediatric primary care using the best evidence available may not always be in the best interests of a particular child if the interventions or strategies do not take into consideration the child's and family's unique needs, values, and personal preferences.

Content for Pediatric Primary Care: The Three Domains of Healthcare Problems

Pediatric healthcare problems in this book are conceptualized as falling into three domains: diseases, functional and mental health problems, and developmental problems (Burns, 1991a, 1991b, 1992a, 1992b, 2009). These are domains for the *content* of health care, not the *context* for care. The disease domain includes physiological problems, which are diagnosed and managed at the organ system and cellular levels. Pneumonia, anemia, traumatic injuries, and acne are all examples of diseases diagnosed and managed at this level. Functional health problems are significant issues in pediatric primary care. Nutrition problems such as obesity, elimination problems such as encopresis and enuresis, and sleep problems all fall into this domain. Cognitive perceptual problems such as attention deficit hyperactivity disorder and mental health/coping problems also fit into this domain. Problems in this domain are considered primarily as concerns involving daily living and managed through changes in those patterns of daily living. That is not to say physiological issues are not involved, often neurological in nature or with genetic components, but they cannot be treated primarily through cellular treatment modalities. Finally, there are problems of the developmental domain. These are problems that affect the child's developmental trajectory over the long term—issues of motor, language, social, and cognitive development. These problems are just as significant to the child's well-being as many diseases can be. They must be treated through therapies to modify and promote developmental progression.

   This book is organized according to these domains. Units I and II address developmental, functional health, and mental health problems. Unit III concentrates on diseases in all body systems. Depending on the child's developmental age and chief complaint, the clinician should always ask one or two questions in each of the three domains while focusing major attention on the problem at hand. Examples of ancillary questions might include items such as:

- How is he doing in school? or How is school going? (developmental domain)

- How is breastfeeding going now? (functional health domain)
- Is he sleeping through the night? (functional health domain)
- How is toilet training going? (functional health domain)
- What are your plans after you finish high school? (developmental domain)
- What is her mood like most of the time at home? (mental health domain)
- Is she easy or hard to get along with? (mental health or developmental domain)
- Can she do all the things other kids her age are doing? (developmental domain)
- Have you noticed any problems with his health since he was here last? (disease domain)

Such questions can be interjected in a visit while washing hands or doing the physical examination, while waiting for the parent to undress the child, or during the interview process. The provider should always be scanning or conducting surveillance for emerging problems in all three domains.

Context for Pediatric Primary Care: Complicating Factors

The clinician not only needs to provide evidence-based care as much as possible for problems within one or more of the three domains, but also needs to attend to some complicating factors for each client and family.

Developmental Factors

Developmental assessment is an absolutely key element to pediatric primary care. It needs to be considered at every step, not only as content, but also as context. Both the physiology and psychology of children change with age, so one cannot parcel off physical ailments, saying that they are physiologically the same as in adults and therefore can be treated similarly. The infant and young child may not present with symptoms that are easily recognizable due to their immature nervous and physiological systems, limited language skills, limited experiences with illness, and social skills that keep them from being cooperative when needed. Diagnosing problems is difficult. Further, management always needs to consider the developmental level of the child, whether it is choosing a medication form that the child will accept, asking the child and family to change health behaviors, or some other element that best practice would expect to be incorporated into a healthcare plan. Additionally, parents develop along with their children, learning new skills to adapt to their child's forever-emerging new behaviors. Incorporation of developmental factors into daily practice during every pediatric encounter provides the key difference between pediatric experts and those who just provide some care to children.

Family-Centered Care

Another essential factor to consider when providing primary care to children is the child's family. Children come for care in a dyadic relationship with their parents. Even if they are adolescents, the parent is a ghost in the room if not actually present. The parents are the lens through which the child is seen outside of the examining room, and, even within the room, are providing information about changes from normal behavior or physiology as seen by them. The parents know and provide the history, support the child through the physical examination and other tests, and are the ones who must be educated to care for the child after the clinical visit. Without full cooperation and understanding from those caregiving adults, the health care of the child will fall short of its desired goals. Thus, it is in the best interests of child, parents, and the clinician to use the available parent or caregiver to best advantage, listening to and forming an alliance with that essential member of the healthcare team.

Family-centered care involves more than recognizing the parent as essential to the provision of health care for the child. It also involves recognition that families can have problems at the family systems level in addition to the individual child's health problems. In this case, family problems become content, not just context. These, too, must be dealt with because an unhealthy family system often negatively affects the health of the child, both physically and psychologically. Some examples of family problems include social isolation, caregiver role strain, alterations in parenting, family communication problems, absent family members, and inadequate healthcare and financial resources. An example of a family problem is given in one of the case studies, a mother of a newborn whose husband is overseas in the military. She not only does not have the support of the absent parent, but also has additional strains due to anxieties about his safety and perhaps financial problems because military families often receive limited income and perhaps loss of income if a reservist has to put a civilian job on hold. Unless this mother can be adequately supported, she will be unable to provide optimal parenting to her new infant. Divorced families, gay and lesbian parents, single parent families, teen parents, and others may have special needs, too. In any case, the pediatric primary care provider needs to assess for potential family problems even though the family may be functioning well and no concerns emerge. Pediatric primary care occurs on two levels, child and family.

Comorbidities

Another complicating factor relates to comorbidities. Patients often have several problems to address at a given visit. Which problem should be addressed first? Will the management of one problem compromise the status of a second problem or limit the options for treatment? For instance, a child with allergies may not do well with some antibiotics if she has an infection or suggestions of certain foods for diet management if the child is overweight. Or the child with a mental health problem such as anxiety may have greater difficulty coping with a chronic disease that requires aggressive management such as type 1 diabetes. Of course, adults also experience comorbidity problems. Nevertheless, multiple problems affect the pathways that the provider must navigate to provide optimal care. Care is often nonlinear and convoluted, as stated earlier.

Cultural Factors

Cultural differences are the norm in the United States and all other parts of the world these days. Values and beliefs, communication styles, language, healthcare practices, understandings of health and illness causes and cures, food preferences and preparation practices, parenting practices, and other aspects of daily life vary among different people. The clinician must incorporate cultural understandings into assessment and management. Again, adding these factors into the recipe for "best practice" care makes it ever more complex!

The Process of Providing Care As Modeled in This Book

The cases in this book reflect the stories of children and their families who are seen in pediatric primary care settings, and were written by a variety of expert clinicians. In each case, they move from symptom analysis to a mental review of all the possible diagnoses that should be considered and gathering of further data to support or refute the various suppositions, gradually narrowing the list down to the diagnosis that best fits the picture presented by the patient.

Management generally involves three pathways: further diagnostic elements, treatment of the specific condition, and then education to prevent subsequent episodes, limit complications, and promote healthy behaviors and understanding of the problem by the patient and family. The clinician should always consider these three elements, although the plan may not include all elements. In primary care settings, the child's diagnosis is frequently evident from history and physical examination findings alone with no diagnostic testing needed. In some instances, only basic diagnostic tests are required to arrive at a diagnosis or to help determine the management plan. Typically, extensive and/or elaborate additional diagnostic testing is necessary only if the child does not improve or his or her condition worsens. Treatment and education are always required, although sometimes they are delivered over several visits and not all at one time.

Caregiving Teams

Management may also include referrals to other healthcare professionals and then coordination of care across people and/or agencies. Primary care has been defined as comprehensive, continual, and coordinated; however, it is not "solo." No one healthcare provider can be expected to have all the skills, knowledge, and time to provide total care to patients. Rather, care is initiated in the healthcare setting in which a need is identified. Sometimes the initial provider, be it nurse, nurse practitioner, physician, or physician assistant, can manage the case from beginning to end. However, often referrals are made to specialists in the management of specific disease entities, mental health conditions, education problems, or other aspects of unique healthcare needs. The primary care provider role is envisioned as being comprehensive—all body systems and healthcare needs will be evaluated. It is also viewed as continual—care is provided over the long term for a variety of problems and a familiarity with the client and family will be established. Coordination is the element of taking into consideration all the various elements of care necessary for the child and family, setting priorities, and helping the family navigate various specialty services for the resolution of their healthcare problems in a cost-effective, efficient, supportive manner. Sometimes the care can be delivered within the given time slot on the schedule of patients for the day, but sometimes it involves taking other time for phone calls, preparation of papers for consultations and insurance, and even visits with the family to the school or elsewhere. All this work also requires assessment, making a diagnosis of the functionality of the plan given various healthcare systems, and management that may involve providing access to care rather than specialized therapies. The primary care provider uses teams of experts to support his or her work with patients.

Key Points

1. Primary care assessment is linear in broad strokes but convoluted along the pathways from symptom analysis to diagnosis to treatment.
2. Evidence-based practice is easy to conceptualize but difficult to execute.
3. Three domains for primary care practice need to be considered as the provider completes a comprehensive assessment of a patient: disease, functional and mental health, and development.
4. A variety of complicating contextual factors makes assessment and management more difficult: developmental issues, family issues, comorbidities, and cultural variables.
5. Management should consider three basic elements: diagnostic, therapeutic, and educational plans, though not all will be necessary for a given patient.
6. Primary care providers need to use other specialists in a variety of healthcare, mental health, and educational fields to support and provide the care necessary to maximize the health of children and families in their practices.

REFERENCES

Burns, C. (2009). Child and family health assessment. In C. Burns, A. Dunn, M. Brady, N. Starr, & C. Blosser (Eds.), *Pediatric primary care* (4th ed., pp. 12–40). St. Louis: Elsevier.

Burns, C. (1992a). A new assessment model and tool for nurse practitioners. *Journal of Pediatric Health Care, 6,* 73–81.

Burns C. (1992b). Using a comprehensive taxonomy of diagnoses to describe the practice of pediatric nurse practitioners: Findings of a field study. *Journal of Pediatric Health Care, 7,* 115–121,

Burns, C. (1991a). Development and content validity testing of a comprehensive classification of diagnoses for use by pediatric nurse practitioners. *Nursing Diagnosis, 2,* 93–104.

Burns, C. (1991b). Parallels between research and diagnosis: The reliability and validity issues of clinical practice. *Nursing Practice, 16,* 42–50.

Developmental Problems

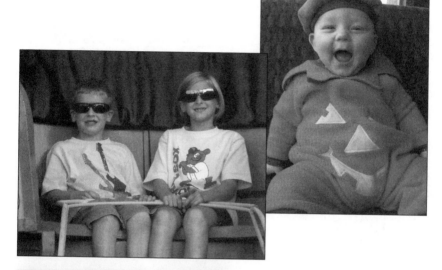

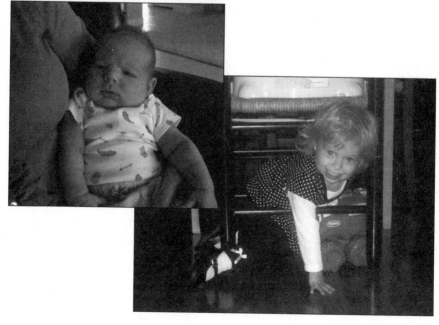

Chapter 2

An Infant with Gross Motor Delays

Elissa Jones-Hua

A child's acquisition of developmental milestones is a dynamic process, and early identification of infants and children with developmental delays is an important facet of primary care practice. Appropriate data collection, consideration of alternative diagnoses, and development of an individualized plan of care are important components, just as with management of diseases. Early identification of at-risk infants and children should lead to early intervention; delays may harm the child. The problem for the provider is deciding when early gaps in developmental progress merit added attention and perhaps referral versus patience with hope for gains that will keep the child within normal limits.

Educational Objectives
1. List the five categories of developmental milestones.
2. Identify at least three risk factors that contribute to developmental delays.
3. Identify abnormal persistence of primitive reflexes.
4. Describe the management of an infant with a motor delay.

Case Presentation and Discussion

Maya Conteh is a 9-month-old African female who comes to your outreach clinic for an initial evaluation. She is accompanied by her mother who speaks Arabic and English. The mother is concerned that Maya is not developing like other children her age. The family emigrated from Sudan one year ago and now lives in low-income student housing because the father is in graduate school. This is their first child. The maternal grandparents are also temporarily living in the household and help out with Maya.

What questions will you ask Maya's mother related to her concerns? ■

Your review of Maya's birth history reveals the following information: Maya was born 11 weeks early and weighed only 2½ pounds. According to the mother, the doctors were surprised to see what a strong and active girl she was. However, when Maya was just a few days old, she stopped breathing and was put on a ventilator. After 24 hours she was able to breathe on her own. According to the mother, the doctors ran a myriad of tests to

11

find out what had happened, but they couldn't find anything wrong. The remainder of Maya's time in the hospital was uneventful and she went home after 2 months.

Once at home, Maya's mother noticed that she drooled and choked easily when she drank from her bottle. As months went by, Maya's mother noticed other things that were odd. Maya couldn't hold her head up straight, roll, or sit with support. In fact, she still can't do these things. She cries a lot and becomes stiff with rage.

What other questions do you need to ask? ■

Before answering this question, here is some more information about child development and acquisition of developmental milestones that you need to consider.

Development of Infants

Development is divided into five categories: gross motor, fine motor, language, cognition, and social/emotional growth. Refer to Table 2-1 for a summary of infant developmental milestones by age in months.

Gross Motor Development

Gross motor skills occur in a typical sequence. The three general patterns of physical development are development occurs in a head to foot progression, strength and coordination of the limbs begin close to the body and move outward, and motor responses proceed from general to specific (Deloian & Berry, 2009).

Reflexes govern much of an infant's behavior during the first 3 months of life. As the newborn reflexes fade, more purposeful movements replace them. Gaining strength and coordination in their muscles allows infants to explore and manipulate objects in their environment. A typical infant follows a known developmental progression, which starts at birth. A summary of primitive reflexes is found in Table 2-2.

Gross motor skills require large muscles or groups of muscles in order to carry out activities. When performing a task, these muscles should act in a coordinated way to accomplish a movement. An important element to consider when assessing gross motor skills is posture. Poor posture makes purposeful movements more difficult to perform. Examples of gross motor tasks in infancy are head control, sitting, rolling over, standing, crawling, and walking.

Tone is an important element in motor skills development. Muscular tone is the basic and constant ongoing contraction or muscular activity in the muscles. The three categories of tone are normal, hypotonic (decreased muscle tone), and hypertonic (increased muscle tone). Infants and children who are hypotonic appear floppy, similar to a rag doll. Hypotonic infants have difficulty maintaining posture against gravity. They often prefer to sit, lie on the floor, or lean against something. In contrast, infants and children with

Table 2–1   Developmental Milestones for Infants (Birth–12 months)

Age (in months)	Gross Motor	Fine Motor	Cognitive	Social
1	Holds head up when prone	Holds hands tightly fisted	Fixes and follows face	Makes throaty sounds
2	Holds chest up when prone	Holds hands unfisted half the time	Tracks horizontally past midline	Shows social smile, coos
3	Head partly lags when child pulls to sitting	Bats at objects; sustains grasp if an object is placed on palm	Regards small objects	Babbles, echoes speaker immediately
4	Rolls front to back; Shows no head lag	Reaches for objects when supine	Mouths objects, shakes rattle; Turns head to localize voice	Laughs out loud, listens to and verbalizes back, makes guttural sounds
5	Rolls back to front; Sits with pelvic support	Transfers objects from hand to mouth to hand	Attains objects he/she reaches for; regards inanimate noise	Makes "raspberries"; smiles/vocalizes to mirror
6	Sits propped on hands (tripod)	Transfers objects from hand to hand; immature rake	Looks for dropped toy; Removes cloth covering face	Discriminates strangers (stranger anxiety begins)
7	Sits without support	Does a commando crawl	Bangs/shakes toys; attempts to hold object in each hand	Imitates speech sounds
8	Gets into sitting position from supine	Shows scissor grasp; Holds block in each hand	Pulls string to pull toy closer; Plays peek-a-boo	Says "dada" inappropriately; Responds selectively to name
9	Pulls to stand; Crawls	Shows inferior pincer grasp; Uncovers hidden objects	Rings bell	Says "mama" inappropriately; Waves goodbye
10	Cruises; Walks with two-hand support	Points with index finger; Shows pincer grasp	Bangs two cubes together; Looks at pictures in book	Says "dada" or "mama" specifically; Comprehends "no"

(continues)

Table 2-1 Developmental Milestones for Infants (Birth–12 months) (Continued)

Age (in months)	Gross Motor	Fine Motor	Cognitive	Social
11	Stands alone Walks with one-hand support		Uncovers toy under cup	Says first word (other than "mama" or "dada")
12	Walks independently	Shows fine pincer grasp Attempts two-block tower		Follows one-step commands, indicates desires by pointing

Source: Adapted from Kimball, R. D. (2001). Healthy growth and development of the newborn/infant. In C. Green-Hernandez, J. K. Singleton, & D. Z. Aronson (Eds.), *Primary care pediatrics* (p. 94). Philadelphia, PA: Lippincott Williams & Wilkins. Used with permission.

Table 2-2   Primitive Reflexes

Reflex	Appearance	Disappearance
Sucking	Birth	3–4 months
Rooting	Birth	3–4 months
Palmar grasp	Birth	3 months
Stepping	Birth	6–8 weeks
Moro	Birth	4 months
Galant	Birth	4–6 months
Babinski	Birth	12 months
Plantar grasp	Birth	8–15 months
Asymmetical tonic neck	2 weeks	6 months
Landau	3 months	15 months to 2 years
Head righting	4–6 months	Persists voluntarily
Parachute	8–9 months	Persists voluntarily

*Different sources vary on the timing of the appearance and disappearance of these primitive reflexes.

Source: Adapted from Feldman, H. M. (2002). Developmental-behavioral pediatrics. In B. J. Zitelli & H. W. Davis (Eds.), *Atlas of pediatric physical diagnosis* (4th ed., p. 59). Philadelphia, PA: Mosby. Used with permission.

hypertonia appear stiff and do not move in a smooth, natural manner. An abnormality in muscular tone is a component of impaired motor skills. Infants and children with abnormal tone expend an enormous amount of energy to carry out movements and maintain postures (Alderman, 2001).

Some causes of gross motor delays include the following conditions: birth trauma, chromosomal abnormalities, inborn errors of metabolism, mitochondrial disorders, brain tumor, hypothyroidism, muscular dystrophies, abuse or neglect, sensory deprivation, shaken baby syndrome, sepsis, malnutrition or starvation, fetal alcohol syndrome, Werdnig-Hoffman disease, and lead or mercury poisoning.

Oro-Motor Development

Oro-motor development sometimes is considered a part of fine motor development because it requires the use of small muscles in a delicately coordinated fashion. Children with problems of drooling, choking, chewing, swallowing, and speech generally have neurological impairments in the area of the brain that controls these functions.

Developmental Delays

Multiple studies have established typical chronological ages at which specific milestones are reached, though with wide ranges. Influences from the social environment, nutrition, disease, and psychologic factors all interact with genetic factors to determine the speed and pattern of development. Individual differences in development are also strongly affected by opportunities to observe and practice specific movements. When children have not reached developmental milestones by the expected time period, they are considered to be developmentally delayed.

Motor delays in children are recognized when the child has a 25% delay in one area of typical development, such as gross motor (Wilson Jones, Morgan, Shelton, & Thorogood, 2007); for example, at 8 months the infant fails to do what a 6-month-old can do. Delays can occur in all five areas of development or may occur in one or two areas. Early motor delays are often a sign of neurological dysfunction.

Epidemiology

At least 8% of all preschool children from birth to 6 years have developmental problems and demonstrate delays in one or more developmental areas (Tervo, 2003).

Prematurity Effects on Development

Infants who are born prematurely are at increased risk for growth problems, developmental delays, and complicated medical problems. Recently, survival rates and outcomes for premature infants have improved. In 2006, nearly 13% of all live births in the United States resulted in infants being born prematurely (U.S. National Center for Health Statistics, 2009). When caring for a preterm child in a primary care setting it is important to account for prematurity by monitoring growth and development according to adjusted age (chronologic age minus weeks premature equals corrected gestational age) (LaHood & Bryant, 2007).

From the above review, some other information you should obtain includes the following:

- Prenatal and neonatal history:
  - Current obstetric history including access to prenatal care, infections or illnesses during pregnancy, and alcohol, cigarette, or drug use during pregnancy
  - Birth history: gestational age, birth weight, length, head circumference, delivery type, APGAR scores, length of stay in hospital
  - Maternal/fetal conditions
  - Complications of labor and delivery
  - Significant neonatal diagnoses
- Past medical history:

- Hospitalizations, surgeries, injuries/illnesses; any MRI, chromosomal, or urine genetic diagnostic tests performed
  - Source of medical care since birth
  - Current medications: over-the-counter, prescribed, supplements, or herbal remedies
  - Immunization status
- Family history:
  - Parents' ages, number of children, medical illness, developmental or psychiatric disabilities, ages and health of siblings, paternal and maternal family history of diseases
- Social history:
  - Insurance coverage, because it may determine where healthcare services can be accessed for developmental problems; educational background; financial and emotional support; dietary considerations
  - Values and beliefs
- Developmental history:
  - At what ages were milestones met: fine motor, gross motor, language, cognitive, and social skills
- Functional health history:
  - Feeding history: breastmilk or formula; introduction of solids; difficulties with eating or drinking; problems with choking, gagging, coughing, or swallowing while eating or drinking
- Any frequent bouts of upper respiratory infections, pneumonias, or chronic upper airway congestion, which could indicate possible penetration and/or aspiration and feeding dysfunction
- Elimination: any problems with urination (retention), having an adequate number of wet diapers, frequency of stooling, problems with constipation
- Sleep: nighttime arousals, snoring, number and length of daytime naps
- Daycare attendance
- Activities the child enjoys

The mother responds that she had limited access to prenatal care. She denies use of alcohol, cigarettes, or drugs. The pregnancy progressed normally with the exception of onset of premature labor and rupture of membranes. Maya spent 2 months in the NICU. Since discharge Maya has not had any hospitalizations, surgeries, or injuries. Maya is frequently congested and easily becomes ill with respiratory infections. The family history of diseases is unremarkable.

The infant is not currently taking any medications. She is behind in her immunizations because Maya has not received her 6-month series. She previously received immunizations at a local health department but medical care has been sporadic because the family moved shortly after Maya came home from the NICU. The family has limited resources and has been unable to locate a primary care physician. Interim care has been obtained at multiple urgent visit clinics or emergency departments.

The mother gives Maya baby formula (20 cal/oz) and offers baby food two to three times daily. She believes that Maya doesn't like the baby food because she frequently pushes it out with her tongue. Maya is difficult to feed because she frequently coughs while eating and/or drinking and drools a lot. As for elimination, the mother reports five wet diapers per day with a bowel movement consisting of balls of stool every other day. Maya's sleep has improved although she continues to wake during the night, crying and arching her back. The mother notes that her legs become stiff.

Developmentally, Maya has a social smile, makes a few vocalizations, and enjoys being held. She is able to pick up small objects with her hands but does not transfer them. The mother feels she makes good eye contact and tracks objects. Her motor and oromotor skills were described earlier.

Maya is cared for by her mother or grandparents during the day. The mother has a few neighbors with children of similar ages but does not share babysitting time or interact socially with them.

What parts of the physical examination will be particularly important for this child? ■

Physical examination. Upon physical examination, you find a thin, normocephalic female infant in no acute distress. Corrected gestational age is noted to be 6 months and 1 week old. Length is between the third and fifth percentile with weight below the third percentile. Ophthalmoscopic examination reveals strabismus. Examination of the oropharynx reveals an intact palate with a positive gag reflex. Drooling is evident. The abdomen is rounded and palpation reveals stool. You focus special attention on the neurological examination. Muscle tone is greater in the lower extremities than the upper extremities, with clonus at the ankles. At times she exhibits hyperextension and adduction (scissoring) of the lower extremities. Deep tendon reflexes are brisk. She exhibits head lag when pulled from sitting and has poor trunk control. Primitive reflexes (asymmetric tonic neck reflex and Moro reflex) are present. The remainder of the physical examination is within normal limits.

Does Maya have developmental delays for a 6-month corrected age infant? If so, in what areas? ■

Considering the milestones for normal children at 6 months of age, Maya has not achieved full head control (4-month skill), rolling (5-month skill), or sitting propped (6-month skill). She also has significant oro-motor problems with her choking, drooling, and tongue thrusting. Although she has some beginning fine motor skills with picking up objects, she is not yet transferring them hand to mouth (5-month skill). Her decreased trunk tone and increased lower extremity tone with ankle clonus are also worrisome observations. The presence of asymmetric tonic neck and Moro reflexes, which should all have been assimilated into more mature movements by 4 to 6 months, is also abnormal.

Are there some laboratory or radiological studies that would be helpful to you at this point in your decision making? ■

Diagnostic Studies

Based on the above history and physical examination, further diagnostic studies are warranted. Maya has problems with feeding, constipation, gross motor skills, and strabismus. Laboratory tests including a complete blood count (rule out infection, anemia), complete metabolic panel (evaluate electrolytes, nutritional status), thyroid-stimulating hormone (thyroid disorder), and lead level (high levels can cause developmental delay) would provide a quick clinical snapshot.

An abdominal X-ray would evaluate stool burden because chronic constipation can cause diminished desire to eat. If there is suspicion of aspiration, the child should be referred for a modified barium swallow or video swallow. Decreased oral motor skills, resulting in prolonged feeding time and ineffective swallowing patterns leading to aspiration, are common and lead to malnutrition or inadequate growth (Wilson Jones, Morgan, & Shelton, 2007).

Due to the abnormal neurologic examination, a computed tomography (CAT scan) or magnetic resonance imaging (MRI) would be indicated to rule out brain damage. In addition, the finding of strabismus would indicate a need for referral to an ophthalmologist. Chromosomal and other genetic studies may be obtained later if needed.

Making the Diagnosis

The neurodevelopmental examination, history and physical, and the child's developmental profile should be combined to formulate a neurodevelopmental diagnosis. Maya's history and physical examination findings are consistent with an upper motor neuron lesion, such as in cerebral palsy. Indications of an upper motor neuron lesion include increased tone, muscle weakness, exaggerated reflexes, and continued primitive reflexes. Atrophy and fasciculations are indicative of a lower motor neuron lesion, although mild atrophy may develop in children with upper motor neuron lesions due to disuse of muscles.

Social isolation and limited economic resources are other factors to consider in providing this family with care.

Cerebral Palsy Information

Pathophysiology

Cerebral palsy (CP) is an umbrella term encompassing a group of *nonprogressive* disorders of posture and movement caused by a defect or insult to the central nervous system (Wilson Jones, Morgan, Shelton, & Thorogood, 2007). In prema-ture infants (< 32 weeks or < 2,500 g), the most likely cause of CP is injury to the periventricular white matter of the brain, which results in intraventricular hemorrhage or periventricular leukomalacia. The motor tracts in the developing brain of a premature infant between 24 and 32 weeks gestation are vulnerable to injury. Postnatal risk factors associated with cerebral palsy include asphyxia, seizures (within 48 hours of birth), cerebral infarction, hyperbilirubinemia, sep-sis, respiratory distress syndrome/chronic lung disease, meningitis, postnatal steroids, intraventricular hemorrhage, periventricular leukomalacia, shaken baby syndrome, and head injury (Wilson Jones et al., 2007).

Some infants are born with CP whereas others acquire it after they are born. Early signs of CP usually appear before 3 months of age. On average, a child with cerebral palsy is not diagnosed until approximately 12 months of age or later. Identifying the predominant motor characteristics is one method of classifying CP. Motor characteristics include the following: spastic, hypo-tonic, athetotic, dystonic, and/or ataxic movements. In addition, it is important to describe the pattern of limb involvement including monoplegia, diplegia, triplegia, hemiplegia, or quadriplegia (Wilson Jones, Morgan, Shelton, & Thorogood, 2007).

When making the diagnosis, the healthcare provider must be cautious of the child who is *losing* developmental milestones, because this may indicate a degenerative process (spinal muscular atrophy or mitochondrial myopathy) and not CP. A diagnosis of CP is often easier if there is known brain damage, which is documented by CAT scan or MRI. Although CAT scans identify brain malformations, structures and abnormalities that are closer to bony structures can be visualized more clearly with an MRI (Blosser & Reider-Demer, 2009). If a metabolic syndrome or genetic disorder is suspected, high resolution chromo-somes or biochemical studies would be needed. Therefore, a referral to a devel-opmental pediatrician for a definitive diagnosis is indicated.

Epidemiology
Many studies have shown that cerebral palsy occurs in 1 in 3,000 live births.

Cultural and Ethnic Factors

Maya's family is at a disadvantage when facing the prospect of significant health care for their infant girl, as are many immigrant families. They may have different understandings of healthcare conditions as well as limited expe-rience with the U.S. healthcare system as compared with the system for health care in their country of origin. Culture colors one's views of causation of illness and appropriate treatment regimens. Communication is also difficult, not only because of language differences, but also due to different ways of interacting, expressing one's feelings and thoughts, and being socially appropriate. Finally, economic resources can create barriers to healthcare services. Thus, utilization of medical services by immigrant families is often episodic and frequently occurs in settings such as emergency departments.

Extended families play a prominent role in many immigrant cultures. They are an important source of strength, but they may also create conflicts with use of health services and adaptation to U.S. healthcare customs (American Academy of Pediatrics, 1997). You need to take into account these common issues for immigrants and individualize care for this particular family.

Management

How do you plan to treat this child with probable cerebral palsy? ■

Once a developmental delay has been identified, it is imperative not to adopt a wait-and-see approach. Immediate referral for an initial evaluation and treatment at a multidisciplinary clinic is required. Multidisciplinary clinics use a team approach to provide care for children with multiple medical needs. The team includes developmental pediatricians, orthopedists, physiatrists (rehabilitation), neurologists, nurses, speech pathologists, physical and occupational therapists, and social workers. Services from an ophthalmologist, dentist, geneticist, and registered dietician may be recommended based on the needs of the child. Specialized therapists are often required to educate the family in the use of adaptive equipment such as splints, wheelchairs, walkers, and augmentative communication devises (Blosser & Reider-Demer, 2009; Wilson Jones, Morgan, & Shelton, 2007).

It is essential that the primary care provider coordinate the child's care with the other members of the healthcare team. The multidisciplinary clinic does not replace the role of the primary care provider in providing well or sick child care.

Therapeutic plan: What needs to be done therapeutically? ■

Interventions are aimed at increasing functionality, improving capabilities, and sustaining health in terms of fostering locomotion, cognitive development, social interaction, and independence. The goal of CP management is not to cure or to achieve normalcy (Krigger, 2006), but rather, to help maximize and coordinate movement, minimize discomfort and pain, and prevent long-term complications. The effects of CP can often be reduced with early and ongoing treatment. Children younger than 3 years old can greatly benefit from early intervention services, which is a system of services generally coordinated through educational service districts that support infants and toddlers with disabilities and their families. Referrals can be made by the primary care provider or concerned family members. The referral should be initiated while waiting for an appointment for an initial evaluation in a multidisciplinary clinic.

Associated problems with CP include mental retardation, seizures, vision difficulties, limb shortening and scoliosis, feeding difficulties, dental problems, hearing loss, joint problems, and problems with spatial awareness. The primary care provider, as well as the developmental team, should be involved in surveillance activities of the child and schedule routine assessments to manage emerging comorbidities as early as possible.

Treatment Options

CP is a lifelong condition for which there is no cure. Treatment is focused on improving capabilities. CP doesn't always cause profound disabilities. The earlier treatment begins the better chance children have of overcoming developmental disabilities or learning new ways to accomplish personally challenging tasks. The type and amount of treatment depends on how many problems the child has and the level of severity. Early intervention services (physical, occupational, speech, and developmental therapy) that focus on mobilization, stretching, relaxation, positioning, and bracing are the primary management techniques for spasticity.

Medication management is also a more recent mainstay of treatment. The goal of drug therapy is to reduce the effects of CP and prevent complications by altering muscle tone and/or abnormal movements. Medications may include anticholinergics (trihexyphenidyl, benztropine), oral diazepam (Valium), baclofen (Lioresal), tizanidine (Zanaflex), and dantrolene (Dantrium). Injections of botulinum toxin (Botox) directly into spastic muscles may provide a temporary reduction in spasticity and thus facilitate physical therapy. If the child has a seizure disorder, anticonvulsants will also be prescribed and monitored by a neurologist (Blosser & Reimer-Demer, 2009).

Baclofen is a medication that is used to lessen spasticity. Intrathecal baclofen pump therapy uses an implantable device to deliver a liquid form of baclofen directly to the cerebrospinal fluid surrounding the spinal cord. By delivering baclofen directly to the intrathecal space, an effective level of the medication can be achieved with much smaller doses than with oral administration, thereby reducing the incidence of adverse effects.

Surgical treatment may include soft tissue release to relieve flexion deformities, tendon transfers to optimize functional use of the extremities, and osteotomies to correct deformities. Surgery may also be used to sever overactivated nerves (called a selective dorsal root rhizotomy).

In Maya's case, it would be appropriate to make a referral for early intervention services as well as a consult by a developmental pediatrician through a multidisciplinary clinic. You may also make a recommendation for a swallow study to evaluate for safety of oral feedings. Additionally, you prescribe Miralax for constipation and recommend dietary modification including increasing fluids. You suggest bringing a person from the local Sudanese community with more experience in the U.S. healthcare system if the family is uncomfortable going to the multidisciplinary clinic alone.

Valium may be prescribed for leg spasms but should not be used in infants less than 6 months of age or in children who do not have spasmodic episodes.

Further treatment options will be recommended by the multidisciplinary team. Based on parental report, Maya will need her 6-month immunizations today.

Educational plan: What will you do to educate the family about gross motor delays and suspected CP? ■

Points to make through discussion include:

- Share concerns with parents when you become suspicious of cerebral palsy. Parents may understand and cope better with the eventual diagnosis of cerebral palsy if they feel involved in the diagnostic process from the beginning.
- Explain the possible diagnoses and pathophysiology.
- Learn from the family about their understanding of cerebral palsy or similar conditions in their country, what causes it, and how it is treated. Incorporate their expectations into the plan of care as possible and explain differences in approaches from one country to the other.
- Discuss what to expect from the initial evaluation from early intervention services as well as the developmental pediatrician in the multidisciplinary clinic.
- Explain the reasons behind the recommendation for a swallow study. Discuss causes and symptoms of possible feeding dysfunction.
- Provide informational handouts on newly prescribed medications, such as Miralax and Valium, and discuss directions for administration.
- Provide clear instructions about how to access early intervention services and a developmental multidisciplinary clinic in your area.
- Answer the family's questions.

When do you want to see this patient back again? ■

First, you will need to follow up on the results of the swallow study and determine appropriate interventions based on the findings. Second, you will need to follow up on the developmental team evaluation. The length of time it takes to get a new patient into a multidisciplinary clinic varies and may take several months; however, once the patient is seen, the developmental pediatrician and team will dictate a letter to the provider with further recommendations and follow-up. Based on the above information, it would be feasible to have the patient return to your clinic in 3 to 4 weeks to check on weight and feeding issues, or sooner depending on the results of the swallow study. You may need to adjust the level of care based on the needs of the patient and family. Of course, you will need to make appointments for well child visits and to monitor the child's weight, nutrition, and constipation issues.

Maya's mother verbalizes an understanding of the information and asks appropriate questions. The grandparents are available to provide emotional support. The mother is concerned about conveying the correct information to her husband and asks if it would be alright for him to call with questions. The family does not express any opinions at this point about the cause and management of children with conditions such as cerebral palsy in their country. You happily agree to meet with him if they have additional questions, knowing that the perceptions of disease causation and treatment vary from culture to culture and should be addressed with the family again.

What long-term issues do you need to be aware of for children with cerebral palsy or similar motor disorders? What complications may arise? ■

Children with CP who receive no interventions have poorer functional abilities. Developmentally they make less progress and are at increased risk for contractures and deformities (Blosser & Reider-Demer, 2009). A common secondary complication of CP is hip subluxation. Increased tone causes muscular forces to be unbalanced, which can lead to structural straightening of the femoral neck (Alderman, 2001).

The prognosis of CP is uncertain in nearly all children at the time of diagnosis, particularly with respect to specific outcomes such as functional ability, language, or cognitive ability. CP does not become worse or better over time; however, it poses different kinds of problems at different stages of life. Treatments have to be changed and adjusted as the person grows older. Ongoing medical care is indicated at every stage of the disorder.

CP itself is generally not a cause of death; however, it can shorten a person's life span for other, related reasons. Lung infections that can lead to pneumonia and other diseases are more common among people with CP. Poor nutrition can also contribute to the incidence of infections in this population.

The intellectual potential of a child born with CP often will not be known until the child starts school. People with CP are more likely to have some type of learning disability. The ability to live independently with CP also varies widely depending on the severity of the disability. Some individuals with CP will require assistance for all activities of daily living whereas others can live semi-independently, needing support only for certain activities. Still others can live in complete independence.

Is cerebral palsy preventable? ■

Preventive measures are aimed at improving prenatal care by routinely testing pregnant women for Rh factor in order to prevent blood incompatibility. Additionally, newborn jaundice is being treated by photo therapy in order to prevent severe brain damage from kernicterus. Other preventive programs are focused on preventing prematurity, reducing exposure of pregnant women to infections, and reducing unnecessary exposure to X-rays. Measures also are being taken to control maternal diabetes, anemia, and other nutritional deficiencies.

What resources are available for healthcare providers and families? ■

Parents whose child has been diagnosed with CP often ask questions that involve concern and anxiety about their child's future. Families face many challenging demands, including both emotional and physical. Meeting the challenges of a disability requires families to rely upon their inner strength and the support of others. Equally important are the support and services the family and child receive from educational and other social service agencies.

Services for children with disabilities are now mandated from birth to 21 years under the Individuals with Disabilities Education Act (IDEA). IDEA requires that families be involved with the planning, development, and implementation of services throughout a child's life. IDEA helps families in the development of an individualized family services plan (IFSP). Starting at age 3, an individualized education program (IEP) should be developed for children who previously had an IFSP. The IEP focuses on long-term goals and objectives for educating the child. Children with disabilities (including infants and toddlers) are entitled to receive special education and related services based on their individual needs, which are determined by an assessment and evaluation. Gross motor delays alone may grant eligibility for Supplemental Security Income, which, in turn, may (in most states) provide Medicaid eligibility (United Cerebral Palsy, 2008). The financial resources available for this family, which is only in the country temporarily, is less positive. What support might be available through the home country is an area the family could explore.

Key Points from the Case

1. Recognize delays early through periodic developmental screening.
2. Hear and interpret parental concerns.
3. Coordinate the family's access to services and additional referrals for specialty care and treatment.
4. Be aware of cultural beliefs and practices in regards to treatment.
5. Advocate for the patient and family and offer ongoing emotional support

---

REFERENCES

Alderman, A. (2001). The physically challenged child. In C. Green-Hernandez, J. K. Singleton, & D. Z. Aronson (Eds.), *Primary care pediatrics* (pp. 217–228). Philadelphia, PA: Lippincott, Williams & Wilkins.

American Academy of Pediatrics. (1997). Committee on community health services. Health care for children of immigrant families. *Pediatrics, 100*(1), 153–156.

Blosser, C. G., & Reider-Demer, M. (2009). Neurologic disorders. In C. Burns, A. Dunn, M. Brady, N. Starr, & C. G. Blosser (Eds.), *Pediatric primary care* (pp. 634–672). St. Louis, MO: Elsevier.

Deloian, B., & Berry, A. (2009). Developmental management in pediatric primary care. In C. Burns, A. Dunn, M. Brady, N. Starr, & C. G. Blosser (Eds.), *Pediatric primary care* (pp. 53–70). St. Louis, MO: Elsevier.

Feldman, H. M. (2002). Developmental-behavioral pediatrics. In B. J. Zitelli & H. W. Davis (Eds.), *Atlas of pediatric physical diagnosis* (4th ed., pp. 58–86). Philadelphia, PA: Mosby.

Kimball, R. D. (2001). Healthy growth and development of the newborn/infant. In C. Green-Hernandez, J. K. Singleton, & D. Z. Aronson (Eds.), *Primary care pediatrics* (p. 93–128). Philadelphia, PA: Lippincott Williams & Wilkins.

Krigger, K. W. (2006). Cerebral palsy: An overview. *American Family Physician, 73*(1), 91–100.

LaHood, A., & Bryant, C. (2007). Outpatient care of the premature infant. *American Family Physician, 76*(8), 1159–1164.

Tervo, R. (2003). Identifying patterns of developmental delays can help diagnose neurodevelopmental disorders. *A Pediatric Perspective, 12*(3), 1–6.

United Cerebral Palsy. (2008). *Cerebral palsy—facts & figures.* Retrieved October 19, 2008, from http://www.ucp.org/ ucp_channeldoc.cfm/1/11/10427/10427/447

U.S. National Center for Health Statistics. (2009). Births: Final data for 2006. *National Vital Statistics Reports 57* (7), 1-101. Retrieved March 18, 2009, from www.cdc.gov/nchs/data/nvsr/nvsr57/nvsr57_07.pdf

Wilson Jones, M., Morgan, E., & Shelton, J. (2007). Primary care of the child with cerebral palsy: A review of systems (Part II). *Journal of Pediatric Health Care, 21*(4), 226–237.

Wilson Jones, M., Morgan, E., Shelton, J., & Thorogood, C. (2007). Cerebral palsy: Introduction and diagnosis (Part I). *Journal of Pediatric Health Care, 21*(3), 146–152.

Chapter 3

A Toddler with Language and Social Delays

Brian T. Maurer

The ability to perform a thorough toddler developmental assessment is an essential skill that needs to be cultivated by all pediatric healthcare providers. Particularly disturbing is the child who isn't beginning to talk, because language development provides a window that reflects cognitive development. The provider needs to identify problems as early as possible in order to begin necessary interventions. The farther behind the child becomes, the more difficult it will be to bring him or her into the normal range again because normal children are progressing rapidly at this time. Currently, children with language and social delays are appearing all too often in primary care practices, and many parents are frightened of the possibility of autism as a diagnosis for their once normal-appearing child whose language is now delayed.

Educational Objectives
1. Review the developmental milestones for toddlers.
2. Describe the screening and assessment strategies to identify a child with language and social delays and a child who needs to be screened for autism.
3. Describe the primary care provider's role in coordination of services and family support for children with autism or other developmental delays.

Case Presentation and Discussion

Ms. Jones brings her twin boys into the office for their 18-month well child visit. Peter and James are fraternal twins, born vaginally at 36 weeks gestation. To date, with the exception of several minor colds, both boys have enjoyed good health. A quick review of the records shows that both boys have grown well, although Peter ranks slightly higher in his growth parameters (height, weight, and head circumference) than James.

You greet Ms. Jones as you enter the exam room and begin to explore the boys' developmental progress with several open-ended questions, knowing that developmental surveillance is a recommended part of all well child visits, especially at the 9-, 18-, and 30-month visits. Furthermore, you are aware of the American Academy of

Pediatrics' recommendations to use an autism-specific screen at the 18-month visit (American Academy of Pediatrics [AAP], 2006).

Toddler and Preschooler Development

What specific developmental milestones should be sought out at the 18-month visit? ■

Speech and expressive language skills begin to emerge by 15 months of age. Most toddlers engage in active jargoning, laying down underlying speech patterns through vocal inflection and intonation, by their first birthday. In addition, many 15-month-olds use the words "dada" and "mama" specifically to indicate their father and mother, as well as three other words. They also engage in verbal play, pointing to body parts when named and producing animal sounds when asked. The child with no documented expressive speech at 16 months of age is delayed in this area. By 18 months of age, most toddlers will have a vocabulary of 15–20 words. Additional developmental milestones are delineated in Table 3-1.

Given that these twins are fraternal, would you expect to find any marked differences in their development? ■

Fraternal twins, like other siblings, may demonstrate considerable variation in achieving developmental milestones but the variation should be within the range of normal milestones.

Information About Autistic Spectrum Disorders and Language Delays

Autistic spectrum disorders (ASDs) are neurodevelopmental disorders in which children exhibit a lack of age-appropriate personal-social, adaptive, and communication skills. Children with ASDs demonstrate restricted interests, perseverative behaviors with repetitive activities, and qualitative impairments in sharing interests and enjoyment with others. Insistence on maintaining nonfunctional routines and rituals in daily life are additional hallmarks of these disorders.

Pervasive developmental disorder, not otherwise specified (PDD-NOS) is considered to be a subthreshold diagnosis where the young child exhibits characteristics of autism disorder (AD) but fails to meet the strict criteria to allow a formal diagnosis of AD (Figure 3-1).

Asperger syndrome (AS) is a form of AD found in older children. Children with AS do not exhibit the same degree of speech and language problems as children with AD or PDD-NOS.

Table 3-1 Developmental Milestones for Toddlers 18 Months of Age	
Developmental Area	**Characteristics**
I. Gross motor	Runs and climbs well
	Walks up steps
	Directed throwing
	Climbs into adult chair
II. Fine motor	Uses a spoon and cup
	Stacks three or more blocks
	Imitates scribbling
	Dumps pellet
	Drinks from a cup with little spilling
III. Social	Actively engages in social interaction
	Shows fear, anger, affection, and jealousy
IV. Language	Able to say 15–20 words clearly
	Uses two-word phrases and imitates words
	Follows two-step commands (18–24 months)
	Vocabulary increasing (18–24 months)
	Enjoys simple stories (18–24 months)
	Recognizes pronouns (18–24 months)

Etiology

To date, the etiology of ASDs remains elusive. Researchers have postulated that genetic (Muhle, Trentacoste, & Rapin, 2004) and, to a lesser extent, environmental influences play a role. It is highly likely that the etiology is multifactorial (Barbaresi, Katusic, & Voight, 2006).

Epidemiology

The prevalence of ASDs has increased 10-fold over the past several decades. Earlier studies demonstrated a prevalence of 1 in 2,000; recent figures show a frequency of 1 in 150 (Autism and Developmental Disabilities Monitoring Network, 2007), with males outnumbering females by a ratio of 3.5 to 1. With these odds, it is likely that most clinicians will diagnose or follow a child with ASD in the primary care setting.

A timely diagnosis is imperative for successful intervention for the child with ASD.

A. A total of six (or more) items from (1), (2), and (3), with at least two from (1), and one each from (2) and (3):

   (1) Qualitative impairment in social interaction, as manifested by at least two of the following:

   (a) Marked impairment in the use of multiple nonverbal behaviors such as eye-to-eye gaze, facial expression, body postures, and gestures to regulate social interaction

   (b) Failure to develop peer relationships appropriate to developmental level

   (c) Lack of spontaneous seeking to share enjoyment, interests, or achievements with other people (e.g., by a lack of showing, bringing, or pointing out objects of interest)

   (d) Lack of social or emotional reciprocity

   (2) Qualitative impairments in communication as manifested by at least one of the following:

   (a) Delay in, or total lack of, the development of spoken language (not accompanied by an attempt to compensate through alternative modes of communication such as gesture or mime)

   (b) In individuals with adequate speech, marked impairment in the ability to initiate or sustain a conversation with others

   (c) Stereotyped and repetitive use of language or idiosyncratic language

   (d) Lack of varied, spontaneous make-believe play or social imitative play appropriate to developmental level

   (3) Restricted repetitive and stereotyped patterns of behavior, interests, and activities, as manifested by at least one of the following:

   (a) Encompassing preoccupation with one or more stereotyped and restricted patterns of interest that is abnormal either in intensity or focus

   (b) Apparently inflexible adherence to specific, nonfunctional routines or rituals

   (c) Stereotyped and repetitive motor mannerisms (e.g., hand or finger flapping or twisting, or complex whole-body movements)

   (d) Persistent preoccupation with parts of objects

B. Delays or abnormal functioning in at least one of the following areas, with onset prior to age 3 years: (1) social interaction, (2) language as used in social communication, or (3) symbolic or imaginative play.

C. The disturbance is not better accounted for by Rett Disorder or Childhood Disintegrative Disorder

Source: From *Diagnostic and Statistical Manual of Mental Disorders, Fourth Edition Text Revision (DSM-IV-TR)*. Washington DC: American Psychiatric Association; 2000:75. Retrieved at http://www.cdc.gov/ncbdd/autism/overview_diagnostic_criteria.htm

Figure 3-1 Diagnostic criteria for 299.00 autistic disorder.

Data for the Diagnosis
History

Peter has developed several words: he says "dada" and "mama," as well as "ball," "baba" (bottle), and "juice." He also points or gestures to indicate his wants. James, on the other hand, has no discernible words. Many times he screams when he wants something. Ms. Jones admits that she finds it frustrating to figure out what James wants. She asks for advice on how to stimulate James's speech.

How would you respond to Ms. Jones's question? ▪

You acknowledge Ms. Jones's frustration and offer your support. You tell her that before offering advice on how to stimulate James's speech, you need to obtain additional information about other areas of his development.

What additional questions could be asked to get a better handle on James's language development? ▪

You ask Ms. Jones to what extent James seems to understand her when she talks to him. She reports that many times he will just stand and look at her briefly when she speaks to him, then resume his activity without further acknowledgement. Sometimes he doesn't seem to respond when she calls him by name.

Does James meet the criteria for a language delay? ▪

By parental report, James meets the criteria for developmental delay in both expressive speech and receptive language. Not only is he not using simple words to express his desires, but he also demonstrates a lack of comprehension and engagement when others speak to him.

What other concerns arise with this new piece of information? ▪

Adequate hearing discrimination is necessary for proper speech development. A child cannot learn to mimic speech sounds that he cannot hear. Thus, it is vitally important to ascertain the child's ability to hear, especially at the level of speech frequencies.

An additional concern is that James responds inconsistently when called by name. Ms. Jones reports that sometimes James seems to respond to sounds. For example, he runs to the telephone when it rings and stares at the receiver. He also responds to the doorbell. He watches the television for brief periods of time. Meantime, you flip back through James's chart and verify that he passed his newborn hearing screen evaluation. You also note that James has had no middle ear infections to date.

During conversation with their mother, you have a chance to observe Peter and James as they move about the exam room. Peter has pulled a number of books from the plastic basket in the corner. He opens one, flips through the pages briefly, then brings the book to his mother, pulling on her skirt and holding the book up for her to see. "Oh, you've found a book to read!" Ms. Jones says that "Peter likes books." You note that James is sitting on the floor holding a toy car upside down. He spins the wheels repeatedly with one hand over and over again. When you comment on this behavior, Ms. Jones concurs that James frequently engages in such play at home. "He's mesmerized by a music box carousel that spins round and round," she tells you. Another favorite toy is a pinwheel.

Armed with these data, what additional areas of development should be explored? ◼

Although clinical observations support age-appropriate fine motor skills, there are concerns with James's social development (i.e., how he relates to others). Other developmental skills, such as adaptive and gross motor parameters, should be documented as well. Interest in and perseveration with spinning objects such as pinwheels are behaviors commonly associated with autistic children.

You ask Ms. Jones about James's sociability. Does he like to cuddle? Will he blow kisses? Is he averse to being held? Is there any interactive play with his brother?

Ms. Jones reports that James has never been a cuddler. Even as an infant, when he would cry for hours, he refused to be consoled. "We thought he had the colic," she says. "I was always so thankful when he would finally fall asleep. I know they're twins, but James was always so different from his brother." Ms. Jones also reports that James prefers playing with common objects by himself. "It's almost as if he were in his own little world most of the time," she comments.

Ms. Jones states that both boys began to walk independently by 15 months of age. They are very active physically and now climb the stairs at home. Mealtimes have become a chore, because both boys refuse to allow their mother to feed them. They insist on feeding themselves, although they are quite messy. They can hold a spoon and drink from a cup, but Ms. Jones states that they still need a bedtime bottle for comfort.

What additional information do you need to gather to continue your assessment of James? ◼

You continue to search for relevant data by developing the family, social, and environmental history.

Ms. Jones is 36 years of age and has no medical problems. She left her secretarial position one month before the twins were born to devote herself to rearing them. She has been married for 5 years and describes her husband as a supportive spouse and involved father. He looks forward to interacting with the children when he returns home from work. They reside in a relatively new single family home. No other blood relatives in the extended family have been diagnosed with epilepsy, mental retardation, or genetic syndromes.

Physical Examination

It is now time to proceed with the physical examination. Examining a toddler is often a challenging task for the healthcare provider. Many children will actively struggle during the examination at this age. Peter and James are no exceptions.

> During your approach to the children, you notice that James seems to be particularly averse to touch. He recoils at the slightest attempt to soothe him through subdued interaction. At one point, James seems to be more interested in your stethoscope than in any personal interaction. He screams when held for the otoscopic exam. You note that both ear canals are patent with mobile glistening grey tympanic membranes. His palate is intact. There are no hypopigmented lesions on the skin. Neurologically, he exhibits symmetrical muscle tone and strength. You note no dysmorphic features. On the contrary, James appears to be a beautiful little boy.

At this point, you are considering possible diagnoses for the abnormal development you are identifying in this little boy.

Making the Diagnosis

What specific differential diagnoses should be considered at this juncture, given this constellation of symptoms? ■

- Primary language delay, with associated behavioral issues.
- Additional developmental delays in the personal–social and adaptive categories may indicate mental retardation.
- Emerging autistic spectrum disorder: pervasive developmental disorder, NOS.

What other diagnoses would be considered but are of less likelihood in this case? ■

The clinician may consider other diagnoses delineated in Box 3-1. Given the clinical presentation at hand, these are much less likely.

At this point James exhibits several "red flags" on the list of concerns indicating the possibility of autistic spectrum disorder:

- No babbling by 12 months of age
- No pointing or gesturing to indicate wants by 12 months of age
- No single words documented by 16 months of age
- No spontaneous two-word combinations (usually seen by 24 months of age)
- Loss of language or social skills at any age

Box 3-1   Differential diagnosis for autism.

- Neuro-psychological disorders
  - Elective mutism
  - Obsessive-compulsive disorder
  - Schizophrenia of childhood
  - Conduct disorder
  - Mental retardation
- Neurological disorders
  - Absence seizures
  - Tourette syndrome
- Hearing impairment
- Lead poisoning
- Fetal alcohol syndrome
- Genetic conditions
  - Tuberous sclerosis (3–4% of autism cases) (Barbaresi et al., 2006).
  - Fragile X (7% of autism cases) (Barbaresi et al., 2006).
  - Rett syndrome
  - Cornelia de Lange syndrome
  - Down syndrome
  - Angelman syndrome
  - Smith-Magenis syndrome
- Inborn errors of metabolism (5% of autism cases) (Barbaresi et al., 2006).
  - Phenylketonuria

James also exhibits several early warning signs of autistic spectrum disorder:

- Extremes of temperament and behavior (marked irritability to alarming passivity)
- Lack of meaningful social eye contact
- Inconsistent orienting to his name
- Lack of joint attention
- Lack of motor and expressive reciprocation
- Lack of reciprocation to sounds
- Lack of interactive play

Joint attention, a normal behavior that occurs spontaneously in young children, is manifested as apparent enjoyment in sharing an experience with another person. A deficit in joint attention skills is an important diagnostic clue for ASD in the very young child.

What diagnoses were ruled out through your physical examination? ■

Normal-appearing tympanic membranes suggest the absence of conductive hearing loss, although this finding does not rule out sensorineural loss. The absence of ash leaf spots or café au lait macules make neurocutaneous disorders less likely. A normal neurological examination and absence of dysmorphic features point away from fetal alcohol syndrome or a genetic aberration, such as Down syndrome.

Other Tests for the Diagnosis

At this point, what additional testing is indicated to arrive at a diagnosis? ■

- Recheck the child's head circumference. Twenty-five percent of autistic children exhibit macrocephaly.
- Despite the mother's report and your documentation of normal tympanic membranes, a formal audiological evaluation is warranted to rule out a hearing problem (Filipek et al., 2000).
- Lead testing is indicated if not done previously (Filipek et al.).
- Various screening tools are available to assist the clinician in further evaluation of the child suspected of having an autistic spectrum disorder, such as the Pervasive Developmental Disorder Screening Test (PDDST-II) (Siegel, 2004a, 2004b), Checklist for Autism in Toddlers (CHAT) (Baird et al., 2000), and the Modified Checklist for Autism in Toddlers (M-CHAT) (Robins, Fein, Barton, & Green, 2001). These questionnaires are designed to be completed by the parent and subsequently scored by the clinician. The CHAT includes additional clinical observation questions. In the M-CHAT (Figure 3-2), critical items indicative of autism include:
  - Lack of response when called by name
  - Lack of imitation/reciprocation
  - Failure to "follow a point"
  - Lack of pointing to indicate interest
  - Lack of interest in other children
  - Lack of bringing objects over to parent to "show"

What additional diagnostic testing might be considered? ■

Although routine screening for ASDs in the primary care setting is based on clinical observation, laboratory investigation may be warranted given the child's presentation. More sophisticated testing, if indicated, is usually initiated by a pediatric specialist (e.g., a pediatric neurologist, psychiatrist, geneticist, or developmental pediatrician) (Filipek et al., 2000).

M-CHAT

Please fill out the following about how your child usually is. Please try to answer every question. If the behavior is rare (e.g., you've seen it once or twice), please answer as if the child does not do it.

1. Does your child enjoy being swung, bounced on your knee, etc.? Yes No
2. Does your child take an interest in other children? Yes No
3. Does your child like climbing on things, such as up stairs? Yes No
4. Does your child enjoy playing peek-a-boo/hide-and-seek? Yes No
5. Does your child ever pretend, for example, to talk on the phone or take care of a doll or pretend other things? Yes No
6. Does your child ever use his/her index finger to point, to ask for something? Yes No
7. Does your child ever use his/her index finger to point, to indicate interest in something? Yes No
8. Can your child play properly with small toys (e.g. cars or blocks) without just mouthing, fiddling, or dropping them? Yes No
9. Does your child ever bring objects over to you (parent) to show you something? Yes No
10. Does your child look you in the eye for more than a second or two? Yes No
11. Does your child ever seem oversensitive to noise? (e.g., plugging ears) Yes No
12. Does your child smile in response to your face or your smile? Yes No
13. Does your child imitate you? (e.g., you make a face-will your child imitate it?) Yes No
14. Does your child respond to his/her name when you call? Yes No
15. If you point at a toy across the room, does your child look at it? Yes No
16. Does your child walk? Yes No
17. Does your child look at things you are looking at? Yes No
18. Does your child make unusual finger movements near his/her face? Yes No
19. Does your child try to attract your attention to his/her own activity? Yes No
20. Have you ever wondered if your child is deaf? Yes No
21. Does your child understand what people say? Yes No
22. Does your child sometimes stare at nothing or wander with no purpose? Yes No
23. Does your child look at your face to check your reaction when faced with something unfamiliar? Yes No

Source: © 1999 Diane Robins, Deborah Fein, & Marianne Barton. Used with permission.

Please refer to Robins, D., Fein, D., Barton, M., & Green, J. (2001). The Modified Checklist for Autism in Toddlers: An initial study investigating the early detection of austism and pervasive developmental disorders. *Journal of Autism and Developmental Disorder, 31*(2), 131–144.

Note. The Modified Checklist for Autism in Toddlers (M-CHAT) and supplemental materials are available for free download for clinical research and educational purposes. There are two authorized Web sites that these materials can be downloaded from: www.firstsigns.org and www2.gsu.edu/~wwwpsy/faculty/robins.htm. Users should be aware that the M-CHAT continues to be studied and may be revised in the future. Any revisions will be posted to the two Web sites noted above. The M-CHAT must be used in its entirety. There is no evidence that using a subset of items will be valid.

Figure 3-2   Modified Checklist for Autism in Toddlers (M-CHAT).

Were James to meet the criteria for global developmental delays and mental retardation (GDD/MR), high-resolution chromosome analysis and DNA for fragile X testing would be indicated. Seven to eight percent of children with ASD test positive for fragile X (Muhle et al., 2004).

In children with cyclic vomiting, unusual odor, regression of skills, or dysmorphic features, selective metabolic testing may be considered. In the absence of seizure activity or focal neurological signs, routine EEG and neuroimaging are not indicated.

Many times children suspected of having an ASD are referred to a pediatric developmental specialist for further evaluation.

Management

You express your concerns about James's development to Ms. Jones and suggest that further testing be done. She concurs.

Diagnostic and Intervention Plan

The results of laboratory testing and audiological screening are within normal limits. You refer James to a developmental pediatrician. As part of his evaluation, a Childhood Autism Rating Scale (CARS) (Schopler, Reichler, DeVellis, & Daly, 1980) is administered. Numerical values are assigned given the child's performance on this 15-item assessment tool. A score above 30 on the CARS is suggestive of an autistic spectrum disorder. On the basis of the specialist's assessment, James's profile falls into the category of autistic spectrum, meeting the criteria for autism disorder. Placement in an early intervention program specializing in children with autistic spectrum disorders is recommended. Fortunately, the family's local school district has an excellent center that specializes in children with this disorder.

Educational interventions form the basis for management of children with ASDs. The sooner the intervention is initiated, the better the outcome. Children with ASDs should be actively engaged in an intervention program at least 25 hours per week throughout the calendar year (Myers & Johnson, 2007).

Specific methodologic programs include Applied Behavior Analysis (ABA), highly structured comprehensive early intervention programs, and functional behavior analysis. ABA methods are designed to shape desirable adaptive behaviors, and their effectiveness has been well documented (Barbaresi et al., 2006; Myers & Johnson, 2007). The Treatment and Education of Autistic and Related Communication-Handicapped Children (TEACCH) program emphasizes structured teaching and environmental modification to improve skills of individuals with ASDs.

Other appropriate interventions include speech and language therapy, social skills instruction, and occupational therapy. Primary care providers play a vital role in advocating these services for the child with an ASD as well as the child's need for continuing participation in programs for autistic children throughout childhood.

Educational Plan

One month later Ms. Jones telephones your office to ask what caused James's autism. She is particularly concerned about the vaccines both boys received and whether they should continue to receive any additional vaccines. She heard on the news that some vaccines can cause autism. She wonders if Peter may be at risk as well.

How do you respond to her questions? ■

You inform Ms. Jones that the latest research has not shown a causal relationship between any of the routine childhood vaccines and autism. On the contrary, not vaccinating children places them at higher risk for developing complications secondary to diseases such as rubella, a known cause of autism.

It is most important to monitor the development of younger siblings of autistic children. The incidence of autism in monozygotic twins is 60%, while dizygotic twins and other siblings have a 5–6% risk of recurrence of autism (Bailey, Le Courteur, & Gottesman, 1995; Muhle et al., 2004). Although Peter shows no developmental delays at 18 months of age, he should be screened specifically for autism at 24 months of age. Some children will demonstrate a regression of developmental milestones between 18 and 24 months of age, so you will want to monitor Peter's development carefully during the next year.

What additional information do you want to give James's mother at this time? ■

Because caretakers of children with ASDs are frequently desperate to pursue any intervention that offers hope for improved outcome, it is imperative that providers educate them about unsubstantiated and ineffective therapies. These include sensory integration therapy, auditory integration training, behavioral optometry, craniosacral manipulation, dolphin-assisted therapy, music therapy, and facilitated communication. Likewise, there is as yet insufficient scientific evidence to support the use of biologic therapies such as restrictive diets, chelation therapy, gastrointestinal treatments, and dietary supplementation regimens (Barbaresi et al., 2006). Such ineffective therapeutic approaches offer false hope and may place unnecessary financial burdens on families.

Pharmacologic regimens may be indicated to alleviate disruptive behaviors such as aggression, self-injurious behaviors, sleep disturbance, and mood lability. Practitioners may consider a therapeutic trial of medication in the case of maladaptive behaviors not amenable to behavioral therapy. The U.S. Food and Drug Administration has approved risperidone (Myers et al., 2007; Shea et al.,

2004) for the symptomatic treatment of aggressive and self-injurious behaviors in children with ASDs.

Rearing children with ASDs generates significant stress in families. The primary care provider can provide key support to the family through education and anticipatory guidance, and by serving as an advocate for the child. In some cases, referring family members for appropriate mental health services may be indicated. Longitudinal support can be accomplished by maintaining contact with the family through periodic health maintenance visits.

Expected Outcomes

What is the long-term outlook for children diagnosed early with ASD? ■

A diagnosis of ASD is usually confirmed with clear behavioral indicators by 2 to 4 years of age. The earlier the diagnosis is made, the better the long-term outcome, assuming the child is placed in an early intervention program tailored to meet the needs of children with ASDs.

Key Points from the Case

1. All children should be screened for development at well child visits, with special attention given at the 9-month, 18-month, and 30-month visits (AAP, 2006).
2. Survey all children at every well child visit for early subtle signs of ASD, especially younger siblings of a child already diagnosed with an ASD.
3. Screen specifically for ASD at 18 and 24 months of age, consistently using at least one standardized screening tool.
4. If screening results are negative but concerns by parents or the clinician persist, schedule an early targeted visit to reassess the child.
5. Take action if the results of a screening test are positive or if the child demonstrates two or more risk factors. Rather than adopting a "wait-and-see" approach, refer the child for a comprehensive ASD evaluation, an audiologic evaluation, and an early intervention program in a timely manner.
6. Maintain a supportive, coordinating role as the primary care provider for the family with an autistic spectrum disordered child.

(See additional resources in Box 3-2.)

Box 3-2   Autism Resources for Providers

Journals:

Choueiri, R., & Bridgemohan, C. (2005). To make the biggest difference, screen early for autistic spectrum disorders. *Contemporary Pediatrics, 22,* 54–67.

Johnson, C. P. (2008). Recognition of autism before age 2 years. *Pediatrics in Review, 2,* 86–96.

Mauk, J. E., Reber, M., & Batshaw, M. L. (2007). Autism and other pervasive developmental disorders. In M. L. Batshaw (Ed.), *Children with disabilities* (5th ed., Chapter 21). Baltimore: Brooks.

Zwaigenbaum, L., Bryson, S., Rogers, T., Roberts, W., Brian, J., Szatmari, P. (2005). Behavioral manifestations of autism in the first year of life. *International Journal of Developmental Neuroscience, 23,* 143–152. Available at: http://www.ncbi.nlm.nih.gov/pubmed/15749241

Internet Resources:

Autistic Spectrum Disorders: Best Practice Guidelines for Screening, Diagnosis and Assessment, California Department of Developmental Services: http://www.ddhealthinfo. org/documents/ASD_Best_Practice.pdf

Autistic Spectrum Disorders (Pervasive Developmental Disorders), National Institute of Mental Health: http://www.nimh.nih.gov/health/publications/autism/summary.shtml

First Signs, a Web site dedicated to the early identification and intervention of children with developmental delays and disorders. This site also contains an ASD video glossary that clinicians can access to view video recordings of diagnostic signs demonstrated by autistic children: http://www.firstsigns.org

Learn the signs. Act early, Centers for Disease Control and Prevention: http://www.cdc.gov/ ncbddd/autism/actearly/

REFERENCES

American Academy of Pediatrics Council on Children with Disabilities. (2006). Identifying infants and young children with developmental disorders in the medical home: An algorithm for developmental surveillance and screening. *Pediatrics, 118,* 405–420. Retrieved March 2, 2009, from http://pediatrics. aappublications.org/cgi/content/full/118/1/405

American Psychiatric Association. (2000). *DSM-IV-TR diagnostic criteria for the pervasive developmental disorders.* Retrieved November 23, 2008, from http://www.CDC.gov/ncbddd/autism/overview_diagnostic_criteria.htm

Autism and Developmental Disabilities Monitoring Network Surveillance Year 2000 Principal Investigators. (2007). Prevalence of autism spectrum disorders—autism and developmental disabilities monitoring network, six states, United States, 2000. *Morbidity and Mortality Weekly Report,* 56(SS01), 1–11.

Bailey, A., Le Courteur A., & Gottesman, I. (1995). Autism as a strongly genetic disorder: Evidence from a British twin study. *Psychological Medicine, 25,* 63–77.

Baird, G., Charman, T., Baron-Cohen, S., Cox, A., Swettenham, J., Wheelwright, S., et al. (2000). A screening instrument for autism at 18 months of age: A 6-year follow-up study. *Journal of the American Academy of Child and Adolescent Psychiatry, 39,* 694–702.

Barbaresi, W., Katusic, S., & Voight, R. (2006). Autism: A review of the state of the science for pediatric primary health care clinicians. *Archives of Pediatric and Adolescent Medicine, 160,* 1167–1175.

Filipek, P., Accardo, P. J., Ashwal, S., Baranek, G. T., Cook, E. H., Dawson, G., et al. (2000). Practice parameter: Screening and diagnosis of autism. *Neurology, 55,* 468–479.

Muhle, R., Trentacoste, S., & Rapin, I. (2004). The genetics of autism. *Pediatrics, 113,* 472–486.

Myers, S. M., & Johnson, C. P. (2007). Management of children with autistic spectrum disorders. AAP Council on Children with Disabilities. *Pediatrics, 120,* 1162–1182.

Robins, D. I., Fein, D., Barton, M. I., & Green, J. A. (2001). The modified checklist for autism in toddlers: An initial study investigating the early detection of autism and pervasive developmental disorders. *Journal of Autism and Developmental Disorders, 31*(2), 149–151.

Schopler, E., Reichler, R. J., DeVellis, R. F., & Daly, K. (1980). Toward objective classification of childhood autism: Childhood Autism Rating Scale (CARS). *Journal of Autism and Developmental Disorders, 10,* 91–103.

Shea, S., Turgay, A., Carroll, A., Schultz, M., Orlik, H., Smith, I., et al, (2004). Risperidone in the treatment of disruptive behavioral symptoms in children with autistic and other pervasive developmental disorders. *Pediatrics, 114*(5), e634–e641.

Siegel, B. (2004a). Early screening for autism using the PDDST-II. *AAP Society for Developmental and Behavioral Pediatrics News, 13,* 4.

Siegel, B. (2004b). *Pervasive Developmental Disorders Screening Test-II (PDDST-II): Early Childhood Screeners for Autistic Spectrum Disorders.* San Antonio, TX: Harcourt Assessment.

Chapter 4

A School-Age Child with School Failure Problems

Ann Marie McCarthy
Sharon Yearous

School-age children spend a significant portion of their lives in school; therefore, it is crucial that they be in school, healthy, and ready to learn. When a child is having a problem related to school, families often seek help from their primary care provider. It is important for primary care providers to know how to distinguish physical versus psychosocial etiologies for school absences.

Educational Objectives
1. Identify the characteristics of school refusal in a school-age child.
2. Discuss the management of a 12-year-old child with school refusal.

Case Presentation and Discussion

You have been caring for 12-year-old Katie Murphy since she was 9 months old. Ms. Murphy has brought Katie and her older brother to you for their routine health supervision visits and other minor acute illnesses. To date, Katie has never been diagnosed with any chronic health concerns. Katie's last examination was for her 10-year-old well child visit. She was healthy and her development was progressing normally.

Ms. Murphy calls the health clinic concerned about Katie and tells the receptionist that Katie has been absent from school sporadically during the last 3 weeks. According to Ms. Murphy, Katie has complained of stomachaches intermittently during that time. Over the last week Katie's absences from school have increased, all related to the stomachaches. Ms. Murphy states that Katie has not had a fever or any other signs of gastrointestinal distress such as nausea, vomiting, or diarrhea. Her stomachaches occur primarily in the morning and subside later in the day. The receptionist schedules a next day appointment for Katie to be evaluated by you. When you review Katie's record prior to seeing her, your plan is to evaluate her first for an underlying physical cause for her stomachaches. If there isn't a physical etiology, you then will evaluate her for school refusal related to a psychosocial problem.

What information do you need to rule out a physical etiology for Katie's stomachaches? ■

When primary care providers see a child or adolescent who has missed a number of days of school, accompanied by a physical complaint, it is important to rule out any potential underlying physical problems. Thus, an assessment of a child with somatic complaints that may be psychosocial in etiology first requires a thorough assessment of potential physical etiologies, including a complete medical history and physical exam. The history plus a physical examination with medical tests, if indicated, should provide the data needed to rule out a physical etiology in children, like Katie, who present with somatic complaints and increasing school absences.

The child's medical history should involve a prenatal to current age review of body systems, including any associated illnesses, hospitalizations, or surgeries related to a body system, accidents or injuries, current medications (prescription and nonprescription), and any alternative therapies used. Further exploration of any areas that may pertain to presenting health issues should be completed as necessary. In addition, the medical history should include a functional assessment of the child's self-esteem, nutritional habits, sleep habits, involvement in activities, and screening for any type of abuse. The next step after completing a thorough medical history is to review the family medical and social history. A family medical history includes physical and psychological health concerns such as premature death, heart disease, stroke, diabetes, cancer, mental illness, or other inheritable conditions of siblings, parents, and one prior generation of family members (Jarvis, 2007).

Information on school performance should be routinely obtained on all school-aged children. Primary care providers typically screen children before the age of 5 years for developmental and behavioral problems; however, many healthcare providers no longer do this type of screening once children enter school. Recent recommendations suggest that primary care providers should transition from routine developmental screening to screening school performance for school-age children and adolescents. This approach will help with early identification of problems and interventions to improve the child's success in school (Kelly & Aylward, 2005). If concerns are identified, contact with school personnel and review of school attendance and achievement records may be warranted (Fremont, 2003). For example, in evaluating school absence, in addition to the documented school absences, discussion with the school nurse may reveal a student who is frequently seen in the school nurse's office for somatic complaints, essentially being absent from class while still in school.

Psychosocial information should also be obtained to identify behavioral concerns and possible underlying factors contributing to the somatic concern. Screening for emotional problems should be a routine part of all health maintenance visits for children (McCarthy & Eisbach, 2006). An example of a screening instrument that may be appropriate for use in primary care settings is the Pediatric Symptom Checklist (PSC) (Jellinek et al., 1988, 1999). The PSC is one page, with 35 items, completed by parents or children, and designed to help clinicians in outpatient practice screen for school-age children with difficulties in psychosocial functioning. The PSC is included in *Bright Futures in Practice: Mental Health* and the Bright Futures Web site (http://www.brightfutures.org/mentalhealth/pdf/professionals/ped_sympton_chklst.pdf) along with information on reliability and validity, scoring, and cutoff scores for referral.

The final area of history that requires review involves a history of the presenting symptom(s) by starting at the point the symptoms presented until the current time. This review of symptoms can be remembered using the PQRSTU mnemonic (Jarvis, 2007).

- *Provocative or palliative:* What brings on symptoms? What makes them better or worse?
- *Quality or quantity:* How intense are symptoms? What do the symptoms feel like?
- *Region or radiation:* Where do they start? Do the symptoms spread?
- *Severity scale:* Use an age-appropriate rating scale and ask what makes symptoms better or worse.
- *Timing:* This includes onset, duration, and frequency of symptoms.
- *Understanding:* Understand the child's perception of the problem of concern.

Your review of Katie's medical history shows that she does not have any chronic conditions and, except for otitis media as a preschooler, she has been seen only for routine preventive health care. As noted earlier, you last saw her for her 10-year-old health maintenance visit, and no physical or psychosocial problems were noted. She lives with her nuclear family—her father, who is an engineer; her stay-at-home mother; and an older brother who is in ninth grade. No other individuals live in the home. There have been no changes in the family health history. Her school screening questionnaire completed by her mother at the 10-year-old health visit indicated that she was receiving A's and B's in all subjects and enjoyed school. Her behavioral assessment with the PSC, also completed by her mother, fell within the normal range at that time, although Ms. Murphy reported that sometimes Katie worries, is afraid of new situations, and acts younger than her age.

Katie and her mom are present for the appointment. Katie sits close to her mom and seems distant with a flat affect. Upon questioning the reason for their visit today, initially Katie does not respond, and her mother answers your questions. Katie occasionally offers responses to direct questions but her responses are brief, single-word responses, usually yes or no, and with limited eye contact.

You then ask questions specific to the presenting complaint of stomachaches. Ms. Murphy reports that Katie has missed many days of school over the last 3 weeks due to stomachaches. The stomachaches begin in the morning but often appear to resolve by late afternoon. Katie reports some nausea, but denies vomiting or diarrhea with the stomachaches. Her mother states she has not had any fevers over the last 3 weeks. Katie explains that her appetite is normal, yet her mother interrupts and reports that she does not seem to eat very much. You learn that Katie's maternal grandmother passed away about 2 months ago from lung cancer but Ms. Murphy says that everyone seems to be coping well. No other recent family stressors were identified.

During the physical examination you ask Katie some more questions. Katie is hesitant to respond but states she started her menses 6 months ago and denies cramps that prevent her from doing her normal activities. Her mother confirms this information. Katie states that she feels tired at times, especially in the morning, but otherwise denies any other symptoms. She describes her stomachaches as hurting all over, but after she's been up for awhile the pain goes away. She rates her pain as a 4 on a 0–10 pain scale where 0 is no pain and 10 is the worst imaginable pain.

Today's physical exam reveals no fever, normal heart rate (HR) and blood pressure (BP), height is 59 inches, weight 95 pounds, and BMI 19.2 (64th percentile). Her abdomen is flat and nondistended with bowel sounds present in all quadrants, soft and negative for guarding with light and deep palpation. The remainder of the examination is negative. There are no indications for further lab or diagnostic tests at this time.

Your initial assessment suggests that Katie's stomachaches are related to a psychosocial concern and her school absence behavior is possibly school refusal. You decide that you need to obtain further information.

What additional questions will you ask Katie and her mother as you consider the possibility of school refusal due to a psychosocial etiology? ■

Before answering this question, here is some information about school-age children who miss school that should be considered.

School Absence

Laws mandate school attendance. Children and adolescents are typically absent from school for reasons such as illness, appointments, special family events, religious holidays, or school-sanctioned activities. The National Center for Health Statistics (Bloom & Cohen, 2007) reports that in 2006 approximately 29% of students, 5 to 17 years of age, missed no school in the past year due to illness or injury, 29% missed 1 to 2 days of school, 36% missed 3 to 10 days, and 5% missed 11 or more days.

In addition to school absence due to legitimate reasons, children also miss school for reasons that are not acceptable to school and/or parents or guardians. Children who refuse to attend cause problems for themselves and concerns for parents, guardians, and school personnel. There has been some controversy over how to classify unauthorized school absences. Typically, unauthorized school absences have been categorized into two groups: 1) students who intentionally do not attend school, referred to as truancy; and 2) students who have difficulty attending school associated with emotional distress (King & Bernstein, 2001), usually anxiety or fear, referred to as school avoidance, school refusal, or school phobia (Marcontel-Shattuck & Gregory, 2006). Truancy refers to absence from school that is initiated by the student and is not condoned by school officials, parents, or guardians. Truant students typically are not anxious, but instead, display a lack of interest in school and school rules, antisocial behaviors, and conduct problems (King & Bernstein; Marcontel-Shattuck & Gregory; Sewell, 2008). Students who do not attend school due to emotional distress have been further divided into three main clinical groups: anxious/depressed school refusers, separation-anxious school refusers, and phobic school refusers (Egger, Costello, & Angold, 2003; King & Bernstein). However, not all children who refuse to attend school are truant or anxious (Plante, 2007), and some have mixed school refusal behaviors (Egger et al.).

Kearney and colleagues define school refusal behavior as "child motivated refusal to attend school and/or difficulties remaining in classes for an entire day" (Kearney & Albano, 2004, p. 147). This term thus encompasses all students who refuse to go to school, truants, those with anxiety-related disorders, and other unidentified reasons for school refusal, and does not focus on etiology but instead on behaviors. School refusal behavior occurs in all age groups, in boys and girls equally, and is reported to occur in from 1–5% of students (Fremont, 2003) to as many as 28% of students at some point in their school career (Kearney, 2006). Peak ages appear to be 5–7 and 10–14 years of age (Kearney; King & Bernstein, 2001; Marcontel-Shattuck & Gregory, 2006; Plante, 2007; Sewell, 2008). Transitions and changes from one school to another (Kearney; King & Bernstein) or from an extended time at home and a return to school (e.g., vacations, brief illness) (Marcontel-Shattuck & Gregory), as well as stressful experiences at home (e.g., death of a grandparent or pet) or at school (e.g., a bullying episode or exams), can all be triggers for school refusal behavior (Marcontel-Shattuck & Gregory).

Clinical Presentations
School refusal is complex, with various patterns of physical complaints/somatization, behaviors, and emotions displayed by children with school refusal behaviors. If a physical complaint is associated with school refusal, complaints may include headaches, abdominal pains, nausea and vomiting, fatigue, and dizziness (Egger et al., 2003; Kearney & Bensaheb, 2006). Both internalizing and externalizing behavior problems are seen in school refusal, such as anxiety, fear, depression, physical complaints, noncompliance, aggression, and temper tantrums. School refusal behavior is not a *Diagnostic and Statistical Manual of Mental Disorders,* 4th edition, text revision (DSM-IV-TR) diagnosis, but is seen as a behavioral symptom in children with a number of DSM-IV-TR diagnoses (Egger et al.). In one study, the most common

diagnoses associated with students with school refusal behaviors were separation anxiety disorder (22.4%), generalized anxiety disorder (10.5%), oppositional defiant disorder (8.4%), depression (4.9%), specific phobia (4.2%), social anxiety disorder (3.5%), and conduct disorder (2.8%) (Kearney & Albano, 2004).

Children who are truants do not typically tell their parents that they are missing school. These children often do not report physical complaints but often display more externalizing behaviors such as delinquency, lying, and stealing in addition to not attending school (Fremont, 2003). In contrast, parents of children with anxiety-related school refusal behavior typically know about the absences, and parents are usually concerned about the child's absences. The child either may completely refuse to attend school or may attend but leave early. These children often report physical complaints and display behaviors related to problems such as fears, anxiety, separation anxiety, social phobia, post-traumatic stress disorder, panic disorders, and depression (Fremont). These behaviors may include crying, panic, temper tantrums, threats of self-harm, and, as noted in Katie's case, somatization complaints such as stomachaches or headaches (Fremont). Children with anxious school refusal behaviors may have a fear of school that is based in reality (not phobic), such as a fear of being bullied or teased (Egger et al., 2003), an unrecognized learning problem (King & Bernstein, 2001), or a recent life-changing event such as a death in the family or relocation. For many of these children, they feel safer staying at home (Fremont).

Family Dynamics
Dysfunctional family interactions may be noted in children with school refusal behaviors (Fremont, 2003; Marcontel-Shattuck & Gregory, 2006). Family and social stressors such as poverty, unemployment, frequent moves, family conflicts, and a parent with a mental health problem are often found in children with school refusal behaviors (Egger et al., 2003; King & Bernstein, 2001). A study of family functioning in children with school refusal found that single-parent families were overrepresented in this group and that single mothers reported more family problems, particularly role performance and communication (Bernstein & Borchardt, 1996). In a study of 46 adolescents with school refusal behavior and anxiety and major depressive disorders, both parents and children reported low family cohesion or engagement and low adaptability/high rigidity (Bernstein, Warren, Massie, & Thuras, 1999). Parents of children with anxiety-related school refusal have been found to have an increased prevalence of similar symptoms. For example, parents of children with phobic school refusal were found to have an increased prevalence of social phobia, and parents of children with separation anxiety and school refusal have an increased prevalence of panic disorder (Martin, Cabrol, Bouvard, Lepine, & Mouren-Simeoni, 1999).

Consequences

The consequences of school refusal behaviors are both immediate and long term. Immediate consequences are problems with academic achievement, peer relationships, and family functioning. Long-term consequences include ongoing underachievement, employment problems, social difficulties, and an increased risk of psychiatric problems (Fremont, 2003; King & Bernstein, 2001; Sewell, 2008). More negative outcomes are associated with long episodes of school refusal occurring when the student is an adolescent, when the student is depressed, and/or when the student has a lower IQ (Elliot, 1999; Sewell).

You ask Katie and her mother to provide further details about school and the history of absences from school. Katie is in the seventh grade in middle school. Prior to the last 3 weeks, Katie often missed a day or two a month from school for some type of problem that seemed legitimate to mom. During the first week when Katie's school absences began 3 weeks ago, she was home ill on Monday due to the stomachaches. She returned to school on Tuesday and midway through the morning she called her mother saying that her stomach hurt again. Ms. Murphy picked Katie up from school at 11:15 a.m. Katie went back to school on Wednesday but was reluctant about going and voiced her concerns that she didn't want to have to leave school with a stomachache again. She was able to attend a full day on Wednesday, but didn't go to school on Thursday until 10 a.m., and was home on Friday due to stomachaches again. The second week Katie was absent from school on Monday, Thursday, and Friday. Katie's complaints were the same each day—stomachache and intermittent nausea, no vomiting, diarrhea, or fevers. The third week of absences included full days of being absent from school on Monday, Tuesday, Wednesday, and Friday. In order to recognize patterns of school absence and summarize her school absence, you document it in a calendar format.

This week, the school attendance secretary contacted Ms. Murphy because the school was concerned about Katie's recent attendance. Ms. Murphy states that she is also concerned about all the days of school that Katie is missing but does not know what she should do. Ms. Murphy is at home with Katie during these days of school absence and enjoys spending the extra time with her. Ms. Murphy acknowledges Katie's stomachaches and encourages Katie to go to school but she also knows that Katie will most likely report to the school office stating that she doesn't feel well and they will call and ask Ms. Murphy to pick her up. Katie reports that her stomachaches improve during the day. When asked what she does when she stays home, Katie says she watches TV, plays on the computer, and helps her mother with cooking and chores around the house.

Next, you explain to Katie and Ms. Murphy that you often talk with children alone at this age and following approval from both Ms. Murphy and Katie, Ms. Murphy goes to the waiting room while you interview Katie in private.

An approach for interviewing adolescents is to follow the acronym HEADSS(W), and ask questions about home, education, activities, drug use, sexual behaviors, suicide/depression, and weight (Cohen, Mackenzie, & Yates, 1991; Roye, 1995). Asking questions in this order allows the interviewer to begin with presumably less stressful topics and move to more sensitive areas. You start with general questions about how Katie feels about home and school. Katie denies any problems at home. She gets along well with her parents and brother, although she reports that she sometimes doesn't want to be around her family. Katie states that she has several friends in school and two best friends that she has known since kindergarten. During the last 3 weeks, her best friends have only called her twice to see why she was not in school. On both occasions Katie told her friends that she just had a stomachache and did not mention anything else. When you ask more about her two best friends, Katie starts to have tears in her eyes and states that she is hurt that they have only contacted her twice in the last 3 weeks. "It's like they don't care that I'm not in school," she says. Katie states she does not participate in any extracurricular activities other than a church youth group. Katie denies any alcohol or other substance use; she reports that she has never tried alcohol or drugs and is not interested in experimenting. She also denies that she is sexually active and reports that no one has ever touched her in a way that has made her uncomfortable.

Making the Diagnosis

Katie's history and negative physical examination are consistent with school refusal behavior, probably initially related to anxiety and now being reinforced by the response to her staying at home. Having ruled out any physical etiology for Katie's stomachaches, you determine that Katie's pattern of school absences appear to be anxiety-related school refusal behavior. This diagnosis needs to be explained to the family, with support provided in helping them understand the connection between mind and body.

> You explain to Ms. Murphy and Katie that there does not appear to be a physical cause for Katie's stomachaches, but people's emotions, such as anxiety, can result in physical symptoms, such as stomachaches. In addition, the rewards of staying at home and spending time with her mother are now reinforcing Katie's stomachaches.

Management

What information do you need about the management of school refusal in order to help Katie successfully return to school? ■

The first step in developing a management plan for a student with school refusal behavior is to perform a complete assessment of multiple areas including:

- History of factors that may contribute to, trigger, or maintain school refusal behavior
- Physical exam to rule out health problems and reassure child and family
- School information related to achievement, attendance, behavior, and social interactions

- Behavior screening tools completed by parents and teachers (Sewell, 2008)

In this case, you have carried out a physical exam and obtained background information and a description of the school absence behaviors, but will need more on school performance, social interactions, and psychosocial adjustment in order to develop a comprehensive management plan.

The goal of the management plan for a child with anxiety-related school refusal is to return to school, without unauthorized absences, "happy, healthy, and ready to learn." This requires a multidisciplinary team approach that will likely include the primary care provider, teachers, school personnel such as the school nurse and the counselor, and the child's family. The primary care provider rules out organic causes for the physical symptoms and provides information to the team about the link between stress and physiological symptoms; school personnel work with the family on making up missed class work and developing a plan for the child to return to school; and mental health providers may be needed to provide support to manage the school refusal behavior and to help the child and family cope with anxiety and related concerns. The plan needs to be well coordinated, agreed on by all members including the child, and supportive of the family.

The primary care provider needs the parent's permission to contact the school and to obtain information about school performance. Information to obtain includes course grades; standardized test scores; school attendance history; frequency and reasons for visiting the school nurse; any disciplinary actions; Individualized Education Programs (IEPs) or 504 plans, if there are any; and other pertinent records. An IEP or 504 plan would identify any accommodations needed in the school to help the student succeed (U.S. Department of Education, n.d.). The primary care provider may want the principal, teacher, or other school professional to interpret some of these documents. Some of the questions to be answered through school records include whether the student is performing at grade level or as expected and whether any specific learning disorders have been identified.

Both the student's parents and teachers may be asked to complete instruments that assess behavior and emotional concerns in general and school refusal behavior specifically. Behavioral questionnaires are helpful in assessing a child's emotional adjustment and overall behavior (Achenbach & Ruffle, 2000; Glascoe, 2000; Perrin & Stancin, 2002). These instruments often are available in several versions that allow the child, a parent, and/or a teacher to complete similar versions of the instrument and for responses to be compared. As noted earlier, an example of a screening instrument that may be appropriate for use in primary care is the Pediatric Symptom Checklist (PSC) (Jellinek et al., 1988), which has both parent and child versions available. However, when diagnosis is the goal, behavioral assessment instruments, such as the Child Behavior Checklist (CBCL) (Achenbach & Ruffle, 2000) and more specific instruments such as the Children's Depression Inventory (Kovacs, 2003), may be used. For students with school refusal behavior, the use of an assessment instrument (such as the School Refusal Assessment Scale) that specifically evaluates school refusal behavior and clarifies the motivation for the behavior would be particularly valuable.

School Refusal Assessment Scale (SRAS)

Kearney and colleagues developed a model of school refusal behavior based on what motivates the child to avoid school; such motivators are what reinforce the child's behavior (Kearney & Albano, 2004). Four reasons are identified, two based on negative reinforcement (avoid or escape anxiety-provoking situations) and two based on positive reinforcement (gaining pleasurable activities or rewards). Table 4-1 summarizes these four motivating situations for school refusal behavior (Plante, 2007). In general, children with separation anxiety are motivated primarily by positive reinforcement such as attention from a parent; children with anxiety issues of various types are motivated by negative reinforcement such as escape from school teasing; and children with externalizing behaviors, who are often truants, are motivated by positive reinforcements such as obtaining drugs or video time (Kearney & Albano). There is often an overlap across the functions. A child may start with anxiety/negative reinforcement from being able to escape from school problems, but then as they stay home, also may begin to have positive reinforcers such as television or computer time that also maintain the school refusal behaviors.

Based on this model of what motivates school refusal behavior, Kearney and colleagues developed the School Refusal Assessment Scale (SRAS) (Kearney, 2002, 2006, 2007; Kearney & Albano, 2004). The SRAS measures the four functional areas that are thought to motivate school refusal behavior. There are two versions of the SRAS, one for children (SRAS-C) and one for parents (SRAS-P). Each version has 24 items on Likert scales, scored from 0

Table 4-1 Motivations for Avoiding School	
Maintained by Negative Reinforcement	**Maintained by Positive Reinforcement**
To avoid school-based stimuli that trigger anxiety, depression, or both (e.g., teachers, peers, bus, cafeteria)	To pursue increased time and attention from significant others
To escape aversive social or evaluative situations (e.g., anxiety associated with socializing with peers or taking tests)	To pursue tangible reinforcers associated with missing school (e.g., sleeping late, increased TV and video game time, delinquent behavior or substance abuse)

Source: Adapted from Kearney (2002), Kearney (2007), Kearney & Albano (2004), and Plante (2007).

(never) to 6 (always). The highest scoring functional area is most likely the main reason for the school refusal behavior. The scales and further information can be found on the Internet.

Once information on the child's school performance and behavioral concerns are obtained, in addition to the physical examination and medical history information, and the function of the school refusal behavior is identified, you can then develop an appropriate intervention strategy. This will require a team meeting of key individuals, including the family, school personnel, school nurse, mental health personnel, and primary care provider. The meeting may take place at the school and is an opportunity for the primary care provider to experience the child's school environment and have direct interaction with school staff.

> In Katie's case, school attendance records verify that despite her recent increase in absences, her grades have not changed, and she visited the school nurse on the days she was in school with the primary complaint being nonspecific stomachaches. Behavioral assessments were not completed prior to Katie's appointment with you. Your contact with the school results in an appointment arranged for the next day with Katie, her mother, and the school psychologist. Based on the results of the parent and child versions of the CBCL, and the discussion with the family, the psychologist notes that Katie has increased anxiety but no other identified behavior concerns. Completion of the SRAS reveals that Katie's school refusal behavior is related to a desire to avoid school due to anxiety from some peer conflicts and, secondary to that, to obtain attention or positive reinforcement from her mother. A team meeting is scheduled for the following Monday to include both her mother and father, you as the primary care provider, the school psychologist, the school nurse, and Katie's teachers.

Therapeutic plan: What will you do therapeutically? ■

As stated earlier, the immediate goal for children and adolescents with school refusal behavior is for the student to return to school (Fremont, 2003). Primary care providers should not provide excuses for school absences unless there is a medical reason for not attending school (Freemont). Treatment will vary based on the age and developmental and emotional needs of the child and the functional analysis of the school refusal behavior. In addition to assisting the child to return to school, the treatment plan may need to include ongoing mental health counseling for the child and/or parents if any family members need treatment for anxiety, depression, phobia, post-traumatic stress disorder, or other mental health concerns. Interventions may concentrate on the child and/or parents and involve school support personnel. The following discussion focuses on approaches for children with anxiety-related school refusal.

The plan to return the child to school often involves systematic desensitization (a gradual return to school) (Fremont, 2003; Kearney, 2006; Plante,

2007). Attending school for part of a day may be less stressful than attending for a full day. It is important that the parents and school personnel be consistent in carrying out the approach of gradual reintroduction. However, if the school refusal episode has not been long, it may be possible to have the student return to school full time immediately (Sewell, 2008).

Cognitive-behavioral approaches may help the child with school refusal behaviors (Fremont, 2003; Kearney & Albano, 2004). Children with anxiety may benefit from relaxation training, both muscle relaxation and controlled breathing. Children with difficulties with peers may benefit from social skills training. Positive reinforcement (e.g., verbal praise, earning time with a valued adult in the school such as a teacher or principal) for school attendance can support the child's return to school. For older children, contingency management and developing a contract with parents and school personnel can be valuable tools. Older children and adolescents may benefit from understanding the patterns of their own emotional responses and resultant behaviors, such as school avoidance, through the use of diaries, discussions, and counseling. Cognitive restructuring therapy that assists the individual in identifying negative thoughts and modifying these thoughts can be helpful for students with illogical thinking related to their experiences at school. In conjunction with these cognitive-behavioral and counseling approaches, medication for the child's underlying anxiety or depression problems may need to be considered (Fremont, 2003; Heyne, King, Tonge, & Cooper, 2001; Kearney, 2006).

Parents play a key role in the treatment of school refusal, and must work closely with school personnel to address the student's school refusal behavior. Behavioral approaches such as systematic desensitization and contingency contracting require intense involvement from parents. Children who require counseling need the support of their parents as they learn how to cope with their anxiety. Parents may need support in recognizing that they are positively reinforcing the child's school refusal behavior and in addressing their own behavior by learning to provide incentives to the child for coping and disincentives for maintaining the sick role and missing school (Plante, 2007). Parents may need treatment for their own anxiety or other mental health concerns.

School personnel, in partnership with the child's family and often the child's primary care provider, will typically develop a detailed management plan for the child's return to school including how the child's gradual return to school is to be carried out. For example, will the child take the bus or be brought to school by a parent? Who will meet the child at school? Which classes will the child attend? When will the amount of time at school be increased? Are rewards included for successful attendance? In addition to the management plan, other issues need to be addressed by school personnel. If the child has had an extended episode of school absence, plans for completing missed school work may need to be made. If the motivation for the school refusal behavior was to avoid some aspect of school, such as teasing by other students or learning problems, school personnel need to address these difficulties.

> At the team meeting, Katie's parents learned about Katie's general anxiety, and Ms. Murphy acknowledged that she now realized that while she enjoyed having Katie at home with her, that this was not in Katie's best interest. A plan for gradual reintroduction to school was developed, with her attending half days for the next 3 days and then moving to full days the following week. Katie's homeroom teacher would meet her each morning and provide support as needed. Missed coursework was discussed and a plan to make up missed assignments agreed on. The school psychologist planned to meet with Katie frequently in the next few weeks and to adjust the need for ongoing sessions as appropriate. Sessions with the school psychologist would focus on relaxation techniques and exploring some of the concerns that Katie has related to school, including assistance with peer relationships. Ms. Murphy decided that she would reward Katie with a special activity when Katie had completed a full week of school, and discussed ways to support Katie interacting more with her peers. In consultation with Katie's parents, you recommend that at this point Katie does not need medication for her anxiety. However, you will reassess this decision at a follow-up visit. The decision was made that Ms. Murphy and the school psychologist will meet with Katie the next morning to discuss the plan. You plan to call the family and meet with Katie after that discussion to see if she will agree to counseling and the plan as arranged.

> ***When do you want to see this patient back again?*** ▪

The primary care provider may initiate follow-up with the student's parent via telephone or written communication within a week to inquire about the effectiveness of the reintroduction plan and with an office visit scheduled in the next few weeks to confirm that the child has returned to school and to follow up on the family's needs for counseling services. Children who are treated with medications will need to be monitored.

> Katie returned for a follow-up visit in one month. She had returned to school, although she still reported stomachaches periodically. Ms. Murphy reported that she did not see any other physical symptoms so encouraged Katie to go to school. She had met with the school psychologist and had learned how to recognize the signs that she was becoming increasingly anxious and how to use some relaxation techniques in response to her anxiety. All of her missed schoolwork had been completed, and her grades seemed to be good. She was interacting more with her close friends, and Ms. Murphy felt that overall Katie seemed happy. Katie spoke more with you and said that she still worried at times, but that school was "OK" and that she was doing more things with her two best friends, including a sleepover planned for the next weekend.

Key Points from the Case

1. School refusal is a common problem that must be addressed immediately using a variety of assessment strategies.

2. School refusal may arise for a variety of reasons; the assessment needs to identify the appropriate causes for the individual child.

2. Management of school refusal requires a team effort, including the child, parents, healthcare provider, and school educators and counselors.

4. The primary care provider needs to be a part of the team, including visiting with the school personnel, attending a team meeting, and following up both with the healthcare and the total management plan to get the child back into school and functioning in a happy and healthy way.

REFERENCES

Achenbach, T. M., & Ruffle, T. M. (2000). The Child Behavior Checklist and related forms for assessing behavior/emotional problems and competencies. *Pediatrics in Review, 21*, 265–271.

Bernstein, G. A., & Borchardt, C. M. (1996). School refusal: Family constellation and family functioning. *Journal of Anxiety Disorders, 10*(1), 1–19.

Bernstein, G. A., Warren, S. L., Massie, E. D., & Thuras, P. D. (1999). Family dimensions in anxious-depressed school refusers. *Journal of Anxiety Disorders, 13*(5), 513–528.

Bloom, B., & Cohen, R. A. (2007). Summary health statistics for U.S. children: National Health Interview Survey, 2006. National Center for Health Statistics. *Vital and Health Statistics 10*(234). Retrieved July 25, 2008, from http://www.cdc.gov/nchs/data/series/sr_10/sr10_234.pdf

Cohen, E., Mackenzie, R. G., & Yates, G. L. (1991). HEADSS, a psychosocial risk assessment instrument: Implications for designing effective intervention programs for runaway youth. *Journal of Adolescent Health, 12*(7), 539–544.

Egger, H. L., Costello, E. J., & Angold, A. (2003). School refusal and psychiatric disorders: A community study. *Journal of the American Academy of Child and Adolescent Psychiatry, 42*(7), 797–807.

Elliot, J. G. (1999). School refusal: Issues of conceptualization, assessment, and treatment. *Journal of Child Psychology and Psychiatry, 40*, 1001–1012.

Fremont, W. (2003). School refusal in children and adolescents. *American Family Physician, 68*, 1555–1560.

Glascoe, F. P. (2000). Detecting and addressing developmental and behavioral problems in primary care. *Pediatric Nursing, 26*(3), 251–258.

Heyne, D., King, N. J., Tonge, B. J., & Cooper, H. (2001). School refusal epidemiology and management. *Pediatric Drugs, 3*(10), 719–732.

Jarvis, C. (2007). *Physical examination and health assessment* (5th ed.). St. Louis, MO: Elsevier/Saunders.

Jellinek, M. S., Murphy, J. M., Little, M., Pagano, M. E., Comer, D. M., & Kelleher, K. J. (1999). Use of the Pediatric Symptom Checklist to screen for psychosocial problems in pediatric primary care. *Archives of Pediatric and Adolescent Medicine, 153*, 254–260.

Jellinek, M. S., Murphy, J. M., Robinson, J., Feins, A., Lamb, S., & Fenton, T. (1988). Pediatric symptom checklist: Screening school-age children for psychosocial dysfunction. *Journal of Pediatrics, 112*, 201–209.

Kearney, C. A. (2002). Identifying the function of school refusal behavior: A revision of the school refusal assessment scale. *Journal of Psychopathology and Behavioral Assessment, 24*(4), 235–245.

Kearney, C. A. (2006). Dealing with school refusal behavior, a primer for family physicians. *Journal of Family Practice, 55*(8), 685–692.

Kearney, C. A. (2007). Forms and functions of school refusal behavior in youth: An empirical analysis of absenteeism severity. *Journal of Child Psychology and Psychiatry, 48*(1), 53–61.

Kearney, C. A., & Albano, A. M. (2004). The functional profiles of school refusal behavior. *Behavior Modification, 28*(1), 147–161.

Kearney, C. A., & Bensaheb, A. (2006). School absenteeism and school refusal behavior: A review and suggestions for school-based health professionals. *Journal of School Health, 76*(1), 3–7.

Kelly, D. P., & Aylward, G. P. (2005). Identifying school performance problems in the pediatric office. *Pediatric Annals, 34*(4), 288–298.

King, N. J., & Bernstein, G. A. (2001). School refusal in children and adolescents: A review of the past 10 years. *Journal of the American Academy of Child and Adolescent Psychiatry, 40*(2), 197–205.

Kovacs, M. (2003). *Children's Depression Inventory: Technical manual update.* Toronto: Multi-Health Services.

Marcontel-Shattuck, M., & Gregory, E. K. (2006). Dealing with controversy in the practice of school nursing. In J. Slekeman (Ed.), *School nursing: A comprehensive textbook* (pp. 1113–1142). Philadelphia: F.A. Davis.

Martin, C., Cabrol, S., Bouvard, M. P., Lepine, J. P., & Mouren-Simeoni, M. C. (1999). Anxiety and depressive disorders in fathers and mothers of anxious school-refusing children. *Journal of the American Academy of Child and Adolescent Psychiatry, 38*(7), 916–922.

McCarthy, A. M., & Eisbach, S. (2006). Supporting emotional health. In M. J. Krajicek & M. Craft-Rosenberg (Eds.), *Nursing excellence for children and families* (pp. 113–134). New York: Springer.

Perrin, E., & Stancin, T. (2002). A continuing dilemma: Whether and how to screen for concerns about children's behavior. *Pediatrics in Review, 23*(8), 264–276.

Plante, W. A. (2007, December). Anxiety, somatic symptoms, and school refusal in children and adolescents. *The Brown University Child and Adolescent Behavior Letter,* (pp. 3–6).

Roye, C. F. (1995). Breaking through to the adolescent patient. *American Journal of Nursing 95*(12), 18–24.

Sewell, J. (2008). School refusal. *Australian Family Physician, 37*(4), 406–408.

U.S. Department of Education. (n.d.). *Individualized education program.* Retrieved October 24, 2008, from http://idea.ed.gov

Chapter 5

An Adolescent with Fatigue

Dawn Lee Garzon

Fatigue is one of the most common adolescent complaints in primary care settings. A number of medical, behavioral, and psychosocial factors can produce this subjective complaint; therefore, pediatric healthcare providers must be able to differentiate among common causes of fatigue and determine the need for medical intervention for adolescents with this complaint.

Educational Objectives

1. Consider adolescent development issues affecting both the diagnosis and treatment of fatigue.
2. Describe the lifestyle factors that affect the incidence of adolescent fatigue.
3. Describe the objective and subjective findings needed to establish a differential diagnosis in an adolescent with fatigue.
4. Formulate a tailored plan of care to manage an adolescent with fatigue.

Case Presentation and Discussion

Jennifer Styles is a 17-year-old who presents to your office with a complaint of "being tired all the time." Jennifer admits that her fatigue has worsened significantly over the summer and is worried that she won't make it through the day once school starts in a few weeks. She reports that she has two summer jobs, one at the community pool as a lifeguard and one where she helps babysit two school-age children. Jennifer is not accompanied by anyone else, but she says she can call her mother on the cell phone if "anyone needs her." "But," she tells you, "my mom thinks I have mono."

What are the most common causes of fatigue in adolescents? ■

Fatigue as a Symptom

Fatigue is a common somatic complaint that often presents with other symptoms like sleepiness, altered ability to focus, irritability, and weakness. By definition, fatigue is a sense of abnormal or excessive tiredness that results in a need for rest and results in an impaired ability to perform normal activities. It is one of the most common complaints in pediatrics and is especially prevalent during adolescence. Most teenagers complain of "being tired" at one time or another, and parents often complain that their adolescents seem exhausted or have very low energy. National studies show that 67% of adolescent females in 6th through 10th grade complain of morning fatigue at least once a week (Ghandour, Overpeck, Huang, Kogan, & Scheidt, 2004). The challenge of this condition is that fatigue can result from a self-limiting situation like staying up all night studying for final examinations, be a symptom of a mental illness like depression, or indicate the presence of a significant medical condition like anemia or cardiomyopathy.

Pathophysiology
There are multiple conditions that cause fatigue. It is the normal result of physical exertion or energy use that exceeds the body's normal capacity (Ozuah & Sigler, 2001). Physiologic reasons for fatigue appear when the level of cellular metabolic need is greater than the cell's adenosine triphosphate (ATP) stores, the body's glucose or glycogen stores are depleted, metabolism is altered, or cerebral oxygenation is compromised. Busy school schedules, participation in extracurricular activities, inadequate sleep, inadequate caloric intake, substance use/abuse, and dysfunctional sleep patterns can all result in abnormally tired teens.

Many adolescents with fatigue experience symptoms as an abrupt complaint following an acute infection (Carter, Kronenberger, Edwards, Michalczyk, & Marshall, 1996). However, postinfectious fatigue can last for weeks to years. Illnesses that are known to cause fatigue include acute and chronic Epstein-Barr infection, cytomegalovirus, herpesvirus, human immunodeficiency virus (HIV), histoplasmosis, *Mycoplasma* pneumonia, toxoplasmosis, tuberculosis, rheumatoid arthritis, diabetes mellitus, cancer, Lyme disease, and hepatitis (Feins, 1999; Ozuah & Sigler, 2001; Tunnessen & Roberts, 1999).

Fatigue can also be a response to stress and is considered a symptom of depression.

Cultural Influences of Fatigue
Culture shapes and influences how individuals experience health symptoms and whether or not they seek medical attention. Fatigue is a universal human complaint and, therefore, occurs in all populations; however, there are some significant cultural variations that are worth noting. Some cultures value achievement and activity or "doing," whereas others value just "being" (Giger & Davidhizer, 2004). Individuals from "doing" cultures may be less tolerant of fatigue symptoms and, therefore, are more likely to present to healthcare providers for treatment (Lubkin & Larsen, 2005; Ware & Kleinman, 1992). The belief that altered energy states should be treated to increase energy is also important. There are many homeopathic and complementary medical treatments used to combat fatigue that range from the use of herbal medications

and dietary modification to guided imagery, meditation, and cognitive behavioral therapy.

Ghandour and associates (2004) conducted a population-based investigation of 8,250 U.S. teens and found racial/ethnic variation in the report of morning fatigue. In this study, the authors found that non-Hispanic white and Hispanic adolescents reported morning fatigue at least one to three times a week at higher rates than their Asian, non-Hispanic black, and Native American peers (38.3% and 34.2% versus 31.2%, 30.8%, and 26.5%, respectively).

Adolescent Development Factors

Adolescence has traditionally been described as a time to achieve four major milestones—separation from parents, establishment of peer relationships, achievement of sexual identity, and establishment of vocational goals for adulthood. Many authors have further broken down this 7 year or more phase of human development into three subunits—early, middle, and late adolescence—because teens do not achieve the four major goals along parallel trajectories. Rather, early teens are characterized as working on issues of physical development and comfort with one's sexually maturing body and emerging sexual interests and behaviors, whereas middle teens are working to achieve parental separation and peer relationships with the opposite sex, and late teens are focused on development of intimate relationships with the opposite sex (or a single partner) and vocational choices and plans. The average 17-year-old is transitioning from middle to late adolescence.

Cognitively, following the traditional Piagetian characterizations, the adolescent can deal with abstract concepts, thoughts of the future, and goals rather than just dealing with concrete or current issues.

Gathering Key Data

History

When obtaining a patient history for a fatigue complaint, the primary care provider should carefully try to determine the presence of underlying illness and also to establish the degree of impairment caused by fatigue. Ideally, the health history should be obtained from the teen and parent separately. Especially important is the need to distinguish among senses of tiredness, activity intolerance, weakness, and lethargy (Tunnessen & Roberts, 1999). The health history should include the following:

Diseases:

- History of present illness/symptom analysis
  - Ranked scoring of energy level (scale of 1–10 sufficient)
  - Onset of and duration of symptoms (acute symptoms defined as less than 2 months whereas chronic is 2 months or more)

- Associated symptoms including fever, rash, vomiting, abdominal pain, sore throat, myalgias, headache, back pain, polydipsia, polyuria, heart palpitations, and painful or swollen lymph nodes
- Feelings of sadness, loss of interest in normal activities, impaired concentration, quality of affect, interaction with others, and stress levels
- Alleviating/aggravating factors
- Pharmacologic and nonpharmacologic treatments used and effectiveness of these therapies (special care should be paid to note medications that are known to cause tiredness, e.g., first-generation antihistamines)
- Degree of impairment of normal activities (extracurricular, school, social) and presence of activity intolerance
- Past medical history
  - Anemia, allergies, CNS disorders
  - Recent travel, insect/tick bites, or exposure to infectious disease
- Review of systems
  - Menstrual history and sexual history (to determine likelihood of pregnancy)
  - Significant head injury, presence of dizziness, clumsiness
  - Alcohol, tobacco, and illicit drug use
- Family history of diseases

Functional health patterns:

- Nutrition: Appetite and 24-hour diet recall (note type and frequency of carbohydrate intake, caloric restrictions, caffeine use)
- Sleep and rest: Thorough sleep history including normal sleep habits and the presence of insomnia or parasomnias
- Psychosocial history
  - Job history and occupational exposures (note numbers of hours worked, time of day worked, and chemical/infectious exposures)
  - Family life issues
  - School issues

Developmental history:

- Independence from parents
- Peer relationships
- Sexual patterns
- Vocational issues
- Cognitive level

Jennifer reveals that she has had no recent travel except for a weekend trip to the beach with her family. She denies fever and is able to keep up her daily routines despite her fatigue. There is no history of recent tick, mosquito, or other insect bites. No one at home is ill, and she has no known sick contacts. She denies feelings of sadness, impaired concentration, and alcohol, tobacco, or other substance use. Jennifer's mom has hypothyroidism and takes "some pill once a day" to treat it.

Routine medications include daily use of a multivitamin with iron and ibuprofen 600 mg every 6 hours as needed for menstrual discomfort. She has seasonal allergies but is not currently taking medication for them. Jennifer reports that she is not currently sexually active and that she is currently menstruating so her last dose of ibuprofen was this morning. Her 24-hour diet recall is listed in Table 5-1. Jennifer states that she keeps a water bottle with her at work and she drinks at least 36 ounces of water a day. She denies constipation and diarrhea. She has no polyuria or dysuria.

Jennifer has an active social life and tries to get together with her friends "at least two to three times a week" but she has been "hanging out" with her closest circle of friends "most nights since summer is almost over." Hanging out usually consists of meeting at a friend's house, watching TV or playing video games, and listening to music. She is a senior in high school and achieves A and B grades without difficulty and anticipates going to college next year, though without a vocation in mind.

Jennifer has two jobs over the summer. She works 4 days a week at the local swimming pool. Her workday typically begins at 10 a.m. and ends around 6:30 p.m. Three days during the work week and one day on the weekend she babysits her neighbor's two children in the evening. During the week, she goes from the pool directly to her neighbor's and works until 10 p.m. On Saturday, she babysits from 7:30 a.m. until 4 p.m. She is allowed to sleep after the children go to sleep, but she is usually awake when the mother comes home because "their sofa is too uncomfortable to sleep on and I am usually chatting with my friends online." Most evenings, Jennifer falls asleep around midnight, "but there are nights I watch movies until 2 a.m." She sets her alarm to wake her at 7:30 a.m. but admits she often uses the snooze button three to four times before getting up. Jennifer falls asleep listening to her MP3 player, and she reports often awakening 2 to 3 hours after falling asleep to find her lights are on and her music is still playing.

Given these history findings, what is the most likely cause of Jennifer's fatigue? ■

Table 5-1   Jennifer's 24-Hour Diet Recall

Breakfast	Lunch	Dinner	Snacks
½ cup egg substitute	Grilled cheese sandwich	Small steak	Midmorning:
Fruit yogurt	Chips	Baked potato with	Glazed donut
Coffee with nondairy	Fruit cup	sour cream	Afternoon:
creamer and sugar	2% milk	Salad with lettuce,	Small apple
		cucumber, carrot,	Evening:
		and sesame seeds	Popsicle
		Diet soda	

What additional questions regarding Jennifer's sleep habits would help establish the diagnosis? ▪

Physical Examination Findings

Jennifer is a well-groomed adolescent with a normal affect. Her mental status is normal. Her height is 5'6", and her weight is 145 pounds (BMI 23.4). There are no rashes or lymphadenopathy and her vital signs are normal. Skin tone is nonjaundiced and capillary refill is less than 2 seconds in all extremities. There is no nasal turbinate edema, her conjunctiva are noninjected, and her tympanic membranes and oropharynx are normal. Jennifer's thyroid is nontender, normal sized, and without palpable lesions. There are no heart murmurs, and her heart rate is regular. Lung sounds are clear, and there are no signs of allergy, cyanosis, or clubbing. Both liver and spleen are nonpalpable, and the other abdominal exam findings are negative. Neurologic exam reveals 2+ deep tendon reflexes (DTRs) in all extremities with normal movement, strength, and sensation. All other exam findings are normal. Pelvic examination is deferred.

Is it possible Jennifer's fatigue is caused by a significant medical condition? ▪

What diagnostic testing can be used to determine the cause of Jennifer's fatigue? ▪

While performing the physical examination, Jennifer's cell phone rings, and her mother asks to speak with you. The mother requests that you test Jennifer for mononucleosis and hypothyroidism because she first showed symptoms of hypothyroidism during her junior year of high school. You talk to Jennifer about her mother's request, and Jennifer agrees to the testing. Laboratory findings are as follows:

- Complete blood count (CBC): WBC $6.2 \times 10^3/mm^3$ (normal), RBC 4.7 million/mL (normal), hematocrit 40% (normal), and hemoglobin 13.2 g/dL (normal).
- Thyroid function tests: T4 7.2 µg/dL (normal), TSH 1.9 µIU/mL (normal).
- Urinalysis: pH 5.0, specific gravity 1.020 and negative for nitrites, blood, sugar, bilirubin, and protein (normal UA).
- Epstein-Barr titers and heterophile antibody: negative for acute and chronic infection.

Making the Diagnosis

In order to determine if the root of Jennifer's symptoms is behavioral or physical, it is important to understand the clinical presentations of the most common causes of adolescent fatigue. In many instances, a detailed history and physical examination are all that are needed. Laboratory testing should be used to rule out serious illness and help narrow the differential diagnosis in cases where history and physical examination data prove inconclusive. Table 5-2 contains a list of commonly used laboratory tests with clinical indications.

Table 5-2 Commonly Used Laboratory Tests Used to Establish the Diagnosis of Adolescent Fatigue	
Laboratory Test	Indication
Complete blood count (CBC) with differential	Ill-appearing teens; unexplained fever; pallor, pica, or poor iron intake; suspected cancer; abnormal bleeding
Thyroid function testing (T4 and TSH)	Enlarged or tender thyroid, unexplained weight loss/gain, constipation/diarrhea, heat/cold intolerance
Throat culture	Cervical adenopathy, fever, exudative pharyngitis
Epstein-Barr titers or heterophile antibody test	Cervical adenopathy, exudative pharyngitis, splenomegaly, known contact with EBV-infected individual
Erythrocyte sedimentation rate	Chronic inflammation and suspected autoimmune disease, chronic infection, inflammatory bowel disease
Routine urinalysis	Dependent edema, oligouria, polyuria, polydipsia, polyphagia
Liver function tests	Jaundice, chronic abdominal pain, hepatitis exposure
Pregnancy test	Missed menstrual period, unprotected sexual activity
Drug screen	Suspected substance abuse, confusion, erratic behavior

Several common differential diagnoses and clinical presentations should be considered when adolescents present with fatigue. Mononucleosis, or Epstein-Barr virus (EBV) infection, is one of the most common causes of adolescent fatigue. Acute mononucleosis is characterized by marked sore throat, anorexia, anterior and posterior cervical adenopathy, fever, malaise, and myalgias. Approximately half of all cases may be accompanied by splenomegaly. Chronic mononucleosis follows acute symptoms and most often presents with marked fatigue, painful glands, and loss of appetite, although mild presentation of acute symptoms is possible (White, Sullivan, & Buchwald, 2004). Chronic EBV symptoms can last for up to 6 months following an acute episode. Positive EBV titers and heterophile antibody test (Mono Spot) indicate acute EBV infection, although up to 10% of adolescents with this disease will have a negative Mono Spot (Ozuah & Sigler, 2001). Complete blood counts indicate elevated white blood counts and may demonstrate the presence of atypical lymphocytes. In this case, Jennifer's history, physical examination, and laboratory results are not consistent with this diagnosis. Because she has had symptoms all summer and the white blood cell counts are normal, it will not be necessary to repeat the EBV titer.

Depression impacts the lives of up to 5% of teens and is one of the most common causes of chronic fatigue (American Academy of Child and Adolescent Psychiatry, 2004; Green, 1998). The classic symptoms of depression include marked loss of interest in activities and feelings of sadness. However, also common are irritation, agitation, impaired concentration, decreased school performance, substance use, and risk taking. Jennifer does not report any of these symptoms, thus making this diagnosis unlikely.

Allergies can disrupt sleep, and many of the medications commonly used to treat allergies (especially first-generation antihistamines) cause drowsiness. Pale, boggy nasal turbinates; clear rhinorrhea; pharyngeal cobblestoning; nonexudative conjunctivitis; sneezing; and increased tearing are signs of allergic disease. Even though Jennifer does have seasonal allergies, she is not currently taking antihistamines and her physical examination does not support this diagnosis.

Anemia may occur secondary to dietary restriction (especially iron intake), infection, chronic illness, and idiopathic causes. Most older children and teens with anemia are asymptomatic, although complaints of fatigue, activity intolerance, and pallor are common. Adolescents are especially susceptible to iron-deficiency anemia because of increased metabolic needs and dietary habits. Jennifer's CBC indicates that she is not anemic.

Behavioral causes of fatigue include excessive exercise, overscheduling, and caloric restriction. Adolescents often have busy academic lives, social obligations, sports activities, and jobs that, in combination, result in physical and mental fatigue. Adolescents are very body conscious and will commonly use caloric restriction as a means of losing weight quickly. Skipped meals, high caffeine intake that impacts sleep, and diets that are often too high in carbohydrates, both simple and complex, also cause fatigue. Jennifer's 24-hour diet recall does not support caloric restriction as a cause of her fatigue, but her work schedule is rigorous and may be contributing to her symptoms.

Despite the need for 9 to 9½ hours of sleep each night, most teens sleep for only an average of 7 to 7½ hours (Mindell & Owens, 2003). The epidemic of fatigue caused by inadequate sleep is so great that as many as 68% of high school students report excessive daytime sleepiness (Kothare & Kaleyias, 2008). Work schedules, busy social calendars, and the need to finish school assignments often result in late bedtimes and fragmented sleep. Most high schools begin before 8:00 a.m., resulting in very early wake-up times, often as early as 5:00 a.m. (Mindell & Owens). Puberty causes increased sleep needs secondary to rapid growth and metabolic needs, and a resetting of the circadian sleep rhythms that result in teens actually becoming sleepy 2 hours later than their prepubertal peers (Mindell & Owens; Kothare & Kaleyias).

Based upon the history and physical findings in this case, the most likely cause of Jennifer's fatigue is sleep deprivation.

Management

What additional information needs to be considered prior to making a management plan for Jennifer? ■

Jennifer is actively working on her adolescent developmental milestones. In her case, she has achieved some degree of independence from her parents in that they trust her to visit your office unaccompanied and allow her to schedule her own activities fairly independently of the family. She is obviously very involved with peer relationships given her many phone, texting, and "hanging out" hours per week. Although not directly working on a future vocation, her two jobs indicate that she is working on issues related to employment— employee roles and responsibilities and financial gain. Her involvement with school indicates that she is a goal-directed young woman who is cognitively developing as predicted.

Given these characterizations, your plan will need to:

- Acknowledge that she is the primary decision maker related to her problem, not her parents. (independence from parents developmental task)
- Peer time needs to be assumed, though with adjustments. (peer relations task)
- Her involvement with employment as well as school is important to maintain to some degree. (cognitive and vocational goals)

Therapeutic Management Plan

Sleep Hygiene Measures

Management of fatigue caused by poor sleep hygiene and insufficient sleep primarily focuses on behavioral modification and promotion of healthy sleep habits. Medications should be used for only brief periods of time and are not indicated for the majority of children.

The first step in forming an appropriate management plan is the determination of each adolescent's practices that increase arousal and/or disrupt sleep cues (Mindell & Owens, 2003). Behaviors that arouse include caffeine intake, engaging in exercise in the late evening, watching television or playing video games while in bed, or trying to sleep in a nondarkened room. Behaviors that disrupt normal sleep cues include falling asleep while watching television or listening to music, spending long periods of time in bed while not sleeping, taking late naps, and sleeping in too late. Altered sleep cues are quite common during adolescence because most teens sleep too little during the work week, thus causing their "sleep clock" to be readjusted. This causes them to not feel sleepy until late evening to early morning (11:00 p.m. to 1:00 a.m.). Then, because they are so tired, they attempt to "make up" sleep on the weekends, thus resetting their sleep cycle even later. Sleep diaries are an excellent way to determine sleep patterns and behaviors and provide for greater depth of information than sleep recalls.

When you call Jennifer to give her the laboratory results, you ask her to keep a sleep diary and request a follow-up visit in 10 days. Jennifer's sleep diary reveals that she routinely gets 5 to 6 hours of sleep on weekday nights, she naps for 4 to 5 hours on weekends, and rarely falls asleep until after midnight. Her diary also reveals that her sleep is disrupted at least twice a week by friends who call her cell phone or send text messages after 1:00 a.m.

Medications

There is little scientific evidence for best approaches to pharmacologic treatment of sleep problems in children and adolescents. Most medications used to treat sleep problems are prescribed without Food and Drug Administration (FDA) approval, also known as off label use (Pelayo & Dubik, 2008). Most teens do not require medications, but pharmacologic therapies should be considered in cases where there is significant trouble initiating or maintaining sleep. Because prescription hypnotics are not indicated for use in children younger than 18 years, primary care therapies for insomnia should be used for only brief periods and should focus on use of two types of medications: antihistamines and melatonin.

The first generation antihistamines are known for causing drowsiness. Diphenhydramine is the most common ingredient in over-the-counter sleep aids and has been shown to decrease time to sleep and number of night-time awakenings when taken shortly before sleep (Pelayo & Dubik, 2008). Peak blood levels typically occur within 2 hours of dosing, and average duration of activity is 4 to 6 hours (Pelayo & Dubik). Normal adult doses are 25 to 50 milligrams. Common side effects include dizziness and daytime drowsiness, although significant side effects are rare and diphenhydramine is considered to have a good safety profile. A small but significant number of children will actually have paradoxical arousal from this medication, so caution should be used with the first dose.

Melatonin is available over the counter and is given to mimic the normal secretion of melatonin by the pineal gland. Melatonin levels cycle in a circadian rhythm and are generally highest at night and lowest during the day (Pelayo & Dubik, 2008). Blood levels typically increase 1 to 2 hours prior to bedtime and are considered to be the final trigger for sleep (Wagner, Wagner, & Hening, 1998). Melatonin is indicated for use in jet lag, in blindness-induced circadian rhythm disturbances, and in delayed sleep patterns (Mindell & Owens, 2003). Adult doses of melatonin are 1 to 3 mg and demonstrate best response when taken 2 hours prior to sleep (Pelayo & Dubik). There are two important issues to consider with melatonin. First, it is considered a diet supplement and therefore is not regulated by the FDA for safety, purity, or efficacy (Wagner et al.). Second, the National Sleep Foundation warns against melatonin use in individuals with immunodeficiencies, lymphoproliferative disease, and those taking corticosteroids or immunosuppressants because of its effect of enhancing immune function (Toitu, 2001). Side effects include nausea, headache, and lightheadedness (Mindell & Owens).

How would you manage Jennifer at this time? ■

Patient Education

The cornerstone of treatment for inadequate sleep is patient and family education about sleep needs and good sleep hygiene. Parents and adolescents must be taught that teens need 9 to 9½ hours sleep at night and that naps, when taken, should be brief (no longer than 30 to 45 minutes). Naps should only take place in the early afternoon. Sleep hygiene instruction should focus on developing good sleep schedules, making the bedroom "sleep friendly," encouraging health habits, promoting bedtime routines, and avoiding sleep disturbances (Table 5-3).

You help Jennifer recognize that her sleep patterns are the most likely cause of her fatigue. Your education begins by talking to Jennifer about ways she might make her bedroom more sleep friendly. You teach her to turn off her cell phone and computer before going to bed. You suggest that she only go to bed when sleepy and that she listen to music before getting into bed. Jennifer agrees to go to bed once she feels sleepy and to not try to "fight" her sleep. She agrees to set routine sleep and awake times and to not deviate more than one hour from these times. You review healthy nutrition and suggest a routine exercise program in the mid to late afternoon. Jennifer's mother commits to making sure she does not schedule evening activities and promises to help Jennifer wake up in the morning.

Once school starts, she will no longer work her lifeguard job. When babysitting, Jennifer decides to make phone calls and work on homework after her neighbor's children go to sleep so that she can go to bed within 30 minutes of arriving home.

Lastly, you decide to have her try melatonin 3 mg PO at bedtime for the next week until her sleep routines are better regulated.

Is there anything else you would add to the plan at this time? ■

Jennifer may need to make some adjustments in the time she spends with friends and the hours in which she talks with them. You and Jennifer need to agree upon a plan to inform her mother of the diagnosis and the plan that has been established.

When do you want Jennifer to follow up with you? ■

Follow-Up Parameters and Expected Outcomes

Adolescents with fatigue should be followed closely until a cause of their fatigue is found. Parents and adolescents should be asked to keep in close contact with the healthcare provider and should return for re-evaluation if symptoms change or worsen. Most critical for prompt evaluation is the development of fever, activity intolerance, abnormal bleeding or bruising, or fatigue that suddenly worsens or persists beyond a few weeks. Psychiatric referral for evaluation is indicated for fatigue that lasts more than 3 months in afebrile adolescents with normal physical findings and laboratory results (Feins, 1999). Referral to sleep specialists is indicated for failure to respond within 1 month of establishing sleep routines, if primary care pharmacologic intervention fails

Table 5-3 Good Sleep Hygiene for Adolescents	
Hygiene Goals	Steps to Improve Sleep Area
Make the bedroom "sleep friendly"	Bed should be comfortable with clean sheets and adequate covers and blankets.
	Temperature should be cool (less than 75 degrees).
	The room should be quiet and dark.
Establish good sleep schedules	Teens should go to bed and awaken at approximately the same time each day.
	Don't move bedtimes more than one hour a day.
	Limit naps to 30 to 45 minutes in the early afternoon.
	Never let teens sleep past 10:00 a.m.
	Don't use "all nighters" when studying—learning is processed during sleep and memory is best after "sleeping on it."
Encourage health habits	Routine exercise can help promote deep sleep, but vigorous exercise after 7:00 p.m. should be discouraged.
	Don't use caffeine, tobacco, and alcohol.
	Eat a well-balanced diet and avoid eating less than 2 hours before sleep.
Promote bedtime routines	Only engage in "quiet" activities like reading, listening to calm music, and watching television for 30 to 60 minutes before sleep.
	Eat a light snack or drink a glass of milk before bed, if hungry.
Avoid sleep disturbances	Turn off cell phones, computers, video games, televisions, and music prior to going to sleep.
	Use shades, blinds, or sheets to darken east-facing bedroom windows.
	Close doors and windows when noise might interrupt sleep.

Source: Table adapted from Mindell & Owens (2003) and Howard (2001).

or if prolonged pharmacologic treatment is required (Howard, 2001; Mindell & Owens, 2003).

You call Jennifer 2 weeks after her recheck appointment. She informs you that her fatigue is significantly decreased and she is no longer using the melatonin. She eliminated caffeine after 6:00 p.m. and implemented the sleep hygiene plan you created with her. You schedule a well examination in 3 months and tell her to call you if her symptoms recur or if she has questions or concerns.

Key Points from the Case

1. Fatigue is a complex symptom that is influenced by a number of factors.
2. Fatigue is a universal complaint that is especially common during adolescence.
3. It is essential that the evaluation of fatigue focuses on the diagnosis of underlying medical conditions that result in fatigue.
4. The most common cause of adolescent fatigue is insufficient sleep and poor sleep hygiene.
5. Adolescent sleep problems are best managed with behavioral modification and the development of good sleep habits. Medications should not be used in most cases and should be limited to use of antihistamines and melatonin in primary care settings.
6. The management plan needs to consider the adolescent's developmental level and milestones currently being achieved in order to support those important activities of their age.

REFERENCES

American Academy of Child and Adolescent Psychiatry. (2004). *Depression in children and adolescents.* Washington, DC: American Academy of Child and Adolescent Psychiatry.

Carter, B. D., Kronenberger, W. G., Edwards, J. F., Michalczyk, L., & Marshall, G. S. (1996). Differential diagnosis of chronic fatigue in children: Behavioral and emotional dimensions. *Developmental and Behavioral Pediatrics, 17*(1), 16–21.

Feins, A. (1999). Fatigue. In R. A. Dershewitz (Ed.), *Ambulatory pediatric care* (3rd ed., pp. 913–915). Philadelphia: Lippincott-Raven.

Ghandour, R. M., Overpeck, M. D., Huang, Z. J., Kogan, M. D., & Scheidt, P. C. (2004). Headache, stomachache, backache, and morning fatigue among adolescent girls in the United States. *Archives of Pediatric and Adolescent Medicine, 158,* 797–803.

Giger, J. N., & Davidhizer, R. E. (2004). *Transcultural nursing: Assessment and intervention* (4th ed.). St. Louis, MO: Mosby.

Green, M. (1998). *Pediatric diagnosis: Interpretation of symptoms and signs in children and adolescents.* Philadelphia: WB Saunders.

Howard, B. J. (2001). Sleep disturbances. In R. A. Hoekelman, H. M. Adam, N. M. Nelson, M. L. Weitzman, & M. H. Wilson (Eds.), *Primary pediatric care* (4th ed., pp. 858–868). St. Louis: Mosby.

Kothare, S. V., & Kaleyias, J. K. (2008). The clinical and laboratory assessment of the sleepy child. *Seminars in Pediatric Neurology, 15*(2), 61–69.

Lubkin, I. M, & Larsen, P. D. (2005). *Chronic illness: Impact and interventions.* Boston: Jones and Bartlett.

Mindell, J. A., & Owens, J. A. (2003). *A clinical guide to pediatric sleep: Diagnosis and management of sleep problems*. Philadelphia: Lippincott, Williams & Wilkins.

Ozuah, P. O., & Sigler, A. T. (2001). Fatigue and weakness. In R. A. Hoekelman, H. M. Adam, N. M. Nelson, M. L. Weitzman, & M. H. Wilson (Eds.), *Primary pediatric care* (4th ed., pp. 1079–1084). St. Louis: Mosby.

Pelayo, R., & Dubik, M. (2008). Pediatric sleep pharmacology. *Seminars in Pediatric Neurology, 15*, 79–90.

Toitu, Y. (2001). Human aging and melatonin: Clinical relevance. *Experts in Gerontology, 36*, 1083–1100.

Tunnessen, W. W., & Roberts, K. B. (1999). Fatigue. In Tunnessen & Roberts (Eds.), *Signs and symptoms in pediatrics* (3rd ed., pp. 46–52). Philadelphia: Lippincott, Williams, & Wilkins.

Wagner, J., Wagner, M. L., & Hening, W. A. (1998). Beyond benzodiazepines: Alternative pharmacologic agents for the treatment of insomnia. *Annals of Pharmacotherapy, 32*, 680–691.

Ware, N. C., & Kleinman, A. (1992). Culture and somatic experience: The social course of illness in neurasthenia and chronic fatigue syndrome. *Psychosomatic Medicine, 54*, 546–560.

White, P. D., Sullivan, T. P. F., & Buchwald, D. (2004). The nosology of sub-acute and chronic fatigue syndromes that follow infectious mononucleosis. *Psychological Medicine, 34*, 499–507.

Functional Health and Mental Health Problems

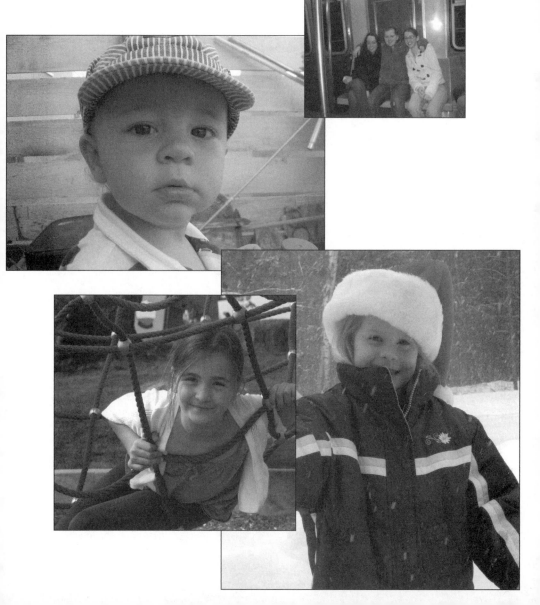

Chapter 6

The Well Infant

Anna Marie Hefner

A newborn baby, whether it is the first or last child, is unique and brings changes to family dynamics. The initial newborn visit provides a special opportunity for the healthcare provider to discuss the mother's pregnancy and delivery, immediate postpartum mother and infant issues, and plans for individualized care of both the baby and family. For the discharge of a mother and her newborn occurring within 24 to 48 hours after childbirth, the American Academy of Pediatrics recommends that the first office visit occur as early as 2 days after discharge. Factors that determine the timing for scheduling this first visit include the healthcare needs of the newborn, the date of discharge of the mother and infant, and the concerns of the family.

According to the American Academy of Pediatrics (2004, p. 1435), the purpose of the initial visit is to:

- Weigh the infant; assess the infant's general health, hydration, and degree of jaundice; identify any new problems; review feeding pattern and technique, including observation of breastfeeding for adequacy of position, latch-on, and swallowing; and obtain historical evidence of adequate urination and defecation patterns for the infant
- Assess quality of mother–infant interaction and details of infant behavior
- Reinforce maternal or family education in infant care, particularly regarding infant feeding
- Review the outstanding results of laboratory tests performed before discharge
- Perform screening tests in accordance with state regulations and other tests that are clinically indicated, such as serum bilirubin
- Verify the plan for health care maintenance, including a method for obtaining emergency services, preventive care and immunizations, periodic evaluations and physical examinations, and necessary screenings

Educational Objectives

1. Apply the guidelines for management of newborn health care, including prenatal history and childbirth, assessment of infant's general health, reviewing feeding patterns and technique, preventive care and immunizations, physical examination, and necessary screenings.

2. Assess the quality of mother–infant interaction.
3. Identify the strengths of the family and reinforce family education in infant care.
4. Consider the cultural factors that might affect the healthcare plan and the family's understanding and compliance with the plan of care.

Case Presentation and Discussion

Lauren Calzada is a 4-day-old Mexican American female born to a 34-year-old gravida 2 para 2 Mexican American mother in a common law marriage. She has a previous male child, Anthony, born 3 years ago. She explains that her newborn daughter is breastfeeding every 2-4 hours and is healthy; however, the 3-year-old is whining all the time. She has noticed Lauren is more "yellow" than Anthony was at birth. Ms. Calzada is concerned about the jaundice Lauren is exhibiting.

What initial questions need to be asked of Ms. Calzada? ■

The healthcare provider should establish a baseline history that includes information about the following:

- *Pregnancy:* Para and gravida status, when she first sought prenatal care, any maternal health problems (e.g., toxemia of pregnancy or gestational diabetes), any fetal health issues.
- *Labor:* Length and complications.
- *Delivery:* Type of delivery, use of instruments, any maternal or fetal complications.
- *Hospitalization:* How soon after birth was the infant discharged home?
- *Neonatal course or issues since discharge:* Feeding, voiding, sleeping, and any worrisome symptoms or signs or parental concerns.

Ms. Calzada says she remained healthy during her pregnancy. Her labor was unremarkable, with a spontaneous vaginal delivery 6 hours after the first contractions, just 2 days before her due date. Ms. Calzada had a small labial laceration requiring sutures with no further complications. Lauren had a "small lump on the left side of her head" (cephalohematoma) at delivery, but no other problems were noted after delivery or during the hospital stay. Ms. Calzada breastfed Lauren in the delivery room and experienced no breastfeeding problems. She and Lauren were released from the hospital 36 hours after delivery, and since then Lauren has been breastfeeding every 2-3 hours and voiding adequately.

Last evening she noticed Lauren had "yellow cheeks," and by morning the jaundice appeared on the baby's chest. She called the healthcare provider and made a late morning appointment.

What additional questions will you ask Ms. Calzada related to the jaundice? ■

Before answering this question, here is essential information about jaundice in the newborn that you need to consider.

Pathophysiology of Newborn Jaundice

Jaundice results from the deposition of unconjugated bilirubin in the skin and mucous membranes. It is a result of the shortened life span of the red blood cells, declining hematocrit, immature liver uptake and conjugation of bilirubin, and increased reabsorption of bilirubin in the intestines. The common risk factors include ABO incompatibility, prematurity, breastmilk jaundice, and a previously affected sibling.

Additionally, cephalohematomas, bruising, and trauma from an instrumented delivery may increase the risk for elevation of serum bilirubin. **Ms. Calzada told you about Lauren's "bump" and the hospital record noted a cephalohematoma on the left temporal area.** In a cephalohematoma, there is a collection of blood under the periosteum. This blood breaks down into heme, which becomes bili and may contribute to jaundice, and iron, which is recycled into new red blood cells. However, jaundice is present to some degree in most newborns and is known as physiological jaundice (De Almeida & Draque, 2007).

Jaundice can be detected when blanching of the skin reveals a yellow color. It starts on the face and progresses caudally. The higher the total bilirubin, the further it progresses down the body (Johnson, Bhutani, & Brown, 2002). Jaundice is difficult to detect in dark-skinned newborns. The examination should always occur in a well-lit room.

Other information you should obtain includes the following:

- What is the mother's blood type and baby's blood type?
- What is the Rh factor of the mother?
- Has the baby had a fever?
- Has the baby or the mother been exposed to any person or persons with an infection in the 2 weeks prior to delivery?
- What have the baby's feeding and voiding patterns been since discharge from the hospital?
- What was the mother's first pregnancy experience like and was she able to successfully breastfeed her first child?

Your further questioning reveals the following additional information:

According to Ms. Calzada, Lauren breastfeeds every 3–4 hours, 5 minutes on each breast. She has approximately four to five wet diapers a day; the urine is dark yellow in color. Ms. Calzada reports that Lauren has had one green stool since discharge. There were no exposures to individuals with infectious diseases in the 2 weeks prior to her delivery or since then. Her first pregnancy resulted in a healthy, term male infant without complications. She was successful in breastfeeding Anthony for his first year of life.

You review the results of the laboratory studies conducted during their hospital stay.

The laboratory reports note that Ms. Calzada's blood type is O+, Lauren is A+, direct Coombs negative. Lauren's total bilirubin at 12 hours was 1.8 mg/dL.

The healthcare provider should also discuss Lauren's sleeping schedule. Ms. Calzada tells you that Lauren is sleeping longer stretches of time, almost 4 hours at times, allowing her to get the housework done.

Social History

Lauren's father is deployed in Iraq and will be on leave in 4 months. Ms. Calzada's mother is expected to arrive in 1 week and will stay with her daughter for 1 month. They live in two-bedroom military base housing, and Ms. Calzada has a few friends who come by when they can. Her church provides her meals since she has been home each evening. She says, "I'm coping OK. My church friends are a big help but I'll be happy to have my mother come and help me."

Physical Examination

The vital signs are T 37° Celsius, pulse 142, respiratory rate (RR) 48, weight 3.2 kg (45th percentile), length 50 cm (75th percentile), and head circumference 34 cm (75th percentile). The infant is jaundiced to the abdomen. The anterior fontanel is flat and slightly sunken; oral mucosa is moist. No cephalohematoma or bruising is present. The sclera of both eyes are clear. Muscle tone and activity are normal. Reflexes: suck and swallow strong and coordinated, rooting intact. The remainder of the physical exam is normal.

Making the Diagnosis

Differential Diagnosis

The differential diagnoses for jaundice in the newborn include ABO incompatibility, infection, physiological jaundice of the newborn, and breastmilk jaundice.

This history and physical examination are consistent with a diagnosis of physiological jaundice and may be exaggerated with breastfeeding jaundice. She has jaundice to the abdomen, breastfeeding every 3–4 hours, and a history of a cephalohematoma.

Other problems that need to be addressed include:

- Breastfeeding techniques
- Military family with husband deployed

How do you plan to treat the jaundice? ■

Do you need to do anything to confirm the diagnosis, such as laboratory studies? ■

At this time, a total and direct bilirubin would need to be done. The laboratory results for Lauren are total bilirubin of 6.8 mg/dL with a direct bilirubin of 0.1 mg/dL. Additional testing would need to be done if there were additional symptoms such as a fever, listlessness, increased irritability, or poor feeding. A complete blood count, reticulocyte count, and serum albumin levels may also need to be checked.

Therapeutic plan: What will you do therapeutically? ▪

Treatment is not usually necessary with physiological jaundice. However, Lauren would need to be kept hydrated. Mother can increase the frequency of breastfeeding to every 2–3 hours during the waking hours and allow baby to sleep up to 4 hours at night. Physiological jaundice usually resolves within 1 to 2 weeks.

Educational plan: What will you do to educate Ms. Calzada about breastfeeding and its management? ▪

Jaundice

Ms. Calzada needs to bring Lauren back to the healthcare provider if the baby develops a fever, becomes listless, or is not feeding well. Jaundice is usually not dangerous in the term healthy newborn. Additionally, Ms. Calzada should call the provider if the jaundice becomes more severe, lasts longer than 2 weeks, or if other symptoms develop.

Nutrition: Breastfeeding

Breastfeeding should be for a minimum of 10 minutes on each breast or until the baby is content. Watch Ms. Calzada breastfeed her infant. Review how to hold the baby and correct latching on, if you note problems with her technique. Discuss that newborn infants typically demand feedings 8 to 12 times per day for the first 4 to 6 weeks of life. Lauren can also receive sunlight through adequate exposure to indirect sunlight. Lauren's mom can place the baby by a window that has sun exposure, but not in such a position that the sun is directly shining on the infant. Mom can also take the baby outside with her to sit in the shade on a warm day. Discussion of bowel movements—frequency and transitional stools, voiding patterns of six to eight wet diapers per day—should also be addressed.

What other areas of education and anticipatory guidance are needed for the family? ▪

Bright Futures: Guidelines for Health Supervision of Infants, Children, and Adolescents (Hagan, Shaw, & Duncan, 2008) identifies three key areas of anticipatory guidance that should be addressed at each well child visit. Because this sick visit is focusing on the assessment and management of Lauren's jaundice, you will not want to overwhelm the mother with extensive healthcare teaching. The healthcare provider should mainly use this time to address the issue of jaundice brought forth by the mother. However, the healthcare provider should also discuss at least one to two anticipatory guidance issues (e.g., car seat use and limited outings) at this visit and explain to Ms. Calzada that they will be discussing anticipatory guidance issues at future wellness visits. The clinician will need to identify what anticipatory guidance topic or topics should be a priority issue addressed at this time. The focus could be a safety, sleep, or general infant care issue that emerged from information obtained during the history and examination of the infant. Keep in mind that a discussion about safety, such as the use of an infant car seat, is always an appropriate issue to address at every healthcare encounter.

Subsequent visits will address the following areas of anticipatory guidance:

- Promotion of healthy and safe habits
  - *Car seat safety:* Position the newborn in the back seat of a car, facing backwards, following manufacturer's instructions and the vehicle's owner manual. The infant needs to remain in the car seat at all times during travel.
  - *Crib safety:* Slats in the crib should be no further than 2⅜ inches apart.
  - *Smoke-free environment:* Families should make their home and car nonsmoking zones.
  - *Home safety:* The baby should never be left alone in water or on high places such as changing tables, beds, chairs, or sofas. Keep one hand on the baby.
  - *Hygiene:* Caregivers' should wash their hands with soap and water frequently, especially after diaper changes and before feeding the baby.
- Infant care
  - *Outings:* The newborn is susceptible to illness and needs to be protected from anyone with a cold or illness. Consider carefully the necessity of bringing the newborn on outings such as trips to the grocery store, faith-based activities, and restaurants in order to avoid persons with colds or flu.
  - *Cord care:* Air dry the cord by keeping the diaper below the cord until the cord falls off (about 10–14 days). There may be some slight bleeding for a day or two when the cord falls off.
  - *Prevent diaper rash:* Clean baby and air dry after each diaper change. Change diaper frequently.
  - *Bathing:* Baby's skin does not need to be washed daily with soap. Tell the mother to wipe the baby's genital area with each diaper change and to avoid detergent-based soaps. Newborn infants need to be bathed every few days and as needed.
  - *Cradle cap prevention:* Wash scalp (every other day to daily) with baby shampoo or mild soap such as Dove. Demonstrate washing the scalp to the parent to reassure and decrease fear of touching the "soft spot."
  - *Temperature taking:* Review the procedure of taking a temperature with the parents.
- Feeding

- *Feeding times:* Feed the baby when hungry. Signs of hunger include sucking, rooting, fussing, and putting hand to mouth.
- *Burping and spitting up:* Burp baby by gently rubbing or patting their back while holding the baby against your shoulder and chest or supporting the baby in a sitting position on your lap. Burp midway through feeding and at the end of feeding. Babies can have "wet burps" up to 30 minutes after feeding.

Military Family Needs

The military family has unique needs based on deployment in times of war, training assignments, and potential reassignment to another base. Children of military personnel have universal access to Tricare, the military health insurance. Parents can then secure health care for their dependents in military facilities or through civilian options (Budzik, 2008).

Military deployments, whether to war torn areas or just for training sessions outside of their home base station, are often stressful times for these families, some of whom may be temporarily displaced when such assignments occur. The ability of a military family to acclimate to deployments and family separation may vary from those who have an affinity to cope well with the cycle of military moves and/or deployment to those whose lives are thrust into turmoil. Although, Ms. Calzada's children are very young, the healthcare provider should be alert to potential problems that children may also experience. Research focusing on the effect of deployment in children reveals that children can be impacted by the separation caused by deployment for extended periods of time. Budzik (2008) noted that research conducted with military families during Operation Desert Storm demonstrated that children of deployed soldiers experienced increased symptoms of depression; however, their symptoms were rarely pathological. Lamberg (2004) noted that some children became more confident and independent during times of deployment for their parent. Gibbs and colleagues (2007) investigated the incidence of maltreatment of children of enlisted soldiers during times of deployment and noted an increase in the incidence rate during times of deployment. Thus, the implications of these studies clearly validate the need for families left behind, like the Calzadas, to receive the emotional, psychosocial, and sometimes financial support they need.

Ms. Calzada now has two children with a husband in Iraq and is awaiting help from her mother. A study by Giles (2005) found that Army wives appear to suffer from high levels of stress, and their coping mechanisms were affected by constant turbulence and isolation. He noted that Army dependents require more support from their healthcare provider than the average civilian family.

Because of the isolation Ms. Calzada may feel, the healthcare provider needs to be alert for the development of postpartum depression and symptomatology of isolation. Assessing for postpartum depression should be an integral part of well child visits during the next 6 to 12 months. Healthcare providers must be proactive in providing support and alternative services. In Ms. Calzada's situation, you should discuss whether there are services on base for new mothers. She is currently using her church support system to help care for her children until her mother arrives. Additionally, when her husband returns in 4 months, the healthcare provider should encourage her to seek out military services that are available to them to promote a positive integration of the family after his experiences in Iraq. Proactive intervention can help the family better cope with "after effects" of potential postdeployment stressors. In addition, acknowledge Ms. Calzada's decision to utilize resources such as her church family during the fourth trimester.

The military has an Operation Homefront program (accessed at http://www.operationhomefront.net) that is an excellent resource that provides emergency assistance and morale to troops, to the families they leave behind, and to wounded warriors when they return home. The Department of Defense has a Web site called Military Homefront dedicated to providing information to help troops and their families and service providers (http://www.militaryhomefront.dod.mil). Civilian healthcare providers may find this Web site beneficial when caring for military families.

When do you want to see this patient back again? ■

This patient should be scheduled to come back in a week to be rechecked. However, if Lauren develops any symptomatology (as identified in the educational plan), she will need to be seen earlier.

Key Points from the Case

1. Treatment of jaundice depends on the cause of the jaundice. In Lauren's case, it was physiological jaundice. She needs to be kept hydrated and the jaundice should resolve in 10–14 days.

2. Breastfeeding every 2 to 3 hours, nursing 8 to 12 times in a 24-hour period, is expected during the first few days of life. By 1 week of age, the newborn should be breastfeeding every 2 to 3 hours with longer stretches up to 4 hours for sleeping.

3. The role of the provider is to help the new family deal with specific issues, health issues, and the needs of the mother and baby. It is a supportive role as the family makes adjustments to the new family member. Education and anticipatory guidance can help alleviate unnecessary anxiety.

4. Military families have special needs as parents that need to be addressed.

REFERENCES

American Academy of Pediatrics, Committee on Fetus and Newborn. (2004). Hospital stay for healthy term newborns. *Pediatrics, 113*, 1434–1436.

Budzik, C. (2008). Providing well child care for military families: What every provider needs to consider. *Pediatric Annals, 37*(3), 185–188.

De Almeida, M. F. B., & Draque, C. M. (2007). Neonatal jaundice and breastfeeding. *Nurse Research, 8*(7), 282–288.

Gibbs, D. A., Martine, S. L., Kupper, L. L., & Johnson, R. E. (2007). Child maltreatment in enlisted soldiers' families during combat-related deployment. *Journal of the American Medical Association, 298*, 528–535.

Giles, S. (2005). Army dependents: Childhood illness and health provision. *Community Practitioner, 78*(6), 213–217.

Hagan, J. E., Shaw, J. S., & Duncan, P. (Eds.). (2008). *Bright futures guidelines for health supervision of infants, children, and adolescents* (3rd ed.). Elk Grove Village, IL: American Academy of Pediatrics.

Johnson, L. H., Bhutani, V. K., & Brown, A. K. (2002). System-based approach to management of neonatal jaundice and prevention of kernicterus. *Journal of Pediatrics, 40*(4), 396–403.

Lamberg, L. (2004). When military parents are sent to war, children left behind need ample support. *Journal of the American Medical Association, 292*(13), 1541–1542.

Chapter 7

The Overweight Preschooler

Margaret A. Brady

Childhood overweight is an increasing health problem that the primary health-care provider (PCP) often faces on a daily basis when seeing pediatric patients. Rarely do parents of young children bring their child to the PCP for either sick or well child visits with expressed concerns of overweight. Typically, parents think in terms of "baby fat" that will magically disappear as the child grows or believe that comorbidities linked to obesity are issues seen only during adulthood. Because childhood overweight often becomes a chronic problem, the PCP must be vigilant in identifying risk factors and in assessing weight, nutrition, and physical activity issues when caring for children. The PCP must also remember that nutrition and weight are likely culturally bound. Therefore, a family-centered approach is needed because the child typically is not the only obese member of the family unit.

Educational Objectives

1. Describe how genetic inheritance and environmental factors impact the development of obesity in young children.
2. Explain the diagnostic criteria used to determine whether a child is at risk for overweight or obesity.
3. Describe the common clinical manifestations and comorbidities associated with pediatric obesity.
4. Apply physical activity and nutrition management guidelines for prevention of overweight and obesity to a toddler who is at the 85th percentile for BMI.
5. Integrate knowledge of culture, development, nutrition, physical activity, and behavioral approaches to develop a treatment plan for the toddler who is obese.

Case Presentation and Discussion

Maria Smith is a 3-year-old girl who is brought in by her mother, Margarita Smith, for her 3-year-old health supervision examination. Mrs. Smith says that the family just moved from out of state and that Maria and her younger 22-month-old brother, Bobby, are now going to be receiving care at your clinic. Mrs. Smith says that Maria has been a healthy child and she has no real concerns at this time except that Maria needs to see a dentist because she has lots of cavities. Mrs. Smith pauses and then says, "Maria's preschool teacher says Maria needs to go on a diet because she is too fat." You acknowledge that it is important for Maria to see a dentist and that her growth and development are important issues that you will be discussing with Mrs. Smith as part of this health supervision visit.

The Health Supervision Visit and Areas of Concern Identified by the Mother

The *Bright Futures: Guidelines for Health Supervision of Infants, Children, and Adolescents* (Hagan, Shaw, & Duncan, 2008) outlines 10 themes that should be promoted when children are seen for health supervision visits: the promotion of family support, child development, mental health, healthy weight, healthy nutrition, physical activity, oral health, healthy sexual development and sexuality, safety and injury prevention, and community relationships and resources.

Mrs. Smith has already identified issues related to oral health and healthy weight. You decide that you need some introductory family background and then will investigate these oral health and healthy weight issues next because they are the concerns she has listed as her priority items.

What questions should you ask Mrs. Smith about family support and mental health issues? ■

You begin by asking general questions about the family and learn the following. Mrs. Smith is married to Maria's father, who was recently discharged from the Army and now works as an auto mechanic. She proudly tells you that they bought their first home and are happy to have two healthy children, Maria and her 22-month-old brother, Bobby. The maternal grandmother, grandfather, and 18-year-old uncle live around the corner from them. The grandparents watch the children 2 days a week while Mrs. Smith works at a fast food restaurant during the day. Money is tight but they are doing OK and are happy to now have health insurance through Mr. Smith's job. Mrs. Smith smiles and tells you that her husband is very loving with the children and loves to read to them before bedtime. The children and Mr. Smith like to go to the local park on the weekends so Maria and Bobby can play on the swings with the other neighborhood children. Mrs. Smith is Hispanic and Mr. Smith is African American. Mrs. Smith said that she and her husband are happy in their marriage. While they were dating, it was a tense situation for both families at first because of their different ethnicities, but their respective families now like each other.

During the visit, you note that Mrs. Smith communicates in a loving manner with the children and gives them appropriate choices. When either one of them misbehaves (e.g., when Maria reached for a tongue blade), her response was appropriate.

Developmental Surveillance and Promotion of Safety and Injury Prevention

Your clinic routinely uses a developmental screening checklist for all health supervision examinations. The list was developed from *Bright Futures* materials.

> Maria does well in all areas (social-emotional, communicative, cognitive, and physical development), and Mrs. Smith is pleased. She reports that Maria is toilet trained for bladder and bowel during the day and wet her bed only once this past month. Maria has been attending Head Start for the past 6 weeks and "is doing well" socializing with the other children.
>
> After asking Mrs. Smith questions about car safety seats, pedestrian safety, fall risks, and guns, you are comfortable that both Maria and her brother are well supervised and the appropriate safety precautions have been implemented to prevent unintentional injuries in the home and car environment.

Oral Health

> Maria has not yet seen a dentist despite obvious caries in her frontal incisors. Mrs. Smith says that she was told by her last primary care provider that the cavities were from drinking too many bottles of milk. She says, "I was so tired with two babies that I let Maria have a bottle of milk to carry around the house. I feel badly now because that is why she has all those cavities. I know that I need to take her to the dentist." Upon further questioning, you are told that Mrs. Smith took the bottle away from Maria at 22 months of age and that she often had 50 ounces of whole milk a day when she was a toddler. She has not had a bottle for the past 10 months and drinks 24 ounces of whole milk a day from a cup and only with her meals and snacks. Mrs. Smith brushes Maria's teeth with a soft toothbrush and toothpaste twice a day, "but it is a struggle." Maria drinks tap water daily; their water has the recommended amount of fluoride.

Healthful Nutrition, Physical Activity, and Healthy Weight

Culture and food are often interconnected, so you start off by asking questions about Maria's typical eating pattern—number of meals, snacks, portion sizes, and food preferences.

> You are told that Maria eats three meals and two snacks daily. Maria likes cheese but isn't good about eating vegetables. She also likes apples and strawberries. She prefers the "kids' meals" from the fast food restaurant that mom works in and eats them four times a week. The Smiths enjoy a family meal on Saturdays and Sundays at either the maternal or paternal grandparents' home, having either Mexican food or "soul" food depending on the relative they are visiting. Maria's favorite vegetable is a "french fry"; she has sodas about three times a week as a treat and has about 12 ounces of juice a day. The grandparents like to give Maria and Bobby candy treats on the weekends, but Mrs. Smith doesn't give them candy otherwise.

You ask about the physical activities Maria likes to do. Mrs. Smith says, "Maria loves to draw her pictures," and she prefers interacting with other children by sitting down as she "isn't a runner." You also ask Maria what she likes to do best with the other children at preschool or home. She says, "I like to color and play with my dolls." You ask Maria how fast she can run, what her favorite games are, and whether she likes to play inside or outside. She replies, "I can't run as fast as the other kids. I like to stay inside with teacher and watch videos. I like *The Little Mermaid*." When asked how long Maria watches videos, TV, or participates in other screen time activities on a daily basis, Mrs. Smith says, "about 3 hours, but more like 5 hours when grandma is babysitting."

You ask whether Mrs. Smith remembers being shown Maria's growth grids or given information about her height and weight during her prior health supervision visits. She said, "Yes, Maria has been over the 95th percentile in height and weight since she was 6 months old. But our families are big people."

Here is some information about the problem of obesity in children that you need to consider as you continue your data collection.

Obesity in Children

Epidemiology of Obesity

The rapidly increasing prevalence of childhood obesity has become an escalating problem and is considered a major public health issue in the United States. The National Health and Nutrition Examination Survey (NHANES) reported that 14% of children ages 2–5 years were overweight (National Center for Health Statistics, 2007), and in 2006 17% of children ages 6 to 17 in the United States were overweight (Federal Interagency Forum, 2008). A national study of 3-year-olds reported that 35% of the children in this study were overweight and that Hispanic children were twice as likely as black or white children to be overweight or obese (Kimbro, Brooks-Gunn, & McLanahan, 2007).

Etiology

Simply stated, obesity results when energy intake from food exceeds energy expenditure. Factors that cause this imbalance are numerous and influence both the prevalence and severity of overweight in an individual (Anderson & Butcher, 2006). Genetic inheritance factors are estimated to account for anywhere from 16% to 85% of body mass index (BMI) and from 35% to 63% of body fat percentage (Yang, Kelly, & He, 2007); however, the exact mechanism of how genes contribute to the prevalence and severity of obesity is unknown. All ethnic minorities in the United States are at higher risk for overweight than whites regardless of socioeconomic status (Freedman et al., 2008). Gene regulation involved in energy homeostasis, thermogenesis, adipogenesis, leptin, insulin levels, or a combination of these factors is thought to contribute to obesity (Lagou et al., 2008; Yang et al., 2007).

Genes interact with diet via digestion and absorption of nutrients to regulate energy metabolism and cellular growth. Genes also affect expenditure of energy through physical activity by regulating cellular maximal oxygen uptake and skeletal muscle metabolism. Thus, some individuals perform better in their athletic activities because of their genetic inheritance. However, the impetus to become involved in physical activity and the level of involvement largely occur through positive rewards for performance, which is a significant factor. In contrast, engaging in sedentary activities (watching television, excessive screen time activities) is associated with energy conservation with low metabolic demands. Television or screen time activities combined with food intake are particularly problematic. This hypothesis is now supported by studies demonstrating that excessive energy consumption with television viewing may be a greater problem than the lack of activity per se (Epstein et al., 2008; Matheson, Killen, Wang, Varady, & Robinson, 2004).

Intrauterine environment is now viewed as one of the most potent factors in determining risk for future overweight and obesity based on studies with large and small for gestational weight infants (Gillman, Rifas-Shiman, Berkey, Field, & Colditz, 2003; Simmons, 2004). An overly nutrient-rich intrauterine environment appears to impact fetal metabolism, which puts the child at risk for later overweight by creating demand for excessive energy intake after birth (Rasmussen & Kjolhede, 2008). Hence, maternal preconception overweight and excessive weight gain during pregnancy are issues associated with childhood overweight. The converse to this is the small for gestational age infant who is now thought to be programmed by a nutrient-poor environment to function with a "thrifty gene" that may forever alter the child's level of nutrient needs. Overfeeding such a child is also problematic.

Certain environmental and lifestyle changes are directly linked to the increasing prevalence of childhood obesity in almost every part of the world; these result in children being raised in an obesogenic environment. When meals are not prepared at home and fast food is the meal of choice, there is a significantly greater risk for childhood overweight (Larson et al., 2008; Pereira et al., 2005). Likewise, the lack of neighborhood safety for outdoor play, increased sedentary screen time activities (> 2 hours per day) as part of a child's everyday life events, and the reduction of physical education in schools are factors that reduce the opportunities of children to perform physical activities. Larger proportions of food servings, increased consumption of foods higher in total fat and saturated fats, decreased consumption of fruits and vegetables, and increased sweetened beverage intake are related to unhealthful food choices and eating patterns that are now more often the norm than not.

Parents provide both the genetic and environmental factors which are important to the weight of their children. Strong predictors of childhood overweight that continues throughout childhood are having either one or both parents overweight and low income status (Danielzik, 2004; Dorosty, Emmett,

Reilly, & ALSPAC, 2000; Gahagan, 2004; Sothern & Gordon, 2003; Whitaker, Wright, Pepe, Seidel, & Dierz, 1997).

Diagnostic Criteria for Childhood Obesity

The American Academy of Pediatrics (AAP) Expert Committee (Barlow & Expert Committee, 2007) and the Centers for Disease Control and Prevention (CDC) use body mass index (BMI) percentile classification based on age and gender to define childhood overweight and obesity. BMI measurements are used beginning at age 2 years. If a child's BMI is equal to or greater than the 95th percentile for age and gender, the child is considered obese. A child is termed overweight if the BMI is at the 85th to less than the 95th percentile. The AAP and CDC recommend the use of weight-for-length in children younger than 2 years, with values above the 95th percentile indicating overweight. Although the BMI is not a perfect measure, it is currently considered the measurement of choice to determine overweight in children (Krebs et al., 2007; Kuczmarski et al., 2002).

Comorbidities Linked to Childhood Obesity

The problems associated with childhood obesity are numerous and include hypertension; lipid profile abnormalities; polycystic ovary syndrome; fatty plaque development within the arterial intima; type 2 diabetes mellitus (Libman & Arslanian, 2007), which occurs more commonly after 10 years of age; asthma (Glazebrook et al., 2006); more fractures and musculoskeletal conditions (Taylor et al., 2006); nonalcoholic fatty liver disease (Riley, Bass, Rosenthal, & Merriman, 2005); sleep-disordered breathing and obstructive sleep apnea (Muzumdar & Rao, 2006); and academic performance and social/emotional well-being issues (Gable, Britt-Rankin, & Krull, 2008). The pathophysiologic consequences of childhood obesity related to the comorbid conditions just identified are linked to such underlying processes as metabolic overwork due to insulin resistance, hyperglycemia, excessive adipose tissues, stress on bones, and negative self-esteem.

From the above review, what additional questions should you ask? ▉

What other areas do you want to explore in the history which might be related to the obesity problem? ▉

History

Pregnancy, Labor, and Delivery

Mrs. Smith reports that she had high blood pressure during her last 4 months of pregnancy with both of her children and was on insulin for gestational diabetes. She was induced at 38 weeks with Maria because of her hypertension and diabetes. Maria weighed 8 pounds 15 ounces at birth, had no problems, and went home with mom on day 2.

Family Medical History

You ask about the weight status of other family members, cardiovascular risk factors (heart attacks before the age of 50 years, hypertension, hyperlipidemia), and diabetes.

Mrs. Smith tells you that Maria's maternal and paternal grandmothers have type 2 diabetes and her paternal grandfather had a heart attack at age 52. Mrs. Smith relates that both sets of grandparents are very overweight with blood pressure and cholesterol problems. She tries to watch her own weight and considers herself to be a little overweight, wearing "large women" clothes. She ends by saying, "I come from big boned people." Mrs. Smith said that her blood sugars have gone back to normal after both of her pregnancies. She says, "I don't want to get diabetes like my mom and dad." She reports that her husband has maintained his army weight since his discharge 3 months ago because he exercises a lot.

Additional Nutrition Questions

You start out by saying, "Let's talk about what Maria ate yesterday for her meals and snacks."

Mrs. Smith relates that Maria had a large bowl of sugar puffs for breakfast with milk and a piece of toast and fruit juice (6 ounces). For lunch, she ate at the fast food restaurant where mom works and had a kid's meal—cheeseburger, fries, a yogurt, and a regular soda as a treat (because she was a good girl). Grandma cooked cheese enchiladas for the family dinner, and Maria had one, and a scoop of ice cream for dessert. She thinks Maria had her usual glass of whole milk (about 8 ounces) but doesn't know for sure because her mom fed the kids because she had to work until 8 p.m. Her snacks were apple slices around 10 a.m. and a chocolate chip cookie before bed with 8 ounces of whole milk.

You note to yourself that her diet is high in carbohydrates and Maria's portion sizes are excessive.

Past Medical Problems and Review of Systems

- *Illnesses:* Maria has been healthy but was diagnosed with "low iron" anemia at age 15 months. She was treated with iron and was told to limit her milk intake. Maria has never been hospitalized or taken to the emergency room for illnesses or injuries and has no known allergies to foods or medications.
- *Sleep:* A review of systems is positive for loud snoring at night and some restlessness with sleep. However, Maria does not seem sleepy during the day and takes an occasional 20- to 30-minute nap. She sleeps about 10 to 11 hours a night.

- *Immunization history:* A review of Maria's immunization history reveals that she is up to date with all required immunizations for a child of 3 years.
- *Physical activity:* You ask about the type of physical and play activities Maria did yesterday. Mrs. Smith took the kids for a walk around the block before she went to work and then grandma babysat. Maria told her mom that she and her brother and grandma watched her grandma's "soaps," played with their toys and dolls, and then watched her favorite videos in the afternoon until her dad picked the children up. Maria and her dad played his favorite video games after they went home from grandma's house at 7 p.m. Mrs. Smith got off from work at 8 p.m.

Psychosocial History

- *School adjustment:* Maria seems happy at school and is doing well. The only issue has been that some of the kids call her "fatso," which prompted the teacher to call Mrs. Smith and talk to her about Maria's weight.
- *Discipline:* You ask Mrs. Smith how she disciplines Maria when her behavior is not appropriate and how she rewards Maria for good behavior. Mrs. Smith says that Maria has a short time-out in her room and that she rewards Maria with praise. When asked whether she uses food as a reward, Mrs. Smith said, "I try not to reward her with candy like her grandparents do, but I've been giving her a piece of chocolate every day that she doesn't fight with her baby brother. That seems to be the only way to control the fighting between Maria and Bobby."

What aspects of the physical examination will be important in this case? ■

A developmentally appropriate approach to conducting the physical examination of a 3-year-old such as Maria involves approaching her slowly and keeping her mother close to her, gaining her involvement in the examination process, and giving attention to issues of modesty that may now surface as an area of concern for some preschoolers. A complete physical examination is needed, with the primary care provider being diligent to investigate for signs of secondary complications associated with obesity (e.g., obstructive sleep apnea, hypertension, orthopedic issues, etc.).

Physical Examination

Maria is in the 75th percentile in height and well above the 95th percentile in weight. Her BMI places her in the 97th percentile; her BP is normal for age, sex, and height percentile. Her general appearance is that of a happy but noticeably overweight preschooler. The general physical examination is within normal limits for age with the following positive findings: multiple caries involving the upper incisors and lower molars, and purple striae on her thighs. Chafing marks of her inner thighs are noted, and her vulvar area is erythematous, but without discharge. Inspection for acanthosis nigricans is negative.

The cardiovascular examination is within normal limits for age and reveals a normal S1 and S2 with no murmurs noted. She has full range of motion in all joints with bilateral symmetry and good strength in all extremities. A waddling gait is noted when she walks back and forth in the room. The EENT (eyes, ears, nose, and throat) exam is normal for age with 3+ tonsils bilaterally.

Making the Diagnosis

Do you need to do anything else, such as laboratory studies, to confirm the diagnosis? ■

Routine urine and hemoglobin screening is a standard practice in your clinic at the 3-year health supervision visit. **Maria's urine dip is negative for glucose and ketones and all other urine parameters are negative. Her hemoglobin is 11 g/dL, which is normal for her age.** These results provide baseline data to help you rule out anemia as well as glucosuria and ketonuria. A baseline fasting lipid profile for triglycerides, total serum cholesterol was ordered because of the paternal grandfather's history of a heart attack at age 52 years. In addition, a thyroid screen was ordered because Mrs. Smith wanted reassurance that Maria's overweight was not due to hypothyroidism. Otherwise, thyroid testing is not necessary at this age if the only symptom is overweight with no other symptoms such as goiter, brittle hair, stunted growth, or fatigue consistent with hypothyroidism present (Libman, Sun, Foley, & Becker, 2008). Although type 2 diabetes in children is predominantly seen after 10 years of age, you order a fasting blood glucose because Maria is at high risk due to her family history and ethnic background.

What are your diagnoses? ■

Maria's Hispanic/African American ethnic status puts her in a high risk category for obesity. Her history and physical examination with a BMI > 95th percentile are consistent with the diagnosis of obesity due to poor nutritional practices and an inactive lifestyle. Obesity is a family issue that must also be addressed. She has multiple caries. In addition, the possibility of obstructive sleep apnea needs further assessment and monitoring of symptoms. You will await the results of her lipid, thyroid, and fasting glucose readings to determine whether additional problems are identified. Maria's cognitive, gross and fine motor skills, and language development are appropriate for age. Her thigh and vulvar skin irritation can be easily treated with topical barrier agents. In summary, your diagnoses are:

- Obesity with a BMI at the 97th percentile
- Normal cognitive, language, social, and fine and gross motor development for age
- Caries
- Thigh and vulvar skin irritation secondary to obesity

Management

Overview of Nutrition and Physical Activitiy Guidelines

The U.S. Department of Agriculture provides guidelines and recommendations for structuring a healthy diet for children 2 years of age or older at http://www.mypyramid.gov/KIDS/. The healthy diet emphasizes fruits, vegetables, whole grains, and fat-free or low-fat milk and milk products and is low in saturated fats, trans fats, cholesterol, sodium, and added sugars. Appropriate food portion size for age is stressed. This Web site contains information about developing personal MyPryamid goals and planning meals. Another important point to stress with parents of young children is the need to limit fruit juice to ≤ 4 ounces per day at any age (Spear et al., 2007), excessive milk intake, and sweetened beverage intake.

Sixty minutes or more of daily moderate to vigorous intense physical activity is recommended to maintain weight. For preschool children, this is interpreted as active play. The benefits of moderate and intense levels of physical activity also include improved mood and attention (Berkey, Rockett, Gillman, & Colditz, 2003) and reduction of cardiovascular risk factors, whether or not weight loss occurs (McGavok, Sellers, & Dean, 2007; McMurray, Harrell, Creighton, Wang, & Bangdiwala, 2008). Limiting a child's daily screen time to no more than 2 hours is important. Sedentary activities are often a way of life for obese children or adults who may find physical activity difficult. Thus, the obese child will need to start with shorter periods of moderate to vigorous physical activity and gradually increase to these recommended levels over time. To lose weight, at least 90 minutes of vigorous daily physical activity are needed.

Culture has a significant impact on attitudes about foods, food choices, and eating practices and must be addressed as part of the management plan (Lumeng, 2008). The goal is to work within the culture to adopt culturally-appropriate healthier eating habits. Because the obese child is part of a family unit with other members who typically also have weight management issues, changes to more healthful nutrition and physical activity practices should focus on both the child and the family; family meals and healthier eating practices should be emphasized for all members of the unit. Likewise, physical activities should be encouraged for all members of the family, with physical activities scheduled as a family unit together whenever possible.

A Staged Treatment for Obesity

Using an evidence-based approach to the management of childhood obesity provides guidance to help children, adolescents, and their family to return to healthier nutrition and physical activity practices. In addition, the treatment of secondary complications (e.g., type 2 diabetes and obstructive sleep apnea) that are now more commonly found in younger obese children and adolescents also becomes an area that requires attention in order to avoid resulting negative personal and societal consequences. The AAP Expert Committee (Barlow & Expert Committee, 2007) recommends a four-stage approach for the prevention and management of overweight. Highlights of these stages are identified by Gottesman et al. (2010):

- *Stage 1: Prevention Plus:* The goal of this stage is to move the child's BMI to the 85th percentile; it will take 3–6 months for a noticeable change in BMI. Key concepts are to encourage family meals, eating at the table, adding more daily servings of fruits and vegetables, daily breakfast, and no sweetened beverages. Vigorous physical activity daily for $\geq$ 60 minutes needs to be planned with $\leq$ 2 hours of daily screen time per day allowed for the child. The provider should see the patient every 3 to 6 months. The goal of this stage is to increase physical activity, decrease physical inactivity, and improve the nutrition quality of the child's meals and snacks and develop better eating practices (e.g., not eating in front of television or grazing on food throughout the day).
- *Stage 2: Structured Weight Management:* Stage 2 includes all components of stage 1 with the addition of behavioral counseling. The key components of healthy eating in this stage are to emphasize foods with low calorie density, structured meals with one to two healthy snacks, and no sweetened beverages. The child should have 60 minutes of planned and supervised daily physical activity, and screen time should be limited to $\leq$ 60 minutes daily. A daily recording of physical activity and TV time, with a 3-day food log between visits, should be submitted for review. The parent or child should identify and use planned reinforcements which are not food related for desired behaviors. Schedule monthly visits to the PCP, and use of the services of multidisciplinary team members should be considered including referrals to family counseling, dietitian, physical therapy, and/or exercise therapist.
- *Stage 3: Comprehensive, Multidisciplinary Intervention:* The strategies for stage 3 include those listed in stages 1 and 2 plus a diet and daily physical activity plan to achieve a negative energy balance for weight loss. A multidisciplinary team approach is essential for both the child and family. More frequent follow-up visits are needed, with visits scheduled every 2 to 3 weeks. If comorbid medical issues are present, they must be monitored closely.
- *Stage 4: Tertiary Care Intervention:* Older children and adolescents who are severely obese and have failed stage 3 need to be referred to a pediatric obesity expert for stage 4 intervention. Management strategies may include very low calorie meal and snack plans, pharmacotherapy (e.g., Sibutramine or Orlistat), and/or bariatric surgery. A multidisciplinary team approach is essential.

Prevention

Prevention of overweight and obesity is of paramount importance, and every pediatric health supervision visit beginning at birth should provide anticipatory guidance about healthful nutrition practice, a healthy weight, and the promotion of age-appropriate physical activities and goals. When a child is found to be at risk for overweight or is obese, management of this problem and secondary complications, if present, become the focus of treatment to get the child "back on track." Once obesity is established it is difficult to reverse. Therefore, the prevention of childhood overweight must focus on health promotion and anticipatory guidance activities that emphasize healthful nutrition and optimal feeding and eating behaviors. The National Association of Pediatric Nurse Practitioners in their Healthy Eating and Activity Together (HEAT) Initiative developed clinical practice guidelines entitled *Identifying and Preventing Overweight in Childhood*; these can be accessed via the National Guideline Clearinghouse at http://www.guideline.gov. They are an excellent resource for PCPs.

Strengthening Parenting Skills and Family Motivation for Change

Strengthening parenting skills and family motivation to embrace healthful nutrition practices and inclusion of physical activity into a daily life plan are strategies the PCP must employ for both the prevention and treatment of obesity. The tenets of motivational interviewing techniques stress the need for self-management of healthcare problems and/or a return to healthier lifestyles and choices. The steps of motivational interviewing include assessing the importance, confidence (using a scale of 0–10 to rate confidence in the ability to change), and readiness for change; exploring the importance of making a behavior change; building confidence in the ability to change; and planning for change. For children, motivational interviewing requires the healthcare provider to work with the child and/or parents, who are the ones who determine what practices and interventions for change can be implemented in their lives. The emphasis is on patient values and preferences rather than telling the child or parent exactly what they "must do" (Gance-Cleveland, 2007). Information about motivational interviewing can be found at http://www.motivationalinterview.org.

Therapeutic Plan: What will you do therapeutically to manage this child? ▪

Maria's BMI is at the 97th percentile, which requires stage 1 weight management—prevention plus—as identified for this category. Reducing Maria's sedentary activities by decreasing her daily screen time, increasing her daily physical activities through increased opportunities for active play, and providing more healthful meals and snacks with appropriate portions as identified in http://Mypyramid.gov/KIDS/ are the three areas to address with Mrs. Smith. Because Maria has been teased about her weight by her preschool friends, you address the problem of negative self-esteem, which could become an issue for her. Furthermore, Mrs. Smith has indicated a readiness for change regarding nutrition and physical activity for her whole family. Building Mrs. Smith's confidence that she can identify changes that will work considering her family's lifestyle and personal preferences is essential.

Mrs. Smith identified the following plan for Maria. She will be allowed only 2 hours of screen time per day, and they will walk to preschool and the grandparents' home rather than going in the car. She will encourage more play time. Mrs. Smith is going to talk with the grandparents about providing Maria with more nutritious snacks and will also discuss with her husband ways they can increase the entire family's physical activity time together. Mrs. Smith says that she is going to try to reduce the number of times Maria has fast foods and will reduce Maria's soda drinking to two half-cans per week. She is also going to talk with Maria about her schoolmates calling her "fatso" and how best to respond to them.

Caries

A dental referral is initiated for Maria, and you provide her mother with pamphlets and teaching about healthy dental practices including daily brushing, fluoride sealants, and dental visits.

Skin Issues

You recommend a topical over-the-counter barrier cream to be applied twice a day.

When do you want to see this patient back again? ▮

You want to initially see Maria back in a month to 6 weeks. You will review the laboratory studies that were ordered, discuss the effectiveness of the treatment plan, and support the family in the new treatment management at this time. As the family develops self-care skills, further appointments can be spread further apart.

How should you close today's visit? ▮

You end by saying that Maria will be scheduled for a follow-up visit in 6 weeks to check her weight and review how Maria and her family are doing with the increased emphasis on healthy food choices and practices and increasing their daily activity. You ask Mrs. Smith to tell you how comfortable she is with implementing some of the suggestions that either you have given her or she has identified on her own to increase Maria's daily physical activity and to promote more healthful nutrition practices for her daughter. You write the plan down in Maria's chart and identify that, on a scale of 1 to 10, Mrs. Smith is a 5 in her comfort level that this plan will help both Maria and her family. You praise Mrs. Smith for her willingness to address the family's issue of being overweight and provide Mrs. Smith with a list of local community recreational programs that focus on increasing physical activities for young children and their parents.

The Follow-Up Visit

Maria and her mother return in 6 weeks for a weight recheck and follow-up counseling regarding nutrition and physical activity. Her weight is a ½ pound lower and she has seen the dentist and begun dental treatment for her multiple caries. You review her laboratory results. Her fasting blood glucose is 90 mg/dL (normal) and her thyroid and lipid panels are also within normal limits for age. Mrs. Smith is pleased with Maria's normal laboratory results.

Mrs. Smith says that the entire family is walking twice every day for a total of 30 to 45 minutes. The grandparents have also been receptive to reducing the portion sizes they give Maria when they provide her meals and are giving her healthier food choices by providing more fruits and vegetables. Maria still asks for candy rewards but Mrs. Smith is limiting this to only once a week as compared to five or six times, which she had done in the past.

You decide to wait to order polysomnography based on the data that Maria's loud snoring has not worsened and she remains awake and cheerful during the day.

Key Points from the Case

1. Obesity results when there is an imbalance between energy intake from food and energy expenditure from physical activity. Therefore, healthful nutrition practices and behaviors such as improved nutrition quality, appropriate portions, daily breakfast, and a daily plan of physical activity are key elements in the prevention and treatment of childhood obesity.

2. Heritability is a critical correlate regarding the prevalence and severity of obesity, with ethnic minorities at higher risk for overweight.

3. An obesogenic environment starting during prenatal development has a significant impact on the development of childhood obesity.

4. The primary care provider should address nutrition and physical activity at every well child visit by consistently monitoring growth parameters (height and weight percentiles) starting at birth and charting BMI beginning at age 2 years.

5. Childhood overweight and obesity typically do not occur as a single family member issue, but rather also as a health issue for other family members. Thus, a family-centered approach is needed as part of the management plan.

6. Motivational interviewing is a technique that establishes a collaborative relationship in the prevention, treatment, and management of a health problem. Offering management options and involving the caregiver and older child with decisions related to types of physical activity to engage in and adopting more healthful food choices encourages the practice of self-care management of the child's overweight problem.

7. Excessive screen time and food portions, lack of daily physical activity, fast food consumption, and using food as a reward are unhealthful behaviors that should be discussed with parents.
8. The emotional toll of childhood overweight and obesity, such as poor self-esteem and victimization by bullying, should also be addressed.
9. Some parents do not believe their child is overweight or at risk for comorbidities that they erroneously believe are adult onset problems.
10. Because of the increased prevalence of childhood overweight and obesity, primary care providers must assume an active role in the prevention and management of childhood obesity.

REFERENCES

Anderson, P. M., & Butcher, K. F. (2006). Childhood obesity: Trends and potential causes. *Future of Children, 16*, 19–45.

Barlow, S. E., & Expert Committee. (2007). Expert committee recommendations regarding the prevention, assessment, and treatment of child and adolescent overweight and obesity: Summary report. *Pediatrics, 120*, S164–S192.

Berkey, C. S., Rockett, H. R. H., Gillman, M. W., & Colditz, G. A. (2003). One-year changes in activity and in inactivity among 10- to 15-year old boys and girls: Relationship to change in body mass index. *Pediatrics, 111*, 836–834.

Danielzik, S. (2004). Parental overweight, socioeconomic status and high birth weight are the major determinates of overweight and obesity in 5–7 year old children. Baseline data of the Kiel Obesity Prevention Study (KOPS). *International Journal of Obesity and Related Metabolic Disorders, 28*, 1494–1502.

Dorosty, A., Emmert, P., Reilly, J., & ALSPAC Study Team. (2000). Factors associated with early adiposity rebound. *Pediatrics, 105*, 1115–1118.

Epstein, L. H., Roemmich, J. N., Robinson, J. L., Paluch, R. A., Winiewicz, D. D., Fuerch, J. H., et al. (2008). A randomized trial of the effects of reducing television viewing and computer use on body mass index in young children. *Archives of Pediatric and Adolescent Medicine, 162*, 239–245.

Federal Interagency Forum on Child and Family Statistics. (2008). *America's children in brief: Key national indicators of well-being, 2008.* Retrieved January 18, 2009, from http://www.childstats.gov/americaschildren

Freedman, D. S., Wang, J., Thornton, J. C., Mei, Z., Pierson, R. N., Jr., Dietz, W. H., et al. (2008). Racial/ethnic differences in body fatness among children and adolescents. *Obesity, 16*(5), 1105–1111.

Gable, S., Britt-Rankin, J., & Krull, J. L. (2008). *Ecological predictors and developmental outcomes of persistent childhood overweight.* Washington, DC: U.S. Department of Agriculture. Contractor and Cooperator Report No 42.

Gahagan, S. (2004). Child and adolescent obesity. *Current Problems in Pediatric and Adolescent Health Care, 34*, 6–43.

Gance-Cleveland, B. (2007). Motivational interviewing: Improving patient education. *Journal of Pediatric Health Care, 21*, 81–88.

Gillman, M. W., Rifas-Shiman, S. L., Berkey, C. S., Field, A. E., & Colditz, G. A. (2003). Maternal gestational diabetes, birth weight, and adolescent obesity. *Pediatrics, 111*, e221–226.

Glazebrook, C., McPherson, A. C., MacDonald, I. A., Swift, J. A., Ramsay, C., Newbould, R., et al. (2006). Asthma as a barrier to children's physical activity: Implications for body mass index and mental health. *Pediatrics, 118*, 2443–2449.

Gottesman, M. M., Brady, M. A., Gance-Cleveland, B., & Duderstadt, K. G. (2010). Obesity. In P. Jackson Allen, J. A. Vessey, and N. A. Schapiro (Eds.), *Primary Care of the Child with a Chronic Condition* (5th ed.). St. Louis, MO: Mosby.

Hagan, J. F., Shaw, J. S., & Duncan, R. M. (Eds.). (2008). *Bright futures: Guidelines for health supervision of infants, children, and adolescents* (3rd ed.). Elk Grove Village, IL: American Academy of Pediatrics.

Kimbro, R. T., Brooks-Gunn, J., & McLanahan, S. (2007). Racial and ethnic differences in overweight and obesity among 3-year-old children. *American Journal of Public Health, 97*, 298–305.

Krebs, N. F., Himes, J. H., Jacobson, D., Nicklas, T. A., Guilday, P., & Styne, D. (2007). Assessment of child and adolescent overweight and obesity. *Pediatrics, 120*, S193–S228.

Kuczmarski, R. J., Ogden, C. L., Guo, S. S., Grummer-Strawn, L. M., Flegal, K. M., Mei, Z., et al. (2002). CDC growth charts for the United States: Methods and development. *Vital Health Statistics, 11*, 1–190.

Lagou, V., Scott, R. A., Manios, Y., Chen, T. J., Wang, G., Grammatikaki, E., et al. (2008). Impact of peroxisome proliferator-activated receptors γ and δ on adiposity in toddlers and preschoolers in the GENESIS study. *Obesity, 16*, 913–918.

Larson, N. I., Neumark-Sztainer, D. R., Story, M. T., Wall, M. M., Harnack, L. J., & Eisenberg, M. E. (2008). Fast food intake: Longitudinal trends during the transition to young adulthood and correlates of intake. *Journal of Adolescent Health, 43*, 79–86.

Libman, I. M., & Arslanian, S. A. (2007). Prevention and treatment of type 2 diabetes in youth. *Hormonal Research, 67*(1), 22–34.

Libman, I. M., Sun, K., Foley, T. P., & Becker, D. J. (2008). Thyroid autoimmunity in children with features of both type 1 and type 2 diabetes. *Pediatric Diabetes, 9*(4Pt 1), 266–271.

Lumeng, J. C. (2008). Mother knows best? Feeding styles and child obesity. *Contemporary Pediatrics, 25*, 32–48.

Matheson, D. M., Killen, J. D., Wang, Y., Varady, A., & Robinson, T. N. (2004). Children's food consumption during television viewing. *American Journal of Clinical Nutrition, 79*, 1088–1094.

McGavok, J., Sellers, E., & Dean, H. (2007). Physical activity for the prevention and management of youth-onset type 2 diabetes mellitus: Focus on cardiovascular complications. *Diabetes and Vascular Disease Research, 4*, 305–310.

McMurray, R. G., Harrell, J. S., Creighton, D., Wang, Z., & Bangdiwala, S. I. (2008). Influence of physical activity on change in weight status as children become adolescents. *International Journal of Pediatric Obesity, 3*, 69–77.

Muzumdar, H., & Rao, M. (2006). Pulmonary dysfunction and sleep apnea in morbid obesity. *Pediatric Endocrinology Reviews, 3*(Suppl 4), 579–583.

National Center for Health Statistics. (2007*). Health, United States, 2007 with chartbook on trends in the health of Americans.* Hyattsville, MD: U.S. Government Printing Office.

Pereira, M. A., Kartashov, A. I., Ebbeling, C. B., Van Horn, L., Slattery, M. L., Jacobs, D. R., et al. (2005). Fast-food habits, weight gain, and insulin resistance (the CARDIA study): 15-year prospective analysis. *Lancet, 365*, 36–42.

Rasmussen, K. M., & Kjolhede, C. L. (2008). Maternal obesity: A problem for both mother and child. *Obesity, 16*, 929–931.

Riley, M. R., Bass, N. M., Rosenthal, P., & Merriman, R. B. (2005). Underdiagnosis of pediatric obesity and underscreening for fatty liver disease and metabolic syndrome by pediatricians and pediatric subspecialists. *Journal of Pediatrics, 147*, 839–842.

Simmons, R. (2004). Fetal origins of adult disease: Concepts and controversies. *NeoReviews, 5*(12), e511.

Sothern, M., & Gordon, S. (2003). Prevention of obesity in young children. A critical challenge for medical professionals. *Clinical Pediatrics, 42*, 101–111.

Spear, B. A., Barlow, S., Ervin, C., Ludwig, D. S., Saelens, B. E., Schetzina, K. E., et al. (2007). Recommendations for treatment of child and adolescent overweight and obesity. *Pediatrics, 120*, S254–S288.

Taylor, E. D., Theim, K. R., Mirch, M. C., Ghorbani, S., Tanofsky-Kraff, M., Adler-Wailes, D. C., et al. (2006). Orthopedic complications of overweight in children and adolescents. *Pediatrics, 117*, 2167–2174.

Whitaker, R. C., Wright, J. A., Pepe, M. S., Seidel, K. D., & Dierz, W. H. (1997). Predicting obesity in young adulthood from childhood and parental obesity. *New England Journal of Medicine, 337*, 869–873.

Yang, W., Kelly, T., & He, J. (2007). Genetic epidemiology of obesity. *Epidemiologic Reviews, 29*, 49–61.

Chapter 8

The Breastfed Infant Who Is Not Gaining

Pamela J. Hellings

Breastfeeding is a learned skill. Not infrequently, mothers encounter feeding difficulties that may result in slow weight gain for the baby. The challenge is to separate the common problems from the more complex issues. Slow weight gain cannot be dismissed as simply poor feeding technique in the early post-partum days. The provider must consider and eliminate other possibilities through a knowledgeable and thoughtful history and physical examination process.

Educational Objectives

1. Recognize issues associated with slow weight gain in a newborn infant.
2. Manage the feeding issues to maintain breastfeeding whenever possible.
3. Provide appropriate follow-up to assure adequate nutrition and weight gain in the infant and to support the family.

Case Presentation and Discussion

You pick up a message that Mrs. Jackson called one hour ago. She gave birth 8 days ago to her first child, a male infant, Peter. She did not keep her 3-day follow-up appointment at the clinic because she was "too exhausted" after delivery. She is breastfeeding but is worried that he is not getting enough to eat.

What further information would be helpful at this point? ■

In order to make the decision regarding the need for follow-up, a description of the feeding frequency and duration as well as a wet diaper and stool count would be helpful.

You call her back and she reveals that Peter is eating five to six times per day for 20 to 30 minutes total and is sleeping most of the rest of the time. He has had four wet diapers in the last 24 hours and no stool in 72 hours. You ask her to bring Peter in for a status check.

Table 8-1   After Breastmilk Comes In: How to Tell If Infant Is Getting Enough
Infant should:
Nurse at least 8 times in 24 hours, although 10–12 times is more common
Seem satisfied after feeding
Have at least six wet diapers with light yellow or colorless urine
Have four or more bowel movements per day
Have yellow and curdy, cottage cheese–like stool
Swallow loudly
Breasts should:
Feel full before a feeding and softer after a feeding

Your criteria for adequate breastfeeding are as follows: At 8 days old, a baby should be feeding 8 to 12 times in 24 hours for a minimum of 10 to 15 minutes per side. In addition, he should be stooling three to four times daily and voiding light yellow urine at least six to eight times (see Table 8-1).

> You are concerned so you fit them into the day's schedule. She arrives one hour later with Peter and her husband. You do not have any information on this patient because this will be their first visit to your practice.

Breastfeeding Support

In addition to the indicators that Peter is not feeding adequately, there are also other reasons for bringing in the Jackson family at this point. The transition to successful lactation often requires providing support and information for families. Even in the absence of significant problems, a review of technique and expectations for breastfeeding and evaluation for maternal breast comfort are warranted. Among the most common reasons given for stopping breastfeeding are perception of inadequate milk production and sore nipples (Schwartz et al., 2002). The 3-day visit provides an important opportunity to address these issues. However, the Jackson family missed that appointment, so now is the time to assess the situation and provide needed support and/or intervention.

Professional healthcare organizations recommend exclusive breastfeeding for 6 months (American Academy of Pediatrics, 2005; National Association of Pediatric Nurse Practitioners, 2007); the Healthy People 2010 goal (Healthy People, 2000) is for 50% of babies to continue to be breastfed at 6 months of age.

First Visit

What information do you want to collect now? ■

The history-taking process for breastfeeding problems needs to include gathering key information about the baby, the mother, and breastfeeding activities in areas where problems may interfere with adequate weight gain.

The measurements were taken and the baby weighs 6 pounds 6 ounces today. You now enter the room and find a sleeping baby in the arms of a worried looking mother. Mr. Jackson also appears somewhat somber. Mrs. Jackson provides you with the following information.

Infant, Mother, and Breastfeeding History

Birth History. The baby was born at 37 weeks and was a 6-pound 13-ounce male infant. There were no complications for mother or baby after a vaginal birth and an uneventful first pregnancy for this 27-year-old woman. Mother and baby were discharged together at 48 hours. The baby was sleepy during hospitalization, but nurses observed two feedings and did not report any problems. The discharge weight was 6 pounds 6 ounces (7% weight loss). The family was given a follow-up clinic appointment for 3 days after discharge but they did not attend.

Key information in this history: Peter's history to date has been uncomplicated by any notable problems. However, his birth at 37 weeks (near preterm) and his 7% weight loss, although within normal limits, are important to note. (See Table 8-2.)

Feeding history. Mr. Jackson has been trying to help keep Peter awake during feeding attempts. They have to wake the baby for feedings and stimulate him to keep him awake. They are successful every 4+ hours. Peter generally feeds for 20–30 minutes but a lot of that time is spent in waking him up. Mrs. Jackson reaffirms that he has had four to five wet diapers (disposable) in the last 24 hours and no stool for 3 days. The last stool was green, pasty, and smooth in texture. She has seen him urinate during a diaper change and describes a strong stream. Mrs. Jackson thinks maybe she feels her let-down but does not hear any loud swallows from Peter during feeding. She has leaked breastmilk occasionally but not as much in the last 48 hours. On the second day home, she experienced some engorgement but Peter continued to nurse and her breasts became less hard. Her nipples are a little sore but she has not experienced any cracking or bleeding.

Table 8-2   Infant Problems That May Affect Weight Gain
Infections
Endocrine/metabolic problems
Abnormalities of mouth or throat
Congenital heart disease
CNS problems
Near preterm status

Table 8-3   Technique Problems That May Affect Weight Gain
Infrequent feeds
Inadequate postejection suckling time
Ineffective suckling (poor latch or flutter sucking)

The parents have been grateful that Peter has been such a great sleeper for the past few days because they now are getting more sleep than they expected. However, in the last 2 days they have begun to worry that he may not be getting enough to eat. Peter's maternal grandmother says he looks "skinny" and has recommended that they supplement with formula. They want to breastfeed and have resisted supplementation so far. Peter's last feeding was 2.5 hours ago.

Key information in this history: The infrequent and less than vigorous feedings are important to note. The lack of audible sounds of swallowing are also concerning. Finally, the absence of stool for 72 hours provides an indication that Peter is not getting enough breastmilk to gain weight. (See Table 8-3.)

Mother's related history. Mrs. Jackson has some allergies to pollens and dust but takes no prescription or over-the-counter medication on a regular basis. She denies any other chronic illnesses or conditions. She has not had any surgery other than an appendectomy at age 13 years. The pregnancy was uneventful and uncomplicated with routine prenatal care beginning in the first trimester. Her vaginal bleeding has stopped. She plans to use progestin-type birth control pills beginning at 6 weeks postpartum. She has been drinking lots of fluids and eating well in order to provide milk.

Key information in this history: Mrs. Jackson is healthy by history. The lack of any chronic illnesses or surgery to the breasts or thorax is encouraging. In addition, she is not using any medications routinely and there is no evidence of hormonal influences from retained placenta or contraceptives. (See Tables 8-4 and 8-5.)

Other than the feeding concerns, Mr. and Mrs. Jackson have no other questions about Peter at this time.

What will you look for on the physical examination given the history to this point? ■

Table 8-4   Drugs That May Decrease Milk Supply
L-dopa derivatives
Ergot compounds such as bromocriptine
Large doses (> 600 mg/day) vitamin B_6 (pyridoxine)
Estrogen
Nicotine

Table 8-5   Maternal Problems That May Affect Infant Weight Gain
Chronic illnesses
Certain medications (see Table 8-4)
Drug or alcohol abuse
Smoking
Endocrine problems, especially involving the thyroid
Breast surgery
Anatomical problems including inadequate mammary gland development
Fatigue or stress
Inability to "let down"
Inadequate diet
Retained placenta

Physical Examination

You move on to the physical examination of Peter. Your examination reveals a baby with decreased fat distribution over his face, abdomen, and extremities but no evidence of dehydration. He is quietly alert at this time. He appears somewhat pale without any signs of jaundice. He weighs in at 6 pounds 6 ounces. His temperature taken in the axilla is 98°F. He has good tone and responds to light and sounds. His heart rate is regular, and no heart murmur is heard. Femoral pulses are palpable and equal. His lungs are clear. His mucous membranes are moist, his suck is strong, and his palate intact. His umbilical cord stump has fallen off, and the area is clean and dry. In addition, his circumcision is healing well. He has voided in his disposable diaper and the urine is a light golden color. There is no "brick dust," an indicator that a baby is not getting enough milk. ("Brick dust" on the diaper results from uric acid crystals forming in concentrated urine). Otherwise his physical examination is unremarkable.

Mr. and Mrs. Jackson become very upset at his weight as they realize he has not gained any weight since discharge. They wonder if they should go and get some formula immediately.

What do you say at this point? ■

Peter's exam is within normal limits with the exception of weight. In addition, there are indicators supporting inadequate weight gain but not the more serious failure to thrive. You share this information with the Jacksons in a supportive manner and urge them to stay calm while you proceed with the breastfeeding evaluation.

What will you look for on your breastfeeding evaluation? ■

Breastfeeding Observation

Prior to observing a feeding, you examine Mrs. Jackson's breasts. Her breasts are slightly firm with nipples that appear somewhat flat but evert with tactile stimulation. There are no cracks or bleeding visible. You are able to hand express drops of milk from both breasts.

Observation of a breastfeeding session reveals that Peter latches on successfully but starts to get drowsy fairly quickly. Positioning is adequate in the "cradle" position but Mrs. Jackson is reminded to keep him "tummy to tummy" as Peter falls away from the breast as he goes to sleep. Mr. Jackson attempts to help by talking to Peter and stroking his back. Meanwhile, Mrs. Jackson makes a few attempts to wake him but then gives up and shrugs her shoulders as if to say that this is typical. When removed from the breast and stimulated with a cold wet washcloth on his trunk, Peter wakes up again. Regular stimulation with gentle but persistent scratching to the soles of his feet and top of his head helps him stay with feeding. Periodically Peter is taken off, given additional stimulation, and switched to the other side if he does not respond to wakening techniques at the breast. He ends up at the breast for more than 30 minutes—most of which is alert feeding. He has gone back and forth twice to each breast. Some loud swallows are heard briefly at the beginning on each side. After feeding, he weighs 6 pounds 8.5 ounces on the same scale he was weighed on prior to your seeing him, a gain of 1.5 oz. Mom and dad are somewhat relieved by this news.

Making the Diagnosis

Given the histories of the mother and baby as well as the feeding history, the physical examination, and breastfeeding assessment/observation, the problem appears to be slow weight gain.

In assessing slow weight gain, a helpful way to approach the evaluation is to identify risk factors that are mother-related, infant-related, and/or technique-related (Lawrence & Lawrence, 2005). In this case, the mother has no chronic illness, takes no medications routinely, and her vaginal bleeding has stopped. Her breast exam reveals no significant issues as her nipples evert with stimulation, there are no cracks or bleeding, she is not engorged, and breastmilk is expressible from both breasts. There are no red flags for maternal health issues other than that she is a first-time mother and seems unclear about expected feeding frequency and output. She is producing milk for her baby.

The baby is afebrile and not visibly jaundiced. Key information obtained includes the following:

- Special attention should be paid to evaluation of the heart to rule out congenital heart disease that may not have been apparent before hospital discharge. There is no murmur and his pulses are normal.
- The suck is strong, and the palate is intact. Submucosal clefts can result in poor weight gain and need to be ruled out.
- This baby has no evidence of positive physical findings related to infection, hyperbilirubinemia, or dehydration.

- However, this baby was born at 37 weeks and should be considered a "late preterm infant." Sleepiness and slow feeding are common in the slightly preterm infant, despite a healthy birth weight and absence of other problems associated with prematurity (Meier, Furman, & Degenhardt, 2007).

The technique issues are primarily related to feeding frequency and duration, although inefficient suckling with inadequate milk transfer must also be considered. Mrs. Jackson is using proper positioning and gets latch-on with little difficulty. Peter gained 1.5 ounces after an alert and persistent feeding. That is very good news, and seems to confirm that his lack of weight gain is likely not related to health problems for him or his mother.

Successful breastmilk production is based on supply and demand. Regular, frequent stimulation with a successful latch, routine emptying of the breast, and the release of maternal hormones aid in the establishment of an adequate milk supply to sustain infant growth (Hellings, 2009). Peter has not been feeding the expected 10–12 times in 24 hours, and quality feedings have been of short duration.

After consideration of the possibilities, the most likely expanded diagnosis is slow weight gain due to inadequate feeding frequency and duration.

Management

The Jacksons are sent home with instructions to feed Peter every 2–3 hours for the next 24 hours and to use the awakening techniques demonstrated. They are reminded to set an alarm if necessary to wake themselves and to count the interval between feedings as the time from the start of one feeding to the start of the next. They are asked to keep a diary of feedings—time feeding started, duration, and a statement about quality of the feed—and number of voids and stools. Finally, they are asked to return tomorrow to check on progress. Mr. and Mrs. Jackson indicate that they think this is something they can do for 24 hours and they both state they really want the baby to be breastfed.

Important Considerations in Making the Management Plan

It is good that the parents came in so soon and that the mother's supply does not appear to have markedly decreased at this time. The weight gain associated with the feeding in the clinic also provides support for sending the family home with clear instructions regarding feeding. Supplementation is not necessary at this time; however, early follow-up to make sure that Peter continues to gain weight is very important.

Follow-Up Visit #1

The Jacksons return the next afternoon. They look tired and state they did not get much sleep last night. However, they think Peter has been doing better with feedings. In reviewing their diary, you note the feeding frequency and duration, wet diaper counts, and stool output. They still have to stimulate him a bit, but he has fed nine times in the last 24 hours. He had one large, loose, curdy, slightly greenish stool at 5 a.m. You commend them for their efforts. Mrs. Jackson does state that her nipples are sorer than yesterday. They are anxiously awaiting his weight check to see if their feeding efforts have been successful.

Important considerations in the follow-up examination: Peter's general appearance is important to note. In addition, he should be weighed on the same scale as yesterday. A full physical examination was completed yesterday and need not be repeated today.

Physical Examinations of Infant and Mother

Peter is alert and responsive. His cheeks look fuller. He weighs 6 pounds 9 ounces, an overall gain of 2 ounces in 24 hours. Mrs. Jackson says that her breasts feel fuller between feedings.

As Mrs. Jackson prepares to feed Peter, you examine her breasts again. You note some redness and a chapped appearance on the nipples. There is no cracking or bleeding. You review positioning and latch-on techniques with her as she puts Peter to breast. She states that she can feel the difference between a good latch and a poor one as you take him on and off several times to secure a good latch. You advise her to reposition him if the latch is painful rather than trying to ignore the pain. She finishes feeding Peter before they return home with another scheduled weight-check appointment in 2 days and instructions to call with any questions.

Peter has gained 2 ounces in 24 hours and has stooled once. The frequent feedings with poor technique at times has resulted in some increased nipple tenderness and irritation for Mrs. Jackson. With better technique and continued attention to feeding frequency and duration, the parents can go home and continue with the plan.

Follow-Up Visit #2

Mrs. Jackson is smiling and feeling confident that he has gained more weight. She states that her husband had to return to work so she came alone this time with Peter. He is 11 days old and is waking up now on his own to feed and fed 10 times in the last 24 hours. He stooled three times in the last 24 hours and the most recent one was runny, yellow-orange in color, and very curdy. She states that her nipples are less sore and admits that she did not set the alarm last night. Peter awakened on his own every 2 to 2.5 hours, with one stretch of 3 hours during the night.

Physical Examinations of Infant and Mother

Mrs. Jackson's nipples no longer have a chapped appearance but are still a little red. The skin remains intact. Her breasts are full, and she begins to actively leak milk during her exam. She puts Peter to breast with no difficulty, and he begins to feed vigorously with audible swallows.

Peter is awake and alert during the feeding. He requires no stimulation to keep feeding. He weighs 6 pounds 14 ounces, 1 ounce above birth weight and 5 ounces more than 2 days ago.

Because he is feeding well, you go ahead and get the second metabolic screening test done. Mrs. Jackson is really happy and gets out her cell phone to call her husband and share the news.

Peter gained 5 ounces in 2 days, more than the ½ to 1 ounce per day gain usually expected. He has been gaining at a "catch-up" rate. He is likely to continue at this rate for only a few more days and will then slow down to the normal expected daily weight gain. He has reached birth weight, an important milestone. Peter should return in 1 week to make sure he continues to gain weight. The parents should be encouraged to call with questions and are provided with information about how to assess if he is getting enough breastmilk.

What problems were avoided by this quick intervention and what could have been done preventively to avoid this breastfeeding problem? ■

This case study details a common clinical scenario in pediatric primary care. This time, there is a happy ending with a baby gaining weight on exclusive breastfeeding and with more confident parents. The story might have played out differently if the parents had delayed seeking assistance or if the mother's milk supply had been more compromised.

The problems might have been avoided if early assessment at the 3-day postdischarge visit had taken place and the slow feeding identified and managed. It is imperative to emphasize to parents the importance of that early follow-up visit, especially for the breastfeeding family. In addition, providing verbal and written information regarding expectations for breastfeeding and urine/stool output at the time of discharge from the hospital can be very helpful to parents, especially first-time parents, as they begin to care for their newborns (see Table 8-6).

In the assessment process for each individual patient, other problems might be found that suggest more complex health concerns for mother or baby. The need to carefully consider potential risk factors for insufficient infant weight gain is an important part of an initial breastfeeding visit.

Key Points from the Case

1. Early follow-up of breastfeeding families and assessment/identification of problems are important for supporting successful breastfeeding.
2. Common breastfeeding problems do not always require the services of a lactation consultant. However, primary care providers need to have a knowledgeable approach to the assessment and management process.
3. The assessment process includes recognition and identification of problems in the baby, mother, and breastfeeding technique.
4. Management strategies for slow weight gain must take into account issues for the baby, the mother, and breastfeeding technique.

Table 8-6 Guidelines for Breastfeeding in the First Few Days

	First 8 hours	8–24 hours	Day 2	Day 3	Day 4	Day 5	Day 6 on
Milk supply	Express few drops		Milk in between the 2nd and 4th day			Milk in: breasts firm/leak milk	Breasts softer after nursing
Baby's activity	Put to breast in 1st hour. Your baby should have at least 6 or more wet diapers with light yellow or colorless urine. Your baby should have four or more bowel movements per day. Your baby's stool should look yellow and curdy like cottage cheese.	Wake baby to feed	Baby more awake/cooperative	Look for feeding cues: rooting, hands to mouth; listen for regular swallows during nursing			Baby satisfied after feedings
Feeding routine	Baby sleepy after birth	Feed every 1.5 to 3 hours	Feedings at least 8–10 times in 24 hours			May have one longer interval in feedings	
Breast-feeding	Wakes up/responds after deep sleep	Nurse at both breasts	Both sides 10–15 min. per side	Manage engorgement —soften breast for baby	Nurse 10–15 min. per side every 2–3 hours for first few months		Nipple tenderness improved or gone
Baby's urine output		One wet diaper in 1st 24 hours	One wet diaper every 8 hours	4–6 wet diapers in 24 hours	Urine light yellow	6–8 wet diapers of light yellow urine per 24 hours	
Baby's stool		Meconium stool	2nd meconium stool	Stools changing from black green to yellow	Urine light yellow	3–4 seedy yellow stools day	Number of stools may slowly decrease after 4–6 weeks

Source: Adapted from Thilo, E. H. & Townsend, S. F. (1996). Early newborn discharge: Have we gone too far? *Contemporary Pediatrics, 13,* 29–46.

REFERENCES

American Academy of Pediatrics. (2005). Breastfeeding and the use of human milk. *Pediatrics, 115*, 496–506.

Healthy People 2010. (2000). *National health promotion and disease prevention objectives.* DHHS Pub. No. 91-50213. Washington, DC: Government Printing Office.

Hellings, P. (2009). Breastfeeding. In C. Burns, A. Dunn, M. Brady, N. Starr, & C. Blosser (Eds.), *Pediatric primary care* (4th ed., pp. 235–252). St. Louis, MO: Saunders Elsevier.

Lawrence, R. A., & Lawrence, R. M. (2005). Normal growth, failure to thrive, and obesity in the breastfed infant. In R. A. Lawrence, R. M. Lawrence (Eds.) *Breastfeeding: A guide for the medical profession* (pp. 436–447). Philadelphia: Elsevier Mosby.

Meier, P., Furman, L., & Degenhardt, M. (2007). Increased lactation risk for late preterm infants and mothers: Evidence and management strategies to protect breastfeeding. *Journal of Midwifery and Women's Health, 52*, 579–587.

National Association of Pediatric Nurse Practitioners. (2007). NAPNAP position statement on breastfeeding. *Journal of Pediatric Health Care, 21*(2), A39–A40.

Schwartz, D., Arcy, H., Gillespie, B., Bobo, J., Longeway, M., & Foxman, B. (2002). Factors associated with weaning in the first 3 months postpartum. *Journal of Family Practice, 51*(5), 439–444.

Thilo, E. H. & Townsend, S. F. (1996). Early newborn discharge: Have we gone too far? *Contemporary Pediatrics, 13*, 29–46.

Chapter 9

The Constipated 8-Year-Old

Tamra D. Kehoe

Undoubtedly, the primary care provider will encounter patients with concerns related to constipation. Childhood constipation accounts for approximately 3% of general pediatric outpatient visits and 25% of pediatric gastroenterology consultations (Baker et al., 2006). Parents often worry that their child's stools are too large, too infrequent, or too hard, or are painful to pass. Children presenting with encopresis may have fecal soiling without painful defecation, which is often perceived to be chronic diarrhea.

Families are often frustrated by multiple trials of ineffective strategies or believe their children are lazy or choose to have fecal accidents. The management of constipation and fecal soiling can be challenging for the child, family, and healthcare provider. To successfully treat these children, a well-organized plan utilizing medication as well as behavioral modification is paramount.

Educational Objectives
1. Discuss the etiology of encopresis including predisposing mechanical and psychosocial factors.
2. Apply the guidelines for management of encopresis to a school-age child.
3. Identify barriers to successful treatment.

Case Presentation and Discussion

Zachary Morris is an 8-year-old male who is brought to your office by his parents with concerns of fecal accidents that have been occurring since 6 years of age. Mrs. Morris reports Zach's school has recommended a medical evaluation because Zach is now being teased by peers for his malodorous smell and because he often wears a pull-up diaper which is occasionally visible. Zachary has loose to peanut butter consistency stools in his underwear or pull-up approximately four to five times daily; he denies any sensation of these stools. He is frequently malodorous and will sit in his soiled underwear until mandated by his parents to clean up. They believe he is quite lazy and elects to stool in his pants rather than excuse himself to the bathroom. Soiling occurs more frequently when he is on the computer, watching TV, or engaged in active play.

Mom expresses great frustration. Soiling was initially infrequent but has escalated to a daily problem. Because of odor and frequent leakage, the family tends to withdraw from outings and social events.

What questions will you ask about strategies the parents have tried? ■

Zachary's parents have utilized various strategies to correct his soiling including sticker charts and reward systems for putting stool in the potty, mandatory toilet sits every 2 hours, time-outs, and punishments. Medical treatment from their pediatrician has included polyethylene glycol 3350 powder (PEG 3350), 1 cap (17 g) orally every day for 2 weeks. This treatment resulted in more accidents, so his parents discontinued the stool softener after 1 week.

At this point, the problem sounds like encopresis so you consider what you know about this condition.

Pathophysiology of Constipation

Encopresis or fecal soiling refers to the repetitive voluntary or involuntary passage of stool in inappropriate places by children 4 years or older, at which time a child may reasonably be expected to have completed toilet training and exercise bowel control. Encopresis is usually associated with chronic constipation and functional fecal retention; however, it may occur in the absence of fecal retention, in which case, it is termed nonretentive encopresis. If a child is under 4 years old, it is termed fecal incontinence. Criteria for the diagnosis of functional constipation in children can be found in Table 9-1.

Encopresis can be termed retentive or nonretentive. Retentive encopresis is associated with constipation. The major difference between retentive and nonretentive encopresis is intent. In nonretentive soiling, the child is *voluntarily* stooling in inappropriate places, and it is usually associated with some degree of psychological disturbance.

Pathophysiology

Functional constipation, meaning constipation without evidence of a pathological condition, is most commonly caused by painful bowel movements with resultant voluntary withholding of feces. This withholding is done to avoid uncomfortable or painful defecation. In the majority of cases, encopresis is thought to occur as a consequence of chronic functional constipation with resulting overflow incontinence (Di Lorenzo & Benninga, 2004). The overflow stool can be pasty to watery, and is often confused with diarrhea.

There are time periods when a child is more vulnerable to developing acute constipation. In infancy, the change from breastmilk to formula or the addition of solids can cause constipation. Toddlers may exhibit magical thinking that results in fearful reactions or have conflict over toileting. School-age children

Table 9-1 Rome III Criteria for the Diagnosis of Functional Constipation in Children	
Infants and Toddlers	Children with Developmental Age 4 to 18 Years
At least two of the following present for at least 1 month:	*At least two of the following present for at least 2 months:*
• Two or fewer defecations per week	• Two or fewer defecations per week
• At least one episode of incontinence after the acquisition of toileting skills	• At least one episode of fecal incontinence per week
• History of excessive stool retention	• History of retentive posturing or excessive volitional stool retention
• History of painful or hard bowel movements	• History of painful or hard bowel movements
• Presence of a large fecal mass in the rectum	• Presence of a large fecal mass in the rectum
• History of large diameter stool that may obstruct the toilet	• History of large diameter stool that may obstruct the toilet

Source: Data from: Hyman, P. E., Milla, P. J., Benninga, M. A., et al. (2006). Childhood functional gastrointestinal disorders: Neonate/toddler. *Gastroenterology, 130,* 1519; and Rasquin, A., Di Lorenzo, C., Fobes, D., et al. (2006). Childhood functional disorders: Child/adolescent. *Gastroenterology, 130,* 1527.

may be too busy to stop play or there may be lack of privacy at school. Events common to all age groups that can lead to painful defecation include changes in diet, routines, stressful events, and/or illness (Baker et al., 2006).

Withholding feces can lead to prolonged fecal contact in the colon with reabsorption of fluids and an increase in the size and hardness of stool (Baker et al., 2006). The passage of these large, hard stools can be quite painful and difficult. The child may then consciously delay the passage of stool with subsequent defecation urges. These withholding behaviors can be subtle with children, especially toddlers, and can be mistaken for attempts to pass stool. Maintaining a rigid posture with clenched fists, hiding in a corner or other room, or excessive grunting and straining are often signs of voluntary fecal withholding. For other children, parents will recognize withholding behaviors as children rise up to their toes and rock back and forth. Many parents call this the "poopy dance."

As the rectum is continually stretched with retained stool, defecation urges subside. Soft or watery stool eventually leaks around the retained fecal mass, resulting in fecal soiling.

Epidemiology

Although few prospective studies have been conducted to examine the prevalence of encopresis in childhood, an estimated 1–2% of children younger than

10 years have encopresis. The range of age at presentation is typically 4–12 years, with a peak at 7–9 years. Approximately 80% of affected children are boys (Borowitz, 2008).

Approximately 80–95% of children with encopresis have a history of constipation or painful bowel movements. The remaining 5–20% are said to have nonretentive encopresis; however, many of these children have a remote history of constipation or painful defecation or demonstrate incomplete evacuation during defecation (Partin, Hamill, Fischel, & Partin, 1992). Little or no evidence indicates that encopresis is primarily a behavioral disorder, and most available evidence suggests that behavioral difficulties associated with encopresis may be the result of the encopresis and not the cause (Joinson et al., 2007). Also, there is no scientific evidence to suggest that encopresis is an indicator of sexual abuse (Mellon, Whiteside, & Friedrich, 2006). Low self-esteem or parent–child conflict as a result of the disorder is not uncommon (Borowitz, 2008).

What information from the history do you need to make the correct diagnosis? ■

History Taking

As with all pediatric complaints, the assessment of a child with encopresis begins with a careful and detailed history.

Questions to be asked during evaluation include:

- What are the frequency and consistency of the stools?
- What are the frequency and timing of the fecal soiling?
- Is there visible blood or mucous in the stool?
- Are there complaints of pain with defecation?
- When did potty training occur and was that a smooth or difficult transition?
- What was the timing for the passage of meconium stool after birth?
- Does the child exhibit any withholding behaviors?
- Have there been any delays in motor milestones?
- Is there a history of urinary dysfunction or recurrent urinary tract infections?
- Is there a family history of constipation or encopresis?
- Are restrooms at school or daycare available when needed and acceptable by the child for use?
- What treatments, medications, and/or strategies have been utilized in the past?

In addition, inquire about dietary history, exercise patterns, and behavioral history—what are normal behaviors for this child. A psychosocial history that includes seeking information about members of the household, alternative caregivers, and interactions with family members and peers should also be obtained.

What other conditions might cause stooling problems? ■

A history of stool withholding behavior reduces the likelihood that there is an organic disorder (Baker et al., 2006). Organic causes account for only 5% of cases of constipation and include anatomic, neuromuscular, metabolic, or endocrine causes (Castiglia, 2001). The most common organic etiology for constipation is Hirschsprung disease. The absence of ganglion cells in the muscle of the rectum does not allow relaxation of the rectal walls, thus not allowing feces to enter into the anal canal. These children are typically identified when there is no passage of meconium stool shortly after birth or upon evidence of bowel obstruction in the newborn period. Interestingly, most children with Hirschsprung disease never have soiling (Castiglia).

Anatomic defects of the spine and anus can also lead to constipation and encopresis. The most common of these include meningomyelocele (spina bifida), tethered cord syndrome, and imperforate anus with fistula (Coughlin, 2003).

Metabolic and endocrine abnormalities that promote constipation and subsequent stool holding include hypothyroidism, hypokalemia, and hypercalcemia, as well as lead intoxication, cystic fibrosis, celiac disease, and diabetes mellitus (Coughlin, 2003).

You talk with Zachary and his mother. The following information emerges from your interview:

Zachary was the full-term product of a normal vaginal delivery. He produced meconium stool in the first hours of life. He has been well and healthy. You also elicit a history of difficulty with toilet training. He had toilet resistance and had bowel movements in his pull-up diapers until he was 4½ years old. Zachary has always had large diameter stools that frequently clogged the toilet, and he typically has a bowel movement every 3 days. No blood has been noted on his stools, and there has been no evidence of anal fissures.

Since he started school, his parents have minimal knowledge of his toileting behaviors and assume he is defecating regularly. However, they really don't know. Zachary can't remember the last time he had a stool in the toilet. The nearest bathroom to his classroom is down the hall. The teacher does not allow students to freely use the restroom; they must raise their hand to get permission and then carry a large red key that signals bathroom permission. Zachary hates to use the bathroom at school.

Zachary had been continent for urine both day and night since 3 years of age. In the past year, he has been incontinent for daytime urine one to three times per week, with urinary dribbling. He insists he does not feel the urge to urinate until it is too late and he wets himself. Zachary is the youngest of three children; both parents work full time. His middle school brother watches him after school for 2 hours until his parents get home. Zachary is quite active at home, enjoying biking, rollerblading, and basketball. He has avoided team sports because he is worried about public soiling. He enjoys the computer and plays computer games for hours at a time.

What aspects of the physical examination will be important in this case? ■

Physical Examination

It is necessary to perform a thorough physical examination as part of the evaluation of the child with encopresis. Examination of the external perineum for skin tags, anal position, and anal tone gives clues to an anatomical or inflammatory condition. Inspection of the lower back for pigmentary irregularities, sacral dimples, tufts of hair, or asymmetry of the spine can give clues to a neurologic abnormality. Digital exam of the anorectal area is recommended. It gives immediate indication of sensation, anal tone, the size of the rectum, and the presence of anal wink. It also determines presence of a fecal mass in the rectum and the amount and consistency of rectal stool.

The abdominal exam requires palpation for assessment of the amount of retained fecal matter. A neurological examination will detect signs of spinal nerve involvement, which can be responsible for abnormal sphincter function from a spinal cord tumor or a tethered cord. Assessment of lower extremity tone, strength, and deep tendon reflexes is warranted as well as evaluating the cremasteric reflex. Detection of a physical abnormality could lead to the identification of an organic disorder (see Table 9-2).

Should you order any laboratory or radiology studies? ■

In most patients, the diagnosis is established with the history and complete physical examination, including the rectal exam (Baker et al., 2006). Generally speaking, diagnostics are not warranted, except in those children who fail medical management or who have a red flag identified on history and/or physical examination. A KUB can be helpful for evaluating the amount of stool in the colon when the history is unclear; when palpation of the abdomen may be difficult, as with obese children; or sometimes to convince a family there is backed up stool in the colon (Baker et al., 2006). Most often a KUB is done to assess the effectiveness of a bowel clean-out or provide clarity once medical management has begun.

Laboratory studies are seldom warranted. These are typically ordered when patients have failed medical management and/or families need further evidence because encopresis is typically a functional disorder. If additional testing is needed, the healthcare provider should consider the need for such studies as a complete metabolic panel (screen for calcium, potassium, and electrolytes), sedimentation rate, thyroid studies (free T4, TSH), IgA and tissue transglutaminase IgA to screen for celiac disease, and a lead level. If indicated, screen for cystic fibrosis with a sweat chloride test.

When considering tethered cord because of persistent urinary dysfunction despite an effective bowel clean-out, a screening radiograph of the lower spine

---

Table 9-2   Red Flags Distinguishing Organic Constipation from Functional Constipation

- Failure to thrive
- Lack of lumbosacral curve
- Pilonidal dimple covered by tuft of hair
- Midline pigmentary abnormalities of the lower spine
- Flat buttocks
- Anteriorly displaced anus
- Patulous anus
- Absent anal wink
- Occult blood
- Absent cremasteric reflex
- Decreased lower extremity tone and/or strength

Source: Baker, S., Liptak, G., Colletti, R., Croffie, J., Di Lorenzo, C., Ector, W., et al. (2006). Clinical practice guideline: Evaluation and treatment of constipation in infants and children: Recommendations of the North American Society for Pediatric Gastroenterology, Hepatology and Nutrition. *Journal of Pediatric Gastroenterology and Nutrition, 43*, e1–e13.

---

looking for spina bifida occulta can be helpful. About 98% of people with tethered cord have spina bifida occulta, but 10–20% of the normal population has spina bifida occulta without adverse sequelae. The most definitive diagnostic test for tethered cord is magnetic resonance imaging (Rosen, Buonomo, Andrade, & Nurko, 2004). Once tethered cord is identified, a neurosurgical referral is necessary. Hirschsprung's disease can be identified by barium enema and/or rectal biopsy.

Upon physical examination, you find Zachary is at the 70th percentile for height and weight with a BMI of 17, which is at the 75th percentile. Vital signs are within normal limits. He is well developed. Head, ears, eyes, nose, and throat are all normal and without palpable lymphadenopathy. His heart has a regular rate and rhythm and no murmur is auscultated. Lungs are clear with good aeration bilaterally. The abdomen is rounded and slightly tense with a hard palpable mass from the suprapubic area to his umbilicus. There are ropey loops of bowel palapated in the left lower quadrant and right lower quadrant, without tenderness. Rectal examination reveals a normotonic, normally placed anus without skin tags or fissures and a positive anal wink. There is pasty thick stool in moderate amounts around the anus. The digital examination reveals a rectum full of hard stool, which is guaiac negative. When the patient is asked to expel the examining finger, there is rectal tightening of the external anal sphincter (EAS) rather than expected relaxation.

No dimples or tufts of hair are noted. The spine is straight. Strength and deep tendon reflexes in the lower extremities are normal and symmetric.

Making the Diagnosis

The history and physical examination are consistent with the diagnosis of retentive encopresis. He has a history of not wanting to use the restroom at school resulting in fecal withholding, fecal accidents, wearing pull-up diapers, no sensation of stooling, and sitting in his soiled underwear until his parents tell him to clean up. His physical examination is normal except for palpable stool in his abdomen and rectal tightening response.

Management

How do you plan to treat this child with encopresis? ■

Are diagnostics warranted at this point in time? ■

No red flags were identified to suggest diagnostics are needed. With frequent soiling and a large amount of palpable stool in the abdomen, treatment can begin.

The management of the encopretic child is within the realm of the primary care provider, as long as treatment is approached in a consistent and physiologically oriented way (Levy, 2001). This approach is cost effective and provides faster results than other treatment modalities based on intensive psychological intervention. Once there is improved function, more normal relationships can flourish. For this reason, it is recommended that, unless there are clearly identified psychosocial dysfunction issues, management should concentrate on effective bowel clean-out with subsequent resolution of the soiling. There is time later to refer for mental health intervention if no progress or slow progress is encountered.

Management is based on four key elements (Levy, 2001):

- *Disimpaction of the rectum and colon:* To stop the soiling and allow normal sensation to return.
- *Daily stool softening:* To keep the colon clear of stool so it can regain normal tone and the ability to propel stool more effectively.
- *Establishment of effective toilet habits:* To achieve the goal of evacuating stool at regular times daily.
- *Parental education:* With the goal of demystification, which allows greater understanding and, hopefully, commitment to treatment.

Disimpaction is necessary before any long-term success can be maintained. It may be accomplished with the use of oral medications or rectal medications. The oral route allows greater sense of control and is less invasive, but compliance can be more problematic. The rectal route is quite invasive and sometimes traumatic for the child, but is faster and allows the parent more control. The choice of treatment can be determined after discussing options with the child and parents.

When the oral route is selected, high-dose oral electrolyte solutions are recommended (Baker et al., 2006). Although there are no controlled trials demonstrating the effectiveness of high-dose magnesium hydroxide, magnesium citrate, lactulose, sorbital, senna, or bisacodyl for initial disimpaction, these laxatives have been used successfully in that role (Baker et al., 2006).

When the rectal route is preferred, phosphate enemas, saline enemas, or mineral oil enemas followed by a phosphate enema are effective (Baker et al., 2006).

Disimpaction is typically completed using oral medications. Dosages of various medications used in treatment of constipation/impaction are found in Table 9-3. Most disimpactions can be completed at home. On occasion, children may have to be admitted to the hospital for disimpaction. A nasogastric tube is placed, and PEG 3350 (Miralax) with electrolytes is administered until rectal effluent is clear.

Following discussion with Zachary and his parents, it was decided to use an over-the-counter electrolyte solution, PEG 3350. Because it has no taste or texture and dissolves readily in fluids, it is easy to administer. Magnesium citrate is quite effective and typically promotes a faster clean-out, but it is quite sour tasting and is difficult for many children to accept. PEG 3350 also tends to have less association with abdominal cramping than magnesium citrate.

Zachary's parents were instructed to mix 17 g of PEG 3350, which is measured easily by the bottle's cap, with 8 ounces of a beverage of choice, which gives about 2 g PEG 3350 per ounce. Beverages can be cold or hot, clear or milk products, and the beverage with PEG mixture is good in the refrigerator for 48 hours. PEG 3350 is not to be mixed with foods. The recommended clean-out dose of PEG 3350 is 1.5 g/kg/day. Zachary weighs 65 pounds (30 kg), so he needs 44 g of PEG 3350 per day in divided doses, which is approximately 22 ounces per day of the PEG 3350/fluid mixture. He is to drink this dose of PEG 3350 daily until his stool is very runny. The amount of time needed to complete a bowel clean-out is quite variable, but commonly takes 4–5 days.

Initially, stool may be quite loose as the softer leakage is cleaned out first. The hard stool then begins to break down and stool will be quite grainy and thick for a number of days, before it finally starts to thin and become a "thin mud puddle." An effective clean-out has not occurred until you reach this point. Because Zachary is in school, his parents have been instructed to begin the clean-out over the weekend and anticipate missed days of school. Teachers should be advised of his absence and have work sent home. To promote faster evacuation of stool, a stimulant, bisacodyl, can be added to the daily regimen giving one 5 mg tablet orally once or twice a day. During the clean-out, many children feel nauseated and have stomachaches and/or emesis; however, the clean-out should not be stopped unless symptoms are severe.

Table 9-3   Medication for Use in Treatment of Encopresis/Constipation

Type of Medication	Selected Medications	Recommended Dosages
Osmotic	Lactulose	1–3 mL/kg/day PO qd/bid; max 60 mL qd
	Sorbital	Same as lactulose
	Magnesium hydroxide (MOM, milk of magnesia)	1–3 mL/kg/day of 400 mg/5 mL; available as liquid 400 mg/5 mL, 800 mg/5 mL, or tablets Max 60 mL/day of 400 mg/5 mL
	Barley malt extract	2–10 mL/240 mL of milk or juice; suitable for infants drinking from bottle
	Magnesium citrate	< 6 years: 1–3 mL/kg/day PO 6–12 years: 100–150 mL/day PO > 12 years: 150–300 mL/day PO
	PEG 3350	Disimpaction: 1–3 g/kg/day divided into 2–4 doses Maintenance dose: 0.5–1.0 g/kg/day QD or divided bid
Lubricant	Mineral oil	< 1 yr: not recommended Disimpaction: 15–30 mL/yr of age, up to 240 mL/day Maintenance: 1–3 mL/kg/day
Stimulant	Sennodies (Senna, Senokot, Ex-Lax)	2–6 years: 2.5–7.5 mL/day 6–12 years: 5–15 mL/day/

Table 9-3   Medication for Use in Treatment of Encopresis/Constipation (Continued)

Type of Medication	Selected Medications	Recommended Dosages
	Bisacodyl (Dulcolax)	Available as syrup, 8.8 mg of sennosides/5 mL; also available in tablets and granules > 2 years: ½ to 1 10-mg suppository PR as a single dose 5–15 mg PO as a single dose
Osmotic enema	Sodium phosphate enema (Fleet enema)	2–11 years: 6 mL/kg/day PR; may administer up to 135 mL qd/bid in older children > 11 years: An adult enema or 4.5 oz (135 mL) PR qd/bid prn Note: 1 pediatric enema = 2.25 oz (67.5 mL)

Source: Data from Baker, S., Liptak, G., Colletti, R., Croffie, J., Di Lorenzo, C., Ector, W., et al. (2006). Clinical practice guideline: Evaluation and treatment of constipation in infants and children: Recommendations of the North American Society for Pediatric Gastroenterology, Hepatology and Nutrition. *Journal of Pediatric Gastroenterology and Nutrition, 43,* e1–e13; Borowitz, S. (2008). *Encopresis.* Retrieved May 2008, from http://www.emedicine.com/ped/TOPIC670.HTM#section~AuthorsandEditors; Tobias, N., Mason, D., & Lutkenhoff, M., et al. (2008). Management principles of organic causes of childhood constipation. *Journal of Pediatric Health Care, 22*(1), 12–23. Retrieved June 2008, from http://www.medscape.com/viewarticle/569470

Once a bowel clean-out is completed and Zachary is having watery stools, stimulant medication is discontinued and the PEG 3350 dose is decreased to half the initial clean-out dose. Zachary's maintenance phase begins with the decreased dose. The maintenance dose of PEG 3350 is about 8 g/kg/day in a single dose or divided. Zachary is instructed to return to the office in 3 weeks and call as needed for assistance.

Maintenance or Daily Stool Softening

Once the impaction has been removed, the treatment focuses on the prevention of another impaction. At this point, soiling should significantly decrease or resolve. It is important to have full evacuation of stool from the colon and that stools be soft and easy to pass, be nonpainful, and be difficult to withhold. This is especially paramount for the toddler with active stool withholding related to pain with defecation. There is no correct dose of daily stool softener, but rather enough daily medicine should be given to produce one to three soft, mushy, milkshake-consistency stools. During the first month of maintenance, a stooling calendar charting all stools and their consistency should be logged.

Dietary changes are commonly advised. Recommendations have focused on increasing fluids and fiber in the diet to promote passage of stool; however, the literature is mixed on this issue. A balanced diet that includes whole grains, fruits, and vegetables is recommended as part of the treatment for constipation in children (Baker et al., 2006; Levy, 2001). Milk and cheese should be eaten sparingly because they can cause constipation. Forceful implementation of a high fiber diet is undesirable and often not worth the power struggle it invites.

Next Visit

Zachary is seen back at the office following a bowel clean-out that took 5 days to reach "dirty water" bowel movements. Bisacodyl is discontinued, and he continues to take 12 ounces of the PEG 3350 mixture daily. He is having two soft, milkshake-consistency stools in the toilet every day and soiling has stopped. Zachary finally smiles as he talks to you. Urinary incontinence has resolved. On exam, his abdomen is soft, nontender, and without palpable fecal mass. Zachary and his parents are pleased.

You then discuss continued maintenance on a daily stool softener for a minimum of 4–6 months and very typically closer to 2 years. Stimulants can be utilized intermittently for short periods as needed to avoid recurrence of impaction. Prolonged use of stimulant laxatives is not recommended. When there has been no soiling for about 6 months, discontinuance of maintenance therapy can be discussed. Relapse is common, and the clean-out regimen can be reinstituted at any time as needed. Zachary is asked to maintain a stooling calendar so that progress can be tracked. Timed toileting routines are discussed along with strategies that promote rectal relaxation with defecation. Zachary is to return to the office in 1 month and call as needed.

Establishing Effective Toilet Habits

The goal of establishing effective toileting habits is to promote stool evacuation from the body at regular times of the day. Because the rectum is stretched from months or years of withholding patterns, many encopretic children may not be able to feel when it is time to go to the bathroom.

Timing of toileting routines should be planned to take advantage of the gastrocolic reflex, a series of propulsive mass peristaltic movements triggered by ingestion of food. Convenient times are in the morning after breakfast and after dinner. Many school-age children benefit from routine timed toilet visits when returning from school. If the stool is kept very soft and the child sits on the toilet 15–20 minutes after meals, a successful bowel movement can occur. It is not necessary to remind the child more than two to three times per day to try to have a bowel movement.

Children with painful defecation, especially those under the age of 5, are often afraid to allow the stool to pass out of their bodies. They will try to hold in the stool to avoid having pain. They can sometimes appear to be straining, but may actually be working hard to keep stool inside. If the legs are bent and the child rests his/her feet on the floor or stepstool, it will be easier to allow the stool to pass out of the body. Other toileting tips that promote rectal relaxation with defecation include:

- Bending forward so your chest is resting on your thighs.
- Pushing while sitting on the toilet. Fun activities to promote muscle relaxation are:
  - Blow bubbles in a glass of water through a straw.
  - Blow hard through your mouth.
  - Blow up a balloon or blow bubbles.
  - Roar like a lion.
  - Put your hand on your child's belly and have them use their stomach muscles to push it away.

Some children have a "eureka" moment as they experience rectal relaxation versus tightening.

Be sure to reward any positive change toward the goal of having bowel movements in the toilet. Sticker charts or reward systems that have failed in the past may now be beneficial as stool is comfortably passed. It is important for parents to talk about bowel movements and monitor output. A stooling calendar for the first month is essential and should include how many stools go in the toilet, how many accidents occur, and the texture of the stool. Adjust stool softeners to maintain one to three milkshake-consistency stools per day.

Parental Education

The successful treatment of encopresis requires a well-organized plan, parental understanding of the underlying effects of chronic stool holding, and patience.

Most often encopresis is the culmination of months to years of dysfunctional bowel habits. Treatment is time consuming, and relapse is common (Pyles & Gray, 1997). Parents often feel guilty about their reaction to fecal incontinence and their misunderstanding of the situation. Frustration and anger are common emotions encountered. Close follow-up by telephone and/or by office visits is recommended. Some families may need counseling to help manage their emotions, expectations, and dysfunctional patterns. Table 9-4 describes the treatment options for encopresis.

Is the child safe on laxatives long term? ■ ***What are potential side effects?*** ■ ***Is it habit forming?*** ■

Numerous pediatric studies confirm that PEG 3350 is a safe and nonhabit-forming stool softener (Gandy, Michaia, Preud'Homme, & Mezoff, 2004; Loening-Baucke, Krishan, & Pashankar, 2004; Pashankar, Lowning-Baucke, & Bishop, 2003; Youssef et al., 2002). It is not absorbed by the body but rather stays in the colon and holds onto the water it is mixed with. Miralax is not a stimulant laxative; it does not cause the colon to contract and does not cause laxative dependence. It simply softens the stools and makes it harder for the child to hold onto the stool.

1 Month Later

Zachary is seen in your office 1 month following the clean-out. His mother presents the stooling calendar. Zach continues to have one to two soft, mushy stools per day in the toilet without soiling. There has been no urinary incontinence. Zachary has routine toilet sits after school and dinner, with a large output of soft stool within 3–4 minutes of sitting. He still needs reminders from his mother to maintain toileting routines. A couple of minor fecal accidents have occurred when Zach has been on the computer for over an hour, so his parents curtailed computer time to 30-minute time periods with resolution. They are instructed to maintain daily stool softening and routine toilet sits. Summer vacation is near, so emphasis on daily routines and the need to sit on the toilet regularly are reiterated. A return visit is scheduled in 3 months.

What would you do if your treatment didn't work? ■

The most common reason for continued encopresis despite medical treatment is an inadequate clean-out. If necessary, a KUB can be obtained to assess for retained fecal material. Children who initially present with a many-year history of encopresis without any previous medical management may take a number of weeks on high-dose laxative before a clean-out is completed. Consider adding a stimulant to the daily regimen for a couple of weeks to enhance motility. Certainly the wrong dose of softener, especially too little, or incorrect administration may thwart clean-out efforts. Lack of buy-in by the parents, child, or school may prevent adherence with treatment. Additionally,

Table 9-4 Treatment for Encopresis

Phase I: Disimpaction (bowel clean-out) 3–5 days until stool output is runny diarrhea

Oral clean-out (preferable)

- PEG 3350 1–3 g/kg/day in divided doses, 2–4/day

  Mix 17 g (4 level tsp. of Miralax) in 8 oz of fluid to equal ~2 g/oz; can be mixed in hot or cold fluids and stored in the refrigerator for 48 hours.

  OR

- Magnesium citrate: < 6 years: 1–3 mL/kg/day PO; 6–12 years: 100–150 mL/day PO; > 12 years: 150–300 mL/day PO

  Serve chilled or mixed with other fluids or syrups to make more palatable.

  PLUS (as desired)

- Stimulant such as Dulcolax or Ex Lax qd to bid as tolerated.

Enema clean-out (infrequently)

- Sodium phosphate (Fleet enema): 2–11 years: 6 mL/kg/day PR; may administer up to 135 mL qd/bid in older children; > 11 years: an adult enema or 4.5 oz (135 ml) PR qd/bid prn

  Note: 1 pediatric enema = 2.25 oz (67.5 mL)

Phase II: Maintenance, daily stool softening (4–12 months)

The goal is to stop re-accumulation of stool in the emptied out rectum. Adjust daily medicine to achieve one to three soft mushy stools/day.

- Oral laxatives
  - PEG 3350 0.5–1 g/kg/day PO qd/bid
  - lactulose 1–3 mL/kg/day PO qd/bid
  - Magnesium hydroxide 1–3 mL/kg/day PO qd/bid
- Behavioral training
  - Establish daily toilet schedule 20 minutes after meals two to three times per day for 5–10 minutes.
  - Promote use of rectal relaxation techniques.
  - Provide positive reinforcement for toilet sitting and stool results.
  - Maintain stooling calendar, recording time and amount.
- Parental education
  - Demystification, which allows greater understanding and, hopefully, commitment to treatment

Phase III: Weaning

- Gradual tapering of laxative
- Continued high-fiber diet, adequate fluid intake, and behavioral modification

if maintenance therapy is aborted too quickly, the child can then revert to holding patterns, which create constipation and continued fecal accidents. Maintenance therapy should be given a minimal trial of 4–6 months and more realistically 1–2 years, especially if the encopresis is centered around potty training issues (Thompson, 2001).

How often should you follow up with children and families with an encopresis problem? ■

Follow-up is very important. It is recommended that the healthcare provider see the patient within 2–4 weeks of the initial clean-out and then monthly until new routines are established and there is good family understanding of the treatment plan and goals. If soiling reoccurs, the child needs to start over again with a new bowel clean-out because the rectum is impacted again.

If a bowel clean-out has been adequate and medical management has been followed, a careful review by the primary care provider of the differential diagnosis of the organic causes of constipation/encopresis should be undertaken. It may be appropriate at this time to consider laboratory or radiologic tests to search for nonfunctional causes of the child's symptoms.

In cases where psychosocial issues are at the foundation of the soiling problem, a referral to a psychiatrist, psychologist, and/or other mental health provider may be appropriate. Unfortunately, the number of therapists who are experienced in the management of encopretic children is small, and many times the primary care provider is left to assume the main role in directing care.

What is the prognosis for encopresis? ■

Even with aggressive medical and behavioral interventions, as many as 30% of children remain symptomatic (Rockney, McQuade, Days, Linn, & Alario, 1996). Consultation with a pediatric gastroenterologist is warranted when therapy fails, when an organic disease is of concern, or when management is complex.

Key Points from the Case

1. Assessment and management of pediatric encopresis is a challenging problem faced by the primary care provider.
2. Because approximately 80–95% of children with encopresis have a history of constipation or painful bowel movements, management usually focuses on disimpaction of stool followed by daily stool softeners to ensure passage of stool without pain.

3. In addition to stool softeners as the mainstay of treatment, behavioral strategies to promote effective toileting routines are recommended.

4. Progress towards the goal of resolution of soiling is typically slow and tedious. Frequent follow-up by the primary care provider that focuses on continued education about medication dosages, toileting routines and strategies that promote rectal relaxation, age-appropriate rewards and consequences, and importance of consistency is paramount.

5. If therapy fails, consider the adequacy of the disimpaction efforts, compliance of medical management, length of maintenance therapy, and psychosocial issues that may thwart progress. Refer or consult as needed with a pediatric gastroenterologist and/or mental health provider.

REFERENCES

Baker, S., Liptak, G., Colletti, R., Croffie, J., Di Lorenzo, C., Ector, W., & Nurko, S. (2006). Clinical practice guideline: Evaluation and treatment of constipation in infants and children: Recommendations of the North American Society for Pediatric Gastroenterology, Hepatology and Nutrition. *Journal of Pediatric Gastroenterology and Nutrition, 43*, e1–e13.

Borowitz, S. (2008). *Encopresis.* Retrieved May 2008, from http://www.emedicine.com/ped/TOPIC670.HTM#section~AuthorsandEditors

Castiglia, P. (2001). Constipation in children. *Journal of Pediatric Health Care, 15*(4), 200–202.

Coughlin, E. (2003). Assessment and management of pediatric constipation in primary care. *Pediatric Nursing, 29*(4), 296–301.

Di Lorenzo, C., & Benninga, M. (2004). Pathophysiology of pediatric fecal incontinence. *Gastroenterology, 126*(1 Suppl 1), S33–S40.

Gandy, E., Michaia, S., Preud'Homme, D., & Mezoff, A. (2004). PEG for constipation in children younger than eighteen months old. *Journal of Pediatric Gastroenterology and Nutrition, 39*(2), 197–199.

Hyman, P. E., Milla, P. J., Benninga, M. A., et al. (2006). Childhood functional gastrointestinal disorders: Neonate/toddler. *Gastroenterology, 130*, 1519.

Joinson, C., Heron, J., Butler, R., Von Gontard, A., Butler, U., Emond, A., et al. (2007). A United Kingdom population-based study of intellectual capacities in children with and without soiling, daytime wetting, and bed-wetting. *Pediatrics, 120*(2), e308–e316.

Levy, J. (2001). *A guide to children's digestive and nutritional needs.* Retrieved May 2008, from http://www.naspghan.org/wmspage.cfm?parm1=104

Loening-Baucke, V., Krishna, R., & Pashankar, D. (2004). PEG 3350 without electrolytes for the treatment of functional constipation in infants and toddlers. *Journal of Pediatric Gastroenterology and Nutrition, 39*(5), 536–539.

Mellon, M., Whiteside, S., & Friedrich, W. (2006). The relevance of fecal soiling as an indicator of child sexual abuse: A preliminary analysis. *Journal of Developmental and Behavioral Pediatrics, 27*(1), 25–32.

Partin, J. C., Hamill, S., Fischel, J. E., & Partin, J. S. (1992). Painful defecation and fecal soiling in children. *Pediatrics, 89*(6 Pt 1), 1007–1009.

Pashankar, D., Lowning-Baucke, V., & Bishop, W. (2003). Safety of PEG 3350 for the treatment of chronic constipation in children with dysfunctional elimination. *Archives of Pediatric and Adolescent Medicine, 157,* 661–664.

Pyles, C., & Gray, J. (1997). Encopresis: An algorithmic approach. *Physician Assistant, 21*(7), 56, 58, 60–62, 67–68, 70–74.

Rasquin, A., Di Lorenzo, C., Fobes, D., et al. (2006). Childhood functional disorders: Child/adolescent. *Gastroenterology, 130*(5):1527–1537.

Rockney, R., McQuade, W., Days, A., Linn, M., & Alario, A. (1996). Encopresis treatment outcome: Long-term follow-up of 45 cases. *Journal of Developmental and Behavioral Pediatrics, 17*(6), 380–385.

Rosen, C., Buonomo, C., Andrade, R., & Nurko, S. (2004). Incidence of spinal cord lesions in patients with intractable constipation. *Journal of Pediatrics, 143,* 409–411.

Thompson, J. (2001). The management of chronic constipation in children. *Community Practitioner, 74*(1), 29–30.

Tobias, N., Mason, D., & Lutkenhoff, M. (2008). Management principles of organic causes of childhood constipation. *Journal of Pediatric Health Care, 22*(1), 12–23. Retrieved June 2008, from http://www.medscape.com/viewarticle/569470

Youssef, N., Peters, J., Henderson, W., Shultz-Peters, S., Lockhart, D., & Di Lorenzo, C. (2002). Dose response of PEG 3350 for the treatment of childhood fecal impaction. *Journal of Pediatrics, 14*(3), 410–414.

Chapter 10

The Teen Needing a Sports Physical

Catherine G. Blosser

The preparticipation sports examination (PPE) is often the only health examination for the majority of youth and adolescents in any given year. One percent to 8% of teens undergoing a PPE will have findings that require further evaluation or referral prior to authorizing sports participation; fewer than 1% will need to be excluded from sports because of a significant finding (Landry & Logan, 2007). The PPE should be performed according to customary and standard practices; all history and physical findings need to be documented, including any perceived risk factors and advice about potential dangers of participation that have been discussed with the youth and his or her family. (A signed consent is warranted in such a case.) Ideally, the PPE is performed by the primary care provider. Massive sports examination screenings (i.e., examination stations) are offered in many communities to allay costs and time for both the youth and parent. However, there is a loss of continuity from the history to the examination and then to follow-up, a lack of privacy and patient–provider familiarity, and little time for health promotion discussions when this process is used.

Educational Objectives
1. Identify the two parts of the PPE.
2. Apply customary and standard practices for performing a PPE, including a thorough assessment of health status, fitness level, maturity level, and detection of injuries and illnesses that might limit participation and/or lead to morbidity or mortality.
3. Discuss the advantages to using a PPE form.
4. Discuss necessary documentation components of the cardiovascular examination.
5. Discuss lifestyle risk factors and ways to promote healthy choices.
6. Discuss risk factors specific to females athletes.
7. Recommend ways to improve athletic performance.
8. Discuss the pros and cons of mass screenings designed with stations for conducting the PPE that are standard within some school districts.
9. Identify opportunities within your practice community for establishing stronger ties with coaches and trainers.

Case Presentation and Discussion

Nikola Avery is a 16-year-old Caucasian female who is planning to try out for the cross-country running team at her high school. She comes today with her 20-year-old sister, who is in the waiting room because their parents both work. Nikola has just transferred into the school district from another state; she relates that this will be her second year of running competitively in high school.

You tell Nikola that before doing the physical examination, you want to review the history form she and her mother completed (it is cosigned). This form was sent out by the clinic to the family at the time the appointment was made.

Assessing Risk Factors for Sports Participation

The assessment of a young person for sports participation needs to include any history or physical findings that would alert the provider about the need for further inquiry or raise concerns regarding the activity appropriate for that particular person. A well-designed preparticipation physical examination form would serve this purpose and also allow for a time-efficient examination. A sample form is available in Figure 10-1.

What risk factors for sports participation come to your mind? ■

Risk factors

Risk factors of note include:

- Previous trauma, especially to the musculoskeletal or central nervous system
- Cardiovascular disease (including congenital heart disease, carditis, dysrhythmia, mitral valve prolapse, hypertension above the 90th percentile, and exertional syncope)
- Prior history of heat intolerance
- Chronic medical conditions, including allergic reactions, respiratory problems, sickle cell disease, diabetes, human immunodeficiency virus (HIV), eating disorders, cerebral palsy, and hemophilia
- Seizures
- Infectious mononucleosis
- Skin infections
- Anatomic abnormalities, including missing paired organs, or Down or Marfan syndromes (or history of Marfan syndrome in family)
- Obesity
- In females, menstrual and eating habit irregularities
- Family history of sudden death

Table 10-1 will help the provider determine whether sports participation should be allowed, whether further evaluation is needed before being allowed, or if the risk factor precludes participation. In some cases, an alternative sport can be proposed that reduces risk and allows participation for the individual.

Ohio High School Athletic Association
Preparticipation Physical Evaluation

Page 1 of 4

DATE OF EXAM:_____

Name _____ Sex _____ Age _____ Date of Birth _____

Grade_____ School _____ Sport(s) _____

Address _____ Phone _____

Personal Physician_____

In case of emergency, contact: Name _____ Relationship _____

Phone (H) _____ (W) _____ (Cell) _____ (Cell) _____

History

This section is to be carefully completed by the student and his/her parent(s) or legal guardian(s) before participation in interscholastic athletics in order to help detect possible risks.

Explain "YES" answers in the space provided. Circle questions you don't know the answer to.

	Yes	No
1. Has a doctor ever denied or restricted you participation in sports for any reason?	☐	☐
2. Do you have an ongoing medical condition (like diabetes or asthma)?	☐	☐
3. Are you currently taking any prescription or nonprescription (over-the-counter) medicines or pills?	☐	☐
4. Do you have allergies to medicines, pollens, foods, or stinging insects?	☐	☐
5. Do you think you are in good health?	☐	☐
6. Have you ever passed out or nearly passed out DURING exercise?	☐	☐
7. Have you ever passed out or nearly passed out AFTER exercise?	☐	☐
8. Have you ever had discomfort, pain, or pressure in your chest during exercise?	☐	☐
9. Does your heart race or skip beats during exercise?	☐	☐
10. Has a doctor ever told you that you have (check all that apply):		
☐ High Blood Pressure ☐ A heart murmur		
☐ High Cholesterol ☐ A heart infection		
11. Has a doctor ever ordered a test for your heart? (for example, ECG, echocardiogram)	☐	☐
12. Has anyone in your family died for no apparent reason?	☐	☐
13. Does anyone in your family have a heart problem?	☐	☐
14. Has any family member or relative died of heart problems or of sudden death before age 50?	☐	☐
15. Does anyone in your family have Marfan syndrome?	☐	☐
16. Have you ever spent the night in a hospital?	☐	☐
17. Have you ever had surgery?	☐	☐
18. Have you ever had an injury, like a sprain, muscle or ligament tear, or tendinitis, that caused you to miss a practice or game? If yes, circle affected area below:	☐	☐
19. Have you had any broken or fractured bones or dislocated joints? If yes, circle below:	☐	☐
20. Have you had a bone or joint injury that required x-rays, MRI, CT, surgery, injections, rehabilitation, physical therapy, a brace, a cast, or crutches? If yes, circle below:	☐	☐

Head	Neck	Shoulder	Upper Arm	Elbow	Forearm	Hand / Fingers	Chest
Upper back	Lower back	Hip	Thigh	Knee	Calf/shin	Ankle	Foot / Toes

	Yes	No
21. Have you ever had a stress fracture?	☐	☐
22. Have you been told that you have or have you had an x-ray for atlantoaxial (neck) instability?	☐	☐
23. Do you regularly use a brace or assistive device?	☐	☐
24. Has a doctor ever told you that you have asthma or allergies?	☐	☐

	Yes	No
25. Do you cough, wheeze, or have difficulty breathing during or after exercise?	☐	☐
26. Is there anyone in your family who has asthma?	☐	☐
27. Have you ever used an inhaler or taken asthma medicine?	☐	☐
28. Were you born without or are you missing a kidney, an eye, a testicle, or any other organ?	☐	☐
29. Have you had infectious mononucleosis (mono) within the last month?	☐	☐
30. Do you have any rashes, pressure sores, or other skin problems?	☐	☐
31. Have you had a herpes skin infection?	☐	☐
32. Have you ever had a head injury or concussion?	☐	☐
33. Have you been hit in the head and been confused or lost your memory?	☐	☐
34. Have you ever had a seizure?	☐	☐
35. Do you have headaches with exercise?	☐	☐
36. Have you ever had numbness, tingling, or weakness in your arms or legs after being hit or falling?	☐	☐
37. Have you ever been unable to move your arms or legs after being hit or falling?	☐	☐
38. When exercising in the heat, do you have severe muscle cramps or become ill?	☐	☐
39. Has a doctor told you that you or someone in your family has sickle cell trait or sickle cell disease?	☐	☐
40. Have you had any problems with your eyes or vision?	☐	☐
41. Do you wear glasses or contact lenses?	☐	☐
42. Do you wear protective eyewear, such as goggles or a face shield?	☐	☐
43. Are you happy with your weight?	☐	☐
44. Are you trying to gain or lose weight?	☐	☐
45. Has anyone recommended you change your weight or eating habits?	☐	☐
46. Do you limit or carefully control what you eat?	☐	☐
47. Do you have any concerns that you would like to discuss with a doctor?	☐	☐
FEMALES ONLY		
48. Have you ever had a menstrual period?	☐	☐
49. How old were you when you had your first menstrual period?	_____	
50. How many periods have you had in the last 12 months?	_____	

Explain "Yes" Answers Here: (Attach additional sheets as needed)

_____
_____
_____
_____
_____
_____

I (we) hereby state, to the best of my (our) knowledge, my (our) answers to the above questions are complete and correct.

Signature: _____ Signature: _____ Date: _____

Athlete Parent or Guardian (If athlete is under 18)

The student has family insurance ☐ Yes ☐ No; If yes, family insurance company name and policy number: _____

NOTE: CONSENT AND HIPAA RELEASE FORMS THAT MUST BE SIGNED BY BOTH THE PARENT AND THE STUDENT ARE ON A SEPARATE SHEET.
NOTE: HISTORY AND ALL CONSENT FORMS MUST BE COMPLETED PRIOR TO PHYSICAL EXAMINATION

Modified from American Academy of Family Physicians, American Academy of Pediatrics, American College of Sports Medicine, American Medical Society for Sports Medicine, American Orthopaedic Society for Sports Medicine, and American Osteopathic Academy of Sports Medicine, 2004. Rev. 03/06

(continues)

Figure 10-1 Preparticipation physical examination form.

Physical Examination Form

The section below is to be completed by physician or staff after history and consent forms are completed.

Students Name_____   Birth Date_____

Height_____ Weight_____ % Body Fat (optional)_____ Pulse_____ BP_____/_____, _____/_____, _____/_____

Vision R 20/_____ L 20/_____   Corrected: Y   N   Pupils: Equal _____ Unequal _____

Follow-Up Questions on More Sensitive Issues (Optional)
1. Do you feel stressed out or under a lot of pressure?
2. Do you ever feel so sad or hopeless that you stop doing some of your usual activities for more than a few days?
3. Do you feel safe?
4. Have you ever tried cigarette smoking, even 1 or 2 puffs? Do you currently smoke?
5. During the past 30 days, did you use chewing tobacco, snuff, or dip?
6. During the past 30 days, have you had at least 1 drink of alcohol?
7. Have you ever taken steroid pills or shots without a doctor's prescription?
8. Have you ever taken any supplements to help you gain or lose weight or improve your performance?
9. Questions from the Youth Risk Behavior Survey (http://www.cdc.gov/HealthyYouth/yrbs/index.htm) on guns, seatbelts, unprotected sex, domestic violence, drugs, etc.

Notes: _____
_____
_____
_____

MEDICAL	Normal	Abnormal findings	Initials*
Appearance			
Eyes/ears/nose/throat			
Hearing			
Lymph nodes			
Heart			
Murmurs			
Pulses			
Lungs			
Abdomen			
Genitalia (males only)			
Skin			
MUSCULOSKELETAL			
Neck			
Back			
Shoulder/arm			
Elbow/forearm			
Wrist/hand/fingers			
Hip/thigh			
Knee			
Leg/ankle			
Foot/toes			

*Multiple-examiner set-up only.
Notes: _____
_____

Clearance

☐ Cleared without restriction
☐ Cleared, with recommendations for further evaluation or treatment for: _____
_____
_____

☐ Not cleared for: ☐ All Sports ☐ Certain sports: _____ Reason: _____
Recommendations: _____
_____
_____

Emergency Information:
Allergies: _____
Other Information: _____
Name of Physician: (print/type/stamp) _____ (M.D., D.O., D.C.) Date: _____
If the Physician's Assistant (P.A.) or Advanced Nurse Practitioner (A.N.P.) performed the exam, name and address of collaborating physician or physician group:
Address: _____ Phone: _____

Signature of Physician: _____

Figure 10-1   Preparticipation physical examination form. (Continued)

Table 10-1   Sports Participation Clearance Based on Medical Conditions

May Clear for Participation	Needs Further Evaluation/Information Before Clearing for Participation	Do Not Clear for Participation
• Diabetes mellitus, as long as diet, hydration, and insulin therapy are monitored, especially if playing time is equal to or greater than 30 minutes	• Down syndrome or other known atlantoaxial instability (radiographic screening once during preschool years is recommended [AAP, 2001b])	• Carditis or those with the following key warning signs for potential sudden death, especially when under exertion (Greene, 2000):
• Congenital heart disease—mild forms	• Bleeding disorder	○ Syncope
• HIV infection as long as health and stamina allow; discuss care of skin lesions and universal precautions needed by others if handling affected person's body fluids. There has never been a documented case of HIV transmission via skin or mucous membrane exposure to body fluids (including blood) during contact or collision sports (CDC, 2006).	• Hypertension, until clearer etiology determined	○ Near syncope
	• Congenital heart disease—moderate/severe forms or those with prior history of surgery to correct defect	○ Palpitations
	• Dysrhythmia	○ Exertional dyspnea
	• Mitral valve prolapse with symptoms of chest pain, possible dysrhythmia, or leaking	○ Excessive, unexplained shortness of breath (fatigue, orthopnea, paroxysmal nocturnal apnea)
	• Heart murmur, if not "innocent"	○ Chest pain with long QT wave, noninnocent heart murmur, increased systolic blood pressure
• Mitral valve prolapse without symptoms	• Cerebral palsy	○ History of death or significant heart disease in family member younger than 50 years old
• Innocent heart murmur	• Mild diarrhea (monitor for dehydration, heat illness)	• Diarrhea (increases risk of dehydration and heat illness)
• Controlled seizures	• Eating disorders (medical and psychiatric evaluation needed prior to clearance for sports)	• Fever: active/chronic
• One ovary	• Eyes (vision 20/40 corrected in worse eye, loss of an eye, detached retina, prior eye surgery, eye injury); determine eligibility to participate on an individual basis and availability of protective eyewear for chosen sport	
• One testicle (protective cup needed for a contact sport)		
• Asthma (severe asthmatics may need to modify participation at times)		

(continues)

Table 10–1 Sports Participation Clearance Based on Medical Conditions (Continued)

May Clear for Participation	Needs Further Evaluation/Information Before Clearing for Participation	Do Not Clear for Participation
• Sickle cell trait • Hernia—refer for repair; instruct person to watch for symptoms of incarceration	• Heat illness history (has a greater chance of recurrence)—determine contributing factors and devise preventive measures prior to clearing for participation • One kidney (choose sport based on minimizing risk of contact or collision) • Enlarged liver or spleen (acute due to illness [e.g., mononucleosis]: can play after resolution to avoid rupture); if chronic, choose sport based on minimizing risk of contact or collision • Malignancy • Musculoskeletal disorders restricting movement or causing pain • Neurologic: history of head/spinal trauma, severe or repeated concussions, craniotomy (all types of sports activities need evaluation) • Seizures, if poorly controlled • Obesity (need strategy to ensure hydration and acclimatization) • Organ transplant recipient • Pulmonary compromise, including cystic fibrosis (evaluate oxygenation during a graded exercise test; ensure hydration and acclimatization)	

Table 10-1   Sports Participation Clearance Based on Medical Conditions (Continued)

May Clear for Participation	Needs Further Evaluation/Information Before Clearing for Participation	Do Not Clear for Participation
	• Acute upper respiratory infection, unless mild	
	• Sickle cell disease: if health status permits, all but high-exertion, collision/contact sports permitted; ensure hydration and acclimatization to avoid heat illness.	
	• Skin boils, herpes simplex, impetigo, scabies, *Molluscum contagiosum* while person is contagious and person is participating in martial arts, wrestling, or other collision, contact, or limited contact sports or if gym mats or equipment is shared (e.g., wrestling, baseball). *H. simplex* lesions should be healed if person wrestles or plays rugby (others can usually cover lesions); impetiginous lesions should be treated for at least 48 hours before resuming play; *Tinea gladiatorum* should be treated for 48–72 hours prior to playing—covering lesions is not acceptable. Scabies, lice, or *Molluscum contagiosum* must be treated prior to contact or collision sports participation, especially when equipment is shared (Blosser, 2009).	

Contact/collision sports: basketball, boxing, diving, field hockey, football (flag and tackle), ice hockey, lacrosse, martial arts, rodeo, rugby, ski jumping, soccer, team handball, water polo, wrestling; *limited contact:* baseball, bicycling, cheerleading, canoeing/kayaking (white water), fencing, field (high jump, pole vault), floor hockey, gymnastics, handball, horseback riding, racquetball, skating (all types), skiing (all types), softball, squash, ultimate Frisbee, volleyball, windsurfing and surfing; *noncontact:* archery, badminton, bodybuilding, canoeing/kayaking (flat water), crew rowing, curling, dancing, field (discuss, javelin, shot put), golf, orienteering, power lifting, race walking, riflery, rope jumping, running, sailing, scuba diving, strength training, swimming, table tennis, tennis, track, weight lifting.

Source: Data from American Academy of Pediatrics (AAP) Committee on Sports Medicine. (1994). Medical conditions affecting sports participation. *Pediatrics, 94,* 757–760; American Academy of Pediatrics (AAP). (2001a). Practice guidelines: Medical conditions affecting sports participation. *Pediatrics, 107*(5), 1205–1209; American Academy of Pediatrics. (2001b). Health supervision for children with Down syndrome. *Pediatrics, 107*(2), 442–449; Blosser, C. (2009). Activities and sports for children and adolescents. In Burns, C., Dunn, A., Brady, M., Starr, N., & Blosser, C. (Eds.). *Pediatric Primary Care.* St. Louis: Elsevier/Saunders; Centers for Disease Control and Prevention (CDC). (2006). *HIV/AIDS questions and answers: Can I get HIV while playing sports?* Retrieved April 13, 2009, from http://www.cdc.gov/hiv/resources/qa/qa30.htm; Greene, P. (2000). Pearls for practice: Recognizing young people at risk for sudden cardiac death in preparticipation sports physicals. *Journal of the American Academy of Nurse Practitioner, 12*(1), 11–14.

Advantages and Disadvantages of Sports Participation

The well-formulated PPE assesses both physical and psychosocial readiness factors. The sporting activity should lead to a reduction in stress rather than induce it. The individual's personality, motivation, or other situational factors contribute to the level of stress experienced. Therefore, the provider should assess the individual's level of awareness of the demands of the sport, the anticipated response to these demands (experiencing defeat), and consequences of participation within the context of the time commitment.

Positive aspects of any sport include an overall increase in fitness, gained social skills, increased self-esteem and confidence, increased coordination and physical skills, enjoyment, recreation, and a chance for increased family involvement. Negative factors can involve the stress of competition or meeting adult goals, potential injuries, and comparison of abilities to those of others.

The following items have been checked "yes" on the form that Nikola returned:

1. She had an injury since her last checkup.
2. She has been hospitalized overnight.
3. She has been told she had a heart murmur "as a child."
4. She has had a head injury.
5. She wears soft contact lenses.

Under the explanation area on the form is written: "Motor vehicle accident 2 months ago; she spent night in hospital after hitting her head; had stress fracture left ankle 6 months ago—OK now."

What other key questions do you need to ask Nikola? ■

You ask Nikola more questions about the motor vehicle accident (MVA) and hospital stay. She reports going to the emergency room 2 months ago after a family motor vehicle accident because "I hit my head against the side of the door, even though I had my seat-belt on. I was pretty dizzy and threw up a couple of times." She stayed in the hospital overnight and then saw a physician a couple of times after that.

Then you ask Nikola about some health-related and lifestyle issues. She replies that she runs every day for an hour (weekends maybe more) and works out at her local gym (to build muscle). She is happy with her current weight. She has always liked to run a lot, but didn't get into track and field at school until the beginning of the last school year. She also likes to play tennis, swim, cycle, and downhill ski.

Health Care

Other than after the MVA, her last physical examination was about 2 years ago.

Medications

She has always had some occasional headaches (have not increased since the MVA); acetaminophen relieves the pain. She has no nausea, vomiting, or photophobia. She takes a store-brand multivitamin daily. "My Mom buys whatever is cheapest for the whole family."

Past Medical History

She had asthma as a child, but has not used her inhaler "in years."

Psychosocial History

She admits to using alcohol and marijuana "a few times, but only if my friends have it." She denies using any steroids or sports-enhancing drugs. She has had sex "off and on" since she was 15 years old, using condoms "most of the time." She was on birth control pills last year, but is not on any birth control method now. She has had only one partner and vice versa with no steady boyfriend at this time.

She gets mostly A's in school and hopes to run throughout high school.

Review of Systems

- Complaints: None; 0/10 pain scale.
- Gynecological: Her menses are mostly regular, with a cycle of 30 days. "Sometimes I skip a month." Menarche at age 12 years. She used to have more irregular, heavy periods until she was on birth control pills last year. Last menstural period was 3 weeks ago, normal flow and duration.
- Head: Occasional headaches (1–2 per month), relieved with over-the-counter (OTC) medications.
- Musculoskeletal: Occasional right knee swelling, relieved with cold packs and OTC pain medications.
- Remainder of systems: No complaints; review of sudden death criteria negative. (See Table 10-1 under Do Not Clear for Participation.)

Family History

Her maternal grandmother has diabetes and high blood pressure; both paternal grandparents have high blood pressure. Her maternal grandfather died last year of a heart attack (age 58). "I think my Mom has high cholesterol—she is always on a diet." Father has high blood pressure. A younger sister has asthma, for which she uses an inhaler. She thinks her 20-year-old sister is "OK."

Nutrition

You ask Nikola about her nutritional habits:
- *Do you skip meals?* "I don't usually eat breakfast; I eat lunch at school." Dinner is usually at home or "I grab a snack if there is a track meet."
- *What do you eat during a typical day?* Breakfast: glass of orange juice; lunch: salad and candy bar; dinner: hamburger and milkshake or salad if she eats out or meat/vegetable/potato at home; snacks: candy bar or power bar. Lots of water or sports drink if running.
- *Who prepares the meals at your house?* "My Mom or Dad usually. We sometimes just go out for a hamburger or pizza on weekends."

· *As a follow-up to the above question, you ask , "Do you ever cause yourself to throw up or do you take laxatives?* "No, I'd never do that." *Have you lost weight over the last year or two?* "Yes, about 5 pounds, after I broke up with my boyfriend and started running more to forget."

Based on the information provided, what else do you need to consider? ■

From the history and answers gleaned from Nikola up to this point, there are further questions you need answered before you could reasonably be expected to clear her for sports participation.

- What was the nature and diagnosis of the head injury after the MVA? Did she exhibit any postconcussive syndrome symptoms? Would running place her at further risk of neurological trauma?
- Does this young lady exhibit risks for the female athlete triad?

Previous Head Trauma

Postconcussive syndrome is a side effect of a minor head injury. The incidence is quite variable, depending upon the definition—29% to 90% (Legome, Alt, & Wu, 2006). Most literature defines this syndrome as comprising the continuation of at least three of the following signs: headache, dizziness, fatigue, irritability, impaired memory and concentration, insomnia, and sensitivity to noise and light. The definition of the syndrome is based upon the onset and duration of symptoms and varies across the literature. It can be defined as occurring within a week of the injury with a duration of a few weeks to 6 months (Legome et al.).

A repeat concussion is often progressively more serious, especially if it occurs before the neurological symptoms from the prior head injury have completely resolved (referred to as *second-impact syndrome*). The sequelae of the second impact—even as minor as a blow to the chest or back—can cause massive brain swelling and herniation; mortality can approach 50% (Cantu, 2003; Stevenson & Adelson, 2003).

Approximately 300,000 second impact or concussion injuries occur annually in the United States from sports or recreational-related activities (Brain Injury Association, 2004). A participant in an organized sport is six times more likely to suffer such trauma than someone performing a recreational sports activity (Browne & Lam, 2006).

Given that Nikola's chosen sport is running, a noncontact sport, you can be reasonably assured that she is less likely to suffer another head injury as a consequence of participating in her organized sport. However, had she chosen a contact or collision sport (e.g., soccer) your advice might be different pending further information regarding the nature of her head injury and return-to-play guidelines. (See Table 10-3.)

You need to know the following to complete Nikola's history regarding her head injury (send for her medical records from the hospital and physician who saw her afterwards):

- Did she suffer from a Grade 1, 2, or 3 concussion? (The definition is based on a recognized set of criteria such as length of loss of consciousness, mental status [impaired orientation, memory, concentration, or delayed information or reaction time], and duration of mental changes.)
- How long did she exhibit headaches or cranial nerve symptoms after the injury (dizziness, vertigo, nausea, tinnitus, blurry vision, hearing loss, diplopia, diminished sense of taste and smell, sensitivity to light and noise)?
- Did she exhibit anxiety, irritability, depression, sleep disturbance, change in appetite, decreased libido, fatigue, or personality changes?
- If she exhibited cognitive changes, for how long after her injury were they experienced?

Female Athlete Triad

Sudden death, one sports-related problem, is less likely to occur in females, but they are more at risk of other conditions. Their risks are altered due to environmental, anatomic, hormonal, biomechanical, and neuromuscular factors (Blosser, 2009). One such condition is referred to as the *female athlete triad,* which is composed of a progressive set of three interrelated conditions. Anorexia (or disordered eating), amenorrhea (including oligomenorrhea), and osteopenia/osteoporosis occur along a continuum rather than in unison. The existence of one of these symptoms, therefore, should serve as a red flag during the PPE. Females engaged in sports where leanness and/or endurance are particularly advantageous are more prone to this disorder (e.g., gymnasts, ballerinas, swimmers and divers, figure skaters, distance runners, and cross-country skiers) (American Academy of Pediatrics [AAP], 2002). Additionally, female runners, cheerleaders, and gymnasts (i.e., those in high impact sports) are at greater risk of suffering a stress fracture than males (Loud et al., 2005). Although the fracture can be an isolated event due to the nature of the exercise itself, footwear, or musculoskeletal factors, it can also be due to osteopenia, osteoporosis, menstrual dysfunction, poor nutrition, or an eating disorder. Common anatomical areas for stress fractures include the foot, tibia, fibula, femur, and pelvis.

The incidence of amenorrhea in athletes can be as high as 66%, depending on the sport. The amenorrhea may be primary (delayed menarche past 16 years), secondary (no menses for 3–6 months after regular menses has been established), or oligomenorrhea (cycle length greater than 35 days but less than 3 months). None of these is a normal response to exercise, and caloric intake will need to be increased and/or exercise will need to be decreased in order to return to a normal body fat-to-lean ratio (AAP, 2002; Griffin et al., 2003).

Serum gonadotropin concentrations are reduced due to reduced hypothalamic pulsatile release of gonadotropin-releasing factor.

Nutritional deficits in an active female athlete can result in an imbalance when energy (caloric) expenditure exceeds energy (caloric) intake. Nutritional intake must meet both growth and activity needs. The adolescent is growing at a rate second only to that of infancy. Disordered eating, such as binging and purging, or the use of laxatives, diuretics, and diet pills for weight control can result in the same energy deficit. The normal hypothalamic-pituitary-ovarian axis necessary for normal menstruation is surmised to be compromised by the caloric input-output imbalance (Griffin et al., 2003).

Osteopenia (with resulting weakened bones) can be a result of the amenorrhea that is in turn due to inadequate body fat and the resultant hypoestrogenemic state. Inadequate bone formation results. Recovery from this state is slow, and whether it is entirely reversible is unclear. Early intervention is crucial because adult bone mineral density is largely determined by the status of bone mass during adolescence and young adulthood (Davidson, 2003; Griffin et al., 2003). Thus, failing to achieve adequate bone mass during this crucial time in life increases the risk of osteoporosis and fractures as an adult. Changes in weight, height, and body mass index (BMI) are good clues to changes in bone mineral density.

In lieu of an eating disorder, hypothalamic amenorrheic female athletes appear fit, their estimated ideal body weight is more than 85%, and their resting pulse is 40–60 beats/minute (Hergenroeder & Chorley, 2004). Early identification, such as that afforded by the PPE, is imperative so preventive interventions can be instituted. This will ensure that the female may be able to return to a high performance level and enjoy good health in the future.

Fractures or Other Musculoskeletal Disorders in the Female Athlete

As stated earlier, an array of factors can lead to stress fractures. When there is an imbalance between bone resorption and bone deposition, the bone may not be physiologically capable of holding up under repetitive loads. The PPE affords the opportunity to explore the underlying risk factors that contribute (or contributed) to the fracture, conduct a pertinent examination, and implement strategies to prevent recurrence.

The female is 2 to 10 times more likely to experience a noncontact sports anterior cruciate ligament injury than a male. These injuries commonly occur during deceleration, landing, or cutting activities (Griffin et al., 2003).

The anatomy and biomechanics of the patellofemoral joint also put the female athlete at greater risk of having a problem with this joint. Malalignment or an imbalance between muscles of the pelvis, hip, knee, ankle, and foot; articular cartilage lesions; instability; soft tissue factors; and psychosocial factors can contribute to pain and dysfunction of this joint. Additionally, improper training, overuse, or injury can contribute to the pathophysiology. Runners can be afflicted with a painful knee condition known as *runner's knee*; it results from overuse and causes micro-trauma to the sleeve of the knee joint.

Distinguishing factors include pain *around* the knee joint (rather than *inside* it) and initial minor discomfort that progresses to increased pain after running.

The Use of Medroxyprogesterone (Depo-Provera) by the Female Athlete

Since 2004, the Food and Drug Administration has required a "black box" warning about the use of medroxyprogesterone as a contraceptive for adolescents and young adults. Some studies had found that prolonged use resulted in loss of bone mineral density; the loss was duration dependent. Current prescribing recommendations, therefore, advise not using this method of contraception in this age group for longer than 2 years *unless* there is no other alternative (American Society of Health-System Pharmacists, 2008).

What parts of the physical examination do you want to emphasize? ■

Physical Examination

The PPE should consist of two parts, the musculoskeletal and general physical examinations. The simple, standardized 90-second musculoskeletal screening (Figure 10-2) reliably detects 90% of significant injuries, and has a 51% sensitivity and 97% specificity (McCarthy, 2006). Limitations or dysfunction in alignment, flexibility, and proprioception will be detected. Table 10-2 shows the components of an appropriate general organ examination. You want to pay special attention to assessing Nikola's mental status because of her prior head injury, her musculoskeletal examination because of her prior stress fracture history, and her growth parameters and pulse because of concerns regarding her nutrition and eating habits.

Nikola's examination reveals the following:

- Height: 67 inches (slightly under 90%)
- Weight: 127 pounds (approximately 60%)
- BMI: 20 (between 25% and 50%)
- Blood pressure: 115/68, Pulse: 60
- Snellen: 20/20 OD/OS/OU with glasses
- Appearance: Alert, cooperative, good historian, good eye-to-eye contact, smiles frequently, slender

The examination is negative except for a Grade I/VI, short, musical, midsystolic murmur best heard at the apex without radiation, increased slightly when supine.

What diagnostic studies would you consider? ■

The only routine diagnostic test for a PPE is a hemoglobin/hematocrit for females, unless there is a particular risk factor for the individual. Females are more at risk for iron deficiency anemia. Urine drug screening and human immunodeficiency virus (HIV) testing may be required by some organizations.

ACTIVITY 1

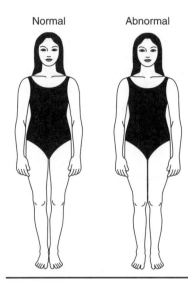

Normal   Abnormal

- Appropriate for interscholastic, intramural, and extra-mural sports activities.
- A screening evaluation created to direct attention to problems but not evaluate the problems.
- Identifies the following conditions that might be adversely affected by athletic participation:
  a. Congenital problems
  b. Acquired problems

Questions such as the following are to be answered by the athlete and signed by BOTH the athlete and parent:
- Have you ever had an illness, condition, or injury that required you to go to the hospital, either as a patient overnight or in the emergency room for X-rays; required an operation; caused you to see a doctor; caused you to miss a game or practice?
- Are you now or have you been under the care of a physician for any reason?
- Do you currently have any medical problems or injuries?
- Have you ever had a broken bone, joint sprain or liga-ment tear, muscle pull, head injury, neck injury or nerve pinch, dislocated joint, back trouble or problems?

Instructions to patient:
"Stand up straight and face me."

What is screened:
Acromioclavicular joints, symmetry of extremities

ACTIVITY 2

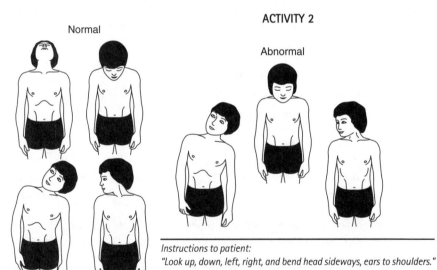

Normal

Abnormal

Instructions to patient:
"Look up, down, left, right, and bend head sideways, ears to shoulders."

What is screened:
Cervical spine range of motion

Figure 10-2   Illustration of the 90-second sports musculoskeletal examination.
From *For the practitioner: Orthopaedic screening examination for participation in sports.* © 1981 Ross Products Division, Abbott Laboratories. Text adapted from Garrich, J. G. (1977). Sports medicine. *Pediatric Clinics of North America, 24,* 737–747.

ACTIVITY 3

Normal

Abnormal

Instructions to patient:
"Shrug your shoulders." (Against resistance by examiner)

What is screened:
Trapezius strength

ACTIVITY 4

Normal

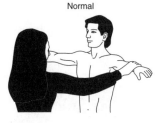

Abnormal

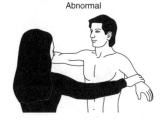

Instructions to patient:
"Hold arms outstretched from your sides and lift them" (Against resistance as examiner pushes down)

What is screened:
Shoulder range of motion

ACTIVITY 5

Normal

Abnormal

ACTIVITY 6

Normal

Abnormal

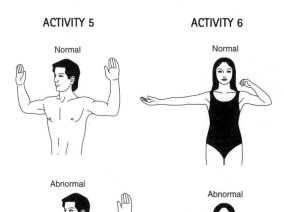

Instructions to patient (Activity 5):
"Raise your elbows at your sides 90 degrees. Rotate your hands backwards."

What is screened:
Deltoid strength
Shoulder rotation

Instructions to patient (Activity 6):
"Hold arms straight out from sides, palms up. Flex and extend your elbows."

What is screened:
Elbow range of motion

(continues)

Figure 10-2   Illustration of the 90-second sports musculoskeletal examination. (Continued)

ACTIVITY 7

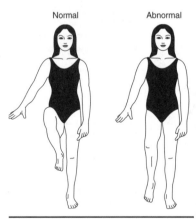

Normal   Abnormal

Instructions to patient:
"Let your arms down again. Flex your elbows so that your hands reach straight out. Rotate your wrists, palms facing up, then down.

What is screened:
Wrist range of motion (pronation/supination)

ACTIVITY 8

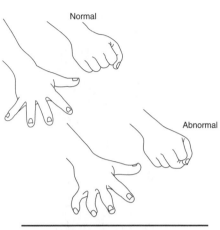

Normal

Abnormal

Instructions to patient:
"Show me your hands. Spread your fingers out (examiner resists spreading). Make a fist and squeeze.

What is screened:
Hand/finger range of motion and strength

ACTIVITY 9

Normal   Abnormal

Instructions to patient:
"Lift your right leg up, bent at the knee. Repeat using the other leg."

What is screened:
Leg symmetry, knee or ankle effusion

ACTIVITY 10

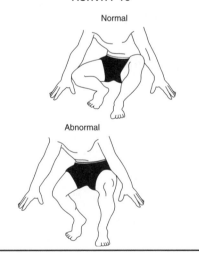

Normal

Abnormal

Instructions to patient:
"Squat like a duck, and walk four steps away from me."

What is screened:
Hip, knee, and ankle range of motion

Figure 10-2 Illustration of the 90-second sports musculoskeletal examination. (Continued)

ACTIVITY 11

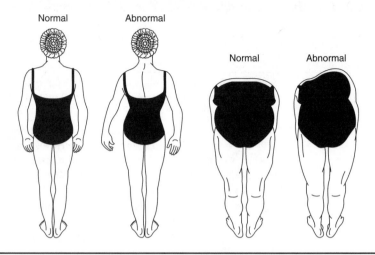

Instructions to patient:
"Stand up straight. Keep your knees as straight as you can, and try to touch your toes. Straighten slowly."

What is screened:
Shoulder symmetry, scoliosis, hip range of motion, hamstring tightness

ACTIVITY 12

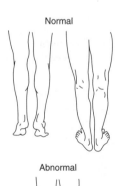

Instructions to patient:
"Stand up on your tiptoes."

What is screened:
Calf symmetry, leg strength

Figure 10-2   Illustration of the 90-second sports musculoskeletal examination. (Continued)

Table 10-2	Example of an Appropriate Preparticipation Physical Examination
Examination Feature	**Comments**
Height and weight	Establish baseline and monitor for eating disorders, steroid abuse.
Blood pressure	Assess in the context of participant's age, height, and sex.
General appearance	Excessive height and excessive long-bone growth (arachnodactyly, arm span greater than height, pectus, excavatum) suggest Marfan syndrome.
Eyes	Important to detect vision defects that leave one of the eyes with < 20/40 corrected vision. Lens subluxations, severe myopia, retinal detachments, and strabismus are associated with Marfan syndrome. Note any anisometropia for the record. Absence of one eye will limit some sport choices.
Cardiovascular	Palpate the point of maximal impulse for increased intensity and displacement, which suggest hypertrophy and failure, respectively. Note heart rate, rhythm. Check for murmurs. A murmur that worsens with standing or Valsalva suggests hypertrophic cardiomyopathy.
	Perform auscultation with the patient supine and again with the patient standing or straining during Valsalva maneuver.
	Check femoral against radial pulses; femoral pulse diminishment suggests aortic coarctation.
Respiratory	Observe for accessory muscle use or prolonged expiration and auscultate for wheezing. Exercise-induced asthma will not produce manifestations on a resting examination and requires exercise testing for diagnosis.
Abdominal	Assess for masses, tenderness, organomegaly (especially liver and spleen). In females, assess for any pain and/or enlargement over hypogastric area or pelvis that might suggest pregnancy or gynecologic problem; proceed with further work-up as indicated.
Genitourinary	Hernias and varicoceles do not usually preclude sports participation. Check for single, undescended testicle, masses. Discuss testicular cancer and provide information about the self-testicular exam.
Musculoskeletal	Use the 90-second musculoskeletal examination (see Figure 10-2). Consider supplemental shoulder, knee, and ankle examinations as indicated specific to the chosen sports injury-prone areas.
Skin	Evidence of *Molluscum cotagiosum*, herpes simplex, impetigo, tinea corporis, or scabies would temporarily prohibit participation in sports where direct skin-to-skin compositor contact occurs (e.g., wrestling, martial arts).
Neurologic	Gross motor assessment with attention to equality of strength, especially with a history of recurrent stingers or burners, head injury. Usually sufficiently grossly assessed during the 90-second musculoskeletal exam.

Source: From Kuravski, K., & Chandran, S. (2000). The preparticipation athletic evaluation. *American Family Physician, 61,* 2683–2690, 2696–2698.

Nikola's hemoglobin is 12.6. Because this is a female runner with a history of stress fracture, weight loss, questionable adequate caloric intake, and transient oligomenorrhea, you are suspicious for early female athlete triad, but also want to rule out thyroid dysfunction. She has also been sexually active. You add the following tests:

- TSH: 3.6 UIU/mL (normal: 0.7-6.4 UIU/mL)
- T4: 1.20 ng/dL (normal: 0.8-2.7 ng/dL)
- Nucleic acid amplification test (NAAT) urine screen: negative (NAATs have high sensitivity and specificity for chlamydia and gonorrhea with the exception of the PCR type NAAT, which does not detect gonorrhea as well as the other two (Cook, Hutchinson, Ostergaard, Braithwaite, & Ness, 2005).

Making the Diagnosis

What other diagnoses will you consider? ■

Differential Diagnoses

The differential diagnoses are secondary to the underlying features of the female athlete triad and include anorexia (malnutrition), leukemia, thyroid disorder, depression and other psychological conditions, osteopenia, osteoporosis, menstrual dysfunction, inadequate sports footwear, anatomical (joint or muscle) factors, osteogenesis imperfecta, early onset juvenile idiopathic arthritis, and overuse. If the amenorrhea continues despite nutritional and weight correction, you would proceed to explore other diagnostic differentials for this condition covered in other references.

Nikola's PPE is reassuringly normal, as far as any residual effects from her head injury. She is at risk of second-impact syndrome should she receive another head trauma. If this should happen, it is not likely it would be a result of her noncontact running sport, but could be a result of recreational activities. Before clearing her for sports you need to obtain the prior head injury treatment records, as previously stated. However, based on the criteria listed in Table 10-3, you surmise it will be doubtful that she would be limited in her ability to run.

Because she is female, she is not as likely to suffer from sudden death as are males, and her review of systems and cardiac examination were all normal. Your review of the criteria suggestive of potential sudden death was also negative. Her murmur is typical of that of an innocent murmur, and no further workup is required.

Aspects of Nikola's examination prompt you to weigh heavily her need to ensure she is obtaining adequate nutritional calories to meet her energy and sex steroids needs, and thus avoid full-blown manifestations of the female athlete triad. Her headaches are controlled; no further workup is necessary unless they worsen or become more debilitating.

Table 10-3 Recommendations for Management of Concussion[a] in Sports

Definition	First Concussion	Second Concussion	Third Concussion
Grade 1 No LOC; transient confusion, duration of mental status abnormalities[b] of < 30 minutes	No sports activities for 7 days; RTP if asymptomatic on mental status parameters after resting and exerting self. Should be taken to the ER if mental status abnormalities last more than 1 hour.	No sports activity for 4 weeks; RTP if asymptomatic after resting and exerting self on the last 7 days of the 4 weeks off.	No further sports activity in current season.[c] May RTP after the third season.
Grade 2 LOC < 5 minutes; duration of mental status abnormalities ≥ 30 minutes but < 24 hours	No sports activity for 4 weeks; RTP if asymptomatic on mental status parameters after resting and exerting self in the last 7 days of the 4 weeks off.	No sports activity for rest of season; RTP following season if asymptomatic in all parameters.	Terminate contact sports for 1 year; RTP in noncontact sports after that.
Grade 3 LOC greater than 5 minutes; mental status abnormalities > 24 hours.	No sports activity for 4 weeks; RTP if asymptomatic on mental status parameters after resting and exerting self in the last 7 days of the 4 weeks off.	No sports activity for rest of season. No further contact sports after following season; may participate in noncontact sports.	Terminate contact sports for 1 year; RTP in noncontact sports after that.

[a] A concussion is defined as head-trauma-induced alteration in mental status that may or may not involve loss of consciousness. Concussions are graded in three categories. Definitions and treatment recommendations for each category are presented.

[b] Mental status abnormalities include impairment in orientation, memory, concentration, or delayed recall.

[c] Season refers to a playing season, not a year. Examples: football season is one season. If followed by a baseball season, that is the second season, etc.

Note. LOC, Loss of consciousness; RTP, return to play.

Question: *Can the athlete return to the field in the same game?* In collegiate sports: YES, if the athlete meets the criteria of (a) Grade 1 concussion, (b) has no headache, dizziness, posttrauma amnesia, and can recall events of the game and, (c) the athlete, after doing exertion testing with sprints and push-ups on the sidelines, still has no symptoms as assessed by the team physician. NO, if in middle or high school sports.

Adapted from Stevenson K. L., & Adelson, P. D. (2003). Pediatric sports-related head injuries. In DeLee, J. C., Drez, D., Miller, M. D. (Eds.). *DeLee and Drez's orthopaedic sports medicine: Principles and practice* (Vol. 1, 2nd ed., pp. 775–787). Philadelphia: WB Saunders.

Source: From Burns, C., Dunn, A., Brady, M., Starr, N., & Blosser, C. (Eds.). *Pediatric Primary Care*. St. Louis, MO: Elsevier/Saunders.

Management

General Management Strategies
The prevention of injury is not necessarily the most important aspect of PPE management. There are a myriad of health-related topics that should be taken into consideration, as discussed earlier. The provider will need to perform an assessment regarding developmental readiness and the type of preseason conditioning needed. Table 10-4 lists training (conditioning) and other management strategies the provider can recommend.

Educating coaches, parents, and the individual about heat illness (hyperthermia) prevention is important, especially for those participating in high performance recreational activities. See Table 10-4.

Active teenagers need to exceed their baseline caloric needs by 1,500 to 3,000 calories, depending upon the sport. Children require an intake of 60 kcal/kg of ideal body weight per day to maintain normal growth. The daily caloric needs consist of:

- Carbohydrates (CHO): 55% to 75%
- Fats: 25% to 30%
- Protein: 15% to 20%

Women need to ensure adequate iron and calcium intake and may need supplements to achieve adequate levels of both. Calcium intake should be 1,200–1,500 mg/day for all youth.

Different sports involve the use of different fuel sources. Short-term, high-intensity sports (e.g., high jumping, diving) use anaerobic fuel sources, such as carbohydrates. Long-term activities (e.g., running, cross-country skiing) involve aerobic fuel sources, such as carbohydrates (both an aerobic and anaerobic source), protein, and fats. The carbohydrates should come from fruits, vegetables, whole grains, and milk sugars rather than from processed sugar sources. Carbohydrate loading prior to an activity has not been studied in children nor has it proven to enhance performance (Blosser, 2009). However, for activities that last longer than one hour, performance has shown improvement with carbohydrate intake. Additionally, muscle glycogen resynthesis is improved with the intake of CHOs if taken 30 minutes and 2 hours after strenuous activity. Additional protein may be efficacious for intense endurance sports and strength training (1,500 to 3,000 kcal above the recommended daily allowance of 1 g/kg/day). It is important to counsel that eating additional protein should not replace necessary CHOs and fats; extra fat will be stored from excessive, unused protein.

Some athletes (notably wrestlers) may practice weight cycling (weight loss). This practice has not been shown to lead to long-term adverse effects or to affect height and weight; however, it can deplete electrolytes; affect glycogen stores, hormones, and nutrition status; impair mental and academic performance; reduce immunity; and cause pulmonary emboli and pancreatitis

Table 10–4 Management Strategies for the PPE

Injury Prevention	Daily Living	Readiness	Benefits	Training

• **Control symptoms of specific diseases or disorders**
• Rehabilitate injuries
• Counsel regarding:
  ∘ Dehydration
  ∘ Protective equipment approved for that sport; some sports have higher injury rates
• Supportive footwear
• Educated coaching (knowledge of first aid, can recognize head injury or other trauma, can administer CPR)
• Safe environment (floors, fields, equipment)
• Parents need to model equipment safety (ride with bicycle helmets, etc.)
• Highest eye trauma risk from hockey, fencing, boxing, full-contact martial arts, racquetball,
	• Nutrition
	  ∘ Balanced diet
	  ∘ Adequate calories
	  ∘ Hydration
	• Stress management
	  ∘ Expected outcomes
	  ∘ Realistic expectations based upon physical capabilities
	  ∘ Supportive coaching
	  ∘ Parents that support rather than identify with athleticism of child
	  ∘ Emphasize participation rather than winning
	• Balance among home, school, and recreational activities
	• Drug-free participation[c]
	• Family planning
		• Noncontact sports can begin at 7 years old; organized sports at 10 years old (Luebbers, 2003)
		• Understanding of competitiveness comes at 9 years old (Patel, Pratt, & Greydanus, 2002)
		• Understanding the complex nature of tasks for a given sport is understood better at 12 years old (Patel et al.)
		• Emphasize positive health effects of sports
		• Social and psychological maturational levels may lag behind ability of an athletically gifted child exposed to competition; balance is important
		• Take into consideration child's ability and physical stature with
			• Children with physical limitations should be encouraged to participate; help them choose the right sport[a]
			• Can build self-esteem for those academically challenged; find the balance
			• Maintaining a high level of everyday physical activity increases whole body and trochanter bone mass (Janz et al. 2006), particularly in prepubertal through pubertal years (Clinical Advisor, 2005)
				• Overtraining symptoms include feeling "burned out," repeated injuries, lack of enthusiasm and joy for sport
				• Adequate warm-up and stretching exercise before and after playing
				• Conditioning can lessen overuse injuries and duration of rehabilitation, strengthen bone, help with weight control, aid reaction times, and improve performance
				  ∘ Preparatory muscle conditioning, such as warm-up programs to establish motion patterns (can start as young as 10 to 12 years old); improves strength, flexibility, and endurance (not to be confused with
				(continues)

Table 10-4 Management Strategies for the PPE (Continued)

Injury Prevention	Daily Living	Readiness	Benefits	Training

lacrosse, squash, basket-ball, baseball; moderate risk: tennis, badminton, soccer, volleyball, water polo, football, fishing, golf; low risk: swimming, diving, skiing, noncontact martial arts, wrestling, bicycling, track and field, gymnastics
• Prepubertal boys and girls can play contact sports together; after puberty, it can be unsafe for smaller females or males to compete in contact sports with boys or girls of greater age and weight
• Different sports have different injury rates
• Prevent heat illness:
  ○ Do not use salt tablets
  ○ Wear lightweight, dry, "wicking" clothing
		a realistic and safe sport-achievement goal
		• Females are more likely to participate if: compe-tition is not emphasized, sport is composed of small groups versus larger teams, sport is directed towards their stated goal, and their father models physical activity (ACSM, 2003)
		• For those with health problems, overall health needs to be assessed and reviewed within the boundaries of the requirements and risks for any given sport; deci-sion for participation made in consultation with a medical specialist familiar with that child and his or her parents.
				weight training) (Olsen et al., 2005)
				  ○ Plyometric training exercises[b]

Table 10-4 Management Strategies for the PPE (Continued)

Injury Prevention	Daily Living	Readiness	Benefits	Training
◦ Drink cool water rather than warm every 20 minutes at 5 oz (weight under 40 kg); 9 oz (if 60 kg); 10–12 oz (over 60 kg)—Stay hydrated! ◦ Schedule rest periods in shade every 20–30 minutes (remove helmets if worn) ◦ Acclimatize to heat over 8–12 days ◦ Risk factors include obesity, cystic fibrosis, hyperthyroidism, prior heat illness, diabetes, kidney disorders, medications (diuretics, antihistamines, antidepressants, and others), poor health or conditioning				

[a] Children with disabilities have lower levels of physical fitness and are prone to obesity. Encourage families of children with intellectual and developmental disabilities (e.g., Down, fragile X, Turner, Klinefelter, autism, etc.) to advocate for "adapted" PE in schools and regularly encourage their children to participate in sports activities that are fun and make use of physical abilities. The Special Olympics Healthy Athletes program is a resource in many communities throughout the world.

[b] Exercises that combine strength with movements (e.g., hops, jumps); conditions the body to react quickly to stretching and shortening and decreases injuries.

[c] Includes freedom from the use of anabolic-androgenic steroids, steroid precursors (androstenedione and DHEA), growth hormone, creatine, ephedra alkaloids, and performance-enhancing nutritional supplements. (These have been know to contain steroids; amino acid supplementation does not increase muscle mass nor decrease body fat.) Enhanced performance has not been demonstrated for the precursors, ephedra, growth hormone, or nutritional supplements; they can have serious side effects. Street names: gym candy, pumpers, weight trainers, stackers, and Arnolds (Blosser, 2009).

Sources: American College of Sports Medicine (ACSM). (2003, September 4). *Girls more likely to be active when parents participate. News Release.* Retrieved April 20, 2009, from *www.acsm.org/AM/Template.cfm?Section=Home_Page&Template=/CM/Content Display.cfm&ContentID=4249;* Clinical Advisor, Editorial Staff. (2005). Newsline: Childhood exercise increased bone mass. *The Clinical Advisor 8*(11), 21; Janz, K. F., Gilmore, J. M., Burns, T. L., Levy, S. M., Torner, J. C., Willing. M. C., et al. (2006). Physical activity augments bone mineral accrual in young children: The Iowa Bone Development Study. *Journal of Pediatrics, 148*(6), 793–799; Leubbers, P. E. (2003, Spring). The right time for kids to exercise. In: American College of Sports Medicine: *Fit society: Youth sports and health.* Retrieved April 20, 2009, from *http://www.acsm.org/AM/Template.cfm?Section=Search&section=20033&template=/ CM/ContentDisplay.cfm&ContentFileID=40;* Olsen, O. E., Myklebust, G., Engebretsen, L., Holme, I., Bahr, R. (2005). Exercises to prevent lower limb injuries in youth sports: Cluster randomized controlled trials. *British Medical Journal, 330,* 449–452; Patel, D., Pratt, H., & Greydanus, D. (2002). Pediatric neurodevelopment and sports participation. When are Children ready to play sports? *Pediatric Clinics of North America, 49,* 505–531.

(Housh & Johns, 2001). The practice should be discouraged; it is a risk factor for longer term dysfunctional eating. Other rapid weight loss measures practiced by athletes may include removing fluids from the body via sauna or a sweat suit, laxatives, diuretics, diet pills, licit or illicit drugs, nicotine, prolonged fasting, overexercising, or vomiting (Blosser, 2009).

Those who are using drugs to enhance their performance should receive as much information as possible about their side effects. Such information is beyond the scope of this case study, but is available from a plethora of references and community resources. A referral for alcohol and drug assessment and counseling is in order.

Management Considerations for the Female Athlete Triad

The PPE provides an opportunity for the provider to be vigilant for features of the triad in female athletes. The presence of an eating disorder, rapid and progressive weight loss, change in menses patterns with either irregularity or loss of periods, and repeated stress fractures should prompt a team approach for management. This team of specialists often includes a nutritionist, medical provider, and psychiatrist or psychologist. The parents, athletic trainer(s), and athlete are included as part of the team. Exercise may need to be limited until the negative energy balance and unhealthy weight are corrected. If the individual is frankly amenorrheic, gaining weight through reduced training (exercise decreased to 3 days/week only if less than 85% of the estimated ideal body weight; otherwise, no change is necessary) would be part of the management strategy (Landry, 2007). If the amenorrhea has been prolonged and increasing calories is problematic, estrogen/progesterone replacement should be considered (AAP, 2002; Landry, 2007).

The female athlete may neither recognize she has a problem nor be aware of the serious physical consequences. Your education should focus on the benefits of treating the disorder in order to enhance her athletic performance—increasing strength, endurance, and concentration.

How do you plan to manage this adolescent? ■

Female Athlete Triad Issues

Nikola's history and PPE have some elements that suggest early female athlete triad (stress fracture, poor nutrition, oligomenorrhea). Correction of any inadequate calorie consumption should resolve her issues completely. Therefore, you arrange for her to talk with a nutritionist (a sport nutritionist is preferable). If you had discerned a frank eating disorder, then you would also refer her to a specialist in this field in order to deal with the psychological aspects of this condition. You prescribe a calcium supplement of 1,200–1,500 mg/day and ensure that her multivitamin contains iron and vitamin D. You schedule a recheck examination for Nikola in 3 months to recheck her weight and menstruation status.

Second-Impact Syndrome Issues

You also address her risk for second-impact syndrome. Any potential contact/collision activities should involve her using a helmet (e.g., while cycling or for any aggressive downhill skiing). You get permission from her (and note it in her chart) to notify her parents about the dangers of a second head injury.

Family Planning and Lifestyle Issues

You provide her with a pamphlet on birth control options, emphasize the continued use of condoms, and encourage her to return for a prescribed method should she resume sexual activity. You also emphasize the benefits to her health, academics, and sport success of abstaining from drugs and alcohol. Additionally, you advise her to seek medical attention should she have worsening or persistent bone or joint pain during daily activities, because she would need to be evaluated for a stress fracture, runner's knee, or other musculoskeletal disorder. Track and field sports activities have a small risk of eye trauma, but she needs to be wearing any specific recommended eyewear for her sport.

Preparticipation Permission

You give her a quantitative "yes" clearance for sports pending review of her medical records pertaining to the MVA. You receive these records a week later. They reveal that Nikola was given a diagnosis of Grade 1 concussion with some mental confusion to date, time, and event; she was watched overnight in the hospital as a precaution. She demonstrated limited recall about the event and had a mild headache a week later at the clinic; by the second recheck appoint (week 2 post-MVA), she was fully oriented, her headaches had resolved, and no further follow-up was advised. You note in her record receipt of these records, give her a diagnosis of "cleared for sports," and mail off a copy of the sports examination form (the second side of the form in Figure 10-1) to Nikola.

What follow-up care do you want to plan for Nikola? ▆

Nikola needs to return for her weight check in 3 months. You place a note in the system you use in your clinic for important recall purposes.

Additionally, you call her parents and discuss second-impact syndrome with them and Nikola's risk factors for another head injury. You note your call in her chart.

Key Points from the Case

1. The PPE is often the only health examination for the majority of youth and adolescents in any given year. There are two parts: the musculoskeletal and general physical examinations.

2. A standard PPE form should be used.

3. All history and physical findings need to be documented. Findings will help the provider determine whether sports participation should be allowed, whether further evaluation is needed before being allowed, or if risk factors preclude participation.

4. Psychological and physical well-being need to be assessed in order to ascertain the individual's level of awareness of the demands of the sport, the anticipated response to these demands (experiencing defeat), and consequences of participation within the context of the time commitment.

5. Adequate nutritional intake is crucial for maintaining normal growth and meeting the added demands of the physical activity.

6. Postconcussive syndrome/second impact syndrome can be a side effect of a minor head injury; any history of a head injury needs to be fully explored before allowing participation in contact or collision sports.

7. The female athlete's health risks are altered due to environmental, anatomic, hormonal, biomechanical, and neuromuscular factors.

8. The *female athlete triad* is comprised of a progressive set of three interrelated conditions that occur along a continuum rather than in unison: anorexia, amenorrhea, and osteopenia. The existence of one of these symptoms serves as a red flag during the PPE. Management involves a team approach.

9. Medroxyprogesterone (Depo-provera) has a "black box" warning as a contraceptive for adolescents and young adults because of a chance of prolonged bone mineral density loss; careful consideration is indicated before prescribing.

10. General counseling topics should also include preparatory training and warm-ups, heat illness prevention, eye protection, caloric needs, added minerals that may be necessary, drug and alcohol avoidance (including performance enhancing drugs), and risky behaviors.

REFERENCES

American Academy of Pediatrics. (2002). Guidelines for pediatricians: Female athlete triad. *Sportsshorts, 8.* Retrieved April 13, 2009, from https://www.aap.org/sections/sportsmedicine/PDFs/SportsShorts_08.pdf

American Society of Health-System Pharmacists. (2008). *American Hospital Formulary Service (AHFS) Drug Information 2008.* Bethesda, MD: American Society of Health-System Pharmacists.

Blosser, C. (2009). Activities and sports for children and adolescents. In C. Burns, A. Dunn, M. Brady, N. Barber, & C. Blosser (Eds.), *Pediatric primary care* (4th ed., pp. 262–303). St. Louis: Elsevier/Saunders.

Brain Injury Association. (2004). *Fact sheet: Sports and recreation.* Retrieved July 15, 2008, from http://www.biausa.org/BIAUSA.ORG/word.files.to.pdf/good.pdfs/factsheets/SportsAndRec.pdf

Browne, G., & Lam, L. (2006). Concussive head injury in children and adolescents related to sports and other leisure physical activities. *British Journal of Sports Medicine, 40,* 163–168.

Cantu, R. (2003). Head injuries. In J. DeLee, D. Drez, & M. Miller (Eds.), *DeLee and Drez's orthopaedic sports medicine: Principles and practice* (Vol. 1, 2nd ed., pp. 772–773). Philadelphia: WB Saunders.

Centers for Disease Control and Prevention (CDC). (2006). *HIV/AIDS questions and answers: Can I get HIV while playing sports?* Retrieved April 13, 2009, from http://www.cdc.gov/hiv/resources/qa/qa30.htm

Cook, R., Hutchinson, S., Ostergaard, L., Braithwaite, R., & Ness, R. (2005). Systematic review: Noninvasive testing for *Chlamydia trachomatis* and *Neisseria gonorrhoeae. Annals of Internal Medicine, 142,* 914–925.

Davidson, M. (2003). Pharmacotherapeutics for osteoporosis prevention and treatment. *Journal of Midwifery and Women's Health, 48*(1), 39–54.

Griffin, L., Hannafin, J., Indelicato, P., Joy, E., Kibler, W., Lebrun, C., et al. (2003). Summary: Team physician consensus statement: Female athlete issues for the team physician: A consensus statement *Medicine and Science in Sports and Exercise, 35*(10), 1785–1793. Retrieved July 15, 2008, from http://www.acsm.org/AM/Template.cfm?Section=Clinicians1&Template=/CM/ContentDisplay.cfm&ContentID=1617

Hergenroeder, A., & Chorley, J. (2004). Sports medicine. In R. Behrman, R. Kliegman, & H. Jensen (Eds.), *Nelson textbook of pediatrics* (17th ed., pp. 2302–2320). Philadelphia: Elsevier/Saunders.

Housh, T., & Johns, G. (2001). *Current comments: Report on growth in young wrestlers.* Retrieved July 13, 2008, from http://www.acsm.org/AM/Template.cfm?Section=Current_Comments1&Template=/CM/ContentDisplay.cfm&ContentID=8020

Landry, G. L. (2007). Female athletes: Menstrual problems and the risk of osteopenia. In R. M. Kliegman, R. E. Behrman, H. B. Jenson, & B. F. Stanton (Eds.), *Nelson textbook of pediatrics* (18th ed., p. 2865). Philadelphia: Elsevier/Saunders.

Landry, G. L., &, Logan, K. (2007). Sports medicine. In R. M. Kliegman, R. E. Behrman, H. B. Jenson, & B. F. Stanton (Eds.), *Nelson textbook of pediatrics* (18th ed., pp. 2848–2867). Philadelphia: Elsevier/Saunders.

Legome, E., Alt, R., & Wu, T. (2006). *Postconcussive syndrome.* Retrieved July 13, 2008, from http://www.emedicine.com/emerg/topic865.htm

Loud, K. J., Gordon, C. M., Micheli, L. J., & Field, A. E. (2005). Correlates of stress fractures among preadolescent and adolescent girls. *Pediatrics,* 115(4), e399–e406.

McCarthy,V. (2006). Getting to the big game: Keys to performing an efficient sports physical. *Advanced Nurse Practitioner, 14*(6), 67–69.

Stevenson, K., & Adelson, P. (2003). Pediatric sports-related head injuries. In J. DeLee, D. Drez Jr., & M. Miller (Eds.), *DeLee and Drez's orthopaedic sports medicine: Principles and practice* (Vol. 2, 2nd ed., p. 781). Philadelphia: Elsevier/WB Saunders.

Chapter 11

The Infant Not Sleeping Through the Night

Lynne Henry

Sleep, or lack of it, is often not discussed at routine health maintenance visits and is typically not discussed at all until the child's sleep disturbs the parents' sleep. The quality of an infant's sleep can affect an entire family's well-being, resulting in parental fatigue and mood disturbances, which lead to less effective parenting. Furthermore, studies have shown that infant sleep problems can reoccur or persist into early childhood (Chamness, 2008). Many concerns regarding sleep disturbances are related to the infant's or child's developmental level, whereas other sleep-related concerns are associated with habits or behaviors that parents unintentionally support.

Assessment of sleep habits should be addressed at every well child and health maintenance visit. In order to avoid common sleep disturbances, it is important to establish healthy sleep patterns as early as infancy. A sleep assessment should begin with an understanding of normal sleep physiology and knowledge of how the child's developmental stage affects sleep physiology.

Educational Objectives
1. Understand the normal physiology of sleep.
2. Apply developmental factors of the child to the physiology of sleep.
3. Understand the parental role in sleep disturbances.
4. Apply the cultural factors that may influence the normal physiology and management of sleep hygiene issues in the family

Case Presentation and Discussion

Natalia Fernandez is an 8-month-old female who presents today at your rural health clinic with her mother and her paternal grandmother. Mom is concerned because Natalia, who had been sleeping through the night, is now awakening at around 2 a.m. and crying as though something is wrong. This has been going on for about 4 weeks. Mom worries that Natalia may have an ear infection because she pulls at her ears while she is crying. Mom also notes that when she gets Natalia out of the crib, she stops crying and seems to want to play. When this happens, Mom gives Natalia a bottle of formula to calm her down but she drinks only 1–2 ounces. Mom admits that her baby's night waking really frustrates her, and she becomes very irritable with Natalia in these early morning hours.

Assessment

What questions will you need to ask the family related to the presenting complaints? ■

A thorough history can often elicit the underlying issue. As you assess this concern of the mother, there are some detailed questions you should ask. These include:

- A description, from the parent's perspective, of the disturbing behavior
- The baby's usual sleep and feeding patterns
- The length of time the child stays and sleeps in bed relative to the entire day
- The time the parent puts the baby to bed throughout the day
- The parent's expectations of when, where, and how long the baby should sleep
- Exact details of the manner in which the parent puts the baby to bed
- What the parent has tried to do to help stop the sleep disturbance
- How the parent usually responds to the sleep disturbance
- Baby's temperament
- Household routines (who is the primary caregiver)
- Changes in the household (stressors, e.g., new job)
- Family history of sleep problems
- Family history of depression

Obtaining a thorough and accurate history is the key to delineating the problem and developing a differential diagnosis of likely causes.

Upon further review of Natalia's chart and additional questioning of her mom, you learn that Natalia was born via spontaneous vaginal delivery at 40 weeks gestation to Nicole, age 22 years, and Roberto, a 22-year-old Hispanic man. They have no other children. Roberto works full time at a car dealership and Nicole recently returned to work at Starbucks 12 to 15 hours per week. Natalia was diagnosed with GERD (gastroesophageal reflux disease), but the spitting up never interrupted her sleep. In fact, the symptoms of reflux dissipated after she began eating solids by spoon. Natalia's mother is the primary caretaker and usually gives Natalia a bottle about 1 hour before she puts her in her crib at around 8:00 p.m. every night, practicing the "Back to Sleep" recommendations. Natalia uses a silk blanket, called her "meese," to help soothe herself to sleep and usually falls to sleep around 8:15 p.m. or so. Natalia's mother gets her up around 8:30 a.m. when Dad is leaving for work. She began sleeping all night at around 4 months of age. She naps twice a day, 1 hour in the morning around 10:00 a.m. and approximately 2 hours in the afternoon, around 2:00 p.m.

At this point, Natalia begins to fuss and you observe her mother's attempts to comfort her. Mom appears frustrated and hands her off to her paternal grandmother.

Observing this interaction, you ask if there have been any changes in the family's routine at home or any new or different stressors, good or bad, that the family is currently experiencing. Natalia's mother admits that approximately 1 month ago, Natalia's dad's company downsized and he suffered a decrease in his pay. These events required the family to move into the paternal grandmother's home. Grandma interjects that when Natalia cries at night, she goes to her and gives her a bottle, then rocks her back to sleep. Natalia's mother says that a week ago they moved Natalia into their bedroom to avoid waking the grandmother.

The Normal Physiology of Sleep

In order to develop a plan of care for this family, it is important to understand the sleep cycle. There are two sleep states: nonrapid eye movement (NREM) and rapid eye movement (REM). NREM sleep cycles predominate during the first third to half of nighttime sleep, and are divided into four stages (Pohl & Renwick, 2002). In stage 1, the sleeper is drowsy, but responsive, but by stages 3 and 4, it is difficult to arouse the sleeper. The sleeper may be very confused if aroused during this time. Stages 3 and 4 are when the sleeper may experience sleep terrors and sleepwalking, behaviors characterized by dramatic body movements with no awareness of the environment (Pohl & Renwick). During NREM sleep, blood supply to the muscles is increased, energy is restored, tissue growth and repair occur, and growth hormone is released for growth and development (National Sleep Foundation, 2009).

REM sleep cycles predominate in the latter half or third of the night (Pohl & Renwick, 2002). In this stage, muscle tone is inhibited in all systems except the ocular and respiratory systems, and there is loss of ability to regulate body temperature. The sleeper has episodic bursts of eye movement, irregular pulse, and tachypnea but no movement of the extremities. During this cycle, sleepers usually dream and can be easily awakened (Nativio, 2002).

The human body cycles between these NREM and REM phases all through the night. Furthermore, there are very brief arousal periods with transitions from one phase to another (Chamness, 2008). Newborns sleep 16 to 17 of 24 hours a day, with approximately 50% REM cycles, and have one to two cycles per sleep period (Nativio, 2002). Term newborns have four to six evenly distributed sleep-wake periods daily with consolidation of daily sleep into the nighttime period occurring by about 6 weeks of age (Pohl & Renwick, 2002). At approximately 3 months of age, a baby averages about 5 hours of sleep during the day and 10 hours at night, with brief interruptions. About 90% of babies this age sleep through the night (KidsHealth, 2007). Sleep time decreases to about 13 hours per day by 2 years of age, 11 hours per day by 5 years, 10 hours per day by 10 years, and 9 hours per day during adolescence.

By about 3 to 5 years of age, children move to a more adult-like sleep cycle. In addition, daytime sleep decreases to three naps a day by about 6 months, two naps per day between 6 and 12 months, and no naps by 3 to 5 years of age (Pohl & Renwick).

Normal Infant Development

Several major developmental tasks are occurring during infancy that can affect sleep patterns. According to Erikson, by about 2 to 4 months, infants accomplish the emotional developmental task of basic trust (Boynton, Dunn, & Stephens, 1994). With the security of trust, the baby is now aware that differences exist in people and certain people are more important to him or her than others (i.e., primary caretaker). Therefore, infants can experience stranger anxiety by about six months. The infant can feel anxiety if he or she awakens and mother is not there, or comfort if she is there. Infants who have more body contact during the day sleep better at night (Schultz, 2001). It is important to understand that separation anxiety is a normal developmental task for all children, and bedtime is a time of separation. According to Piaget, infants at around 6 months of age accomplish the intellectual task of memory or object permanence (Boynton, Dunn, & Stephens). Thus, the baby may awaken as a normal part of sleep, remember mother, and experience separation anxiety (Nativio, 2002). This developmental process can interfere with sleep for a period of weeks. Thus, between 6 and 12 months of age, separation anxiety can become a major sleep disturbance issue. This is due to the cognitive development of object permanence. Natalia is in this developmental age range.

What about the theory of a trained night feeder? ■

Baby wakes between sleep cycles and needs to learn to put him- or herself back into the next sleep cycle. If fed, he or she learns that food is the way to self-soothe and get back to sleep.

Is a complete physical examination necessary? ■

A complete physical examination should be performed, but probably will not yield much information unless the baby's history points to organic or functional disease. However, the provider needs to identify signs of illness or areas of discomfort that may be interfering with the child's ability to get appropriate levels of sleep. Most experts agree that the clinician should focus on the respiratory and nervous systems for clues to sleep disturbances (Nativio, 2002; Pohl & Renwick, 2002).

Physical Examination

In this particular case, the infant is alert, active, and smiling while sitting in her mother's lap. She has good eye contact with you. The rest of the examination is unremarkable.

During the physical examination, you need to observe the child's behavior (she was smiling) and the parent–child interaction (handed her off to grandma). This can provide clues as to the nature of the maternal–child bond as well as the family dynamics.

Cultural and Ethnic Aspects of Sleep

How might the family's beliefs and expectations affect their perceptions of sleep problems and how they should be managed? ▨

What other cultural influences in this family may affect the baby's sleep behavior as well as the decision to seek medical care? ▨

The family's ethnicity is Hispanic American. An understanding of some of the traditional health beliefs and practices within the Hispanic culture can be helpful in assessing and understanding the concerns presented here. Many families in the Hispanic culture will seek the help of other family resources such as a *señora/abuela* (grandmother), *yerbew* (herbalist), *sobador* (massage therapist), or *portera* (midwife who also treats children) (Kemp, 2005). Family involvement in health care is common among Hispanics, and it is common for a female relative such as a grandmother to accompany mothers to healthcare visits. In the Hispanic culture, childrearing is primarily the woman's responsibility, but the decision-making is left to the man. It is also important to note that traditionally, neither disease prevention nor health promotion visits are valued (Kemp). According to Schachter et al. (1989), there is an increased incidence of all-night co-sleeping (sharing a bed) in Hispanic American children versus white children. Hispanic children are 8 times more likely to share a parental bedroom and 3.5 times more likely to co-sleep than their white cohorts. Schachter found that multiple families sharing a house and crowding, which are more common factors in the Hispanic culture as compared to whites, may be a factor in families' healthcare practices.

In addition, differences noted in family values may play an important role in the sleep habits of the Hispanic culture. There is a greater emphasis on family interdependence and intimacy in Hispanic cultures as compared to white cultures, where the emphasis is on independence and individualism (Schachter et al., 1989).

In this case, several cultural factors may be affecting the sleep habits of this family. As with all families, healthcare providers must be respectful of cultural differences and consider these differences when developing and communicating a plan of care with the family. Thus, the plan of care must be driven by evidence-based practice and the values and preferences of the family.

Making the Diagnosis

Based on your detailed history and physical examination, infection and disease states are ruled out. This case study is a fairly classic presentation of the normal developmental level of an 8-month-old and normal sleep physiology and how the factors of family and environment interact and impact sleep hygiene. The familial expectations of what are normal sleep and feeding patterns may also be factors in this sleep arousal disorder. The history and physical examination are consistent with the diagnosis of: 1) sleep arousal with the development of sleep-onset association disorder, 2) family stress, 3) inappropriate expectations regarding sleep, and 4) a trained night feeder.

Management

How do you plan to treat the child's sleep disturbance? ■

Therapeutic Plan

The plan of care must address the four sleep problems that you have identified:

- Sleep-arousal disorder
- Sleep-onset association disorder
- Family stress
- Inappropriate sleep expectations

To address these issues, you review some of the main points you want to make in your counseling. You also are aware that sleep patterns are very family and culture dependent. For example, some families keep infants and children in the same bed or bedroom with parents until they are several years old. Feeding children in the night may be the norm. Letting infants cry rather than consoling them immediately may vary, too. And, there are issues around generational differences in the ways that sleep and other child-rearing issues are managed. In this case, Grandma must also be integrated into the plan for it to be successful. Parents must define what is problematic for sleep in their infants. In most cases, the infant is happy and rested. It is the parents and household that have the problem. Given these values, you decide that you will want to do the following:

- Counsel and discuss physical findings with Mom and Grandma.
- Counsel regarding normal developmental tasks of the 8- to 12-month-old, including separation anxiety and object permanence.
- Counsel regarding appropriate nutrition for an infant 6 to 12 months old.
- Counsel regarding the lack of nutritional need for a nighttime feeding.
- Counsel on changing the learned behavior of sleep-onset association including use of a transitional sleep object.
- Counsel on how to establish a routine for a healthy sleep pattern in children. (See Box 11-1.)

Box 11-1   Developing a Routine Should Begin Around Two Months of Age

- Consider feeding baby ahead of bedtime rather than just before bedtime.
- Get into a regular routine at bedtime, such as a bath and quiet time approximately 1 hour before bedtime.
- Put baby to bed drowsy, but not asleep.
- Distinguish nighttime from daytime—use a soft voice to talk to baby when putting her to bed at night.
- Never put a baby in bed with a bottle of milk, juice, or any liquid.
- Make sure the sleeping environment is quiet, dark, and not too hot or cold.
- Put infants on their backs to sleep.
- Expect crying; do not reward the baby for awakening (i.e., do not pick up).

From a nutritional standpoint, normal term infants do not need a nighttime feeding after 4 to 6 months of age. Being rocked or fed teaches the baby to associate that activity with going to sleep. This learned behavior occurs in as many as 40% of 6- to 24-month-olds (Nativio, 2002). The last waking memory the baby has needs to be of the crib, not the bottle.

The Ferber method (2006) is a progressive approach in which the parent allows the baby to cry for gradually longer periods of time before returning to him or her briefly. This method recommends putting your infant, after 6 months of age, in the crib drowsy, but still awake. This will help the baby fall asleep on his or her own. You decide to present this plan as an option the family might want to consider, knowing that it might not fit with the family's beliefs about management of infants.

The plan begins with a routine that ends with the baby placed in the crib with her transitional object, in this case, Natalia's "meese." The parent should then leave the room. If the baby cries, wait 5 minutes before re-entering the room. The parent can speak to the baby briefly and touch her stomach, but avoid picking her up or rocking her. After 2 to 3 minutes, the parent should leave and not return until 10 minutes have passed; then they can repeat the reassurance. The next interval should be about 15 minutes, with 15-minute intervals for the rest of the night. Natalia should be awakened at the routine time the next morning. The next night, the first wait increases by 5 minutes, to 10 minutes. Each night the first wait increases by another 5 minutes. She eventually will learn that it is not worth crying for 20 to 30 minutes if the gain is just a few minutes of attention. Falling to sleep on her own is an important developmental task to learn.

Implementing the Plan

> You proceed with your plan. First, you reassure this mother that there are no signs of illness (e.g., ear infection). You continue on to say that although many experts agree that GERD is a medical problem that can interfere with sleep (Chamness, 2008; Pohl & Renwick, 2002), Natalia's GERD symptoms seem to have resolved at around 6 months of age. Therefore, GERD, or any other disease state, does not appear to be a factor in this child's sleep arousal issues.
>
> Next, you tell Mom and Grandma about the normal developmental tasks that Natalia is trying to accomplish. You begin by asking whether the crying begins when she leaves the room or if, when others like Grandma try to hold her now, does this seem to upset Natalia? Mom replies that Natalia seems to cry when she leaves the room and she will look around for Mom, even when held by someone else. You explain that these are indicators that Natalia is beginning to experience some separation anxiety, which is normal. Natalia has learned that Mom is someone special and misses her when she is not within sight.

Experts agree that one way to help babies with separation anxiety is to offer a transitional object like a blanket, doll, or other favorite thing as baby begins to sleep (National Sleep Foundation, 2009; Pohl & Renwick, 2002; Schmitt, 1992; Schultz, 2001). **In this case, Natalia uses a silky blanket called her "meese." Mom may want to also give Natalia something that smells like Mom or Dad to ease this separation. This should help her to return to sleep and comfort her.**

What Grandma unknowingly did was to add a transitional object, the bottle. You need to develop a plan to discontinue the bottle as a transitional object. In addition, she and Mom may have trained Natalia to be a nighttime feeder.

You also consider the family's stressful situation and the changed sleep environment as you further develop the plan of care. The fact that the baby's crib has been moved into the parent's room may be a factor in the sleep arousal of this infant. Children appear to be more distracted by environmental disruptions than are adults (Pohl & Renwick, 2002). However, parents who are accepting of co-sleeping report less sleep problems compared to those who are not. It is known also that families living under stress have babies and children less likely to sleep through the night. Finally, maternal depression may be playing a role in this child's nighttime awakening. Research does not show that mom's depression causes sleep problems, only that children with moms who are depressed have more night waking (National Sleep Foundation, 2009).

Establishing a routine will help change the learned behavior of having a bottle as a transitional object. First, all family members need to be committed to this plan. Families need to be prepared, because the first night without a bottle is usually the most difficult. The family should realize that Natalia will continue to cry until she unlearns the old pattern of the parent and bottle putting her to sleep. Grandma should be committed to the plan and agree not to intervene. You need to reinforce that all children, especially babies, cry when their schedule and environment change. Crying is their only way to communicate before they are able to talk (Pediatric Advisor, 2008a; Pediatric Advisor, 2008b). Crying for brief periods is not harmful. Furthermore, increasing touch, physical contact, and affection during the day can help Natalia adjust to this new task.

You recommend that Nicole offer Natalia a bottle approximately 1 hour before bedtime. It is important to establish a nightly routine that Natalia can count on. This can include a bath, then bottle, then being read a book, and then laying her in the crib under the same conditions that she will wake up to in the nighttime.

One challenging factor with this family is the fact that the parents and baby share a bedroom. Hanging a blanket on the side of the crib that faces the parents' bed can be helpful with separation, because then Natalia cannot see her parents upon awakening. You should remind this family that Natalia may open her eyes and make other movements during the partial awakenings that occur as she cycles through the phases of sleep. This is normal and not a signal to intervene. These awakenings are especially common in children 6 to 12 months of age (Pediatric Advisor, 2008b; Pohl & Renwick, 2002).

The most important fact that needs to be impressed on the family is that Natalia's sleep behaviors may take several nights to weeks to change. Also, this new plan should be started at a time when one or the entire family can afford to lose some sleep for about a week. This helps with consistency with the plan.

You make these recommendations and the mother agrees that the plan is worth trying. Grandma agrees and they leave, saying they are hopeful that it will work as planned.

When should you see this family again? ◼

You ask the family to return in about 2 to 3 weeks. You reassure them that when following a consistent plan, most infants show improvement in a few days and will be sleeping through the night in 1 to 2 weeks.

What complications might occur? ◼

The family should be encouraged to return sooner if:

- They feel that the sleep disturbance is due to a physical cause.
- Someone in the family cannot tolerate the crying at night.
- The steps outlined do not improve the baby's sleep habits within 2 weeks.
- Any other questions or concerns arise.

At follow-up in 2 weeks, Dad accompanies Nicole and Natalia. He does not have any questions and relays to you that the first few nights were fairly sleepless. But, the couple continued with the plan and put a blanket on the side of the crib so Natalia could not see them. They admit to continuing to be awakened by Natalia's movements and verbalizations through the night. They feel certain their movements may also disturb Natalia. They have discussed this with the paternal grandmother and are currently converting a room for Natalia. Mom is aware that this will change Natalia's sleeping environment once again and is taking steps to place familiar items and materials in that room to help with this transition. She also acknowledges that she may have to start back at the beginning to help re-establish good sleep hygiene in Natalia.

Key Points from the Case

1. Sleep assessment should be a part of every well-child visit. The healthcare provider should ask the caregiver if he or she is satisfied with their child's current sleep pattern and follow up on any concern that is expressed (Nativio, 2002).

2. Sleep problems are common in children.

3. Counseling families with anticipatory guidance regarding what is a normal sleep pattern as their child grows can give parents the tools they need to intervene as situations arise with their children.

4. Education about the effect on sleep of temperamental style, developmental stages, and changes in the environment will empower parents and enhance the parent–child relationship.

5. Families need to decide if the plan is workable for them and adapt it as necessary.

REFERENCES

Boynton, R. W., Dunn, E. S., & Stephens, G. R. (1994). *Manual of ambulatory pediatrics* (3rd ed.). Philadelphia, PA: JB Lippincott.

Chamness, J. A. (2008). Taking a pediatric sleep history. *Pediatric Annals, 37*(7), 502–508.

Ferber, R. (2006). *Solve your child's sleep problems.* New York: Simon & Schuster.

Kemp, C. (2005). *Mexican & Mexican-Americans: Health beliefs and practices.* Retrieved April 14, 2009, from http://bearspace.baylor.edu/Charles_Kemp/www/hispanic_health.htm

KidsHealth. (2007). *All about sleep.* Retrieved July 7, 2008, from http://kidshealth.org/PageManager.jsp?dn=KidsHealth&lic=1&ps=107&cat_id=190&article_set=10233

National Sleep Foundation. (2009). *Understanding children's sleep habits.* Retrieved April 14, 2009, from http://www.sleepfoundation.org/site/c.huIXKjM0IxF/b.2419295/k.5AAB/Childrens_Sleep_Habits.htm

Nativio, D. G. (2002). Behavioral sleep problems in childhood. *American Journal for Nurse Practitioners, 6*(3), 30–32.

Pediatric Advisor. (2008a). Sleep patterns in babies. Retrieved July 23, 2008, from http://www.cpnonline.org/CRS/CRS/pa_sleepbab_pep.htm

Pediatric Advisor. (2008b). Awakenings from being held until asleep (trained night crier). Retrieved April 14, 2009, from http://www.cpnonline.org/CRS/CRS/pa_nightcr_hhg.htm

Pohl, C., & Renwick, A. (2002). Putting sleep disturbances to rest. *Contemporary Pediatrics, 19*(11), 74–95.

Schachter, F., Fuchs, M., Bijur, P., & Stone, R. (1989). Co-sleeping and sleep problems in Hispanic-American urban young children. *Pediatrics, 84*(3), 522–530.

Schmitt, B. D. (1992). *Instructions for pediatric patients.* Philadelphia, PA: W. B. Saunders.

Schultz, J. R. (2001). Sleep and bedtime behaviors. In R. C. Baker (Ed.), *Pediatric primary care: Well-child care* (pp. 283–290). Philadelphia, PA: Lippincott Williams & Wilkins.

Chapter 12

The Child Who Is Very Busy and Doesn't Listen

Larry W. Lynn

The incidence of attention deficit hyperactivity disorder (ADHD) has increased dramatically in the past two decades. Current studies estimate up to 8.7% of individuals under 18 years of age are affected by ADHD (Froelich, Lamphear, & Epstein, 2007). Parents of children with ADHD and other individuals are concerned these children are unable to function well at home and in the community, unable to maximize their own potential, and certainly strain their parents' satisfaction and joy in parenting. Practitioners must be vigilant to thoroughly evaluate and appropriately treat patients presenting with possible ADHD. This includes performing a detailed history and physical examination, utilizing behavioral screening tools, ordering appropriate laboratory tests, closely working with psychologists, and titrating medications to an optimal dose.

Educational Objectives
1. Use DSM-IV-TR criteria to develop conversational questions with parents and child as part of the assessment process when screening patients for possible ADHD.
2. Develop differential diagnoses to rule out other behavioral problems.
3. Identify strategies to collaborate with parents, teachers, and psychologists as a treatment team to assist in patient management.
4. Identify strategies to best utilize follow-up appointments in person or by telephone to assist in treatment decisions.
5. Understand the appropriate use of various psychoactive medications for the treatment of ADHD.
6. Know the warnings about treating children and adolescents with stimulant and nonstimulant medications to control ADHD symptoms.
7. Consider the implications of ADHD as a lifelong condition that can possibly lead to problems throughout the lifetime for affected individuals.

Case Presentation and Discussion

Jason Black is an 8-year-old male child who presents to your office accompanied by his mother for a behavioral consultation. He began third grade 3 months ago and is having academic and behavioral problems at school. Despite the efforts of his parents and teachers to help him organize, Jason remains unorganized with his work and belongings. He often fails to bring homework home and frequently forgets to turn in completed assignments at school. He is restless and impulsive. He often blurts out answers in class, interrupting the teacher or his classmates. He tends to violate the personal space of his peers and interferes with their play and interaction during recess and physical education. As a result, he is being socially isolated by peers.

At home, he fails to follow through with parental instructions. He often loses important items such as homework and even his favorite toys. His room is described by his mother as "looking like a tornado came through." The parents have tried time out, restricting activities, and spankings but have seen no improvement in his behavior. He is beginning to see himself as different and describes himself as "dumb" and states, "I have no friends." His teacher suggested the parents seek medical advice and "get some medicine to calm him down." The mother knows there is a problem with Jason's behavior, but is concerned for him to be labeled with ADHD. She is also concerned with the negative comments she reads on various Web sites about treating children with medications to control the symptoms of ADHD. She describes feeling lost because she doesn't know how to help her child.

What questions would you ask Jason and his mother to expand on the information above? ■

It is important to base your questions on the diagnostic criteria for ADHD listed in the *Diagnostic and Statistical Manual of Mental Disorders*, 4th edition, text revision (DSM-IV-TR; APA, 2000). Refer to Table 12-1 and become familiar with these criteria. The child must exhibit six of nine symptoms associated with inattention or six of nine symptoms associated with hyperactivity-impulsivity to consider the diagnosis of ADHD and avoid overidentification and underidentification of the disease. The DSM-IV-TR criteria define three different subtypes of ADHD: 1) ADHD that is predominately inattentive (meets six of nine inattentive behaviors); 2) ADHD that is predominately hyperactive-impulsive (meets six of nine hyperactive-impulsive behaviors); 3) combined type ADHD (has six of nine behaviors in both the inattention and hyperactive-impulsivity behavioral realms).

Are there guidelines to help clinicians deal with ADHD problems? ■

A combination of open- and closed-ended questions based on DSM-IV-TR criteria (APA, 2000) will provide insight into the patient's behavioral history and current problems. The clinician needs to develop questions that are a part of a conversation with parents and children to uncover these issues. The American

Table 12-1   DSM-IV Criteria for ADHD

I. Either A or B:

   A. Six or more of the following symptoms of inattention have been present for at least 6 months to a point that is disruptive and inappropriate for developmental level:

   Inattention
   1. Often does not give close attention to details or makes careless mistakes in schoolwork, work, or other activities.
   2. Often has trouble keeping attention on tasks or play activities.
   3. Often does not seem to listen when spoken to directly.
   4. Often does not follow instructions and fails to finish schoolwork, chores, or duties in the workplace (not due to oppositional behavior or failure to understand instructions).
   5. Often has trouble organizing activities.
   6. Often avoids, dislikes, or doesn't want to do things that take a lot of mental effort for a long period of time (such as schoolwork or homework).
   7. Often loses things needed for tasks and activities (e.g., toys, school assignments, pencils, books, or tools).
   8. Is often easily distracted.
   9. Is often forgetful in daily activities.

   B. Six or more of the following symptoms of hyperactivity–impulsivity have been present for at least 6 months to an extent that is disruptive and inappropriate for developmental level:

   Hyperactivity
   1. Often fidgets with hands or feet or squirms in seat.
   2. Often gets up from seat when remaining in seat is expected.
   3. Often runs about or climbs when and where it is not appropriate (adolescents or adults may feel very restless).
   4. Often has trouble playing or enjoying leisure activities quietly.
   5. Is often "on the go" or often acts as if "driven by a motor."
   6. Often talks excessively.

   Impulsivity
   1. Often blurts out answers before questions have been finished.
   2. Often has trouble waiting one's turn.
   3. Often interrupts or intrudes on others (e.g., butts into conversations or games).

II. Some symptoms that cause impairment were present before age 7 years.

III. Some impairment from the symptoms is present in two or more settings (e.g., at school/work and at home).

IV. There must be clear evidence of significant impairment in social, school, or work functioning.

V. The symptoms do not happen only during the course of a pervasive developmental disorder, schizophrenia, or other psychotic disorder. The symptoms are not better accounted for by another mental disorder (e.g., mood disorder, anxiety disorder, dissociative disorder, or a personality disorder).

(continues)

Table 12-1   DSM-IV Criteria for ADHD (Continued)

Based on these criteria, three types of ADHD are identified:

1. ADHD, *Combined Type*: if both criteria 1A and 1B are met for the past 6 months
2. ADHD, *Predominantly Inattentive Type*: if criterion 1A is met but criterion 1B is not met for the past 6 months
3. ADHD, *Predominantly Hyperactive-Impulsive Type*: if criterion 1B is met but criterion 1A is not met for the past 6 months.

Source: American Psychiatric Association. (2000). *Diagnostic and Statistical Manual of Mental Disorders* (4th ed., text rev.). Washington, DC: American Psychiatric Association.

Academy of Pediatrics (AAP) developed clinical practice guidelines for ADHD in 2000 that highlight the importance of obtaining input from parents, teachers, other caregivers, and professional consultants when evaluating a child for possible ADHD (American Academy of Pediatrics, 2000). Working with these individuals as members of a team will provide information to assist in making the diagnosis of ADHD to help guide you in effective patient management.

Further questioning provides the following information about the history of these behaviors. Jason has always been a very active boy. The mother describes him as "on the go and all boy since he could walk." He attended a preschool class 2 days each week for 3 hours per day at age 4 years and got along well except for trouble sharing and an occasional disagreement with peers. At that time he was described as "energetic" and "loud" on caregiver reports. There has been some concern about behavior since he began kindergarten. He has always been more loud and restless than his peers. Teachers have complained that Jason requires frequent redirection in the classroom. He has performed well academically until this year. Though he was always disorganized and messy, he made A's and B's on most papers in first and second grade. He had no problem learning to read, but does not enjoy sitting and reading because he would rather do something active. This has become a problem area because more reading has been required at school this year. Currently, there is less directed study and more independent study expected within the classroom. Jason cannot keep on task and often interrupts other students while they are working. When asked to complete assignments, he often gets up from his seat. He runs in the hall when the class moves between classrooms. He rarely completes an assignment unless there is one-on-one encouragement from the teacher. His work contains many careless mistakes despite his ability. He has academic potential, as suggested by his scoring above the 90th percentile on the state standards test last spring; however, he has fallen behind this school year in reading and mathematics. He is currently making all D's on his report card. He usually makes B's on tests, but only turns in half his homework assignments, which has a negative impact on his overall grades.

What additional information might be helpful in evaluating this patient? ■

It is important to rule out other medical and psychological causes of inattention and poor behavior when evaluating a child for ADHD. A thorough medical history and review of systems should be performed to exclude other conditions in the differential diagnosis. Table 12-2 provides a differential diagnosis list to consider when evaluating a child for possible ADHD. The history should include questions about:

- Pregnancy, delivery, and developmental milestones
- Sleep and dietary habits
- Family dynamics to rule out family stress or dysfunction as the cause of behavioral problems.
- Possible environmental relationships such as lead poisoning or Lyme disease, if the history warrants consideration.

As you listen to parents and children discuss pertinent information about behavior, consider comorbid disorders being present that may obscure or make the diagnosis less clear. They include conduct disorder, oppositional defiant disorder, and bipolar disorder, which are more common in children with ADHD (Biederman, 2004). These comorbidities can result in incorrect diagnoses and/or inappropriate treatment. For example, treating a bipolar child with a stimulant medication can cause behavior to deteriorate. Comorbid conditions must be considered alone and as potentially existing in conjunction with ADHD for the child to receive appropriate treatment.

Table 12-2   Differential Diagnosis of ADHD
Sleep disorder
Thyroid disease
Autistic spectrum disorder
Psychiatric disorder
• Anxiety disorder
• Oppositional defiant disorder
• Mood disorder
• Adjustment disorder
Family dysfunction
Physical or emotional abuse
Developmental disorder/learning disability
Seizure disorder
Substance abuse
Central auditory processing disorder
Visual or hearing impairment

Jason perceives himself in a negative way, as his earlier comments suggest. Some children with ADHD become depressed to some degree because of the recurring negative interactions or consequences brought about by their behavior. This depression and low self-esteem often improve when the symptoms of ADHD are treated. Persistent depression warrants referral to a psychologist.

What findings are important on the physical examination?

The first part of any thorough physical examination is to simply observe the patient. Get a feeling for the gestalt of this patient. Appreciate any abnormal physical, movement, or behavioral findings as you enter the room and begin to speak with the patient and parents. Is there any syndromic appearance to the patient? Is there evidence of an organic disease such as thyroid disease? Evaluate the pattern of speech and word selection for age appropriateness. Direct questions to the patient and observe the content of responses. Observe how the patient interacts during the interview and examination. Is restlessness, hyperkinetic behavior, or excessive talking present during the interview?

The clinician should perform a thorough physical examination for two reasons. First, one wants to exclude medical conditions from the differential diagnosis. Second, if treatment is necessary, one must be sure there is no underlying medical condition, such as a congenital heart defect or arrhythmia, that might preclude or alter pharmacologic intervention.

Hearing screening should be an initial part of the assessment process.

Jason's physical examination and hearing screening are both normal in all aspects. No neurological, cardiac, sensory, or thyroid abnormalities are identified.

What testing should be done?

Testing falls into two broad and general categories during an ADHD workup: medical and psychological testing. Evaluations should be thorough, but judicious use of potentially expensive tests should be practiced. Order tests based on an adequate index of suspicion.

First, findings during the interview or physical examination might indicate laboratory tests or imaging studies are necessary. For example, if thyroid disease is suspected, then order thyroid function studies. Expensive imaging studies such as MRI or CT scans of the brain should be ordered only if there is a high index of suspicion for neuropathology because these studies do not diagnose or rule out ADHD.

Second, the clinician should administer a DSM-IV-TR–based ADHD screening tool such as the revised Conners' Scales or the Vanderbilt assessment, each of which has teacher and parent versions. Scoring and interpretation of these screening tests is very simple and thoroughly explained in the assessment manual for each tool. Such ADHD rating scales for parents and teachers have been shown to have an odds ratio of 3.0 (equivalent to a sensitivity and specificity greater than 94%) in studies differentiating children with ADHD from normal, age-matched community controls (Green, Wong, & Atkins, 1999).

Additionally, the clinician may want to refer the patient to a psychologist for an extensive evaluation and psychometric testing to rule out low IQ, psychiatric diagnoses, learning difficulties, or developmental problems as contributing factors or as the actual diagnosis. Ideally, when behavioral consultation appointments are scheduled, Conners' Scales or Vanderbilt assessments should be sent to the parents and teachers for completion prior to the appointment. Include a preprinted instruction letter for teachers that requests additional written information she or he believes is important in the evaluation of the child. This allows more information to be discussed at the appointment and also, if indicated, pharmacologic treatment to immediately begin.

> In this case, Conners' Scales were completed by Jason's parents and two teachers prior to the appointment. The results are significant for elevation in measures of hyperactivity-impulsivity and inattention by all four evaluators. The teachers scored Jason significantly higher on the hyperactivity-impulsivity scale than the parents did.

It is common to see children suspected of having ADHD score higher on the scales of hyperactivity-impulsivity and inattention in a structured setting. Often, the behaviors are less noticed or less problematic at home where activities are not as structured and the child is not required to follow group rules. There can be great variation between parental observations as well. Depending on how much time and under what circumstances a parent interacts with a child, this parent may not be exposed to the problem behaviors voiced by teachers and the other parent. It is not uncommon for divorced parents to claim completely different behaviors are observed when the child is in each household. Reviewing the results of these screening tests allows parents to see how their child compares to similar aged peers in the areas of attention and impulsivity from the viewpoint of several adults while the child is in different settings.

Making the Diagnosis

> Based on the interview and information obtained from the Conners' Scales, it appears that Jason meets the criteria for ADHD. His mother has indicated that she has reservations about her son being labeled with a psychiatric diagnosis and is concerned about medical management. Additionally, she explains that his father believes these behaviors are just a part of being a boy, although the father has agreed to a short trial of the medication because Jason is having academic difficulties. However, he remains skeptical about treating for a prolonged period of time. The mother asks how long Jason will be treated and what side effects they should expect to see with medication.

Management

What type of education should you provide to a family when treating a child diagnosed with ADHD? ■

It is extremely important to educate the parents and child about why ADHD is treated, what medications are used, and what follow-up care will be needed in the short term and long term. There is much confusion in the general population about the medications used to treat ADHD. This confusion often results from misinformation obtained through the news media, the Internet, or friends and family members. Clinicians must educate parents and patients about the expected results and potential side effects when treating ADHD with a prescription medication. Free information is available online for parents and clinicians from the American Academy of Pediatrics (http://www.aap.org), the American Academy of Child and Adolescent Psychiatry (http://www.aacap.org), and the organization Children and Adults with Attention Deficit/Hyperactivity Disorder (http://www.chadd.org). During the visit provide an overview of medications used to treat ADHD. Outline the categories of medications, how they work, and what side effects to expect.

The patient will need to be followed up by telephone and in person as the medication is titrated to an effective dose. Inform the parents about titrating the dose based upon the response in their child as an individual. Then, follow-up at various intervals to assess the efficacy of the medication over time. Follow-up visits provide an opportunity for the healthcare provider to assess the patient while giving parents and patients a voice in how the medication is titrated. This type of communication also lessens the likelihood of confusion leading to a medication being unnecessarily discontinued.

A caveat to remember is that if there is no observable change or minimal improvement seen when treating ADHD with medication at a therapeutic dose, then another medication should be considered. If two or more medications have been tried without success, then additional workup and consideration of other diagnoses is indicated. It is important to utilize evidence-based medicine practices when treating ADHD to assure the correct diagnosis is made and an effective treatment strategy is providing desired results (Epstein, Rabinar, & Johnson, 2007; Leslie, Weekerly, Plemmons, Landsvere, & Eastman, 2004).

What medication should be used in the first line of treatment of ADHD? ■

Two classes of FDA-approved medications are used as first-line treatment of ADHD in children and adolescents—stimulants and nonstimulants. The stimulants include the various methylphenidate and amphetamine products; the only approved nonstimulant is atomoxetine. Table 12-3 lists these medications. Note that several medications are used off label for the treatment of ADHD. It is recommended that these medications be prescribed and monitored by a clinician who specializes in treating this disease. Therefore, these medications will not be discussed in this case study.

Table 12–3   Medications Approved to Treat ADHD in Children

Drug	Release and Action	Dosing	Side Effects
Methylphenidate Immediate Release			
Ritalin (methylphenidate)	An immediate release preparation of methylphenidate. Rapid onset of action. Provides 3–4 hours of clinical effect. Must be given 2–3 times per day to adequately control symptoms.	Begin with 2.5–5.0 mg given twice each day, usually upon waking and then 4 hours later. Adjust in increments of 2.5–5.0 mg per day at weekly intervals to a maximum dose of 40 mg per day.	The most commonly seen side effects are decreased appetite, weight loss, and insomnia.
Focalin (dexmethylphenidate)	An immediate release preparation of dexmethylphenidate. Provides 4–6 hours of clinical effect. Typically given twice each day to control symptoms of ADHD.	Begin with 2.5–5.0 mg given as a single a.m. dose or as a twice daily dose. Adjust at increments of 2.5–5.0 mg per dayat weekly intervals to a maximum of 20 mg per day.	The most commonly seen side effects are insomnia, decreased appetite, weight loss, and nausea.
Methylphenidate Extended Release			
Concerta (methylphenidate)	OROS delivery system provides rapid release of methylphenidate with clinical effects noted within 1 hour of administration. The duration of coverage is 8–12 hours.	Begin with 18 mg given as a single daily dose each a.m. Adjust at increments of 9–18 mg per day at weekly intervals to a maximum dose of 72 mg.	The most commonly seen side effects include insomnia, decreased appetite, weight loss, and headache.
Focalin XR (dexmethylphenidate)	SODAS bimodal delivery system provides 50% of dexmethylphenidate released immediately and the remaining 50% released 4 hours later. A single dose can provide 8–12 hours of clinical effect.	Begin with 5 mg as a single daily dose given each a.m. Adjust at increments of 5 mg per day at weekly intervals to a maximum dose of 20 mg per day.	The most commonly seen side effects include insomnia, decreased appetite, weight loss, and nausea.

(continues)

Table 12-3 Medications Approved to Treat ADHD in Children (Continued)			
Drug	Release and Action	Dosing	Side Effects
Methylphenidate Extended Release (continued)			
Metadate CD (methylphenidate)	The extended release capsules are composed of medicated beads, of which 30% are immediate release beads and 70% are extended release beads. The onset of action is rapid. The duration of action is 6–8 hours.	Begin with 10–20 mg as a single daily dose given each morning. Adjust at increments of 10 mg per day at weekly intervals to a maximum dose of 60 mg per day.	The most commonly seen side effects include decreased appetite, weight loss, and insomnia.
Daytrana (methylphenidate transdermal)	An adhesive-based matrix transdermal methylphenidate system applied to intact skin that allows absorption of the drug through the skin. Provides variable amounts of coverage depending on how long the patch is in place. Apply 1.5–2 hours before effect is desired.	Apply a 10 mg patch to the hip each morning 2 hours prior to the desired effect. Continuous delivery of methylphenidate will occur while the patch is in contact with skin. It is recommended to remove the patch 9 hours after application. The effect will persist for 1–2 hours following removal of the patch. Alternate the hip used with each application.	The most commonly seen side effects include insomnia, decreased appetite, nausea, and skin irritation. Skin redness or itching can occur at the application site. If swelling, bumps, or broken skin occur, then the patch should be discontinued.
Amphetamine Immediate Release			
Adderall (mixed amphetamine salts)	Immediate release of mixed amphetamine salts following administration. Has 4–6 hours of clinical effect following a single dose. Can be dosed 1–2 times per day to provide effect over the desired coverage time.	Begin with 2.5–5.0 mg given each a.m. Adjust in increments of 2.5–5.0 mg per day at weekly intervals given as a single a.m. dose or as an a.m. dose with a repeat dose 4 hours later to provide desired coverage.	The most commonly seen side effects include decreased appetite, weight loss, and insomnia.

Table 12-3 Medications Approved to Treat ADHD in Children (Continued)			
Drug	**Release and Action**	**Dosing**	**Side Effects**
Amphetamine Extended Release			
Adderall XR (mixed amphetamine salts)	Two types of drug containing beads deliver mixed amphetamine salts in a double pulsed manner, 50% released immediately and 50% released 4–6 hours later. This provides 8–12 hours of clinical effect in patients.	Begin with 10 mg as a single a.m. dose. Adjust in increments of 5–10 mg per day at weekly intervals to a maximum recommended dose of 30 mg per day.	The most commonly seen side effects include decreased appetite, insomnia, headache, and weight loss.
Vyvanse (lisdexamfetamine)	Lisdexamfetamine dimesylate is a prodrug form of dextroamphetamine. Following administration the prodrug is converted to active dextroamphetamine. It provides 12 hours of clinical effect.	In children 6–12 years of age begin 30 mg as a single morning dose. Adjust in increments of 20 mg per day at weekly intervals to a maximum recommended dose of 70 mg per day.	The most commonly seen side effects include nausea, decreased appetite, insomnia, and abdominal pain.

Source: Vetter, V. L., Elia, J., Erickson, C., Berger, S., Blum, N., Uzark, K., et al. (2008). Cardiovascular monitoring of children and adolescents with heart disease receiving stimulant drugs: A scientific statement from the American Heart Association Council on Cardiovascular Disease in Young Congenital Heart Defects Committee and the Council on Cardiovascular Nursing. *Circulation, 117*(18), 2407–2423.

Psychostimulants are the most frequently used medications for treating ADHD. Stimulants provide an effect in treating ADHD by blocking presynaptic reuptake of the neurotransmitters dopamine and norepinephrine and increasing the release of these monoamines into the synaptic cleft. With more neurotransmitter available at the synapse, signals are transmitted more efficiently. Atomoxetine blocks reuptake of norepinephrine, but does not significantly influence dopamine reuptake. Norepinephrine enhances relevant signals while dopamine suppresses irrelevant signals in the attentional areas of the brain.

Studies have shown that 80% of children treated with a stimulant medication have a good clinical response, with approximately 50% of those responders showing equivalent efficacy with methylphenidate or amphetamine, both of which have been used to treat attention problems for decades (Elia, Borcherding,

Rappoport, & Keysor, 1991; MTA Cooperative Group, 1999). It is important to realize that methylphenidate and amphetamine have different potencies. The typical conversion is 5 mg of amphetamine has potency equivalent to 10 mg of methylphenidate (Elia et al., 1991). Keep this in mind when changing from one of these products to the other.

Timing of Doses

The immediate release forms of these drugs require multiple daily doses. Usually medication is given between 7:00 and 8:00 a.m. and again between 11:00 a.m. and 12:00 noon. Ideally, each dose results in 3–4 hours of positive clinical effect. The problem with immediate release formulations is that patients often have a window of subtherapeutic time prior to the next dose, during which symptoms return. This often occurs during the late morning at school or after school when homework needs to be completed. A third dose is sometimes given after school to allow patients to concentrate on homework. Multiple daily dosing becomes cumbersome for parents and teachers.

In the last decade, extended release formulations of methylphenidate and mixed amphetamine salts providing 8–12 hours of clinical effect following a single dose were introduced to the market. These medications revolutionized the treatment of ADHD with one dose per day providing extended control of symptoms. Studies show 8–12 hours of efficacy with a single morning dose. In 2006, a transdermal patch that delivers methylphenidate in an extended fashion was introduced to the market. Delivery through transdermal methylphenidate patches has allowed flexibility in treating ADHD over the waking day.

Atomoxetine is not a scheduled drug and has shown efficacy in reducing the symptoms of ADHD; it has safety and tolerability similar to that of methylphenidate (Michelson et al., 2002). It also may be given as a single daily dose. Decreased appetite and insomnia are side effects commonly seen in patients treated with atomoxetine (Wernicke & Kratochvil, 2002). Children and adolescents treated with atomoxetine were noted to have minor increases in diastolic blood pressure and heart rate, although there were no differences found on ECG tracings of patients treated with atomoxetine compared to those given placebo (Wernicke & Kratochvil). However, monitoring blood pressure and auscultating the heart should be a part of the routine examination.

A sample treatment plan is outlined in Table 12-4. Remember that feedback from the before-mentioned team is necessary before titrating these medications to their optimum dose. Poor communication between the clinician and parents should not be the reason a child receives less than optimal care for ADHD.

You suggest starting a long-acting medication each morning (5 mg of Focalin XR) and outline follow-up visits or interviews as listed in Table 12-4. The mother reiterates her concern about the safety of stimulant medications. In particular, she has read this class of medication can cause heart attacks and be fatal.

Table 12-4 Sample Treatment Approach for ADHD	
Type of Patient Interaction	Treatment Decisions to Consider
The diagnosis is established and treatment initiated at the first visit.	Education including proper dosing, onset of action, and potential side effects should be discussed prior to the first prescription being written.
A follow-up call from the parents following 1 week of treatment to check for efficacy, tolerability, and potential side effects.	Titrate to a higher dose if indicated. Reassure if typical side effects such as appetite decrease and trouble falling asleep are present.
A follow-up call from the parents following 1-2 additional weeks of treatment.	There should be some noticeable effect obvious to parents and/or teachers at this point. You must decide if an additional dosage increase is warranted now or wait until the next appointment.
1 month *in office* follow-up visit. Weight and blood pressure should be recorded.	Inquire about efficacy at home, in school, and in social situations. Discuss appetite and sleep. Titrate to a higher dose if indicated.
Routine medication checks or maintenance visits every 3-4 months.	It is important to monitor continued efficacy and adverse effects. In particular, appetite and weight gain must be followed over time. Medication should be discontinued if the patient loses $\geq 10\%$ of his or her body weight.

What specific information about potential adverse effects in this class of medication should be given to the mother? ■

Cardiac Problems

There has been concern of an association between sudden death and using stimulant medications (Gutgesell et al., 1999). The American Heart Association (AHA, 2008) released a statement recommending a screening ECG in all children prior to beginning treatment with a stimulant medication (Vetter, Elia, & Erickson, 2008) to rule out any conduction disturbance that could be exacerbated by taking a stimulant medication. The AHA statement has been met with skepticism in the medical community because it contradicts the evidence-based medicine recommendations of the American Academy of Child and Adolescent Psychiatry and the American Academy of Pediatrics (American Academy of Pediatrics, 2000; Pliszka & American Academy of Child and Adolescent Psychiatry, 2007). A policy statement from the AAP published in August 2008 states there is no evidence to demonstrate the likelihood of sudden death is higher in children receiving medications for ADHD than in the general population. Also, the text of this policy statement notes it has not been shown that screening ECGs before starting stimulants have an appropriate balance of benefit, risk, and cost effectiveness for general use in identifying risk factors for sudden death (Perrin, Friedman, & Knilans, 2008).

Despite these warnings, stimulant medications are widely used and historically have a safe profile with regard to adverse events. Many studies have shown participants have no significant cardiac events when treated with a stimulant medication. An important point for parents and patients to understand is that some of the concern is over effects with no clinical significance. For example, a study of one extended release methylphenidate product showed a statistically significant increase in heart rate, systolic blood pressure, and diastolic blood pressure (Quinn, 2005). However, these values were not clinically significant, meaning the changes are not detrimental to otherwise healthy patients using such medications.

It is the obligation of practitioners to ensure that patients are at minimal or no risk when taking medications to treat the symptoms of ADHD. Therefore, prior to prescribing such medications, a thorough physical examination should be performed with emphasis on the cardiac portion of the examination including measuring the blood pressure. Additionally, blood pressure should be measured and the heart should be auscultated at each medication follow-up visit. Caution should be exercised when using stimulant medications in patients with any cardiac abnormality, whether the etiology is structural or is a problem with electrical conduction. In such patients, a cardiology consultation is recommended before initiating therapy.

An important part of treating patients with ADHD is spending time educating parents and patients about the much more likely side effects seen with stimulant medications. The most common side effects seen secondary to using stimulant medications are appetite suppression and insomnia (Efron, Friedrich, & Barker, 1997).

Appetite

Some authors suggest the appetite suppression subsides after 1–3 months of treatment; however, some children will have appetite suppression for the duration of treatment with a stimulant.

Sleep Disturbances

Insomnia is often present in children with ADHD. It can be a basic part of the disease or can be secondary to medications prescribed to control the symptoms of ADHD. A small number of children sleep better after medication is started. Other children will require a medication to help with sleep. The medical literature has scant information about using medications to enhance sleep in children with ADHD. Most clinicians do not want to treat children with sedative hypnotics. Clinicians have a few options when the treatment of insomnia is necessary. Melatonin is used to treat circadian rhythm disturbances and will induce sleep in children with ADHD. It can be purchased over the counter without a prescription. Also, the central alpha agonist clonidine helps induce sleep and has a rapid onset of action; however, clonidine has a variable half-life and should be carefully titrated to avoid "morning hangover" or hypotension in children. Additionally, the antidepressant trazodone effectively induces sleep and is used in patients with ADHD who have insomnia. Consulting with a pediatrician or child psychiatrist experienced in managing insomnia may be the safest and most effective means of achieving good sleep hygiene in patients with ADHD.

Jason's mother agrees that a medication trial is indicated for Jason at this point. Focalin XR (methylphenidate) is started at 5 mg 7:45 a.m. each morning.

First Management Evaluation Visit

The mother phones in 8 days later with a report that Jason seems to be less hyperkinetic at school and pays more attention in the early part of the morning. By 10:00 a.m., however, he is behaving in the typical restless manner.

What is the best treatment intervention at this time? ■

There appears to be some effect early in the morning, which fades away in a few hours. This is typical of a subtherapeutic medication dose. At this point increase the dose of Focalin XR to 10 mg given in the morning. Additionally, have the parents begin behavior modification by slowly integrating various chores and tasks into Jason's daily routine. Keeping his school supplies neat and ready for school the next day is a good starting point. Encourage the parents to visit the Web sites previously mentioned to further their understanding of ADHD.

Second Management Evaluation Visit

Jason presents for the 1-month follow-up appointment with both parents. The father is concerned because Jason has lost 4 pounds of body weight and does not have much appetite. Also, he expresses concern that Jason will "become a zombie because this medicine sedates him so much." Despite these concerns, both parents agree that Jason is behaving better at home and school. The teacher reported that Jason turned in all his homework last week and correctly spelled 19 of 20 words on his spelling test. However, by 2:00 p.m. he becomes restless and continues to be unable to concentrate on homework.

What is the appropriate next step in treating Jason? ■

The following should now be done to treat Jason:

- Increase the dose to 15 mg given as a single morning dose. Tell the parents 15–20 mg appears to be the necessary dose to provide efficacy over time. Observe him on the 15 mg dose for approximately 1–2 weeks, then decide if additional medication is necessary.
- Discuss a strategy for encouraging him to eat more. Some children will eat well at breakfast before taking medication, but then have no appetite the remainder of the day. Drinking or eating a small amount of food with complex carbohydrates and protein is sometimes the best plan at lunchtime. Often it is helpful to have the evening meal as late as possible.
- If he has difficulty following through with tasks at home or he remains oppositional, then referral to a psychologist is necessary.
- Plan to see him for follow-up in 1 month. At that point, if he is stable on medication, visits may be every 3 months.

It is important to provide education at each visit. Behavioral modification through instructions from the clinician prescribing medication or, in more difficult cases, from a psychologist, is necessary for the best clinical results according to the major MTA study (MTA Cooperative Group, 1999). However, stimulant or nonstimulant medications alone are far superior to behavioral modification alone.

What is the long-term prognosis for ADHD?

Parents must understand that ADHD is often a lifelong condition. Parents are often concerned about medicating a child for a prolonged or indefinite period of time. At some point, a controlled wean of the medication can be attempted. This is often requested by middle school- and high school-age patients. However, parents and providers must understand that the symptoms or expression of ADHD change with age. The typical adolescent is not as hyperkinetic as an 8-year-old child. The symptoms may be more subtle in appearance to those involved with these patients, but they nonetheless interfere with life. A prospective study in Wisconsin followed cohorts of teenagers with ADHD who were either treated or not treated with medication to control symptoms of ADHD for more than 13 years as they became young adults. The study found that those with untreated ADHD were more likely to not graduate from high school, be fired from a job, have an STD, have an unwanted pregnancy, be divorced, and be a substance abuser (Barkley, Fische, Smallish, & Fletcher, 2006). This is compelling evidence that ADHD should never be considered cured. Symptoms that have been controlled without medication can return throughout the affected individual's lifetime, especially during times of stress. Keep these points in mind and make patients and parents aware of the potential lifelong nature of this disease.

Key Points from the Case

1. It may take time before the symptoms of ADHD interfere with the child's functioning in a manner that warrants intervention.

2. Symptoms are often more obvious in structured environments.

3. Impairment can be different in different settings, such as home, school, and social situations.

4. Diagnosing ADHD is based on criteria outlined in the DSM-IV-TR.

5. Patient and parent education is mandatory for optimal outcomes. Education should begin with the first visit and be continued at subsequent follow-up visits.

6. ADHD is a lifelong condition and should be considered as influencing any behaviors that interfere with life functioning from the time of diagnosis as a child and continuing throughout adulthood.

7. Refer children with an underlying cardiac problem to a cardiologist prior to treatment with stimulant medications.

8. Use a psychologist to assess for comorbidities and to help with behavior management.

REFERENCES

American Academy of Pediatrics, Subcommittee on Attention Deficit/Hyperactivity Disorder. (2000). Clinical practice guideline: Diagnosis and evaluation of the child with attention-deficit/hyperactivity disorder. *Pediatrics, 105*, 1158–1170.

American Heart Association. (2008). *Cardiovascular monitoring of children and adolescents with heart disease receiving medications for attention deficit/hyperactivity disorder.* Retrieved April 15, 2009, from http://circ.ahajournals.org/cgi/content/full/117/18/2407

American Psychiatric Association. (2000). *Diagnostic and statistical manual of mental disorders* (4th ed., text rev.). Washington, DC: APA.

Barkley, R. A., Fische, R. M., Smallish, L., & Fletcher, K. (2006). Young adult outcome of hyperactivity in children: Adaptive functioning in major life activities. *Journal of the American Academy of Child and Adolescent Psychiatry, 45*, 192–202.

Biederman, J. (2004). Impact of comorbidity in adults with attention-deficit/hyperactivity disorder. *Journal of Clinical Psychiatry, 65*(suppl 3), 3–7.

Efron, D., Friedrich, J., & Barker, M. (1997). Side effects of methylphenidate and dexamphetamine in children with attention deficit hyperactivity disorder: A double-blind, crossover trial. *Pediatrics, 100*(4), 662–666.

Elia, J., Borcherding, B., Rappoport, J., & Keysor, C. (1991). Methylphenidate and dextroamphetamine treatment of hyperactivity: Are there true nonresponders? *Psychiatric Research, 36*, 141–155.

Epstein, J. N., Rabinar, D., & Johnson, D. E. (2007). Presenting implication of evidence based practices for ADHD children among primary care pediatricians. *Archives of Pediatric and Adolescent Medicine, 161*(9), 835–840.

Froelich, T. E., Lamphear, B. P., & Epstein, J. N. (2007). Prevalence, recognition and treatment of attention-deficit/hyperactivity disorder in a national sample of U.S. children. *Archives of Pediatric and Adolescent Medicine, 161*, 857–864.

Green, M., Wong, M., & Atkins, D. (1999). *Diagnosis of attention deficit/hyperactivity disorder: Technical review.* Rockville, MD: U.S. Department of Health and Human Services, Agency for Health Care Policy and Research.

Gutgesell, H., Atkins, D., Barst, R., Buck, M., Franklin, W., Hanes, R., Ringel, R., et al. (1999). Cardiovascular monitoring of children and adolescents receiving psychotropic drugs. *Circulation,* 99, 979–982.

Leslie, L., Weckerly, J., Plemmons, D., Landsvere, J., & Eastman, S. (2004). Implementing the American Academy of Pediatrics attention deficit/hyperactivity disorder guidelines in primary care settings. *Pediatrics, 114*, 129–140.

Michelson, D., Allen, J., Busner, J., Casat, C., Dunn, D., Kratochvil, C., et al. (2002). Once-daily atomoxetine treatment for children and adolescents with attention-deficit/hyperactivity disorder: A randomized, placebo-controlled study. *American Journal of Psychiatry, 159*,1896–1901.

MTA Cooperative Group. (1999). A 14-month randomized clinical trial of treatment strategies for attention-deficit/hyperactivity disorder. *Archives of General Psychiatry, 56*, 1073–1086.

Perrin, J., Friedman, R., & Knilans, T. (2008). The Black Box Working Group and the Section on Cardiology and Cardiac Surgery. Cardiovascular monitoring and stimulant drugs for attention-deficit/hyperactivity disorder. *Pediatrics, 122*, 451–453.

Pliszka, S., & American Academy of Child and Adolescent Psychiatry, Work Group on Quality Issues. (2007). Practice parameter for the assessment and treatment of children and adolescents with attention-deficit/hyperactivity disorder. *Journal of the American Academy of Child and Adolescent Psychiatry, 46*(7), 894–921.

Quinn, D. (2005). Poster presented at the 45th annual meeting of New Clinical Drug Evaluation Unit. Boca Raton, FL.

Vetter, V. L., Elia, J., & Erickson, C. (2008). Cardiovascular monitoring of children and adolescents with heart disease receiving stimulant drugs: A scientific statement from the American Heart Association Council on Cardiovascular Disease in the Young Congenital Heart Defects Committee and the Council on Cardiovascular Nursing. *Circulation, 117*(18), 2407–2423.

Wernicke, J. F., & Kratochvil, C. J. (2002). Safety profile of atomoxetine in the treatment of children and adolescents with ADHD. *Journal of Clinical Psychiatry, 63*(Suppl 12), 50–55.

Chapter 13

The Boy Who Draws a Picture Suggesting an Abuse Situation

Beth Moore
Margaret A. Brady

Sometimes unanticipated psychosocial issues present themselves when children come in for well or sick child examinations. Because the role of the provider includes the protection of children, the provider needs to take the time to collect appropriate data about the child's emotional and physical well-being during the history and physical examination. This includes a thorough social/family assessment to identify potential risks to the physical and psychological well-being of the child.

Educational Objectives

1. Identify the common behavioral signs and symptoms associated with child abuse.
2. Understand how the underlying dynamic factors of culture and socioeconomic status can contribute to child abuse and neglect.
3. Recognize how the age of the child and his or her developmental stage impact the presentation of sexual abuse and what signs the healthcare provider must be alert to when delivering health care to children.
4. Apply the guidelines for the reporting of potential child abuse or neglect.

Case Presentation and Discussion

You are a healthcare provider (HCP) in a busy pediatric practice and are running behind schedule. You enter the room of a family that has waited there for about 45 minutes for routine pediatric health supervision visits for two children. Fortunately, there were some interactive toys and some paper and crayons in the examining room to occupy the children while they waited to be seen. The mother, Susan Jenkins, is there with her 5-year-old son, Tommy, and her 7-year-old daughter, Lucy. She is talking on her cell phone but hangs up when you enter the room. She obviously is a bit irritated and states "I'm going to be late meeting my boyfriend. Can you get us out of here quickly?"

In an effort to build rapport, you apologize for the wait and start to look at the picture her son drew. The boy drew a picture of his house with the mother and the sister in the kitchen and the boy in the bedroom with a man. In the picture the man was very large compared to the boy. The man had a scary face, with large hands. The boy in the picture was quite detailed with a sad face and what clearly looked like genitals. You ask the boy about the picture, and he states that the man is "Roy, my mom's new boyfriend," and identified the boy as "me." The mother becomes upset and passes the picture off as her son's "wild imagination."

Before proceeding, you need to think about the possibility of child abuse for this little boy.

Child Abuse and Neglect

Child abuse includes physical abuse or neglect, sexual abuse, emotional mal-treatment, or threats of injury or harm. Each state has laws that individually define the various types of child abuse and how they are to be interpreted in their state. Acts of commission (inflicting injury) or omission (failure to protect from harm) related to child abuse are both punishable in every state's child abuse statutes. Typically, physical abuse is judged to be the use of unlawful corporal punishment or injury to a child; almost 16% of reported child abuse cases involve the physical abuse of children. General and severe neglect typi-cally account for more than 64% of child victims. Cases of child sexual abuse, sexual assault, or exploitation are responsible for approximately 9% of reported cases. Willfully harming or endangering the mental health of a child is considered emotional maltreatment; approximately 7% of cases fall into this category (U.S. Department of Health and Human Services, 2008).

In 2006, an estimated 3.3 million referrals involving approximately 6 mil-lion children were made to Child Protective Services agencies throughout the United States. Approximately 30% of those reports were substantiated, mean-ing that at least one child was found to be a victim of abuse or neglect (U.S. Department of Health and Human Services, 2008).

Cultural and Socioeconomic Risk Factors for Abuse

Children who live in homes where domestic violence and/or alcohol or drug abuse occurs are at increased risk for abuse and neglect. Stressors for families in crisis can contribute to violence against children, such as struggling to meet financial demands, living in violent communities, or having few social resources. If one child in the family has been abused, it greatly increases the likelihood of siblings also being abused (U.S. Department of Health and Human Services, 2008). Children less than 2 years old and children with physical or mental handicaps are at increased risk for child abuse and are particularly vul-nerable populations for physical abuse. In 2006, more than 80% of children who were killed through abuse were younger than 4 years old; 12% were 4 to 7 years old; 14% were 8 to 11 years old; and 3% were 12 to 17 years old (U.S. Department of Health and Human Services). Likewise, a developmentally chal-lenged teenager, particularly a girl, can become the target of sexual assault.

Because physical abuse commonly leaves visible signs, many individuals who are not healthcare providers consider that physical abuse has the greatest negative implications for the child victim. In addition, the lay public often expresses difficulty in believing that a child could be sexually molested by a family member or trusted adult and, instead, thinks that young children, in particular, fabricate stories of sexual molestation. In actuality, emotional maltreatment and sexual molestation serve to corrupt a child's self-esteem. Thus, the long-term implications for emotional and sexual abuse are just as traumatic for the child as physical abuse.

Who Are the Perpetrators?

Data from reported cases reveal that approximately 75% of perpetrators were parents (40% mothers, 17% fathers, and 18% both parents). Other relatives accounted for 7%, and unmarried partners of parents accounted for 4% of perpetrators. The remaining perpetrators included persons with other or unknown relationships to the child victims. Of all parents who were perpetrators, fewer than 3% committed sexual abuse compared to nearly 75% of sexual perpetrators who were friends or neighbors (U.S. Department of Health and Human Services, 2008).

> Roy is the new boyfriend of Ms. Jenkins. Because Tommy's drawing of his family depicts his sad face and reveals his genitals, and Roy's features are scary, you must consider the possibility of sexual abuse. Your priority concern for this visit has switched from a routine health supervision visit for Tommy to one that will focus on questioning about the possibility of sexual abuse. This drawing and its meaning merit further investigation.

Assessing for Possible Child Abuse

The diagnosis of sexual abuse and the protection of the child from additional harm depend, in part, on the provider's willingness to consider abuse as a possibility. Parents may arrange for their child to be seen in a primary care setting because they have concerns about abuse. More typically, a child is brought in for a routine health supervision visit or minor ill visit and then abuse concerns emerge from either historical information or clinical findings. Primary healthcare providers who suspect that child abuse is occurring or has occurred should conduct a complete healthcare history and elicit key historical information about the presence of behavioral symptoms and signs associated with maltreatment or abuse. Whenever feasible, they should inform the parents of their concerns in a calm, nonaccusatory manner. However, if the parent/caregiver becomes violent or verbally confrontational during the questioning, the clinician may defer informing the parent/caregiver that a suspected child abuse report is being called to child protective services or law enforcement and instead, call these agencies prior to addressing the concerns with the parent (Kellogg & Committee on Child Abuse and Neglect, 2005).

A decision to call law enforcement rather than child protective authorities for an immediate evaluation should be based on whether the child will remain in a continuing abusive or dangerous situation if allowed to return home with the parent or caregiver or if the parent/caregiver is a flight risk. Reporting concerns to the child abuse hotline (Brady & Dunn, 2009) while the child remains in the ambulatory setting allows the provider to receive direction and guidance from child protective services.

What questions will you ask the mother to further evaluate for the potential of child abuse? ■

You determine the need to interview Ms. Jenkins without the children present, and she is in agreement. You tell Tommy and Lucy that you and their mother will be in the next room and then alert the medical assistant to check on the children while you are interviewing their mother. You explain to Ms. Jenkins that you are going to obtain a health history about both children because this is your first visit with this family and you start by obtaining information about Tommy.

In particular, you need to conduct a detailed social history related to living conditions, supervision of the children, and Tommy's school performance. You ask the following questions and receive these answers from Ms. Jenkins:

- *Who lives in the home, where do the children sleep, and who supervises their activities when Ms. Jenkins is not home?* Ms. Jenkins replies "It is just the three of us, Lucy, Tommy, and me. We live in a two-bedroom apartment: Lucy and Tommy share a room. They go to an after school program until I pick them up at 5:30 p.m. I'm with my children all the time."

- *What, if any, is the involvement of Tommy's dad in his life, and do Tommy and Lucy have the same father?* "Lucy and Tommy have the same father, who ran off with another woman about 1 year ago. We never see that jerk!"

- *How is Ms. Jenkins doing financially (does she have a job, does she receive child support from the father) and is she having difficult financial times?* "We get along OK with my job, which just covers the bills. I get an occasional token check from the kids' deadbeat dad. Roy is good and has been giving me some money to help with the kids."

- *When did she first meet Roy, what is their relationship, is he living in the home, and if so when did he move in and what is his relationship with the children?* She replies, "I met Roy in a bar about 3 months ago. He's new to town." She does admit upon further discussion that Roy stays overnight with her, but says, "We're always discrete." She tells you that Roy took care of the kids a couple of times when she went out with her girlfriends to celebrate birthdays. He last babysat about 1 week ago.

- *How is Tommy doing in school and have there been any changes in his grades, performance at school (can't concentrate or is easily distracted), or other behaviors? Has his teacher noted any changes?* "Tommy has been having some problems in kindergarten and the teacher wants me to talk with her. Tommy's been hitting kids lately."

The healthcare provider should seek out information from the parent as to whether there has been a change in the child's general attitude, demeanor, or behaviors at home or with his friends or family members and whether this change was associated with a particular event. In this case, did Ms. Jenkins notice any changes in Tommy or Lucy since Roy entered their lives and home situation?

In addition, the provider should seek information about the presence of behavioral signs that are associated with the various types of child maltreatment, not just sexual abuse, because multiple types of maltreatment may be being inflicted upon the child (Brady & Dunn, 2009). Key questions to ask include:

- *Has Tommy become overly fearful, clingy, shown indiscriminate attachment, or compliance?* Ms. Jenkins replies "No, that has never been a problem for Tommy."
- *Have you noticed extremes or drastic changes in his behavior such as extreme passiveness or aggression lately?* She says, "I've had to give him more time outs the last 2 weeks because he is fighting more with his sister."
- *Does Tommy appear wary of physical contact with adults or frightened of anyone?* In this instance, ask Ms. Jenkins how he relates to Roy. She states, "He isn't frightened of anyone I know. He doesn't seem to like to be around Roy. Tommy is just jealous of Roy now that Tommy doesn't have all of my attention."
- *Has he exhibited signs of being depressed, hypervigilant, withdrawn, or apathetic?* "That's not my Tommy."
- *Have there been any changes in Tommy's bowel or bladder patterns (loss of control such as bed wetting or stool soiling), sleep issues (e.g., nightmares or inability to sleep alone) or eating disorders?* Ms. Jenkins seems to hesitate and says, "He wet the bed last week while I was out with my girlfriends." Upon further questioning, she tells you that Roy was babysitting the kids and she didn't get home until 2 a.m. She noted that Tommy was awake in his bedroom when she went in to check on him. He was crying and said that he was sorry that he wet his bed. This was the first time he had wet his bed at night in the last 12 months.
- *Has Tommy talked about suicide plans or thoughts or made any suicide attempts?* (Suicide and running away are more frequently seen in adolescents. This question is more relevant for the older school age and adolescent age group. Therefore, you focus on issues of depression and sadness). She replies, "No, Tommy's not a sad kid."
- *Does he have any unusual fears, phobias, or compulsive behaviors or has there been a recent negative change in peer relationships?* Ms. Jenkins again ponders for a short time and says, "He got into a fist fight with his best friend at school the other day but wouldn't tell me what it was about." (Ms. Jenkins also said earlier that the teacher wants to talk with her about Tommy's behavior at school.)

In addition, consider the possibility of sexual abuse when the child (Child Welfare Information Gateway, 2007):

- Has difficulty walking or sitting
- Suddenly refuses to change for gym or to participate in physical activities
- Reports pain on urination, urethral discharge, or bleeding or genital bruising

- If female, has atypical vaginal discharge, bleeding, genital bruising, or rashes
- Demonstrates bizarre, sophisticated, or unusual sexual knowledge or behavior
- Becomes pregnant or contracts a venereal disease, particularly if under age 14
- Runs away and/or reports sexual abuse by a parent or another adult caregiver

The healthcare provider must always remember that such behavioral changes are not diagnostic per se of sexual abuse but are often indicative for further thorough investigation by a child abuse expert.

You ask questions that might pertain to Tommy's issues, and Ms. Jenkins denies any such issues with Tommy.

Ms. Jenkins tells you at the end of the interview, "I love my boy, and now wonder if Roy molested him. That drawing of Tommy's isn't like him, and at first I just wanted to ignore the fact that something might have happened. I'll do anything to protect my kids." She then starts crying. You reply, "I'm glad that you are willing to put Tommy's welfare as your first priority."

What other questions do you need to ask Tommy? ■

You talk to Tommy in private. He is reluctant at first and you affirm to him that he has done nothing wrong and is not in trouble. You start off by asking about school, sports, and then ask him to tell you about his drawing. You ask him about the boy, and he says, "It's me." You ask him to tell you about the boy and the people in his picture. He looks down at the floor and says while pointing at the picture, "That's my pee pee, where I go pee." He then identifies Roy, his mother, and sister Lucy. You ask him to tell you about each one of them. He starts with his mother and then his sister; he describes their facial appearance and talks about them in a positive manner. He says nothing about Roy spontaneously, so you ask, "Tommy, who is this person (while pointing to the figure of the adult man)." He says "Roy" and again looks at the floor and avoids eye contact. You start by saying, "He's a tall man. Tell me about your picture of Roy." He says, "Roy scares me when he looks at me. I don't like him. He's got big hands and does bad things with them." You reply, "Oh? Tell me about those bad things." Tommy then continues and says, "Roy came into my bedroom while I was sleeping and pulled down my pjs (pajamas). I woke up, and he was rubbing my pee pee. I didn't like it at all and told him to stop. Roy said, 'This is good for you. It's our secret.'" Tommy pauses, so you ask, "What was he rubbing your pee pee with?" Tommy states, "His big hands." You ask, "And then what happened?" "I told him to stop but he wouldn't." You say, "Oh, and then what happened?" Tommy stated, "He pulled down his pants and told me to kiss his pee pee. I said 'no' and started crying and wet my bed. Lucy woke up and Roy ran out of our room." You end this discussion and ask, "Is there something more you think I should know?" Tommy says, "Roy smelled like beer."

Based on what Tommy said, you have enough data to initiate a report. Tommy will be further examined and interviewed by child protective services and professionals who are expert in the field. Another approach to interviewing children about possible sexual abuse is to talk about "good" and "bad" touches that involve touching the child's private parts. You would use this approach when talking with Lucy to see if she too was a victim.

Should the primary care provider interview the child about the abuse or let the experts do this? ■

Children who are sexually abused are often coerced by the abuser to "keep it a secret." The child must be appropriately questioned without the parent or caregiver present to minimize emotional damage and maximize information retrieval. Although investigative interviews should be conducted by social workers or practitioners specifically trained in child abuse, this should not keep primary care providers from asking relevant questions to obtain a detailed pediatric history and a review of systems. A medical history, past incidents of abuse or suspicious injuries, and menstrual history should be documented (Kellogg & Committee, 2005). Line drawings, dolls, or other aids can be effective tools to help the child to talk about the abuse. It is important for the clinician to avoid leading and suggestive questions or showing strong emotions. Instead maintain a "tell-me-more" or "and-then-what-happened" approach. Document the questions asked and the child's responses as well as his or her demeanor and emotional responses to questioning. Use quotation marks to document the child's exact words and/or your questions. For example, Tommy said, "Roy came into my bedroom and pulled down my pajama pants. I [the HCP] replied, "And then what happened, Tommy?"

The general rule of thumb to remember is that children younger than 3 years of age are generally not interviewed (Kellogg, 2005). Tommy is 5 years old and should be interviewed, beginning by asking him to tell you about the people in his drawings.

What data do you want from the physical examination? ■

Physical Examination

If the routine physical examination of potentially sexually abused children cannot be conducted without additional physical or emotional trauma, the examination should be deferred to professionals from child protective services, who will schedule a detailed forensic examination with a health provider expert in the field of child sexual abuse. If the primary care provider is able to secure the child's cooperation for a physical examination, he or she should conduct the examination mindful of the child's developmental needs for sensitivity, particularly when inspecting the genital and rectal areas. Document all physical finding that are obtained during the regular well or sick child examination. A total body assessment of the skin is important to document. In particular, you are looking for signs of physical abuse such as scarring, burns, or bruising that are suggestive of nonaccidental injury because of their pattern or placement on the body. Features of nonaccidental trauma include any injury that leaves a pattern consistent with an agent of injury (belt or bite marks, rope abrasions, or sock/glove injury pattern with a burn injury) or when the type or degree of injury is inconsistent with the child's developmental capability.

Likewise, the rectal and genital/urinary system should be inspected as you would do for any child. Be sure to have a good light source. Look for any signs of bruising, tears, scars, discharge, or lesions. As is the case for all genital/rectal examinations, inform the child of what you are doing. For the female who is not yet a teen, a frog leg position is the easiest for the child to assume. It allows the girl to comfortably spread her legs apart. With your gloved hand, gently spread the labia majora apart and conduct your inspection. A side-lying position with legs bent at the knees is easiest to inspect the rectal area.

If there has been genital contact by the perpetrator, it is important that forensic evidence, including labs and diagnostics, be collected within 24 to 72 hours after the sexual incident, but only by a forensic expert. This forensic exam will be arranged by child protective services (Kellogg & Committee, 2005). Such examiners frequently use a colposcope to magnify the genital and rectal areas, looking for signs of rectal or genital injuries such as tears, lacerations, abrasions, bruising, scars, scratches, atypical laxity of the anus, anal tags, hymenal trauma, or lesions (e.g., herpes or warts). The examiner will collect specimens for sexually transmitted infections, semen, and pubic hairs depending on the history and age of the child.

Tommy allows you to conduct a complete physical examination, including examining his genital and rectal areas. He doesn't want his mother in the room when this is done. You explain to Tommy that you will need your medical assistant to be there to help you. (This is also done to provide a second person in the room who can verify what occurred during the examination if issues of inappropriate conduct by the provider arise.) Tommy says, "OK, she can be in the room." You do your physical examination, which is essentially normal. You are careful to note, "No bruising, unusual scars, lesions, rashes, or abrasions on the skin or rectal/genital areas. His genital/rectal examination is normal with no anal laxity noted."

Lack of physical findings of sexual abuse is common in young children because of the nature of the abuse (nontraumatic fondling), such as occurred with Tommy. Furthermore, delayed disclosure, quick healing times, and the fact that most sexual abuse of young children does not involve penetrating injury are points the HCP needs to remember (Brady & Dunn, 2009). At this point, no diagnostic laboratory testing for sexually transmitted diseases is needed.

Indicators of Potential Child Abuse in Children's Drawings

When investigating possible abuse in children, art functions as a nonthreatening tool for communication between client and clinician (Stember, 1980). The size and placement of the figure(s) relative to the space available may be indicative of the child's perception of self-importance. Also, many or few details, parts of the drawing emphasized or deemphasized (e.g., heavier or lighter or darker or fainter lines) can indicate how the child feels about him- or herself. The drawing being more advanced or immature than is appropriate for the child's developmental age may be indicative of emotional disturbances. Tears and frowns on a child's face are common indicators of sadness or depression. Smiles may be indicators of happiness, but also may be indicators of repression if inappropriate to the context of the scene. Huge circular mouths are often drawn when oral sex is involved. Similarly, Wohl and Kaufman (1985) suggested that hair is a common representation of masculinity, and that overemphasis on or omission of hair may represent feelings related to sensuality, or sexual anxiety, confusion, or inadequacy. Hands are the most frequently omitted human body part in drawings by persons experiencing significant emotional difficulties. Presumably, omission of hands reflects perceived lack of control.

The assumption underlying the use of art is that, because emotionally disturbed children are believed to reflect their problems in their drawings (Yates, Beutler, & Crago, 1985), the drawings of children who have been abused will differ from those of nonabused children. Free drawings, as well as the House-Tree-Person, Draw-A-Person, and Kinetic Family Drawings are used by psychologists in their assessment of a child who may have been abused. In free expression drawings, the child is asked to make a drawing about whatever he or she wants. The House-Tree-Person Test was originally developed by John Buck as an outgrowth of the Goodenough scale utilized to assess intellectual functioning. The child is asked to draw a house, a tree, and a person the best they can. The child's figure gives some indication of how the child perceives himself or herself in the world (Burns & Kaufman, 1972). For the Goodenough-Harris Draw-A-Person Test, the child is asked to draw a man, a woman, and themselves on separate pieces of paper. Scoring scales are used to examine and score the child's drawings (Harris, 1963). The Kinetic Family Drawings, developed in 1970 by Burns and Kaufman, requires the child to draw a picture of his or her entire family including themselves. The drawing is meant to elicit the child's attitudes toward his or her family and the overall family dynamics (Burns and Kaufman).

The qualitative features of the drawings, such as the colors used, the size and detail of body parts, and the shape of the figures may be interpreted in terms of the presence or absence of sexual abuse. Cantlay (1996) claims that distress and trauma, including sexual abuse, are reflected in drawings. The presence of genitalia is often considered a sign of sexual abuse because it is considered rare for normal, nonabused children to include genitals in their drawings (Di Leo, 1996).

Making the Diagnosis

What is your diagnosis? ■

You determine the following diagnosis for Tommy:

- Suspected sexual molestation by the mother's boyfriend.
- Mother believes son and is willing to cooperate with law enforcement and child protective services.

Based on Tommy's drawing and disclosure of genital fondling and oral copulation by Roy, you suspect that he is the victim of sexual molestation.

You ask your medical assistant to carefully watch the family to ensure that Ms. Jenkins doesn't leave or call anyone while you call child protective services. The supervisor there instructs you to call law enforcement immediately and says the police will come to your office to talk with Tommy and his mother and that they will likely arrest Roy. She also tells you that Tommy and his family will be referred to the local child protection team for further evaluation and follow-up.

Recognizing Child Abuse

You decide to review the signs and symptoms of physical abuse, neglect, and emotional abuse to be sure you have not missed any other forms of child abuse that may be simultaneously occurring with Tommy (Child Welfare Information Gateway, 2007). These include the following: a child shows sudden changes in behavior or school performance; has not received help for physical or medical problems brought to the parents' attention; has learning problems (or difficulty concentrating) that cannot be attributed to specific physical or psychological causes; is always watchful, as though preparing for something bad to happen; lacks adult supervision; is overly compliant, passive, or withdrawn; and comes to school or other activities early, stays late, and does not want to go home.

You need to consider the possibility of physical abuse when the child has unexplained burns, bites, bruises, broken bones, or black eyes; has fading bruises or other marks noticeable after an absence from school; seems frightened of the parents and protests or cries when it is time to go home; shrinks at the approach of adults; or reports injury by a parent or another adult caregiver. Think about the possibility of neglect when the child is frequently absent from school; begs or steals food or money; lacks needed medical or dental care, immunizations, or glasses; is consistently dirty and has severe body odor; lacks sufficient clothing for the weather; abuses alcohol or other drugs; or states that there is no one at home to provide care (Child Welfare Information Gateway, 2007).

Finally, consider the possibility of emotional maltreatment when the child shows extremes in behavior such as overly compliant or demanding behavior, extreme passivity, or aggression; is either inappropriately adult (such as parenting other children) or inappropriately infantile (such as frequently rocking or head-banging); is delayed in physical or emotional development; has attempted suicide; or reports a lack of attachment to the parent (Child Welfare Information Gateway, 2007).

Management

What are the laws regarding reporting of child abuse and neglect? ■

Key Components of Child Abuse and Neglect Reporting Laws

Mandated reporters are any person providing services to a minor child. If a child is not in imminent danger, the individual should call the local child abuse hotline. If the child requires protection and is in imminent danger, both the police and the child abuse hotline should be called. Healthcare professionals such as nurse practitioners, physicians, physician assistants, and nurses are mandated reporters and are protected against civil and criminal action if acting within their professional role (U.S. Department of Health and Human Services, 2008). Every clinical setting that serves children should have the toll-free telephone number of the local child protective services department in an easily accessible location.

More than half of all reports of alleged child abuse or neglect are made by professionals such as educators, law enforcement and legal personnel, social services personnel, medical personnel, mental health personnel, child daycare providers, and foster care providers. Friends, neighbors, relatives, and other nonprofessionals submitted approximately 44% of reports (U.S. Department of Health and Human Services, 2008).

Making a Child Abuse Report

Reports about abuse can be made in all states by calling Childhelp (800-4-A-Child) or the local child protective service agencies. The Childhelp National Child Abuse Hotline is available 24 hours a day, 7 days a week. Counselors are available to answer any questions about child abuse or child neglect. This number can be used by all persons who live in the United States, Canada, Puerto Rico, Guam, or the U.S. Virgin Islands. Mandated reporters must accurately fill out the state-required Suspected Child Abuse Report form online, if available, or mail a hard copy to the address on the form within 36 hours of verbally reporting the abuse (Childhelp, 2006).

Therapeutic plan: What will you do therapeutically to help this child? ■

All children who have been sexually abused should be followed up by a team of healthcare professionals who specialize in child maltreatment. Child protective services and the mental health professionals involved in the care of Tommy will assess the need for mental health treatment and will determine the level of family support needed for the Jenkins family. Unfortunately, there are limited mental health treatment services for abused children. The parents and siblings of the victim may also need treatment and support to cope with the emotional trauma associated with Tommy's sexual abuse. A referral to a mental health professional is essential to the emotional recovery for all child victims such as Tommy (Kellogg & Committee, 2005).

Consequences of Child Abuse and Neglect

Eighty percent of young adults who have been abused meet the diagnostic criteria for at least one psychiatric disorder at the age of 21 years. Abused children are 25% more likely to experience teen pregnancy. Children who experience child abuse and neglect are 59% more likely to be arrested as a juvenile, 28% more likely to be arrested as an adult, and 30% more likely to commit violent crimes. Nearly two thirds of the people in treatment for drug abuse reported being abused as children (Child Welfare Information Gateway, 2008). Thus, failure by the HCP to investigate when there are physical, behavioral, or historic indicators of child abuse and failure to report suspicions to child protective services or law enforcement are breaches of professional ethical conduct. Similarly, these children need to be brought into the social services network so they can secure appropriate mental health counseling that they will need both during the crisis period of disclosure and long term.

What will child protection services do? ▇

A child protective services worker comes to the practice setting with a local police officer who works with child abuse victims. They talk with Ms. Jenkins and explain that they will take the family to the local child protective center for a forensic interview by an expert in the field. They plan to talk with both Tommy and Lucy about Roy. Based on what you and Tommy have told them, the police officer is making arrangements to arrest Roy.

You briefly talk to Ms. Jenkins and she is willing to help in any manner she can. She is upset with herself for what has happened to Tommy. The children are told that they need to talk to some people with their mom about what has happened and have been given assurance by their mom that she is not angry at them, loves them, and will be going with them. The police officer and child protection worker also assure the children that they will be helping the family.

You end by saying that the children will be rescheduled for the routine health supervision examination. Ms. Jenkins tells you that she is glad that you talked to Tommy about the picture because she hadn't really looked at what he was drawing until you asked him about it. She indicates that she will return to you for their health care and will cooperate fully to keep her children safe. You also mention the need for individual counseling for Tommy as well as the need for her to seek mental health assistance, and that the child protection center staff will assist the family in this matter.

Key Points from the Case

1. Recognition of child abuse is dependent on the primary healthcare provider being knowledgeable of the signs and symptoms of abuse and reporting procedures.

2. The primary care provider's initial emotional response to the suspected abuse and finesse in handling the situation with the caregivers and the child can greatly influence whether intervention by child protective services is positive or negative.

3. Accurate documentation of medical history, past incidents of abuse or suspicious injuries, and the child's demeanor and emotional responses to questioning is essential to establishing patterns of abuse.

4. Treatment of child abuse victims by mental health professionals is essential to the child's emotional recovery. The parents of the victim may also need treatment and support to cope with the emotional trauma of their child's abuse.

REFERENCES

Brady, M. A., & Dunn, A. M. (2009). Role relationships. In C. E. Burns, A. M. Dunn, M. A. Brady, N. B. Starr, & C. G. Blosser (Eds.), *Pediatric primary care* (4th ed., pp. 366–394). Philadelphia: Saunders Elsevier.

Burns, R. C. & Kaufman, S. H. (1972). *Action, styles, and symbols in Kinetic Family Drawings (K-F-D): An interpretative manual.* New York: Brunner/Mazel.

Cantlay, L. (1996). *Detecting child abuse: Recognizing children at risk through drawings.* Santa Barbara, CA: Holly Press.

Child Welfare Information Gateway. (2007). *Recognizing child abuse and neglect: Signs and symptoms.* Retrieved October 5, 2008, from http://www.childwelfare. gov/pubs/factsheets/signs.cfm

Child Welfare Information Gateway. (2008). *Long-term consequences of child abuse and neglect fact sheet.* Retrieved April 16, 2009, from http://www.childwelfare. gov/pubs/factsheets/long_term_consequences.cfm

Childhelp. (2006). *Get help now.* Retrieved December 5, 2008, from http://www. childhelp.org/get_help

Di Leo, J. H. (1996). *Young children and their drawings.* New York: Brunner/Mazel.

Harris, D. B. (1963). *Children's drawings as a measure of intellectual maturity.* New York: Harcourt, Brace, and World.

Kellogg, N., & Committee on Child Abuse and Neglect. (2005). The evaluation of sexual abuse in children. *Pediatrics, 116*(2), 506–512.

Stember, C. J. (1980). Art therapy: A new use in the diagnosis and treatment of sexually abused children. In K. McFariane (Ed.), *Sexual Abuse of Children:*

Selected Readings (pp. 59–63). Washington, DC: National Center on Child Abuse and Neglect.

U.S. Department of Health and Human Services, Administration on Children, Youth and Families. (2008). *Child maltreatment 2006, the National Child Abuse and Neglect Data System.* Washington, DC: U.S. Government Printing Office.

Wohl, A., & Kaufman, B. (1985). *Silent screams and hidden cries.* New York: Brunner/Mazel.

Yates, A., Beutler, L., & Crago, M. (1985). Drawings in child victims of incest. *Child Abuse and Neglect, 9*(2), 183–189.

Chapter 14

The 14-Year-Old Who Looks Depressed

Ann M. Guthery

Often primary care providers have adolescents brought to their office with complaints of irritability, decline in school performance, oppositional defiant behavior, withdrawn behavior, and somatic complaints. Deciding whether these symptoms are indicators of depression or are reflective of normal developmental transitions can often be difficult. Determining the persistence, intensity, and impairment caused by these symptoms with regard to home, school, and peers is needed to make the diagnosis of depression.

Educational Objectives
1. Identify symptoms of depression in adolescents.
2. Discuss treatment options including medication management and therapy in setting up a treatment plan.
3. Identify when a referral should be made.

Case Presentation and Discussion

Tom Williams is a 14-year-old male who is brought in by his mother who is concerned about his decreased energy level, frequent headaches, and stomach pains. He often wants to sleep or be alone in his room. He loses his temper easily and at one point punched a hole in the wall after an argument with his father. He just started ninth grade and is struggling with the transition to high school. He used to play baseball, but recently has been ditching his old friends and hanging around with new friends that his mother believes are a bad influence. Since being with these new friends, he has been caught shoplifting cigarettes and one of the peers was suspended for bringing marijuana to school. His mother is worried that he is using drugs, but he denies that he has used any.

You observe during this interaction that Tom's affect is flat and he is tearful as his mother tells you this information. He has dark circles under his eyes and states, "I just don't feel good, I can never get to sleep so I'm tired all the time and everything in my life is bad."

You ask his mother to wait in the waiting room so you can question Tom privately. After his mother leaves he tells you the following:

He has tried marijuana a few times because he wanted to see if it helped him to relax, but he often feels worse after he comes off the high, so has stopped using it. He states he has felt sad for the last year; he often feels that no one likes him and that everyone judges him. His closest friend from the baseball team has a girlfriend whom he spends all his time with, so Tom has had to try and find other friends. He knows that the new friends are not considered the best behaved kids in school, but they at least cause some excitement in his life because he is always bored. He feels he can't ever please his parents because he struggles with academics. He states his parents make him so angry that he feels like he wants to hit them when they are lecturing him for something he has done. He denies suicidal thoughts, but states he feels like he is in a hole and can't crawl out of it. Every day is the same and nothing ever gets better.

In meeting with Tom's mother, you find out that she and Tom's father have been arguing and they have discussed a trial separation and possible divorce. Tom is an only child. His father is diagnosed with bipolar disorder.

What other things do you need to do to further assess this patient? ▉

Before answering this, here is additional information you need to consider.

Description and Etiology of Depression in Children and Adolescents

Definition and Characteristics of Depression

A definition of childhood depression is difficult to find in literature because depression is usually described by symptoms. Depression in children and adolescents may be defined with the same criteria as for adults. It is based on negative cognitions such as hopelessness, negative view of the self, negative self-schema, negative attributions, loss of locus of control, and cognitive distortions. Depression is hard to diagnose in children because many also have comorbid diagnoses such as anxiety. Depression in children appears to be a syndrome with a combination of dysphoria (inappropriately or excessively sad mood) or anhedonia (loss of pleasure in response to previously enjoyed activities) as the two most significant symptoms.

Depression symptoms change with age. For example, in preschool children, decreased appetite, failure to gain weight, sad appearance, irritable mood, feeling bored, GI upset, sleep difficulties, and repetitive behaviors are the most common symptoms. They tend not to report depressed mood or hopelessness feelings (Hankin, 2006). In children ages 3–8 years, aggression and self-endangering behaviors are more common. Negative life events sometimes lead to depressive symptoms in early childhood while a negative explanatory style leads to depressive symptoms in later childhood and adolescence. Major depressive disorder in young people continues into adulthood across many studies (Hankin, 2006; Rice, Harold, & Tharper, 2002). Genetic and biological factors also have been found to contribute to the occurrence of depression in children.

Pathophysiology

Norepinephrine and serotonin are the two neurotransmitters most often implicated in mood disorders. People who are depressed have decreased sensitivity of beta adrenergic receptors for both epinephrine and serotonin; these neurotransmitters are increased with use of antidepressants. In addition to the neurotransmitters, studies have shown that the following areas of the brain are involved with mood regulation: medial and orbital prefrontal cortex, anterior cingulated cortex, amygdale, nucleus accumbens, and hypothalamus (Sadock & Sadock, 2007).

Comorbidities

Depression commonly occurs with other mental disorders including anxiety, conduct/oppositional defiant disorders, and attention deficit hyperactivity disorder (ADHD). Eating disorders and substance abuse are associated with depression in adolescents (Hankin, 2006). In examining comorbid conditions in adolescents, Rice et al. (2002) found that chemical dependency could be a form of depression.

Mesquita and Gilliam (1994) reported that both attention deficit disorder and depression can result in difficulty with concentration, psychomotor agitation, and engagement in self-endangering behaviors. Social withdrawal, guilt, weeping, and dysphoria are key to depression. Thus, it is clear that depressed children are suffering and that their emotional and social well-being and academic progress are at risk.

Depression in Children and Their Families

Depressed children may have a depressed parent. In addition, they may have received hard power-assertive discipline, a rigid and inflexible family structure, and internalized aggression. A family interaction of low conflict and aggression and maternal aversiveness was seen in both depression and conduct disorders. Environmental stressors seem to be less correlated with depression.

Theories of Depression

According to Sadock and Sadock (2007), the causal basis for mood disorders is not known, but many theories have been proposed. These theories have been divided according to biological, genetic, and psychosocial factors, as well as cognitive theories.

Biological

It is important to understand that brain chemistry may affect perception and thinking, which in turn could impact mood. One hypothesis is that mood disorders are associated with heterogeneous dysregulation of the biogenic amines; in particular, depleted levels of serotonin and norepinephrine are most often implicated in mood disorders. The pathology for depression seems to occur in the limbic system, the basal ganglia, and the hypothalamus.

Genetic

Genetic factors for depression have been shown in first-degree relatives. Sadock and Sadock (2007) cited a review of genetic studies showing that children have a 25% higher chance of developing a mood disorder if they have one parent with a mood disorder. If both parents have a mood disorder, then children have a 50–75% chance of developing a mood disorder. Key findings from a review of studies by Rice, Harold, and Tharper (2002) showed an increased familial risk, and that recurrent prepubescent major depressive disorder may be more familial than previously thought.

Psychosocial

Psychosocial factors related to depression include life events and environmental stressors such as early loss and abandonment affecting children's mood. Children who have experienced these stressors can show symptoms of internalized hostility, ambivalence, and loss of self-esteem. These factors can all affect thinking and perception, which, in turn, may be related to depressed feelings.

Cognitive Theories

The cognitive theory of depression has been widely studied. According to this theory, depression results from a negative cognitive set (i.e., a tendency to erroneously view the self, future, and one's experience in a negative manner). Basically, the model reveals that a loss of social reinforcement and disruption of close interpersonal relationships mediate the development and maintenance of depression symptoms; the less interpersonal competence one has, the greater the negative impacts on others and the poorer interpersonal problem-solving performance will be.

Stress and Coping

It is important to understand potential resources for coping because they may be spiritual in nature or they may function in place of spiritual resources for the child. People learn modes of coping from their membership group. Coping involves modification of the stressful situation, modification of the meaning of the problem in order to reduce stress, and then management of the stress symptoms. It includes specific behaviors that vary depending on the problem and the social role one is dealing with. However, coping has its limits. As Pearlin et al. (1981) explained, individuals, faced with an array of problems and hardships as they move through life, do not choose between coping and supports, but use both in an effort to avoid, eliminate, or reduce distress.

Epidemiology of Depression

Prevalence rates vary across studies, which use a variety of measures to identify depression. Twenty-eight percent of the students nationwide completing the Youth Behavior Survey (Centers for Disease Control and Prevention [CDC], 2008) reported feeling so sad or hopeless every day for two or more weeks that they changed their activities; 14.5% reported considering suicide, 11.3% had made a suicide plan, and 6.9% had attempted suicide. In an assessment of children with chronic emotional, behavioral, or developmental problems completed in 2001, 43.5% had depression or anxiety problems (CDC, 2005). Hankin (2006), in his review of many adolescent depression studies, notes that between 20% and 50% of adolescents report subsyndrome levels of depression. Generally, studies of individuals with clinically diagnosed major depression report prevalence rates of about 14% for 15 to 18 year olds and about 16.6% for 18 to 29 year olds. In childhood, rates are more like 1% to 3%.

What instruments could you use in your practice to assist in the diagnosis of depression in children? ■

Assessment

Symptom Analysis

In order to complete a full assessment and evaluation of an adolescent for depression, the healthcare provider will need to integrate information from multiple sources. Children and adolescents tend to be reliable in reporting internal symptoms, whereas parents and teachers are more reliable in reporting external symptoms. It is important to interview both the adolescent and the parents separately. Often, use of a screening questionnaire can help in guiding the interview. The Children's Depression Inventory is one such tool (Kovaks, 2003). This is a 27-item symptoms-oriented scale designed for children and adolescents ages 7–17 years. Questions focus on severity of depression symptoms in the last 2 weeks. Whether using a questionnaire or an interview strategy, questions for adolescents need to focus on the following:

- *Mood:* Does the adolescent feel sad, down, irritable, or grouchy? Does the teen feel this way most of the time? Does he or she often cry? Does the teen get into more arguments with others recently, including parents, teachers, or peers?
- *Anhedonia:* Is the teen able to enjoy things he or she used to enjoy? Does he or she have less interest in doing fun things, often feel bored and tired, or have less energy than usual?
- *Guilty feelings or negative self-image:* Does the teen feel bad about him- or herself or feel bad about things they have done? Does the young person feel worthless? Does the teen have any friends and feel that other kids like them?
- *Neurovegetative signs:* Have changes occurred in sleep patterns—not able to sleep, waking up more, sleeping all the time? Are there changes in appetite—increased or decreased? Are there difficulties concentrating in school? Have grades dropped? Does the child or teen not want to go to school because it takes too much energy?
- *Somatic symptoms:* Does the boy or girl have headaches, stomachaches, or body aches? How often and how severe?
- *Suicidal ideation:* Has the child or teen wished to be dead or made a comment that they wished they were not here? Does he or she have any plans for self-harm? How detailed is the plan? What are the

means? Has the youth tried to hurt him- or herself? How long ago did these feelings arise? What was going on when these feelings arose?

- *Substance use:* Is the youth using any drugs or alcohol, and if so, which ones? For how long? How much? Is this a recent change?

Questions for parents encompass similar areas:

- *Mood/affect:* How do they see the child's mood? Has it changed recently? Is the child sad, angry, irritable? Is he or she arguing more? Does he or she avoid doing things he or she used to enjoy doing? Is he or she more withdrawn?
- *Neurovegetative signs:* Have they noticed changes in the child's sleep patterns? Difficulty getting and staying asleep? Sleeping more? Any changes in appetite? Increased or decreased? Weight changes? Changes in energy level?
- *Suicidal ideation:* Has the child voiced any thoughts about wishing he or she was dead? Has the child tried to hurt him- or herself? Are they worried that the child may harm him- or herself? Have they seen that the child is preoccupied with death? Is he or she listening to, writing, or watching more morbid things?
- *Impaired school or peer functioning:* Have the child's grades declined? Is the child showing less interest in social or after-school activities? Has the child missed a lot of school from not feeling well? Is he or she spending less time with peers? Has the peer group changed?
- *Drug abuse:* Are there any signs of substance use (e.g., lethargy, hyperactivity, hypervigilance, deviant or risk-taking behavior, absences or suspension from school, poorer school performance, withdrawal from family or friends, changes in friends, angry outbursts)? **Tom scores positively for depression on the Children's Depression Inventory which you administer in the office.** This instrument validates the history that you obtained earlier.

Physical Examination and Laboratory Studies

What physical examination data should you collect? ■

As a primary care provider, it is important to complete a physical exam and laboratory screenings to rule out any physical causes for these symptoms, such as anemia; vitamin B_{12} deficiency; Cushing syndrome; connective tissue disorders such as juvenile arthritis or lupus; diabetes mellitus; chronic fatigue syndrome; fibromyalgia; hypothyroidism; infections such as mononucleosis, hepatitis, or human immunodeficiency virus (HIV); inflammatory bowel disorder; multiple sclerosis; seizure disorder; or tumors (Kaye, Montgomery, & Munson, 2002). **Tom's physical examination, including a careful neurological examination considering his headaches, is normal for his age.**

Are any laboratory studies indicated for initial diagnosis and screening of depression in children? ■

Laboratory screenings for thyroid abnormalities, CBC, and toxicology are important. No abnormalities were found on the screening lab work for Tom.

Could these symptoms be the result of medication use? ■

A thorough history of use of other medications is needed. Steroids, thyroid supplements, megavitamins, benzodiazepines, beta-blockers, clonidine, Accutane, and oral contraceptives, for example, can all contribute to mood changes. Tom has not taken any medications or substances.

In addition, it is important to rule out ADHD, bipolar disorder, substance use/abuse, and anxiety disorders.

Making the Diagnosis

The results from the history, the positive results of the Childhood Depression Inventory, and data from both Tom and his parents lead you to make a diagnosis of depression. There is no indication of drug use or chronic illness, physical examination data to support a physical illness, or laboratory work indicating physical ailments that might account for his feelings. He has not had suicidal thoughts or other thoughts about harming himself or others.

Management

As a primary care provider, you want to refer Tom to a mental health specialist for care. However, you also have a role to play in advocating for mental health treatment and arranging for a referral, and need to be acquainted with the care the mental health specialist will provide.

Psychoeducation

The following are actions you can expect from the mental health specialist that you can support (Kaye et al., 2002):

- Review stressors and contributing factors to mood changes.
- Clarify coping strategies that the patient and family have to support the adolescent's capacity to discuss their feelings.
- Destigmatize the acknowledgement of emotional difficulties.
- Normalize developmental struggles.
- Identify self-esteem–enhancing activities and skills such as any school-based activities, sports, or camps.
- Reinforce good self-care habits. (Establishing regular eating, sleeping, and exercise habits help mental health.)

- Rule out maltreatment as a contributing factor.
- Educate the teen and family about signs of increasing depression such as sleep disturbances, changes in appetite, school problems, and argumentativeness.

Cognitive Behavioral Therapy

Psychotherapy is used for mild cases of depression. The largest randomized clinical trial for adolescent depression, the Treatment of Adolescent Depression Study (TADS) (March et al., 2004) showed that moderate to severe adolescent depression is best treated with a combination of an antidepressant and cognitive behavioral therapy (CBT). Other studies demonstrate the effectiveness of CBT (Compton et al., 2004; Hazell, 2004; Powers, Jones, & Jones, 2005).

CBT is often the therapy of choice because depression is considered a cognitive dysfunction. CBT is based on the assumption that the way a person thinks, perceives, and actively interacts within the environment determines his or her feelings and behaviors (Beck, 1976). An individual's emotions and behaviors are, in large part, determined by the way in which he or she cognitively appraises the world. The primary care provider who understands basic CBT concepts can better support the mental health specialist's work.

CBT can be understood best as an integrated theory that links cognitive, affective, social, and developmental processes to behavior. An individual's cognitions are termed *schemas* and are central to thought and perception. They have a fundamental influence on emotion and behavior and can be either positive or negative. They help process and organize complex information into meaningful patterns over time (Beck, 1976).

Beck's theory takes into account metacognitions, which are defined as "thoughts about thinking" that emerge during middle childhood. It is at this time that children become more skilled in identifying information needed to solve problems. The development of metacognitions is necessary for the child to develop a sense of self. By 8 years of age, children have been found to distinguish between thoughts and behavior (Flavell, Green, & Flavell, 2000; Quakley, Coker, Palmer, & Reynolds, 2003).

The goal of CBT is to decrease negative schema and their emotional and behavioral consequences. This is done by: 1) assisting the individual to attempt new behaviors and experiences; 2) acknowledging the individual's past but focusing the intervention on the present desired functioning; 3) viewing the changes in emotions and behavior from both an objective and subjective vantage point; 4) refocusing the individual on recent successful experiences; and 5) redirecting the self-evaluations to reasoned depictions of positive perceptions, beliefs, and attitudes. Problems that are brought to the therapy appointment are broken down into a series of questions, the answers to which gradually reveal the solution. In the session, the teen is asked to begin to question his or her own reactions. For example:

- What other plausible perspective(s) can I take about this matter?
- What factual evidence supports or refutes my beliefs?
- What are the pros and cons of continuing to see things the way I see them, and what are the pros and cons of trying to see things differently?
- What constructive action can I take to deal with my beliefs or schemas?
- What sincere advice would I give to a good friend with the same beliefs?

In any type of therapy it is difficult to understand numerous problems in their entirety. CBT focuses on individual events or problems and allows the therapist to conceptualize connections and solutions. A prioritization needs to occur in CBT, as follows: First, assess and problem solve for suicide risk. Next, address interfering behaviors such as homework noncompliance, medication noncompliance, not working collaboratively in therapy, and missing appointments. Third, address behaviors that are dangerous and that interfere with quality of life such as substance abuse, shoplifting, high-risk sexual behaviors, abusive relationships, or homelessness. These behaviors have to be addressed first or no progress can be made.

Goal setting must be mutually agreed on. The goals should be described concretely and with measurable outcomes. The therapist is trying to teach goal-oriented active problem-solving skills focused on concrete, specific patient problems. Other names for CBT have included goal setting, problem solving, self-statement modification, social perception skills training, self-control training, and cognitive restructuring. Over time, CBT can help the teen to recognize themes that identify specific maladaptive automatic thoughts.

In clinical practice, evaluation of the existing knowledge and beliefs of the individual are determined, appropriate interventions are developed to educate and motivate, and the resulting behavior changes are appraised.

For CBT, a "thoughts log" like that shown in Table 14-1 could be used to help the teen change his or her thinking.

Medications

Often psychotherapy is used first for mild cases of depression. Medications may be warranted if this is not effective, or if the depression is more severe. Selective serotonin reuptake inhibitors (SSRIs) are considered the first-line treatment for depression. Food and Drug Administration (FDA) approved indications for pediatric depression controlled trials support the use of fluoxetine (Prozac), paroxetine (Paxil), and citalopram (Celexa) for children and adolescents with depression. Open trials also support the use of Prozac, sertraline (Zoloft), Paxil, Celexa, and fluvoxamine (Luvox). With respect to dosing of these medications, the rule of thumb is to "start low and go slow." Dosing can be increased every 5–7 days to target dose and then should be held for 4–6 weeks before further dose increases. Table 14-2 shows dosing guidelines. Medications are typically given on a QD (daily) schedule. The primary care provider may be asked by the

Table 14–1   Thoughts Log

Date	Situation (event, memory, attempt to do something)	Behavior	Emotion	Thoughts	Response

mental health specialist to prescribe psychotropic medications if that person does not have prescriptive authority. Even if not prescribing, the primary care provider needs to know which medications are being prescribed and provide surveillance related to safety and effectiveness.

When prescribing, it is important to educate patients about side effects because this seems to help with treatment adherence. Common side effects of SSRIs include agitation or restlessness, apathy or amotivation syndrome, gastrointestinal upset or diarrhea, headaches, insomnia, and sexual side effects (Kaye et al., 2002).

Serotonin syndrome is a serious and possibly fatal syndrome that occurs when serotonin has been overstimulated. Symptoms include diarrhea, restlessness, extreme agitation, hyperreflexia, and autonomic instability with possible rapid fluctuations in vital signs, myoclonus, seizures, hyperthermia, uncontrollable shivering and rigidity, delirium, coma, status epilepticus, cardiovascular collapse, and death. Treatment includes removing the offending agent and referral to the hospital for care (Sadock & Sadock, 2007).

Table 14-2	Dosing Table for SSRIs			
Medications	Initial Dose (1 x per day)	Maintenance and Max Dosing Per Day	Half Life	Common Symptoms to Monitor
Prozac (Fluoxetine)	Ch: 2.5–5mg Adol: 5–10mg	Ch: 10–40mg Adol: 20–40mg Max: 60–80mg	1–3 days	Headache, diarrhea, activation, suicidal ideation
Zoloft (Sertraline)	Ch: 12.5–25mg Adol: 25–50mg	Ch: 25–100mg Adol: 50–200mg Max: 200mg	20–28 hours	Headache, sedation, diarrhea, activation, suicidal ideation
Paxil (Paroxetine)	Ch: 5–10mg Adol: 10–20mg	Ch: 10–30mg Adol: 20–40mg Max: 60mg	20–25 hours	Headache, sedation, diarrhea, activation, suicidal ideation
Celexa (Citalopram)	Ch: 5–10mg Adol: 10–20mg	Ch: 10–40mg Adol: 20–40mg Max: 60mg	24 hours	Headache, diarrhea, sedation, activation, suicidal ideation
Luvox (Fluvoxamine)	Ch: 12.5–25mg Adol: 25–50mg	Ch: 50–150mg Adol: 50–200mg Max: 300mg	14–18 hours	Headache, diarrhea, activation, suicidal ideation
Lexapro (Escitalopram)	Ch: 5–10mg Adol: 10–20mg	Ch: 10–20mg Adol: 20–40mg Max: 60mg	24 hours	Headache, diarrhea, activation, suicidal ideation

Sources: Kaye, D. L., Montgomery, M. E., & Munson, S. (2002). *Child and adolescent mental health.* Philadelphia: Lippincott Williams & Wilkins; Stahl, S. (2006). *Essential psychopharmacology: The prescriber's guide.* Cambridge, MA: Cambridge University Press.

SSRIs and Side Effects

If intolerable side effects emerge or a maximal dosage is reached without improvement after 8–12 weeks, then an alternative SSRI should be cross-tapered and substituted. If a second SSRI trial is unsuccessful, then atypical antidepressants (bupropion, venlafaxine, mirtazapine, and duloxetine) can be tried, although it is important to note that fewer data are available on these agents. Bupropion (Wellbutrin) has stimulant-like properties and has been helpful in some adolescents with symptoms of depression and ADHD. It has been associated with increased risk of seizures and should not be used in patients with a history of substance abuse or eating disorders because it is contraindicated in these cases. Venlafaxine (Effexor) has also been shown to help symptoms of depression and anxiety in adolescents. It can cause blood pressure elevations, and 5–7% of patients on it must be monitored for these changes. Mirtazapine (Remeron) has not been used widely in adolescents. It is highly sedating and, rarely, is associated with agranulocytosis. Duloxetine (Cymbalta) also has not been widely used for adolescents, but is available. Adult data show gastrointestinal side effects. Tricyclic antidepressants are not currently supported as first-line agents for treating juvenile depression. Studies have shown that they have a narrow margin for safety and lack of benefit (Kaye et al., 2002; Sadock & Sadock, 2007).

When adolescents are taking antidepressants, the healthcare provider needs to be vigilant for signs of mania, including increased activity, irritability, aggression, euphoria, giddiness, and decreased need for sleep. If these symptoms are present the antidepressant needs to be discontinued. This can occur with use of any of the antidepressants in adolescents predisposed to bipolar disorder (Sadock & Sadock, 2007). Suicide ideation can also occur.

Both adolescents and their families need to be reminded that antidepressants often take 2–4 weeks to alleviate symptoms. The medication should be continued for 6–12 months once symptoms improve. Adolescents should be symptom-free for at least 3 months before considering tapering off of medication. Antidepressants need to be slowly tapered. This will prevent withdrawal symptoms and allow for rapid retitration if depressive symptoms reoccur (Sadock & Sadock, 2007).

In Tom's case, it would be appropriate to start Prozac 10 mg 1 tablet PO in the morning and refer him to a therapist for CBT. It would be important to have him return weekly for 2 to 4 weeks for follow-up to report on how he is feeling and to assess for suicidal ideation.

What will you do to educate him and his mother about depression and the management of his symptoms? ■

The following are points you include when educating Tom about depression and it's management:

- Explain the diagnosis and its pathophysiology, its chronic nature, and the need for medications and therapy to stabilize the depressed mood.

- Explain the use of the antidepressant prescribed, including efficacy and side effects. Reassure them that the medication may not result in improvement for 4–6 weeks and that the improvement may seem subtle. Often parents and teachers will notice the benefit before the teen may feel it.

- Discuss monitoring for suicidal ideation and that it is important for Tom to tell his parents if he has these feelings. Tom or his parents should call you immediately so it can be determined if he might need to be hospitalized at that point.

- Explain your process to arrange for a mental health specialist to see Tom for therapy and your intention to call the therapist to work out a plan to coordinate management as specialist and primary care provider.

Once his mood is stable, follow-up appointments can be changed to meeting every 4–6 weeks to continue to assess response to medications and to support the patient and his parents. In our case example, Tom begins to feel better after 4 weeks on Prozac. He has started to see a therapist and is starting to work on viewing situations in his life more positively. After 6 months of therapy and medications, he is enjoying high school, his grades have improved, and he is more motivated and has his sense of humor back. He has started to play baseball again and is hanging out with more positive peers. No suspicions of drug use are noted.

Key Points from the Case

1. Guidelines can help to simplify the care of depression, such as how to choose a medication or therapy technique, but often the individual's situation and variables of biology, environment, cognition, and events leading to depression all need to be factored into treatment planning.

2. Treatment of depression with a teen includes understanding his or her pathophysiology, cognitive development, family history, family environment, school environment, social environment, and life experiences.

REFERENCES

Beck, A. (1976). *Cognitive therapy and emotional disorders*. New York: International Universities Press.

Centers for Disease Control and Prevention. (2005). Mental health in the United States: Health care and well being of children with chronic emotional, behavioral, or developmental problems—United States, 2001. *Morbidity and Mortality Weekly Report, 54*(39), 985–989.

Centers for Disease Control and Prevention. (2008). Youth risk behavioral surveillance—United States, 2007. *Morbidity and Mortality Weekly Report, 57*(SS-4).

Compton, S., March, J., Brent, D., Albano, A., Weersing, R., & Curry, J. (2004). Cognitive-behavioral psychotherapy for anxiety and depressive disorders in children and adolescents: An evidence-based medicine review. *Journal of the American Academy of Child and Adolescent Psychiatry, 43*(8), 930–959.

Flavell, J. H., Green, F., & Flavell, E. R. (2000). *Young children's knowledge about thinking: Monographs of the Society for Research in Child Development.* Malden, MA: Blackwell.

Hankin, B. (2006). Adolescent depression: Description, causes, and interventions. *Epilepsy and Behavior, 8,* 102–114.

Hazell, P. (2004). Depression in children and adolescents. *Clinical Evidence, 12,* 427–442.

Kaye, D. L., Montgomery, M. E., & Munson, S. (2002). *Child and adolescent mental health.* Philadelphia: Lippincott Williams & Wilkins.

Kovaks, M. (2003). *Children's Depression Inventory: Technical manual.* Toronto: Multi-Health Systems.

March, J., Silva, S., Petrycki, S., Curry, J., Wells, K., Fairbank, J., et al. (2004). Fluoxetine, cognitive behavioral therapy, and their combination for adolescents with depression: Treatment for Adolescents with Depression Study (TADS) randomized controlled trial. *Journal of the American Medical Association, 292,* 807–820.

Mesquita, P. B., & Gilliam, W. S. (1994). Differential diagnosis of childhood depression: Using comorbidity and symptom overlap to generate multiple hypotheses. *Child Psychiatry and Human Development, 24*(3), 157–172.

Pearlin, L. I., Lieberman, M. A., Menaghan, E. G., & Mullan, J. T. (1981). The stress process. *Journal of Health and Social Behavior, 22,* 337–356.

Powers, S., Jones, J., & Jones, B. (2005). Behavioral and cognitive-behavioral interventions with pediatric populations. *Clinical Child Psychology and Psychiatry, 10,* 65–77.

Quakley, S., Coker, S., Palmer, K., & Reynolds, S. (2003). Can children distinguish between thoughts and behaviors? *Behavioural and Cognitive Psychotherapy, 31,* 159–168.

Rice, F., Harold, G., & Tharper, A. (2002). The genetic aetiology of childhood depression: A review. *Journal of Child Psychology and Psychiatry, 43*(1), 65–79.

Sadock, B. J., & Sadock, V. A. (2007). *Kaplan and Sadock's synopsis of psychiatry* (10th ed.). Philadelphia: Lippincott Williams & Wilkins.

Chapter 15

The Teen Who Thinks She Might Be Gay

Sheran M. Simo

Things aren't always the way they appear. Judgments are made on a daily basis regarding every aspect of a person's life, including lifestyle, religious beliefs, and sexual orientation. As is often the case in the primary healthcare setting, the initial reason that brings an individual in for a health visit may evolve into something completely different as the visit progresses.

Educational Objectives
1. Identify lesbian, gay, bisexual, and transgendered (LGBT)–sensitive questions to ask your patients.
2. Identify and become familiar with health issues specific to adolescent LGBT youth.
3. Identify risk factors such as sexually transmitted diseases (STDs), mental health disorders, and violence that LGBT youth may experience.
4. Become familiar with resources available in the community specific to LGBT youth.

Case Presentation and Discussion

Fifteen-year-old Cassandra Stanley is brought to your office by her mother. According to Mrs. Stanley, she would like you to initiate birth control for her daughter. As the story unfolds, you learn that Cassandra is the youngest of three daughters, 8 years younger than her next older sibling. Mom states that she had initiated birth control for Cassandra's sisters and neither of them became pregnant prior to finishing school and getting married. She hopes to provide the same means of protection for Cassandra. As you look to Cassandra to initiate the conversation, you notice that Cassandra appears very upset. She expresses to her mother that she's already told her that she doesn't want to be on birth control so this visit is pointless!

You realize very quickly that you have a stressful situation on your hands and ask Mom to step out of the room to allow you to get to know Cassandra a little better and talk with her in private as you do with all your teen patients. During the course of your conversation, Cassandra blurts out, "My mom wants me to take birth control because she thinks I want to have sex with boys." As you question her further, she relates, "I'm in love with my best friend, and *she* can't get me pregnant!" Cassandra reveals that she has "always known I liked girls" and "can't imagine ever being with a boy."

What information do you need to recall for this situation? ■

Because of the delicate nature of this situation, it is important for the health-care provider (HCP) to be sensitive to the teen's feelings and concerns. In order to promote this type of communication, the provider is encouraged to ask open-ended questions. Asking open-ended questions promotes conversation more readily and helps the teen to think more clearly about what it is that they want to discuss or what questions they need answered, such as, "What questions about being with your partner have come to mind as you've begun to think about being sexually active?" or "What questions would you like to ask me as you begin your sexual relationship?" Asking adolescents closed-ended questions such as "Do you understand?" or "Do you have any questions?" will limit the discussion.

It is also important for the practitioner to be aware of what it means when a female describes herself as a woman-loving woman or lesbian, or a male describes himself as a male-loving male or gay. Sexual orientation describes the direction a person's emotional connections, attractions, and sexual activity lean toward. Attractions may be toward the same sex (homosexual, gay, lesbian), the opposite sex (heterosexual), or toward both sexes (bisexual). Table 15-1 defines these different sexual orientations.

It is important for the HCP to consider several factors when working with adolescents who are deliberating about their own sexual orientation, especially when they believe they are or may be homosexual.

- Adolescents usually establish their sexual identity by the time they reach adolescence, even if they have not had an opportunity to act on it.
- Sexual orientation cannot be changed; it is deeply ingrained within children's makeup. Very often the fact that children or adolescents are gay remains hidden from family and friends, and is often denied by the teens themselves.
- Sexual orientation appears to be a biological phenomenon. Only rarely, if ever, is sexual orientation caused by personal experiences

---

Table 15-1   Definitions

- *Lesbian:* A woman who finds an emotional, sexual, and romantic connection only with another woman.
- *Gay:* Very often used to describe people attracted to members of the same sex, though *gay* is most often used to refer only to men who are attracted to other men.
- *Homosexuality:* Sexual and emotional attraction to a member of the same sex.
- *Bisexual:* Sexual and emotional attraction by one toward members of either sex.
- *Transsexual:* One who identifies with a gender different from the physical body in which they were born, or were assigned to if there was ambiguity of the sexual organs at birth.

and environment (American Academy of Pediatrics, 1999), although heredity seems to also have a place.
- Despite increased knowledge and information about being gay or lesbian, teens still have many concerns. These include (American Academy of Child and Adolescent Psychiatry, 1997):
  - Feeling different from peers
  - Feeling guilty about their sexual orientation
  - Worrying about the response from their families and loved ones
  - Being teased and ridiculed by their peers
  - Worrying about AIDS, HIV infection, and other STDs
  - Fearing discrimination when joining clubs or sports, seeking admission to college, and finding employment
  - Fearing rejection and harassment by others

What health issues might you see in LGBT adolescents? ■

Health Issues Related to LGBT Adolescents

Health Risk Behaviors

LGBT adolescents are at a higher risk for increased use of tobacco, drugs, and alcohol than their heterosexual counterparts, due to increases in social, identity, legal, and discriminatory stressors.

Sexually Transmitted Disease Risks

Because of certain sexual practices performed by LGBT individuals, they are potentially at risk for STDs. These practices include anal and/or vaginal coitus, oral sex, and casual or multiple sex partners. Sexually transmitted infections can include herpes, chlamydia, gonorrhea, trichomoniasis, syphilis, genital warts (HPV), human immunodeficiency virus (HIV), and hepatitis. Furthermore, even though adolescents identify as LGBT, they may not necessarily limit their sexual practices to those of their identified sexual preference. As such, they may be at risk for any or all of the same consequences as their heterosexual counterparts.

Mental Health and Violence Risks

As a result of perceived or real homophobia and increases in other stressors, LGBT adolescents are more likely to suffer from depression. LGBT adolescents also are at risk for violence, both from society at large and in their partnered relationships. It is a misperception to assume that persons in LGBT relationships do not suffer from intimate partner violence.

Healthcare Needs

LGBT adolescents (and adults) may avoid medical care and appropriate health screenings because of a misperception that they are only necessary for heterosexuals. For example, lesbian or transgendered nonsurgical female to males (FTMs) may avoid getting regular Pap smears because they believe they aren't at risk for cervical cancer or choose to ignore the existence of sexual organs they were originally born with. Lesbians and FTM transgendered individuals may be at higher risk for breast cancer because they may be less likely to bear children or lactate.

Lesbians appear to have a better body image; they are often less concerned with being thin for society's sake and as a result may be *more* inclined to be overweight or obese than heterosexual women. This, in turn, increases the risk of health problems associated with obesity, including diabetes, heart disease, hypertension, and cancers of the uterus, ovaries, breast, and colon.

Lesbians are less likely to use oral contraceptives and other forms of hormonal birth control and so are at greater risk for endometrial, breast, and ovarian cancers.

How will you respond to what Cassandra has told you? ■

When her mother leaves the room, you let Cassandra know that you can see that she and her mom have a difference of opinion on whether she should be on birth control. At this point, you question whether Cassandra has told her mother that she is a lesbian, and encourage her to talk to her mother when she reveals that she has not.

You keep in mind that although teenagers may not respond fully with eye contact or verbally, they "hear" everything said to them. It is important to convey a sense of acceptance of her from the beginning of the encounter.

You reassure Cassandra that people not only have different preferences in sex partners, but also have a variety of ways of enacting their sexual orientation and that you respect people's individuality. It's essential to let her know that you are here to provide the kind of information and support she needs to stay healthy and feel positive about herself, to answer questions, and to provide a place to talk personally about anything that affects her body, just as you do for all of your patients.

What important points would you consider during your discussion with Cassandra? ■

The following points would be important to discuss with Cassandra:

- Identify that you are aware of a conflict between the patient and her mom. Use a respectful, straightforward, "coaching" approach allowing space for thinking between points.
- Stress to the patient that sexuality is a very individual thing; that not only are there varying sexual orientations but that even within those, people have their own personal ways of acting that out and that this must be respected and will be respected by you, the healthcare practitioner.
- Encourage her to keep in mind that others are not always as courageous and honest; for example, a bisexual or lesbian woman may be sleeping with a man or using

needle drugs and not admit it. Stress that this is why same-sex sexual encounters should even include safe sex between women.

· Ask her what she knows about how to have safer same-sex encounters, where to get the supplies, and specifically how to use them. Tell her that if she should need coaching about how to talk to another woman about using safe sex to please come back and talk with you whenever she needs to.

Adolescents may move through several phases of sexual experimentation before settling on an orientation. In addition, you realize that to speak of this directly at this encounter could give Cassandra the impression that you do not take her current choice seriously. Instead, you decide to ask from the standpoint of a routine STD screening and ask her if she has ever had sex with a male partner and whether it was ever sex without a condom. If she has had unprotected sex with a male, then you might ask her if you can test her today for STDs as part of her routine "well woman" exam.

Sexual Expression of Adolescents

Epidemiology

In 2006, the U.S. Census Bureau, through an American Community Survey, established that there are approximately 21.6 to 21.7 million adolescents of both genders between the ages of 15 and 19. When evaluating the percentage of those who may present in primary care clinics with issues related to gay or lesbian sexual health and accompanying psychosocial issues, social scientists frequently use the rule of thumb that 1 in 10 adolescents is LGBT or otherwise nonheterosexually identified (U.S. Census Bureau, 2006). Closely supporting this estimate, the Kinsey Institute for Sexual Research sponsored a national survey in 2005 that identified nonheterosexual percentages in the American population as 1 in 8 (Kinsey Institute, 2005).

Although it is important to consider that many teens experiment sexually and do not necessarily form a complete sexual orientation until adulthood, a substantial percentage of adolescents who experiment with same-sex partners will eventually identify themselves as gay, lesbian, bisexual, or transgendered. According to the 2005 Kinsey Institute study:

- Among men ages 18–44, 2.3% considered themselves homosexual, 1.8% identified as bisexual, and 3.9% indicated that they identified as "something else."
- Among women between the ages of 18 and 44, 1.3% identified as homosexual, 2.8% considered themselves bisexual, and 3.8% identified as "something else."

Based on these data, there are at least 2.7 million teens with potential to be involved with same-sex partners around the United States. It is important for healthcare providers to be aware of the needs of this segment of the population, as well as to be prepared to educate and be a source of healthy role modeling for this substantial primary care patient population.

The Kinsey Institute's (2005) national survey also found that of the teens surveyed, there was about a one in three chance of having engaged in sexual activity with at least one partner at some point in their lives (Kinsey Institute, 2005):

- *The findings for men of all sexual orientations ages 15–19 years old:* 45.1% had not had sexual contact with a partner, 29.7% reported one partner in 12 months, and 21.8% reported two or more partners in the 12-month period. Men in this same age group reported that 2.4% had engaged in same-sex contact in the previous 12 months, and 4.5% had same-sex contact at some point in their history.
- *The findings for women of all sexual orientations ages 15–19:* 42.9% had not had sexual contact with a partner, 30.5% had sexual contact with one partner, and 16.8% had sexual contact with two or more partners in the last 12 months. For women in this same age group, 2.7% reported having engaged in a same-sex contact during the previous 12 months; 7.7% had same-sex contact at some point in their history.

You ask Cassandra if she and this (or any other) female partner have had sexual relations beyond kissing. This will create an opening to ask her what safe-sex practices she knows for woman–woman sex. (If the patient were a male, you would ask what he knows about safe-sex practices for male–male sex.)

What are the risks of contracting a sexually transmitted infection? ◾

STD prevention and identification are factors in the health care and education of all adolescents. Almost half of the 19 million new cases of STDs each year occur among adolescents and young adults between the ages of 15 and 24.

Clinicians need to be able to provide appropriate health screening services and education for LGBT youth in primary care settings because there may be no available resources for LGBT youth within the community that can provide these services in an atmosphere of respect and trust. If the patient fears a breach of confidentiality or feels uncomfortable, she or he may not want to admit having had sexual contact with a same-sex partner or any partner during a health-screening interview. It remains important for providers to anticipate reticence on the part of adolescents, given the epidemiological data available.

Given the level of sexual activity that adolescents in general participate in without proper education and sexual health awareness, there is, as stated earlier, a huge potential for adolescents to become part of the population with what the Centers for Disease Control and Prevention (CDC) terms "widespread" increases. Infections such as herpes, HPV, trichomoniasis and bacterial vaginosis are on the rise, as well as diseases such as chlamydia, especially in areas where screening and treatment are not readily available. STDs such as syphilis, hepatitis B, and chancroid are declining in incidence.

Although the demographics of the lifestyle and needs of LGBT adolescents remain constant in the United States, the provision of health and education services and resources for the LGBT youth population do not. Many communities provide little or nothing to affirm the psychological personhood of LGBT youth, thus passively contributing to depression and suicide. As well, the failure to screen for STDs and to educate this population on health and safer sex practices contributes to the spread of STDs. This is why the primary care provider has such a pivotal role in assisting these teens toward adulthood in a positive, responsible way of living and engaging in healthy, fulfilling, and responsible practices in relationships.

At this point, you can provide Cassandra with available literature, a demonstration of related products such as dental dams, and a gender-specific discussion on how people of alternative lifestyles practice safer sex.

What other areas are important to assess for LGBT youth? ▨

When you have given time in the discussion for Cassandra to think about any other questions or issues she may have related to safe sex, you mention to her that the other part of having a healthy sex life is to be treated respectfully and to treat one's partner respectfully as well. You let her know that, as her healthcare provider, it is important for you to know whether anyone has ever hurt her or tried to hurt her and how she responded to any incident like this. You tell her that many patients have mentioned this sort of thing and then listen carefully, because if she has ever been abused or disrespected in some way, it may take her time to be able to say it. You ask her if she has thought about hurting herself or hurt herself in the past, and if she is depressed or feeling hopeless or helpless. She clearly says no, so you can move on to the next point.

Depression, Suicide, and Violence

Depression and suicide are among the central health issues associated with gay adolescents. Gay male adolescents are two to three times more likely than their peers to attempt suicide (CDC, 2008). Primary factors in this trend include isolation, domestic abuse, and the lack of role models, which contribute to a profound sense of alienation that then exacerbates the difficulties associated with mainstream adolescence for both boys and girls.

In 1993, the American Academy of Pediatrics' Committee on Adolescence reported that LGBT youth very often find themselves stigmatized and the recipients of others' prejudice. They may find themselves in conflict with their families, communities, and schools. If parents react with anger, shock, or guilt upon learning that their child is gay or lesbian, the youth is left to seek understanding and acceptance by others outside of the home. Social and school environments may be even less supportive; gay and lesbian youth have been subject to name calling, ostracizing, or physical abuse. In the face of this rejection, the youth may become isolated, run away, become depressed, or commit suicide. Given such widespread social difficulty, it is particularly important for healthcare providers to offer a level of openness and acceptance to adolescents struggling with sexual identity. The American Academy of Pediatrics report advises healthcare providers that ". . . any youth struggling with sexual orientation issues should be offered appropriate referrals to providers and programs that can affirm the adolescent's intrinsic worth regardless of sexual identity. Providers who are unable to be objective because of religious or other personal convictions should refer patients to those who can" (American Academy of Pediatrics, 1993).

Sexually Transmitted Diseases

You tell Cassandra that no matter what one's orientation, it is important to be free of sexually transmitted diseases. You remind her that it is important for her and her partner to learn to be totally honest about any potential for disease (such as one of them having herpes, bisexuality, needle drug use, or multiple partners) before having sex. They should encourage each other to discuss which activities feel good and which ones do not.

You ask her if she has more questions right now. She does not, so you proceed to the physical exam. You also let her know that she does not need to take birth control unless she feels that it is something she needs, regardless of what her sisters have done in the past.

The Sexual History and Physical Examination

The practitioner is cautioned to obtain a sensitive and comprehensive history in order to define those areas that require a more extensive examination. Identifying high-risk behaviors or substance abuse will direct the practitioner's focus during the exam.

The physical exam should include an evaluation of the sexual organs (women: breasts, external genitalia, vagina, cervix, uterus, and adnexa; men: penis, scrotum, rectum, and prostate), identifying the stage of puberty, and a thorough skin assessment (paying close attention to possible signs of abuse or trauma, and sexually transmitted diseases).

According to the American Cancer Society (2008), sexually active women should begin cervical cancer screening (Pap smears) about 3 years after they start having sexual relations. If she waits to have sex until she is over 18, she should start screening no later than age 21. Regardless of the young woman's sexual orientation, she should have a regular Pap test yearly or the newer liquid-based Pap test every 2 years. Even though human papillomavirus (HPV) and the genital warts it can cause is very common in men, HPV-related cancers are very rare in men. There is currently no approved test for men.

Making the Diagnosis

Cassandra is moving through the steps necessary to manage a homosexual lifestyle. She seems comfortable with her sexual identity but is having difficulty communicating with her mother about her sexual orientation. She also needs healthcare education related to known health risk factors for lesbian youth.

Management

Cassandra is not currently sexually active and is less than 18 years of age, so you don't do a Pap smear. If she had been sexually active, it would have been appropriate to test for sexually transmitted diseases. These would have included chlamydia, gonorrhea, HSV-1, HSV-2, and trichomoniasis. After the exam, which was normal, you tell Cassandra that your impression is that she and her mother love each other and that this is a new stage in their relationship. This transition to being a woman and being responsible for herself will take openness and understanding from both sides. You ask her if she has someone she can confide in about her sexuality, or if she would like a referral for confidential counseling.

You let Cassandra know that this may be a difficult experience for her mother to understand and that Cassandra may have to be patient with her mother and realize that like many people in the world, her mother may not yet understand and accept that some people live different lifestyles. This lack of understanding could cause her mother to be afraid, to be in denial of the facts for a time, and perhaps to react negatively to Cassandra's preferences. You ask Cassandra to consider that out of love, her mother is trying to assure that Cassandra has as much freedom to grow into womanhood as possible; she does not want a baby to interfere with those things right now, not realizing that Cassandra's choices are different from her sisters. You explain that this transition to her mother's acceptance will take time and honesty on Cassandra's part and that this might also be facilitated by a referral with a mental health counselor where they could talk together about their experiences around this issue.

Cassandra tells you that she thinks she can talk with her mother about her sexuality without a counselor, but promises to come back if she is having difficulty or her mother seems to be too upset.

You encourage Cassandra to come back regularly for her yearly well-woman exams or if any issues arise that you may help with. Provide her with information regarding the HPV vaccine and encourage her to be vaccinated to help prevent cervical cancer and genital warts. At the end of the appointment you give her a handout of resources she can access for more information about sexual orientation and LGBT issues.

Key Points from the Case

1. Adolescents usually establish their sexual identity by the time they reach adolescence, even if they have not had an opportunity to act on it.

2. LGBT adolescents (and adults) may avoid medical care and appropriate health screenings because of a misperception that they are only necessary for heterosexuals.

3. Proper health screening and education is especially important in the primary care setting for LGBT teens because there may be nowhere else available in the community for proper screening and education to occur in an atmosphere of respect and trust.

RESOURCES

Parents, Families and Friends of Lesbians and Gays (PFLAG):
   http://community.pflag.org
Gay and Lesbian Medical Association (GLMA):
   http://www.glma.org
Indiana Youth Group (IYG):
   http://www.indianayouthgroup.org
Lesbian & Gay Child and Adolescent Psychiatric Association, resources:
   http://www.lagcapa.org/Resources.htm
The National Coalition for Gay, Lesbian, Bisexual, and Transgender Youth:
   *http://*www.outproud.org

REFERENCES

American Academy of Child and Adolescent Psychiatry. (1997). *Gay and lesbian teens.* Retrieved June 23, 2008, from http://www.puberty101.com/aacap_gayteens. shtml

American Academy of Pediatrics. (1993). *Homosexuality and adolescence.* Retrieved July 26, 2008, from http://www.medem.com/MedLB/article_detaillb_for_ printer.cfm?article_ID=ZZZUHJP3KAC&sub_cat=269

American Academy of Pediatrics. (1999). *Sexual stereotypes and sexual orientation.* Retrieved June 23, 2008, from http://www.medem.com/search/article_display. cfm?path=\\TANQUERAY\M_ContentItem&tmstr=/M_ContentItem/ZZZNZ1L6W7C. html&soc=AAP&srch_typ=NAV_SERCH

American Academy of Pediatrics, Committee on Adolescence. (1993). Homosexuality and adolescence. *Pediatrics, 92*(4), 631–634.

American Cancer Society. (2008). *Cervical cancer: Prevention and early detection.* Retrieved October 6, 2008, from http://www.cancer.org/docroot/CRI/content/ CRI_2_6x_cervical_cancer_prevention_and_early_detection_8.asp?sitearea=PED

Centers for Disease Control and Prevention. (2007). *CDC fact sheet: Genital HPV.* Retrieved October 6, 2008, from http://www.cdc.gov/std/HPV/hpv-fact-sheet-press.pdf

Centers for Disease Control and Prevention. (2008). *Lesbian, gay, bisexual and transgender health.* Retrieved October 6, 2008, from http://www.cdc.gov/lgbthealth/

Kinsey Institute. (2005). *Frequently asked sexuality questions to the Kinsey Institute.* Retrieved October 5, 2008, from http://www.indiana.edu/~kinsey/ resources/FAQ.html#homosexuality

U.S. Census Bureau. (2006). Arizona. S0902. Teenagers' Characteristics. Retrieved April 21, 2009, from http://factfinder.census.gov/servlet/STTable?_bm=y&-qr_ name=ACS_2006_EST_G00_S0902&-geo_id=04000US04&-ds_name=ACS_ 2006_EST_G00_&-_lang=en

Diseases

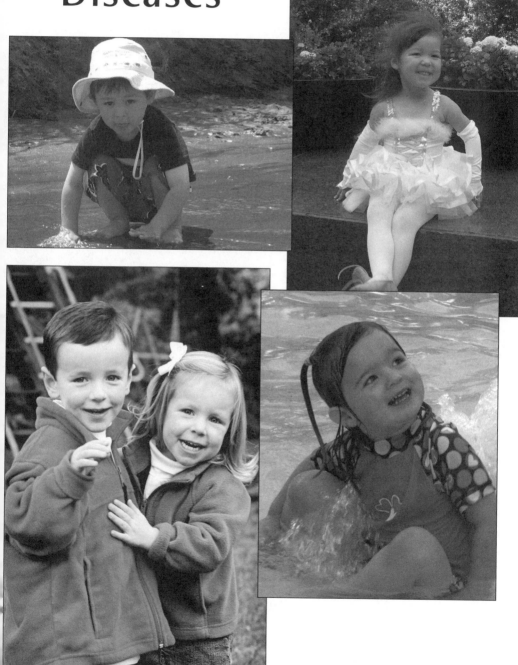

Chapter 16

The Child with a Fever for Six Days

Ritamarie John

Children will often be brought to the primary care provider's office with complaints that seem relatively straightforward and are treated accordingly. The issues for the provider are twofold: maintaining a degree of healthy hesitation in arriving at the diagnosis, and being willing to reevaluate progress, or lack thereof, for the patient who has been sent down a management pathway. The correct diagnosis can sometimes be elusive and require thought and careful consideration of the possible differentials and the most appropriate tests for a problem. In developing a differential diagnosis based on the presentation of the patient, there are sometimes several opportunities where diagnoses can be missed. It is important to use the most specific and sensitive diagnostic tests while keeping in mind their accuracy, precision, and cost. This case will illustrate some of these points.

Educational Objectives

1. Apply key points in the history and physical examination to develop a differential diagnosis.
2. Discuss the variety of pathogens responsible for pharyngitis and infectious mononucleosis.
3. Understand how sensitivity and specificity of laboratory tests aid in the development of the differential diagnosis.
4. Understand how ethnic, cultural, and personal factors play a role in shared decision making when developing a diagnostic and treatment plan.

Case Presentation and Discussion

Maya Santiago is a 7-year-old American with a Peruvian father and a Puerto Rican mother. She presents with a 6-day history of a sore throat associated with fever to 103°F (39.5°C), headache, malaise, painful lymphadenopathy, and overwhelming fatigue. On day three of the illness, Maya was seen for pharyngitis. She was diagnosed with streptococcal pharyngitis after a rapid strep test was positive and was started on Omnicef at 14 mg/kg/day due to a history of rash following Amoxil. The child is worse after 3 days of antibiotic. The mother is concerned that there is something else wrong with the child.

What questions will you need to ask the family related to the presenting complaints? ■

Compliance to medication is an important history point.

The child and mother confirm that they have been taking the antibiotic on a twice a day schedule using a measurer.

In doing a follow-up visit, the healthcare provider can employ the pneumonic NEEDS, which can be a helpful tool to remind the provider about key areas to explore relative to the child's current disposition. NEEDS stands for Nutrition, Elimination, Education/Environment, Development/Daycare, and Sleep/Sexuality.

Nutritionally, the child reports she is able to drink cool liquids, puddings, ice cream, and warm soups. Regarding elimination, she is voiding at least six times a day and has a small, brown, formed stool daily. Education and environment screening indicates that she is in second grade and doing well. She has not been exposed to any sick friends or family members. Concerning development/daycare, she goes to a daycare center for an after-school program as well as being involved in gymnastics 3 days a week, although she has not attended this week. Finally, for sleep assessment, she reports taking at least two naps a day and sleeping 12 hours a night for the past 4 days. Normally she does not take naps and sleeps about 9 hours a night.

Maya's mother reports giving Advil at an appropriate dosage (10 mg/kg/dose) every 6 hours for the persistent fever. She denies the use of any other alternative medication. The child feels worse than she did 3 days ago despite the Advil and the Omnicef. The mother reports that Maya is usually very energetic, and her present behavior is unusual. The mother also denies any history of high persistent fever(s) or serious illnesses in the past.

Due to the lack of response to antibiotic and the presence of lymphadenopathy, fatigue, persistent fever, and tonsillitis, you consider infections such as infectious mononucleosis (IM), which would include signs and symptoms such as Maya's that do not improve with antibiotic treatment.

What other questions do you need to ask Maya and her mother? ▮

Before answering this question, here is some background information about pharyngitis and infectious mononucleosis (IM) that may be helpful to you. Pharyngitis is the third most common complaint in pediatric primary care settings. In this case, the complaint is more complex than a simple pharyngitis and points in the direction of IM with a secondary group A streptococcus infection. You need to consider the pathophysiology, epidemiology, differential diagnosis, and cultural factors before answering this question.

Pathophysiology of Infectious Mononucleosis

A sore throat presents with pain localized to the pharynx, surrounding anatomy, and the neck and is accompanied by dysphasia. The younger the child, the greater the difficulty in identifying the area of painful symptoms. A history of fever and decreased oral intake is one of the signs of pharyngitis in a nontoxic child. There may be accompanying fever, pharyngeal exudates, tonsillar enlargement, uvula inflammation, headache, palatal petechiae, ulcers of the tonsillar pillars, and soft palate, along with anterior cervical lymph node enlargement (Bisno, Gerber, Gwalty, Kaplan, & Schwartz, 2002). The etiology with acute infectious pharyngitis includes bacteria and viruses (see Table 16-1).

IM varies from a simple pharyngitis in that the course is prolonged with fever, lymphadenopathy, and fatigue. Epstein-Barr virus (EBV) is responsible for up to 90% of infectious mononucleosis in adolescent and adults (Hurt & Tammaro, 2007); however, in younger children, the infection is generally subclinical (Hurt & Tammaro; Rezk & Weiss, 2007). The term *IM* indicates a constellation of symptoms that arises from infection with a host of viruses including EBV; however, 10% of IM-like pediatric cases are caused by cytomegalovirus (CMV), human immunodeficiency virus (HIV), or toxoplasmosis infection (Hurt & Tammaro; Smellie et al., 2007). Thus, although the majority of cases of IM are from EBV, other causes need to be considered.

EBV infects the B lymphocytes of the lymphoid-rich areas of the oropharynx, which disseminate the infection in the lymphoreticular system (Rezk & Weiss, 2007). This predilection of EBV to entrench itself within the lymphoreticular system allows for a reservoir of EBV within the B-cells and causes its persistence. The persistence of EBV genes in B-cells results in viral latency and a carrier state (Rezk & Weiss). In addition, EBV-specific cytotoxic T-cell lymphocytes control acute infection and reactivation of infection (Kimura, 2006). This T-cell activation causes production of interleukin 2 and cytokines, causing atypical lymphocytes to appear on a complete blood count (Kimura). The clinical illness of IM may reflect cell damage in the oropharynx caused by viral replication, B-cell proliferation with a rise in cytokine levels, and immunopathology due to the immune response to the virus (Vetsika & Callan, 2004).

CMV has the largest genome size of any virus that infects humans and is a member of the human herpes virus. Human herpes viruses all establish viral latency in the cells they infect; thus, they can reoccur or shed intermittently (Adler & Marshall, 2007). The inner core of viral DNA is contained in a capsid surrounded by a tegument layer and an outer layer composed of glycoproteins. The antigenic glycoproteins trigger an immune response, which includes T-cells (Adler & Marshall). CMV viral DNA can be found in megakaryocytes, monocytes, dendritic cells, and myeloid progenitor cells (Soderberg-Naucler et al., 2001). Reactivation is more likely to occur when the human host is immunosuppressed. Incubation is estimated to be between 1 and 2 months (Adler & Marshall).

Acute infection with HIV was first described as a monolike illness in 1985 (Cooper et al., 1985). After a period of incubation of 2–4 weeks following an acute infection, patients can develop sore throat, malaise, myalgias, arthralgias, nausea, and headache. A nonpruritic maculopapular rash can also be seen (Hurt & Tammaro, 2007).

Toxoplasmosis is the main protozoal cause of a mononucleosis-like illness that can present with rather mild constitutional symptoms of pharyngitis,

Table 16-1   Common Infectious Agents and Acute Pharyngitis

Agent: Bacterial Causes	Clinical Presentation	Most Common Age and Comments
Group A streptococcus	Acute onset with fever Headache Tonsillopharyngitis with exudate Palatal petechiae Nausea and vomiting Abdominal pain Enlarged and tender cervical lymph nodes	5 to 15 years
Mycoplasma pneumoniae	Acute pharyngitis Cough	School age and adolescent
N. gonorrhoeae	Tonsillopharyngitis with erythema, edema or exudate Can appear normal	Relatively rare Sexually active adolescent Sexually abused child School-age child
Non–group A streptococci, usually group C or G	Pharyngitis Fever	
Arcanobacterium haemolyticum	Fever Exudative tonsillopharyngitis Scarlatiniform rash on extensor surfaces that does not peel	Adolescent
Corynebacterium diphtheria	Gradual onset with mild pharyngeal injection and erythema Grey tightly adhering membrane in throat Malaise Low grade fever	Any age Comes from developing countries
Tularemia	Ulcerative-exudative pharyngitis Lymphadenopathy History of ingestion of poorly cooked wild meat or contaminated water	Rare

Agent: Viral Causes	Clinical Presentation	Most Common Age and Comments
Adenovirus	Tonsillopharyngitis If conjunctivitis and high fever, pharyngoconjunctival fever Variable presentation of exudate	Younger children but is highly contagious

Table 16–1 Common Infectious Agents and Acute Pharyngitis (Continued)		
Agent: **Viral Causes**	**Clinical Presentation**	**Most Common Age and Comments**
Influenza	High fever Cough Headache Myalgias Exudative pharyngitis	All ages
Enterovirus	Small vesicles and ulcers in posterior pharynx	1–10 years
Herpes simplex	Exudative pharyngitis with ulcerative lesion on lip Cervical adenopathy Fever	Adolescence
Epstein-Barr virus	Malaise and fatigue Adenopathy Pharyngitis with dysphagia Anorexia with nausea Headache Periorbital edema Palatal enanthem (palatal petechiae) Splenomegaly in up to 60% Jaundice in 5% to 10% Chills with fever Arthralgia and myalgias	Asymptomatic infection in younger children in inner cities Symptomatic infection in adolescents in suburbs
Cytomegalovirus	Fever and fatigue Pharyngitis Diarrhea and abdominal pain Enlarged cervical nodes Splenomegaly Guillain-Barré syndrome	Younger children in daycare Older adolescents who are sexually active
Primary HIV	Acute retroviral syndrome, which mimics IM Occurs days to weeks after exposure	

Sources: Adapted from Fleisher, G. (2008). *Evaluation of sore throat in children.* Retrieved July 3, 2008, from http://www.uptodate.com; Friel, T. J. (2008). *Epidemiology, clinical manifestations, and treatment of cytomegalovirus infection in immunocompetent hosts.* Retrieved July 3, 2008, from http://www. uptodate.com; Hurt, C., & Tammaro, D. (2007). Diagnostic evaluation of mononucleosis like illness. *American Journal of Medicine, 120*(10), 911e1–911e8; Wald, E. (2008). *Approach to diagnosis of acute infectious pharyngitis in children and adolescents.* Retrieved July 1, 2008, from http://www.uptodate.com

maculopapular rashes, nontender cervical or occipital lymphadenopathy, and hepatosplenomegaly. This is a self-limited illness and resolves spontaneously over a few months.

Epidemiology

EBV is transmitted via saliva between individuals and has an incubation period of 4–7 weeks (Vetsika & Callan, 2004). After incubation, pharyngitis, lymphadenopathy, splenomegaly, and fatigue occur. The elevation of transaminases (SGPT, SGOT), indicating a hepatitis, may be evident but jaundice is present in less than 10% of patients (Vetsika & Callan).

CMV is excreted in nearly all body secretions except tears (Adler & Marshall, 2007). Transfusion of CMV-infected blood into a CMV-negative person can cause CMV infection and has been rarely reported as a result of nosocomial contact within a hospital. CMV-caused IM (CMV IM) in children, adolescents, and adults can occur in situations involving close contact with children under age 2 years. Daycare workers and school teachers are at higher risk (Hurt & Tammaro, 2007). Whereas sore throat, fatigue, and malaise are prominent features of IM, CMV IM presents with less prominent lymphadenopathy, pharyngeal erythema, and splenomegaly. Elevated transaminases occur much more commonly with CMV IM.

Toxoplasmosis is found throughout the world, and the members of the cat family are the host. Cats get the infection from eating mice or uncooked meat. The cat sheds the oocyst 3 to 30 days after the ingestion. Transmission also can occur through transfusion or transplantation. Mothers can also transmit the infection to their unborn children. The clinical presentation after the newborn period includes fever, sore throat, lymphadenopathy, and malaise (Pickering, Baker, Long, & McMillan, 2006).

Cultural and Ethnic Aspects

The Hispanic American population is the second largest and fastest-growing population in the United States. To deliver culturally effective pediatric care, the provider needs to understand the beliefs, values, and customs of the population (American Academy of Pediatrics, Committee on Pediatric Workforce, 2004). Flores (2000) identified five normative cultural values that are highly valued by Hispanics and are important to consider in interpersonal interactions:

- *Simpatia*, or kindness expressed to family in times of stress
- *Personalismo*, or formal friendliness
- *Respeto*, or admiration
- *Familismo*, or loyalty to family
- *Fatalsimo*, or the belief that fate cannot be altered

In addition, some Hispanic cultures believe in the "hot–cold" theory and others believe in subtle variations of this theory (Hardwood, 1971). The hot–cold theory of illness is centered on the belief that the body reacts to heat and cold. Some illnesses, often including symptoms of redness or swelling, are classified as hot. Other illnesses such as respiratory infections are cold. Cold illnesses require hot remedies, and hot illnesses are treated with cold foods.

In caring for this family, the provider needs to determine how the parent's ethnic beliefs would affect the care of the child. It is important to show respect for the mother's culture and country as well as formal friendliness by introduction as a primary care provider. It is essential to give an appropriate amount of simpatico about her daughter's illness. **The mother thinks of herself as more American than Puerto Rican and denies belief in the hot–cold theory of disease.**

Differential Diagnosis

The oncological differential diagnosis for infectious mononucleosis includes acute leukemia, Hodgkin's disease, non-Hodgkin's lymphoma, and solid tumors of the neck. The differential diagnosis for pharyngitis includes bacterial, viral, and protozoal causes (see Table 16-1). Many infectious agents have seasonal prevalence, and some infectious agents are more common in different age groups. Allergies can also cause throat pain or pharyngeal tickling, but would not be accompanied by a fever. Acute sinusitis could present with fever, headache, pharyngitis, and cervical adenopathy, but frequently presents with congestion and purulent nasal discharge.

History

From the above review, what other information do you need to obtain? ■

- Are other family members ill or have they been ill in the past 2–3 months?
- Have close friends been ill in the past 2–3 months? (exposure to infectious diseases)
- Is the child in the after-school program involved with the children in the daycare? (exposure to CMV)
- Is the child taking any medication for health? (explores alternative medication use)
- Has the child been in school over the past week? (confirms fatigue and nature of illness)
- Has the child been in contact with pets, especially cats? (looks for toxoplasmosis)
- Has there been any recent travel? (exposure to different infectious agents not seen in the United States)
- Is there any history of sexual assault? (possible HIV exposure)
- Does the child have a history of allergic rhinitis? (allergies)
- Has the family seen any other providers regarding this illness? (integrative medicine approach)

No one has been ill in the household or among the child's close friends. The child is not taking any medications for health and has not been to any other provider. The child is exposed to the daycare children in the after-school program or in her gymnastics class, where the children all use the same equipment. There is no known exposure to cats or other pets. The child has no allergies and has not been sexually assaulted.

What information do you want to collect in your physical examination? ■

Physical Examination: Height, weight, blood pressure, and body mass index are all on the 50th percentile for this Tanner 1 female who has not had any weight loss. The physical examination is remarkable for +3 erythematous tonsils without exudate. There are palatal petechiae on the soft palate. The anterior cervical chain is mildly tender and nodes range in size from 2-2.5 cm. The tonsillar nodes are 2 cm. The nodes are not fixed or mattered. On the right side, there is a 3 cm node on the posterior chain with a few nodes that are less than 1 cm around it. These nodes are not fixed but are tender to touch. There is no axillary, epitrochlear, inguinal, or popliteal nodes. The chest is clear and the heart sounds are normal without murmurs. There is no hepatosplenomegaly or abdominal masses present. The external genitalia is without redness, and the hymenal ring is smooth and without increased redness on gross inspection. The skin is clear without rash or petechiae.

Making the Diagnosis

The history and physical examination are consistent with IM. The family is anxious for laboratory confirmation of the diagnosis.

What initial laboratory diagnostic tests need to be ordered? ■

Laboratory tests are ordered to confirm a suspected diagnosis. Before ordering laboratory tests, consider the following points:

- What is the expense of the test?
- If the patient had no insurance, would you order the test?
- Which test has the lowest cost and will best help you determine the diagnosis?
- Do you know how to interpret the test including sensitivity, specificity, and predictive value for the child's age?
- How will the lab test help you in developing a plan of care for the patient?
- Will the test satisfy the family's concerns and need for further testing?

If the wrong test is ordered, the diagnosis will be delayed. In order to choose a diagnostic test, it is important to consider the test's specificity and sensitivity and to recognize that these can vary with the age of the child. These concepts are explained further in Table 16-2. In trying to determine which test to order, sensitivity, specificity, prevalence, predictive value, and cost must be considered. The main reason to investigate with serology is to confirm the cause of symptoms.

An initial diagnostic strategy would be to do a heterophile antibody test (Bell & Fortune, 2006; Smellie et al., 2007) and a complete blood count (CBC) to look for lymphocytosis and atypical lymphocytes. Each is discussed here.

The Paul Bunnell heterophile antibody is a group of IgM class immunoglobulins that are present when someone has an acute EBV infection. The structurally similar epitropes in the nonhuman RBC (sheep, horse, pig) in the test react

Table 16-2	Understanding Sensitivity and Specificity	
Term	Definition	Memory Mnemonic
Sensitivity	Refers to the number of patients with a condition that test positive. In other words, how effective is this test at picking up patients with the disease compared to a gold standard? • A test with poor sensitivity will miss patients with the condition. Therefore, patients will be incorrectly informed that they do not have a disease. • Also called the true positive rate.	**SNOUT** A high **SeN**sitivity rules **OUT** disease
Specificity	Refers to the number of patients without a condition who correctly test negative when screened. In other words, how effective is the test at accurately excluding people without the condition? • A test with poor specificity will result in a patient being informed that they have a disease, when they are healthy. • Also called the true negative rate.	**SPIN** A high **SP**ecificity rules **IN** disease
Predictive value	Predictive value is determined by the sensitivity and specificity of the test and the prevalence of disease in the population being tested. (Prevalence is defined as the proportion of persons in a defined population at a given point in time with the condition in question.) • The more sensitive a test, the less likely an individual with a negative test will have the disease and thus the greater the negative predictive value. • The more specific the test, the less likely an individual with a positive test will be free from disease and the greater the positive predictive value.	

with the Paul Bunnell heterophile antibody, resulting in red cell agglutination. In adolescents and adults, up to 85% who have clinical IM have detectable Paul Bunnell heterophile antibodies. The antibodies develop during the first week and peak between the second and fifth week of illness (Hurt & Tammaro, 2007). The range of sensitivity for this test is between 71% and 90% (Linderholm, Boman, Juto, & Linde, 1994); however, the results of heterophile antibody testing is lower in children under 12, ranging from 25–50% (Bruu et al., 2000). During the first week of illness, there is a 25% false negative rate (Ebell, 2004).

Rapid Monospot tests are enzyme-linked immunosorbent assay (ELISA) techniques to look for EBV virus infection. Rapid tests may be available in the office depending on insurance reimbursement. Thus, a positive heterophile antibody test or Monospot test indicates that the child has EBV IM; however, a negative Monospot in this girl may mean that the test was done too early in the course of the illness, the child will not react because she is young, or the child has a heterophile-negative mononucleosis-like illness caused by CMV, HIV, or toxoplasmosis. Thus for younger children, this test may not be as helpful.

The CBC during the first week of illness may not show lymphocytosis or increased atypical lymphocytes. As the number of atypical lymphocytes increase, the specificity of the test increases. Remembering the mnemonic **SPIN** helps: A high **SP**ecificity rules **IN** disease. When the number of atypical lymphocytes is greater than 10%, the sensitivity is 75% and the specificity is 92%. When it goes up to greater than 40%, the sensitivity is 25% and the specificity is 100% (Bell & Fortune, 2006). (See Table 16-2.) Thus, the higher the atypical lymphocyte count, the greater the likelihood of IM.

You make a presumptive diagnosis of IM based on Maya's history and clinical findings and begin your discussion with her mother regarding the management plan and laboratory testing that you will do to confirm your IM diagnosis. The reason that a presumptive diagnosis is made at this time is based on the fact that Maya's course of illness is six days in duration and the Monospot test can come back negative during the early course of illness, thus, giving a false negative result.

Management

How do you plan to treat the child's infectious mononucleosis? ■

Therapeutic plan: What will you do therapeutically? ■

The plan is symptom-based and customized to the child's presentation and the family's desires. The goals are to:

- Control fever
- Keep the child hydrated
- Provide enough calories to prevent weight loss
- Allow adequate rest opportunities

- Treat secondary bacterial infections
- Provide opportunities to do school work by coordinating with the school for homework and, if the illness continues, a home tutor
- Avoid splenic rupture by limiting contact play or sports
- Determine the cause of the IM

Treatment Options

Treatment for EBV and CMV IM is symptom based. The use of antipyretics to control fever and keeping the child in light clothing to allow for heat dissipation is important. Appropriate foods and liquids that avoid irritating the throat need to be suggested with cultural sensitivity. Discussing what foods Maya eats and choosing which ones might be tolerated is helpful to the family. Liquids that would be tolerated are selected with input from the family. Because group A streptococcus is a secondary infection for patients with IM, the family is encouraged to finish the Omnicef. At this point, the mother is given a note for the school for school work and the need for a home tutor. Each school system determines the length of time that a child must be out before a home tutor is allowed during a prolonged illness; however, giving the school notice that an illness is likely to be prolonged can help them plan and get the tutor in the house sooner.

There is no medication to treat EBV or CMV IM. The use of acyclovir has not proved to shorten the course of illness (Torre & Tambini, 1999). A recent Cochrane review noted there was insufficient evidence to recommend steroid treatment for symptom control in IM (Candy & Hotopf, 2008). There was also a lack of research on the long-term side effects in patients treated with steroids, including lymphoproliferative disorders (Candy & Hotopf).

Educational plan: What will you do to educate Maya and her family about IM? ■

A discussion with the family about the evaluation for causes and the symptomatic treatment of the IM is important. Points that are raised in the discussion include:

- Explanation of the diagnosis, the variability of the course of IM, and the lack of specific treatment for IM.
- Education regarding dosage of antipyretic and fever management. Discuss fever and keeping the child cool by not using multiple blankets. Also educate regarding the dangers of alcohol baths to reduce fever.
- Explanation of the importance of treating the secondary bacterial infection, despite the fact that it might not make the fever, fatigue, or sore throat disappear.
- Discussion about the possibility of splenic enlargement and that contact play therefore should be avoided, including gymnastics classes.
- Discussion of the importance of hydration, even if the child will not eat food with close monitoring of oral intake and urine output.
- Instructions to monitor for any respiratory problems from enlargement of tonsils and allow for naps as well as a longer sleep period at night.

- You assure the family that you will closely follow up in the office after the laboratory testing is done and will be available by phone for any questions.
- Discuss further laboratory testing to determine the specific infectious agent responsible for the child's IM.

The family wants to know the exact cause of Maya's illness because there are four other children in the household and more than 20 cousins whom the family sees on a regular basis. After discussion of the treatment plan, Maya's mother is instructed to get the lab work done in 2 days to increase the specificity of the testing. The results from day 8 of the illness show a negative Monospot test with a CBC with 78% lymphocytes and 18 atypical lymphocytes. The child returns on day 10 of illness with a predominance of fatigue and fever. The child still complains of a sore throat and painful lymph nodes. The physical examination is unchanged and no hepatosplenomegaly is found. You decide to do additional laboratory testing. Liver function tests and EBV-specific antibodies are ordered to confirm the suspected diagnosis of EBV mononucleosis.

EBV-specific antibodies include IgM and IgG against the viral capsid antigen (VCA), Early antigen (EA) diffuse staining, and EBV nuclear antigen (EBNA). The two tests that are most helpful in diagnosing active and recent infections are the IgM anti-VCA and the EA. IgM levels go up in acute infection and decrease over 3 months. Early antigens are present at the onset of clinical illness and decrease as the infection resolves, usually over 6 weeks. Early antigens are not present once the symptomatic period is ended. Another antibody that can be assayed is IgG antibodies to viral capsid antigen, which will rise 6 to 12 weeks following the EBV infection and remain elevated for life (Ebell, 2004). EBNA are long-term antibodies that do not rise until several weeks to months after the onset of infection. These are not found in acute infection and are a marker of EBV infection in the past (Pickering et al., 2006).

CMV can also cause elevation of the IgM antibodies to VCA. The sensitivities of the tests range from 95% to 100% and the specificities of the test range from 90% to 100%, depending on the laboratory test manufacturer (Bruu et al., 2000).

The results of laboratory testing done on day 10 of Maya's illness are back. The child's tests for IgM VCA, EA, IgG VCA, and EBNA are all negative. The aminotransferases (AST and ALT) are both elevated five times above normal, reflecting a mild hepatitis. The bilirubin and alkaline phosphatase levels are within normal limits, indicating no biliary obstruction. The family is called with the results of the serology and is asked to return in 2 days for reevaluation. At this time, the fever is starting to come down but the fatigue persists. The diagnosis of EBV-negative mononucleosis is considered, and given the attendance at a daycare center after-school program and the predominance of fatigue and fever in the presentation, CMV serology for anti-CMV IgM and IgG is ordered (see Table 16-3). The family persists in wanting to know the exact cause of the illness and wants the additional serology tests done. The plan is to continue to symptomatically treat the child's fever with Advil, allow for rest, provide fluids and foods the child can tolerate, keep the child home from school, limit rough play, and maintain infection control measures to prevent household spread.

Table 16-3 Laboratory Testing in Infectious Mononucleosis (IM)

Name of Test	What You Are Looking For	Sensitivity and Specificity of Test	Comments
Complete blood count with differential	Lymphocytosis with an absolute count > 4,500 cells/mm^3	Depends on when it was drawn during the disease and the clinical presentation consistent with IM.	May be normal in the first week. Likely to have lymphocytosis with atypicals after this.
Atypical lymphocytes	> 10% atypical lymphocytes The higher the number, the more likely the patient has IM.	With a positive heterophile antibody: • Sensitivity ranges from 75% to 25% with an atypical lymphocyte count from > 10% to > 40%. • Specificity ranges from 92% to 100% with an atypical lymphocyte count from > 10% to > 40%. • Specificity and sensitivity of 61% and 95%, respectively, with ≥ 50% lymphocytes and ≥ 10% atypical lymphocytes	The more atypical lymphocytes with a clinical manifestation of IM, the more likely the patient has IM.
Heterophile antibodies	Positive	In adolescents, range of sensitivity is between 71% and 90%. In children under 12, range of sensitivity is from 25–50%.	Depends on age of child
Rapid Monospot test	Positive result	Sensitivity depends on age of child, as seen above.	

(continues)

Table 16-3	Laboratory Testing in Infectious Mononucleosis (IM) (Continued)		
Name of Test	What You Are Looking For	Sensitivity and Specificity of Test	Comments
Early antigen	Elevation	Sensitivities of the tests range from 95% to 100% and specificities range from 90% to 100%, depending on the laboratory test manufacturer.	More accurate test to diagnose EBV IM in younger children, particularly less than 5 years
IgM viral capsid antigen (VCA)	Elevation		
IgG VCA	Can have elevation or no elevation		
EBNA	No elevation in acute infection		

Sources: Adapted from Bruu, A., Hietland, R., Holter, E., Mortensen, L., Natas, O., Petterson, W., et al. (2000). Evaluation of 12 commercial tests for detection of Epstein-Barr virus specific and heterophile antibodies. *Clinical Diagnostic Laboratory Immunology, 7*(3), 451–456; Ebell, M. H. (2004). Epstein-Barr virus infectious mononucleosis. *American Family Physician, 70*(7), 1270–1287; Hurt, C., & Tammaro, D. (2007). Diagnostic evaluation of mononucleosis like illness. *American Journal of Medicine, 120*(10), 911e1–911e8; Linderholm, M., Boman, J., Juto, P., & Linde, A. (1994). Comparative evaluation of nine kits for rapid diagnosis of infectious mononucleosis and Epstein-Barr virus specific serology. *Journal of Clinical Microbiology, 32*, 259–261.

Sources of Diagnostic Error

In developing an initial differential diagnosis, the clinician's past experience plays a significant role in what diagnostic possibilities are considered (Redelmeier, 2005). Other pitfalls include a reliance on initial impression and not reconsidering other diagnoses in light of new data obtained during reevaluations as well as making a decision about a diagnosis based on how the information is presented (framing). Framing effects cause small changes in wording to alter management decisions (Redelmeier). Additionally, clinicians can rely heavily on diagnostic technology or an assertive colleague's opinion. To overcome these possibilities, a person must reconsider their diagnostic options when the colleague is more distant. Lastly, the clinician may prematurely close the diagnostic possibilities; this is known as premature closure (Redelmeier). In this case, the predominance of fever, fatigue, lack of exudative tonsillitis, and significant elevations of transaminases all pointed to CMV (Hurt & Tammaro, 2007). Because most cases of IM are EBV related, the diagnosis needed to be reconsidered in light of the negative serology and the persistent illness.

The serology to diagnose CMV includes anti-CMV IgM, spin-amplified urine culture for CMV with pp65 antigen detection, and CMV PCR. In this case, the least expensive test was ordered because the child was slowly improving. The anti-CMV IgM was significantly elevated.

The results come back on day 21 of illness; the child's fever is effervescing, and the child is starting to take shorter naps. The school is sending in a tutor and the child is able to stay up for longer periods. A reevaluation is done after 7 days. One month after the initial presentation, the child is improved enough to go back to school, but gymnastics classes are not allowed during the first week of resumed school attendance to make sure the child is able to handle school academics before gymnastics is added.

When should the child with IM be allowed to participate in sports? ◼

Splenic rupture is most common within 4 to 21 days after the onset of symptoms (Waninger & Harcke, 2005). Usually during the first few weeks of infection, there is spleen enlargement as a result of lymphocytic infiltration. Although splenomegaly is more common with EBV IM, it can occur with heterophile-negative mononucleosis (Hurt & Tammaro, 2007). Although some authors recommend imaging the spleen prior to return to play, there is variability in the normal size of the spleen in children (Waninger & Harcke). Clearly before an athlete returns to play, he or she should be afebrile, well hydrated, and free from the symptoms of IM. Splenic rupture after 28 days of the onset of illness is rare, but still can occur (Waninger & Harcke). It is important to limit activity in the first 21 days and then, in an asymptomatic athlete, allow a gradual return to play while avoiding activities that put the spleen at risk. The return to full activity should be paced depending on the individual presentation; abrupt increases in exercise should be avoided.

Maya adds one class of gymnastics per week over the next 3 weeks and recovers uneventfully from her CMV IM. The child is followed up 1 month after school was resumed. The family appreciates the concern for the child's condition.

Key Points from the Case

1. When developing a differential diagnosis, it is important to reevaluate your initial impression based on the developing clinical presentation.
2. Diagnostic testing must be done in an organized fashion considering the most likely diagnosis based on history and physical examination.
3. Sensitivity, specificity, and predictive value are important to consider in the interpretation of laboratory testing.
4. Ethnic, cultural, and personal beliefs must be considered in developing a plan of care for the pediatric patient.

REFERENCES

Adler, S. P., & Marshall, B. (2007). Cytomegalovirus. *Pediatrics in Review, 28*(3), 92–100.

American Academy of Pediatrics, Committee on Pediatric Workforce. (2004). *Ensuring culturally effective pediatric care: Implications for education and health policy.* Retrieved August 2, 2008, from http://aappolicy.aappublications.org/cgi/reprint/pediatrics;114/6/1677.pdf

Bell, A. T., & Fortune, B. (2006). What test is the best for diagnosing infectious mononucleosis? *Journal of Family Practice, 55*(9), 799–802.

Bisno, A. L., Gerber, M. A., Gwalty, J. M., Kaplan, E., & Schwartz, R. H. (2002). Practice guidelines for the diagnosis and the management of group A streptococcal pharyngitis. Infectious Disease Society of America. *Clinical Infectious Diseases, 35*, 113–125.

Bruu, A., Hietland, R., Holter, E., Mortensen, L., Natas, O., Petterson, W., et al. (2000). Evaluation of 12 commercial tests for detection of Epstein-Barr virus specific and heterophile antibodies. *Clinical Diagnostic Laboratory Immunology, 7*(3), 451–456.

Candy, B., & Hotopf, M. (2008). Steroids for symptom control in infectious mononucleosis. *Cochrane Database of Systematic Reviews, 2.*

Cooper, D. A., Gold, J., Maclean, P., Donovan, B., Finlayson, R., Barnes, T. G., et al. (1985). Acute AIDS retrovirus infection. Definition of a clinical illness associated with seroconversion. *Lancet, 1*(8428), 537–540.

Ebell, M. H. (2004). Epstein-Barr virus infectious mononucleosis. *American Family Physician, 70*(7), 1270–1287.

Fleisher, G. (2008). *Evaluation of sore throat in children.* Retrieved July 3, 2008, from http://www.uptodate.com

Flores, G. (2000). Culture and the patient-physician relationship: Achieving cultural competency in health care. *Journal of Pediatrics, 136*(1), 14–23.

Friel, T. J. (2008). *Epidemiology, clinical manifestations, and treatment of cytomegalovirus infection in immunocompetent hosts.* Retrieved July 3, 2008, from http://www.uptodate.com

Hardwood, A. (1971). The hot-cold theory of disease: Implications for treatment of Puerto Rican patients. *Journal of the American Medical Association, 216*(7), 1153–1158.

Hurt, C., & Tammaro, D. (2007). Diagnostic evaluation of mononucleosis-like illness. *American Journal of Medicine, 120*(10), 911e1–911e8.

Kimura, H. (2006). Pathogenesis of chronic active Epstein-Barr virus infection: Is this an infectious disease, lymphoproliferative disorder, or immunodeficiency? *Review of Medical Virology, 16*, 251–261.

Linderholm, M., Boman, J., Juto, P., & Linde, A. (1994). Comparative evaluation of nine kits for rapid diagnosis of infectious mononucleosis and Epstein-Barr virus specific serology. *Journal of Clinical Microbiology, 32*, 259–261.

Pickering, L. K., Baker, C. J., Long, S. S., & McMillan, J. A. (Eds.). (2006). *Red book: 2006 report of the Committee on Infectious Diseases* (27th ed., pp. 286–288, 666–670). Elk Grove Village, IL: American Academy of Pediatrics.

Redelmeier, D. (2005). The cognitive psychology of missed diagnosis. *Annals of Internal Medicine, 142*, 115–120.

Rezk, S., & Weiss, L. (2007). Epstein-Barr virus lymphoproliferative disorders. *Human Pathology, 38*, 1293–1304.

Smellie, W. S., Forth, J., Smart, S., Galloway, M. J., Irving, W., Bareford, D., et al. (2007). Best practice in primary care pathology: Review 7. *Journal of Clinical Pathology, 60*, 458–465.

Soderberg-Naucler, C., Streblow, D. N., Fish, K. N., Allan-Yorke, J., Smith, P. P., & Nelson, J. A. (2001). Reactivation of latent human cytomegalovirus in CD14(+) monocytes is differentiation dependent. *Journal of Virology, 75*(16), 7543–7554.

Torre, D., & Tambini, R. (1999). Acyclovir for treatment of infectious mononucleosis: A metaanalysis. *Scandinavian Journal of Infectious Disease, 31*, 543–548.

Vetsika, E., & Callan, M. (2004). Infectious mononucleosis and Epstein-Barr virus. *Expert Reviews in Molecular Medicine, 23*(5), 1–16.

Wald, E. (2008). *Approach to diagnosis of acute infectious pharyngitis in children and adolescents*. Retrieved July 1, 2008, from http://www.uptodate.com

Waninger, K., & Harcke, H. T. (2005). Determination of safe return to play for athletes recovering from infectious mononucleosis: A review of the literature. *Clinical Journal of Sport Medicine, 15*(6), 410–416.

Chapter 17

The Wheezing Child

Deborah A. Bohan

Wheezing is a common presenting symptom of respiratory illness in children. Although the most frequent cause of wheezing in children is asthma, conditions in the respiratory, gastrointestinal, cardiovascular, and other systems can cause children to have problems exchanging air. Problems can range from minimal to life-threatening in severity. The primary care provider needs to sort it all out efficiently, effectively, and inexpensively with the least stress possible to the child and family. Obtaining a detailed history (including family history) and focused physical exam will help in making an accurate diagnosis.

Educational Objectives

1. Describe the prevalence and epidemiology of asthma.
2. Understand the definition of asthma and describe its pathophysiology.
3. Recognize the symptoms of asthma.
4. Establish an appropriate asthma management plan based on new National Heart, Lung and Blood Institute (NHLBI) guidelines.

Case Presentation and Discussion

James Washington is a 4-year-old black male who recently moved to the area with his family. James comes to your office with his mother, Mary Washington, with a chief complaint of difficulty breathing and cough. His symptoms started this morning shortly after waking up, although his mom says he has had some congestion and a runny nose for the past 2–3 days.

History

The important parts of the history in a child with wheezing depend, in part, upon whether a diagnosis such as asthma has been made previously and the reason for the current evaluation. Is this an initial diagnosis, a disease monitoring visit, or an acute exacerbation? In the case of a wheezing child, the history should focus on the presenting symptoms, precipitating factors, and typical symptom patterns.

What other historical data do you need to collect from James? ■

Important additional information to obtain includes:

- Previous history of dyspnea, wheezing, or persistent cough
- Previous office, clinic, or emergency department visits for this same complaint
- Previous hospitalizations or intubations
- Whether steroids were ever prescribed and, if so, last course and for how long
- Precipitating factors
- General medical history, including medications and immunizations

James has had four or five similar episodes over the past 2 years that resulted in unscheduled visits to his former pediatrician's office. Each time, James was sent home with a prescription for an albuterol inhaler to be used as needed. According to Mom, he has a lot of "colds" year round, and they seem to last for a long time. During these episodes, James often wakes up at night coughing. His daycare providers have noticed that he will often start to cough while playing and has to stop his activity to "catch his breath."

James was born at 39 weeks gestational age via a normal spontaneous vaginal delivery. He has no significant medical illnesses other than the wheezing. He has never been prescribed steroids nor hospitalized overnight. He takes no medications other than the albuterol as described, has no known drug allergies, and his immunizations are up to date by record review. He has no complaints of vomiting, heartburn, or hoarseness, and actively engages in vigorous running games with his playmates when "his asthma" is not acting up.

James lives with his parents and an older sister. There is a history of secondhand smoke exposure—Mom smokes in the house. They have one dog, two cats, and a hamster (all house pets).

Dad was diagnosed with asthma as a child but "grew out of it." He still has environmental allergies to dust and pollens and takes an over-the-counter antihistamine as needed.

Wheezing and Asthma in the Child

Many aspects of current and past history as well as physical examination can help the clinician distinguish between transient wheezing and asthma in the young child and confirm asthma in the older child. Although many parents confuse wheezing with upper airway congestion or noisy breathing, a history of previous healthcare provider–diagnosed wheezing is helpful to confirm true wheeze. Most wheezing and coughing in children occurs in association with viral illnesses, but wheezing or coughing apart from obvious infection, such as with exercise, activity, exposure to allergens, or exposure to environmental tobacco smoke, suggests more persistent disease. Additionally, coughing that has responded to bronchodilator therapy is consistent with an asthma cough. Frequent nocturnal coughing may be associated with more severe asthma.

Past medical history, including birth history, prematurity, and history of oxygen requirement or mechanical ventilation, documents important factors that can help differentiate other conditions seen in pediatric patients with recurrent respiratory symptoms. This is especially relevant because often non-atopic infants can have bronchopulmonary dysplasia and airway hyperresponsiveness similar to asthma with a different underlying pathophysiology. Determining the severity of previous respiratory episodes, including urgent or emergent care, hospitalization, and hypoxia, helps the clinician quantify symptom control and potentially predict subsequent episodes. Previous response to therapy, including bronchodilators and steroids (both inhaled and systemic), can also help confirm a diagnosis of asthma. Finally, a prior history of other allergic conditions increases the risk for developing asthma.

The evaluation of a child with recurrent respiratory symptoms should include a thorough review of the family medical history and environmental exposures. A history of healthcare provider–diagnosed asthma in a parent is an important risk factor for persistent wheezing in children. Reviewing the family history for the presence of other atopic disease, such as allergic rhinitis, food allergy, and eczema, can help to establish an atopic genetic background for the patient.

An environmental history should document the presence of potential allergens in the home, including pets and cockroaches; the use of allergen covers for mattresses and pillows; the frequency of cleaning bed linens; and the presence of carpets, upholstered furniture, and stuffed animals. Other potential sources of irritation in the home include tobacco smoke, fireplaces, home heating systems, and home cooling systems. As mentioned earlier, children sensitized to certain allergens are more likely to have asthma.

Overview of Asthma

Asthma is the leading serious chronic illness of children in the United States and the most common chronic disease of childhood. Asthma can be difficult to identify in many cases because of its complexity and heterogeneity; therefore, clinicians need to understand the pathophysiology and natural history of the disease along with the diversity of patient response in order to make an early diagnosis and develop an appropriate management strategy (Centers for Disease Control and Prevention [CDC], 2006a, 2006b).

Epidemiology of Asthma

The following are some pediatric asthma statistics:

- In 2006, an estimated 6.8 million children under age 18 (almost 1.2 million under age 5) were diagnosed with asthma (CDC, 2006b).
- The highest current prevalence rate was seen in those 5–17 years of age (106.3 per 1,000 population), with rates decreasing with age. Overall, the rate in those under 18 years (92.8 per 1,000) was much greater than those over 18 years (72.4 per 1,000) (CDC, 2006b).

- Approximately 12.8 million school days are missed annually due to asthma (CDC, 2006a)
- Asthma has the following impact annually on the medical community (CDC, 2006a):
  - 12.7 million physician visits
  - 1.9 million asthma-related emergency room visits
  - 5,000 deaths
- Asthma has the following annual financial impact:
  - Direct healthcare costs of more than $11.5 billion
  - Indirect healthcare costs of $4.6 billion
  - Prescription drug costs of $5 billion

The statistics on pediatric asthma are quite alarming. More than 9 million U.S. children have been diagnosed with asthma. The prevalence of asthma has increased 75% over the past two decades, and in children under the age of 5 years, asthma rates have increased more than 160%. This has resulted in more than 12 million missed school days annually and a tremendous financial burden in healthcare-related costs (more than $20 billion annually) (CDC, 2006a, 2006b).

The morbidity related to asthma is staggering. People with asthma miss more days at work or school than the average American. Asthma patients and their families spend on average $1,000 per year on medications. The annual cost of asthma in 1998 was estimated to be $11.3 billion, with hospitalizations accounting for most of these costs. The costs associated with asthma continue to increase (Asthma and Allergy Foundation, 2000).

Racial differences in the prevalence of asthma have been demonstrated in the data collected by the National Center for Health Statistics (2002). There continue to be racial and ethnic differences in asthma prevalence and healthcare use and mortality. In 2004, the lifetime prevalence of asthma in persons younger than 14 years of age was highest in the black population with a prevalence of 12.5% in comparison with 7.1% in Hispanics and 7.5% in whites.

An analysis of data from the National Health and Nutrition Examination Survey III (NHANES; CDC, 2002) showed low education status, female sex, current or past smoking history, pet ownership, atopy, and obesity all to be associated with an increased prevalence of asthma. The effect of socioeconomic status on asthma prevalence was further illustrated by this study. There was a statistically significant difference in the prevalence of asthma noted in non-Hispanic black children from families with income less than half the federal poverty level. This difference remained significant even in comparison with non-Hispanic white children from very poor families. The difference in prevalence rates can be postulated to be caused by environmental exposures that are unique to children from poor families that increase the risk of developing bronchial hyperreactivity and asthma. This difference in environmental exposures can be related to the percentage of disadvantaged black children who live in urban areas rather than rural areas. The population at highest risk for asthma is African American children from poor urban neighborhoods (Simon et al., 2003; Smith et al., 2005).

Studies have shown a relationship between parental smoking and childhood asthma. There seems to be an increased risk of early onset asthma in children exposed to tobacco smoke with an increased incidence of wheezing until age 6 years (Strachan & Cook, 1998; Weitzman, Gortmaker, Walker, & Sobol, 1990). The National Health Interview Survey (NHIS) data collected in 1981 show an increased risk of asthma in children under the age of 5 whose mothers smoked at least one half pack of cigarettes per day (odds ratio 2.1, $P = 0.001$) (Weitzman et al., 1990). In addition, the American Academy of Pediatrics (1997) policy statement on the hazards of environmental tobacco smoke to children's health clearly documents the particularly deleterious effect of tobacco smoke on children's lungs. This policy statement notes the negative effect that parental smoking has on both the frequency of exacerbations and the severity of asthma symptoms in their children. Furthermore, when parents reduce the secondhand smoke exposure to their children, the child's asthmatic symptoms are not as severe.

Pathophysiology of Asthma

Asthma is a chronic inflammatory disease characterized by episodic and reversible symptoms. The impact of respiratory infections on asthma incidence is an area of debate. The hygiene hypothesis, proposed by Strachan (1989), is based on the concept that immune responses are mediated by two types of lymphocyte populations: T-helper 1 and T-helper 2 cells. T-helper 1 lymphocytes produce interferon-γ and interleukin-2, and T-helper 2 lymphocytes produce interleukins that can lead to the development of IgE-mediated atopy and allergy. The exposure to airway infections and allergens early in life promotes the maturation of T-helper 1 lymphocytes over T-helper 2 lymphocytes, thereby decreasing the risk of developing allergic conditions (Gore & Custovic, 2005). Persons living in more rural environments may be exposed to allergens early in life with the development of increased T-helper 1 lymphocyte population and less atopy and asthma. There have been several studies supporting this theory as well as studies contradicting these findings (McDonnell et al., 1999; Strachan, Butland, & Anderson, 1996). The varied conclusions may be a result of the intensity, the timing, and the duration of the exposure. The underlying genetic susceptibility of the individual may also contribute to whether a particular exposure in childhood leads to the development of asthma later in life (King, Mannino, & Holguin, 2004). The most frequently cultured infectious pathogens in asthmatics undergoing bronchoscopy with bronchoalveolar lavage are viruses (adenovirus, parainfluenza, influenza, and respiratory syncytial virus), *Mycoplasma pneumoniae*, and *Chlamydia pneumoniae* (Kraft, 2000; Martin et al., 2001; McDonald, Schoeb, & Lindsey, 1991).

Asthma has been suspected to have a strong genetic component, with studies demonstrating increased prevalence of asthma among first-degree relatives of asthmatic subjects (20–25%) versus a general population prevalence (of 4%) (Sandford, Weir, & Pare, 1996; Scirica & Celedon, 2007; Sibbald & Turner-Warwick, 1979). Asthma is regarded as a "complex" disease (i.e., one shaped by many genes and environmental factors that interact to determine susceptibility). The components of the asthma phenotype are passed down through families in complex patterns, but the genes responsible for these inherited components have not yet been identified. The disease appears to result from gene–environment and/or gene–gene interactions; however, it is unknown how many genes may be involved in asthma susceptibility and the strength of their effects. Another possibility is that a large number of genes can contribute to the development of asthma in a population, but that a small subset of genes may shape the disease in affected individuals.

The pathophysiology of asthma involves the following components:

- Airway inflammation
- Intermittent airflow obstruction
- Bronchial hyperresponsiveness

Some of the principal cells identified in airway inflammation include mast cells, eosinophils, epithelial cells, macrophages, and activated T lymphocytes. T lymphocytes play an important role in the regulation of airway inflammation through the release of numerous cytokines (see Figure 17-1). Airflow obstruction can be caused by a variety of changes, including acute bronchoconstriction, airway edema, chronic mucous plug formation, and airway

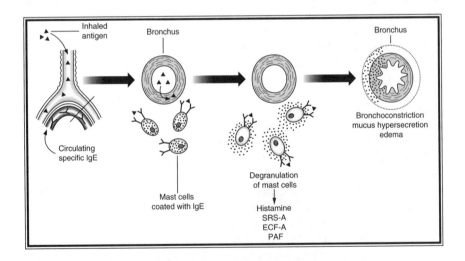

Figure 17-1   Key elements of the pathophysiology of asthma.

From Busse, W. W., O'Bryne, P. M., Holgate, S. T. (2006). Asthma pathogenesis. In: N. F. Adkinson, Jr., J. W. Yunginger, W. W. Busse, B. S. Bochner, S. T. Holgate, F. E. R. Simons, (Eds.), *Middleton's allergy: Principles and practice*, (6th ed., Chapter 66). St. Louis, MO: Mosby. Used with permission.

remodeling. Acute bronchoconstriction is the consequence of immunoglobulin E–dependent mediator release upon exposure to aeroallergens and is the primary component of the early asthmatic response. Airway edema occurs 6–24 hours following an allergen challenge and is referred to as the late asthmatic response. Chronic mucous plug formation consists of an exudate of serum proteins and cell debris that may take weeks to resolve. Airway remodeling is associated with structural changes due to long-standing inflammation and may profoundly affect the extent of reversibility of airway obstruction (Busse, O'Bryne, & Holgate, 2006).

Other Common Causes of Wheezing in Children

Classically, with an acute asthma exacerbation, the child presents with wheezing and respiratory distress. Bronchospasm can also present as cough, chest pain, shortness of breath, and fatigue with exertion.

Asthma is the most likely cause of recurrent wheezing in children younger than 5 years. The most common causes of wheezing in young children are asthma, allergies, gastroesophageal reflux disease, infections, and obstructive sleep apnea. Response to bronchodilators may help differentiate asthma from other causes of wheezing. Chest radiography should be performed in children with recurrent wheezing or a single episode of unexplained wheezing that does not respond to bronchodilators. (See Table 17-1.)

Table 17-1   Causes of Wheezing in Children and Infants

Common	Uncommon	Rare
Allergies	Bronchopulmonary dysplasia	Bronchiolitis obliterans
Asthma or reactive airway disease	Foreign body aspiration	Congenital vascular abnormalities
Gastroesophageal reflux disease		Congestive heart failure
Infections		Cystic fibrosis
Bronchiolitis		Immunodeficiency diseases
Bronchitis		Mediastinal masses
Pneumonia		Primary ciliary dyskinesia
Upper respiratory infection		Tracheobronchial anomalies
Obstructive sleep apnea		Tumor or malignancy
		Vocal cord dysfunction

Sources: Data from Martinati L. C., & Boner, A. L. (1995). Clinical diagnosis of wheezing in early childhood. *Allergy, 50*(9), 701; National Heart, Lung and Blood Institute, National Asthma Education and Prevention Program. (2007). *Expert panel report 3: Guidelines for the diagnosis and management of asthma.* Washington, DC: Author.

Infant Wheezers

Many infants wheeze early in life. Risk factors for persistent wheezing and a predisposition to asthma include:

- Frequent symptoms in the first 12 months of life
- Eczema
- Elevated IgE levels
- Maternal history of asthma
- Maternal smoking

Child Wheezers

More than 85% of wheezing episodes in children are triggered by viral infections. The prevalence of asthma in school-age children in the United States is now estimated to be 9%, having doubled in about 20 years. Wheezing is extremely common, occurring in at least 50% of children, but in the absence of dyspnea or effects on sleep or activities, wheezing is not likely to be caused by asthma. Wheezing in early childhood is associated with bronchial hyperreactivity and reduced lung function in later life, and may be a reason for early intervention and maintenance medication. Children who have severe intermittent wheezing usually develop atopy. There also are transient wheezers, who usually clear by age 3, and nonatopic wheezers who do not seem to develop later asthma, although they may continue to wheeze occasionally when older.

Suspicion of asthma is increased when any one or several historical factors are present (Bush, 2007; Graham, 2006):

- Three or more episodes of otitis media (1.5 times increased risk)
- Pneumonia (1.8 times increased risk)
- Atopic dermatitis (1.9 times increased risk)
- Family asthma history (2 times increased risk)
- Laryngotracheitis (2 times increased risk)
- Allergic rhinitis (2.2 times increased risk)
- Any wheezing in first 3 years (3.3 times increased risk)
- Sinusitis (3.5 times increased risk)
- Family sinusitis history (3.9 times increased risk)
- Recurrent wheezing in first 3 years (4.7 times increased risk)
- Recurrent wheezing in years 4 through 6 (15 times increased risk)

The disease process is variable both from person to person and in each person from episode to episode. At one extreme, sufferers are continuously ill and are frequently in and out of the hospital; at the other extreme symptoms are rare, intermittent, often mild, and sometimes unrecognized. Milder symptoms of asthma often blend into those of allergic bronchitis that often accompanies allergic rhinitis (Akinbami & Schoendorf, 2002; Hopp et al., 1988). This variation can make diagnosis of certain patients extremely challenging, and the history and physical exam should be tailored to exclude other causes of wheezing, as listed earlier.

Despite the myriad causes of wheezing in children, presumptive clinical diagnosis usually is possible by obtaining a thorough clinical history and examination.

What physical examination data do you want to collect? ■

On physical examination, James has a nonproductive cough and some audible wheezing. His height is at the 45th percentile and his weight is at the 50th percentile with a body mass index of 17 placing him just below the 85th percentile. He is afebrile with a heart rate of 92 and a respiratory rate of 24 with mild accessory muscle use but no retractions. His oxygen saturation on room air is 92%. His head, eyes, ears, nose, and throat examination is normal except for boggy turbinates with some clear rhinorrhea and slight postnasal drainage. His tone of his voice is normal with no hoarseness noted; no visible caries nor dental erosion noted and his neck is supple with full range of motion and no lymphadenopathy. On ausculation of his lungs there are expiratory wheezes in all lung fields and an increased expiratory phase. Overall air movement is good. James's cardiac exam reveals a regular rate and rhythm without murmurs or gallops. Radial and femoral pulses are 2+ bilaterally. The abdomen is scaphoid with good bowel sounds and there is no tenderness to palpation, masses, or hepatosplenomegaly. The remainder of the physical exam is normal.

Should you do diagnostic studies? ■

You pause for a moment to consider what, if any, diagnostic studies you should do. Based upon a negative history (no complaints of vomiting, heartburn, painful belching, or recurrent pneumonias) and the lack of physical findings (no hoarseness, tenderness, tooth erosion, or masses), you have no evidence that his wheezing is due to gastroesophageal reflux or a tumor. His cardiac examination is normal, making a cardiovascular condition also unlikely. You are comfortable with your diagnosis of asthma. However, James does have a history of multiple episodes of wheezing and no history of having had a chest X-ray which leaves you somewhat uncomfortable. Thus, the healthcare provider may consider obtaining an initial chest radiograph to rule out other pulmonary pathology. Given this child's history, you decide to order a chest X-ray (PA and lateral), which reveals a normal cardiothymic silhouette, normal orientation of the great vessels, and mild hyperexpansion. Because of the father's history of dust and pollen allergies, you also order a radioallergosorbent test (RAST) along with a total IgE level.

Making the Diagnosis

The 2007 guidelines from the National Asthma Education and Prevention Program (NAEPP); National Heart, Lung and Blood Institute; and National Asthma Education and Prevention Program Expert Panel Report 3 (EPR-3) are moving away from the initial severity classification to a classification based on disease control. Asthma "severity" refers to the underlying intensity of the disease before treatment is initiated, and it is important to remember that severity and control are related.

Based on the EPR-3 guidelines, the provider must first determine the severity of the asthma. After the child's asthma becomes well controlled on medication (plus the elimination of environmental triggers as much as possible), the provider then determines classification based on the lowest level of treatment needed to maintain control. This second classification is made after a period of time in which the provider follows the child. The National Heart Lung and Blood Institute (2007) provides assessment guidelines for the clinician about evaluating components of asthma severity and asthma control (See Tables 17-2 and 17-3).

Classification of the Severity of James' Asthma

Based upon his history, physical examination, and environmental and family risk factors, James was diagnosed with an asthma exacerbation with underlying mild persistent asthma.

Management

Medication Management

Having determined the asthma severity level that James is experiencing based on his history and physical examination findings, you are ready to identify an appropriate medication plan. You prescribe a short burst of oral steroids and an inhaled short acting beta$_2$-agonists (SABA) to treat his acute asthma symptoms and this exacerbation. Oral systemic steroids are used to quickly treat the inflammatory response. A SABA provides quick relief of bronchospasm, relaxing airway smooth muscles, which results in a prompt increase in airflow. A spacer is used so that a higher proportion of small, respirable particles are inhaled rather than having particles from the MDI deposited in the oropharynx. This is particularly important for children who receive inhaled medication via MDI devices.

Inhaled corticosteroids are considered long term control medications and are effective agents to block late reactions to allergens and reduce airway hyperresponsiveness. They also act to inhibit the release of key inflammatory agents.

James was started on oral prednisolone (2 mg/kg divided BID for 5 days) and albuterol 5 mg via MDI (2 puffs) with spacer every 4 hours PRN. Based on the NAEPP guidelines, he will start a low-dose inhaled corticosteroid (0.25 mg budesonide BID) as his daily maintenance medication along with a short-acting bronchodilator (5 mg albuterol via MDI [2 puffs] with spacer) as needed.

Control of Environmental Factors and Other Conditions That Can Affect Asthma

EPR-3 describes new evidence for using multiple approaches to limit exposure to allergens and other substances that can worsen asthma; research shows that single steps are rarely sufficient. EPR-3 also expands the section on other common conditions that asthma patients can have and notes that treating chronic problems

Table 17-2   Classifying Asthma Severity in Children 0-4 Years of Age Not Currently Taking Long-Term Control Medication

Components of Severity		Classification of Asthma Severity (Children 0-4 years of age)			
		Intermittent	Persistent		
			Mild	Moderate	Severe
Impairment	Symptoms	≤ 2 days/week	> 2 days/week but not daily	Daily	Throughout the day
	Nighttime awakenings	0	1-2x/month	3-4x/month	> 1x/week
	Short-acting beta$_2$-agonist use for symptom control (not prevention of EIB)	≤ 2 days/week	> 2 days/week but not daily	Daily	Several times per day
	Interference with normal activity	None	Minor limitation	Some limitation	Extremely limited
Risk	Exacerbations requiring oral systemic corticosteroids	0-1/year	≥ 2 exacerbations in 6 months requiring oral steroids, or ≥ 4 wheezing episodes/ 1 year lasting > 1 day AND risk factors for persistent asthma		

Consider severity and interval since last exacerbation.
Frequency and severity may fluctuate over time.
Exacerbation of any severity may occur in patients in any severity category.

- Level of severity is determined by both impairment and risk. Assess the impairment domain by caregiver's recall of the previous 2-4 weeks. Assign severity to the most severe category in which any feature occurs.
- At present, there are inadequate data to correspond frequencies of exacerbations with different levels of asthma severity. For treatment purposes, patients who had ≥ 2 exacerbations requiring oral corticosteroids in the past 6 months, or ≥ 4 wheezing episodes in the past year, and who have risk factors for persistent asthma, may be considered the same as patients who have persistent asthma, even in the absence of impairment levels consistent with persistent asthma.
- Classifying severity in patients after asthma becomes well controlled, by lowest level of treatment required to maintain control.*

Lowest level of treatment required to maintain control	Classification of Asthma Severity			
	Intermittent	Persistent		
		Mild	Moderate	Severe
	Step 1	Step 2	Step 3 or 4	Step 5 or 6

KEY: EIB, exercise-induced bronchospasm

Note. For population-based evaluations, clinical research, or characterization of a patient's overall asthma severity after control is achieved. For clinical management, the focus is on monitoring the level of control, not the level of severity, once treatment is established.

Source: From National Heart, Lung, and Blood Institute, National Asthma Education and Prevention Program. (2007). *Expert panel report 3: Guidelines for the diagnosis and management of asthma.* Washington, DC: U.S. Department of Health and Human Services.

Table 17-3 Assessing Asthma Control and Adjusting Therapy in Children 0-4 Years of Age

		Classification of Asthma Control (0-4 years of age)		
Components of Control		**Well Controlled**	**Not Well Controlled**	**Very Poorly Controlled**
Impairment	Symptoms	≤ 2 days/week	> 2 days/week	Throughout the day
	Nighttime awakenings	≤ 1x/month	> 1x/month	> 1x/week
	Interference with normal activity	None	Some limitation	Extremely limited
	Short-acting beta$_2$-agonist use for symptom control (not prevention of EIB)	≤ 2 days/week	> 2 days/week	Several times per day
Risk	Exacerbations requiring oral systemic corticosteroids	0-1/year	2-3/year	> 3/year
	Treatment-related adverse effects	Medication side effects can vary in intensity from none to very troublesome and worrisome. The level of intensity does not correlate to specific levels of control but should be considered in the overall assessment of risk.		
Recommended Action for Treatment		• Maintain current treatment • Regular followup every 1-6 months. • Consider step down if well controlled for at least 3 months.	• Step up (1 step) and • Reevaluate in 2-6 weeks. • If no clear benefit in 4-6 weeks, consider alternative diagnoses or adjusting therapy. • For side effects, consider alternative treatment options.	• Consider short course of oral systemic corticosteroids, • Step up (1-2 steps), and • Reevaluate in 2 weeks. • If no clear benefit in 4-6 weeks, consider alternative diagnoses or adjusting therapy. • For side effects, consider alternative treatment options.

KEY: EIB, exercise-induced bronchospasm

Table 17-3   Assessing Asthma Control and Adjusting Therapy in Children 0-4 Years of Age (Continued)

Notes.

- The stepwise approach is meant to assist, not replace, the clinical decision making required to meet individual patient needs.

- The level of control is based on the most severe impairment or risk category. Assess the impairment domain by caregiver's recall of the previous 2–4 weeks. Symptom assessment for longer periods should reflect a global assessment such as inquiring whether the patient's asthma is better or worse since the last visit.

- At present, there are inadequate data to correspond frequencies of exacerbations with different levels of asthma control. In general, more frequent and intense exacerbations (e.g., requiring urgent unscheduled care, hospitalization, or ICU admission) indicate poorer disease control. For treatment purposes, patients who had ≥ 2 exacerbations requiring oral systemic corticosteroids in the past year may be considered the same as patients who have not-well-controlled asthma, even in the absence of impairment levels consistent with not-well-controlled asthma.

- Before step-up therapy:

  - Review adherence to medications, inhaler technique, and environmental control.

  - If an alternative treatment option was used in a step, discontinue it and use the preferred treatment for that step.

Source: From National Heart, Lung, and Blood Institute, National Asthma Education and Prevention Program. (2007). *Expert panel report 3: Guidelines for the diagnosis and management of asthma.* Washington, DC: U.S. Department of Health and Human Services.

---

such as rhinitis and sinusitis, gastroesophageal reflux, overweight or obesity, obstructive sleep apnea, stress, and depression may help improve asthma control.

What kind of follow-up plan is appropriate for a child with a new asthma management plan? ■

Follow-up Visit

James returns for a follow-up visit in 4 weeks. According to Mom, he has been sleeping well with no nighttime awakenings and has not had any difficulty keeping up with the other children at daycare.

He continues to take his budesonide as prescribed and after the first week of treatment, James has not needed to use his albuterol. His RAST testing indicated high reactivity to dust mites and ragweed and moderate reactivity to dog epithelium. Total IgE level was 42. (Normal in reference laboratory is < 35.)

Asthma control can be very complicated and should be tailored to the individual's lifestyle, the individual's history and risk factors, and daytime and nighttime symptoms; the need for "rescue" medications should be used as the best determinant for adjusting therapy. The history obtained at follow-up visits for patients with asthma is helpful in determining if control is adequate. Some examples of pertinent historical questions include current medications and other therapies, how often a short-acting beta$_2$-agonists (SABA) is used, school attendance and performance, and physical activity. You assess that James is well controlled (see Table 17-3 on p. 262).

Key Points from the Case

1. Asthma is a variable disease that commonly begins in early childhood; healthcare providers must learn to recognize the signs and symptoms of asthma in infants and young children.

2. Along with well-known environmental triggers, genetic factors may play a role in disease severity and individual response to treatment.

3. Establishing a diagnosis of asthma involves thorough history taking and physical examination, as well as the exclusion of other possible causes of wheezing. The history should focus on symptoms (i.e., cough or wheeze), precipitating factors or conditions, and the child's typical symptom patterns. Additional history should include a history of atopy, family history of asthma, environmental history, and past medical history. The physical exam is generally normal in the absence of an acute exacerbation. Abnormal findings can suggest severe disease, suboptimal control, or associated atopic conditions.

4. When a diagnosis of asthma is established in a child who is not currently on controller medications, asthma severity should be assessed so that appropriate controller therapy can be started. Treatment should be based on the new EPR-3 treatment guidelines and tailored to the individual needs of the patient because responses to treatment often vary. Asthma control is zero or two or fewer times per week of daytime symptoms or need for SABA; zero limitations on daily activities including exercise; zero nocturnal symptoms or awakening due to asthma (think cough in younger patients); normal or near normal lung function results when available; and finally, no exacerbations.

REFERENCES

Akinbami, L., & Schoendorf, K. (2002). Trends in childhood asthma: Prevalence, health care utilization, and mortality. *Pediatrics, 110*(2 pt 1), 315–322.

American Academy of Pediatrics Committee on Environmental health. (1997). Environmental tobacco smoke: A hazard to children. *Pediatrics, 99*(4), 539–642.

Asthma and Allergy Foundation of America. (2000). *Cost of asthma: A national study.* Retrieved March 26, 2009, from http://www.aafa.org/display.cfm?id=6&sub=63

Bush, A. (2007). Diagnosis of asthma in children under five. *Primary Care Respiratory Journal, 1*(1), 7–15.

Busse, W. W., O'Bryne, P. M., & Holgate, S. T. (2006). Asthma pathogenesis. In: N. F. Adkinson Jr, J. W. Yunginger, W. W. Busse, B. S. Bochner, S. T. Holgate, F. E. R. Simons, (Eds.), *Middleton's allergy: Principles and practice* (6th ed., Chapter 66). St. Louis, MO: Mosby.

Centers for Disease Control and Prevention. (2002). *National Health and Nutrition Examination Survey 2001–2002 data documentation: Household interview questionnaire.* Hyattsville, MD: National Center for Health Statistics.

Centers for Disease Control and Prevention, National Center for Health Statistics. (2006a). *National Health Interview Survey raw data, 2006.* Hyattsville, MD: National Center for Health Statistics.

Centers for Disease Control and Prevention, National Center for Health Statistics. (2006b). *Advance data from vital and health statistics. The state of childhood asthma, United States, 1980–2005.* Number 381.

Gore, C., & Custovic, A. (2005). Can we prevent allergy? *Allergy, 59,* 151–161.

Graham, L. M. (2006). Preschool wheeze prognosis: How do we predict outcome? *Paediatric Respiratory Review, 7*(Suppl 1), S115–S116.

Hopp, R. J., Bewtra, A. K., Biven, R., Nair, N. M., & Townley, R. G. (1988). Bronchial reactivity pattern in nonasthmatic parents of asthmatics. *Annals of Allergy, 61,* 184–186.

King, M. E., Mannino, D. M., & Holguin, F. (2004). Risk factors for asthma incidence. *Panminerva Medicine, 46,* 97–110.

Kraft, M. (2000). The role of bacterial infections in asthma. *Clinics in Chest Medicine, 21,* 301–313.

Martin, R. J., Kraft, M., Chu, H. W., Berns, E. A., & Cassell, G. H. (2001). A link between chronic asthma and chronic infection. *Journal of Allergy and Clinical Immunology, 107,* 595–601.

Martinati, L. C., & Boner, A. L. (1995). Clinical diagnosis of wheezing in early childhood. *Allergy, 50*(9), 701–710.

McDonald, D. M., Schoeb, T. R., & Lindsey, J. R. (1991). Mycoplasma pulmonis infections cause long-lasting potentiation of neurogenic inflammation in the respiratory tract of the rat. *Journal of Clinical Investigation, 87,* 787–799.

McDonnell, W. F., Abbey, D. E., Nishino, N., & Lebowitz, M. D. (1999). Long-term ambient ozone concentration and the incidence of asthma in non-smoking adults: The AHSMOG study. *Environmental Research, 80*(2 pt 1), 110–121.

National Center for Health Statistics. (2002). *National Health Interview Survey.* Hyattsville, MD: Author.

National Heart, Lung and Blood Institute, National Asthma Education and Prevention Program. (2007). *Expert panel report 3: Guidelines for the diagnosis and management of asthma.* Washington, DC: Author.

Sandford, A., Weir, T., & Pare, P. (1996). State of the art: The genetics of asthma. *American Journal of Respiratory and Critical Care Medicine, 153,* 1749–1765.

Scirica, C. V., & Celedon, J. C. (2007). Genetics of asthma: Potential implications for reducing asthma disparities. *Chest, 132*(5 Suppl), 700S–781S.

Sibbald, B., & Turner-Warwick M. (1979). Factors influencing the prevalence of asthma among first degree relatives of extrinsic and intrinsic asthmatics. *Thorax, 34*, 332–337.

Simon, P. A., Zeng, Z., Wold, C. M., Haddock, W., & Fielding, J. E. (2003). Prevalence of childhood asthma and associated morbidity in Los Angeles County: Impacts of race/ethnicity and income. *Journal of Asthma, 40*, 535–543.

Smith, L. A., Hatcher-Ross, J. L., Wertheimer, R., & Kahn, R. S. (2005). Rethinking race/ethnicity, income, and childhood asthma: Racial/ethnic disparities concentrated among the very poor. *Public Health Reports, 120*(2), 109–116.

Strachan, D. P. (1989). Hay fever, hygiene, and household size. *British Medical Journal, 299*, 1259–1260.

Strachan, D. P., Butland, B. K., & Anderson H. R. (1996). Incidence and prognosis of asthma and wheezing illness from early childhood to age 33 in a national British cohort. *British Medical Journal, 312*, 1195–1199.

Strachan, D. P., & Cook, D. G. (1998). Parental smoking and childhood asthma: Longitudinal and case control studies. *Thorax, 53*, 204–212.

Weitzman, M., Gortmaker, S., Walker, D. K., & Sobol, A. (1990). Maternal smoking and childhood asthma. *Pediatrics, 85*, 505–511.

Chapter 18

The Overweight Child with High Blood Sugar

Arlene Smaldone

A child may receive a life-altering diagnosis of a chronic health condition at the time of an acute hospitalization. At follow-up, the primary care provider must review the hospitalization course and laboratory data, perform a history and physical examination, consider family preferences for ongoing care and alternative treatment options, and, perhaps, refine a diagnosis. Most important, the primary care provider can be instrumental in assisting children and families to positively adapt to the new demands imposed by the chronic condition and promoting parent/adolescent shared responsibility for care.

Educational Objectives

1. Apply current guidelines for diagnosis and management of type 2 diabetes to an African American teen.
2. Identify common comorbidities of type 2 diabetes and screening guidelines.
3. Apply appropriate laboratory testing guidelines for an adolescent with type 2 diabetes.
4. Understand the need for a team approach in the delivery of care for a child with type 2 diabetes.
5. Consider developmental and sociocultural factors that may impact the diabetes management plan.

Case Presentation and Discussion

You first meet Mary Smith, a 14-year-old African American female, when she comes to your rural community health center for "follow-up." Three weeks ago while visiting her aunt in another city during summer vacation, she became ill and was hospitalized for 3 days. She was diagnosed with diabetic ketoacidosis (DKA), required intensive care for 2 days, and was told she has diabetes. She was discharged from the hospital on a two injection per day regimen of combined short- and intermediate-acting insulin. During the hospitalization, she and her aunt met with a nutritionist and a diabetes educator. Mary is currently monitoring her blood glucose levels four times per day. She complains of feeling very hungry before lunch and at bedtime. Mary does not bring her blood glucose records but does bring her glucose meter to the visit. Review of blood glucose values stored in the glucometer memory demonstrate readings in the range of 80–100 mg/dL before breakfast and dinner and readings in the range of 60–80 before lunch and at bedtime (Figure 18-1).

Insulin and/or Medications				Blood Glucose Test				
Date	Breakfast	Lunch	Dinner	Bedtime	Breakfast	Lunch	Dinner	Bedtime	Other
8/30	10R/25N		10R/10N		81	50	96	69	
8/31	10R/25N		10R/10N		92	75	85	70	
9/1	10R/25N		10R/10N		100	67	82	100	
9/2	10R/25N		10R/10N		96	102	112	56	
9/3	10R/25N		10R/10N		87	43	76	72	
9/4	7R/25N		7R/10N						

Notes. R=Regular insulin; N=NPH insulin
Blood glucose target range 80-150mg/dL

Figure 18-1   Blood glucose diary highlighting pattern of hypoglycemia before lunch and at bedtime and recommended insulin adjustment.

You obtain a family history and discover that Mary's maternal grandmother and uncle have type 2 diabetes. Mary's uncle receives dialysis for diabetes-associated end stage renal disease. Mary has two younger siblings, an 11-year-old brother and a 5-year-old sister.

You ask Mary's mother to wait in the waiting room while you talk to Mary and complete her physical examination.

What further data do you need to work with Mary and her diabetes diagnosis? ■

History

Your conversation with Mary reveals the following: Menarche occurred 2 years ago; her menstrual periods are irregular and occur every 2 to 3 months. She denies sexual activity, smoking, or drug use. Mary administers all insulin injections and talks about how hard it is to resist eating "junk food." She plays softball on a school team 2 days per week but is inactive on other days. She is in the ninth grade and is a "B" student. She has several friends but has not told anyone about her diabetes. She asks you, "Will I always need to take insulin?" You respond by saying that for now, she needs to continue with injectable insulin to control her hyperglycemia, and that you need additional information before you can answer her question.

Physical Examination Findings

You go on to complete her physical examination before deciding on your plan of care for this long-term diagnosis.

Height: 63 inches (50th percentile); weight 150 pounds (90–95th percentile); body mass index (BMI) 26.6 kg/m² (90–95th percentile); blood pressure 132/86 (> 95th percentile for age and height) (Frazier & Pruette, 2009; National High Blood Pressure Education Program Working Group, 2004); heart rate 78 beats per minute; respirations

14 per minute; office urinalysis pH 7.0, specific gravity 1.010; glucose, protein, and ketones negative. Mary's physical examination is positive for the presence of moderate acanthosis nigricans on the back of her neck and at her axillae.

Diabetes: but what type? ■

Before you can set up the appropriate long-term plan for Mary, you need to have more information about the diabetes diagnosis Mary brings to you. Sometimes it is difficult to distinguish between type 1 and type 2 diabetes in adolescents at the time of diagnosis. Diabetic ketoacidosis (DKA), although a more common presentation of type 1 diabetes, does not exclude a diagnosis of type 2 diabetes (Gahagan & Silverstein, 2003). In one sample of urban youth with type 2 diabetes, 8% presented in DKA at diagnosis (Zdravkovic, Daneman, & Hamilton, 2004). It is important to differentiate between the types of diabetes because treatment options, education approaches, and screening recommendations will differ. The incidence of type 2 diabetes during childhood and adolescence is rising, particularly among adolescents in minority populations. This increase, largely attributed to the rising rate of obesity in childhood, has long-term implications from a public health perspective.

You need to set up a plan for today's visit pending more information, so you ask Mary's mother to authorize release of Mary's hospital records in order to review her hospital record and laboratory evaluation at the time of diagnosis. Today, you note that Mary's blood pressure is elevated and that she is having frequent episodes of hypoglycemia before lunch and at bedtime. Figure 18-1 illustrates the patterns of Mary's blood glucose values. As you await data that will help to clarify Mary's type of diabetes, you decide to decrease Mary's short-acting insulin dose at breakfast and dinner by 10%, and review target blood glucose ranges and identification, as well as treatment of hypoglycemia with Mary and her mother. You also give them a handout from Children's Hospital and Regional Center, Seattle, Washington, entitled "What Is Low Blood Sugar? Hypoglycemia for Children and Families" (this can be accessed online at http://cshcn. org/sites/default/files/webfm/file/WhatIsLowBloodSugar-English.pdf). You also provide information about diabetes for them to give to school personnel (see Table 18-1). You ask Mary to return for follow-up in 2 weeks. In the interim, you instruct Mary to continue to monitor her blood glucose level four times a day and to call you if her blood glucose levels are below 80 mg/dL on two consecutive readings or if her blood glucose levels fall below 80 mg/dL more than four times per week.

Before you see Mary again, you need to review your knowledge of type 1 and type 2 diabetes. It is not clear to you which condition she has.

Diabetes in Children

Pathophysiology of Type 2 Diabetes

Type 2 diabetes is a complex metabolic disorder having a genetic predisposition and characterized by insulin resistance and inadequate insulin secretion by the β cells of the pancreas (American Diabetes Association, 2000). Maintenance of

Table 18-1   Diabetes Educational Resources for Parents, Adolescents, and School Personnel

Resources for Adolescents and Families

1. National Diabetes Education Program (NDEP)[a]:
   http://www.ndep.nih.gov/diabetes/pubs/catalog.htm#ResChildAdol
   - What Is Diabetes (NDEP-63)
   - Be Active (NDEP-64)
   - Stay at a Healthy Weight (NDEPP-65)
   - Make Healthy Food Choices (NDEP-66)
   - Dealing with the Ups and Downs of Diabetes (NDEP-87)
   - Examples of treatments for hypoglycemia:
     http://www.diabetesatwork.org/_files/handouts/I_B_01b_HO(1).pdf

2. American Diabetes Association[a]
   - Wizdom, Type 2 Diabetes: http://web.diabetes.org/wizdom/download/type2.asp
   - Youth Zone: http://www.diabetes.org/youthzone/youth-zone.jsp

3. Children with Diabetes Web site
   - What Is Type 2 Diabetes?:
     http://www.childrenwithdiabetes.com/type2/t2_whatistype2.htm

Resources for School Personnel

National Diabetes Education Program[a]
- Helping the Student with Diabetes Succeed: A Guide for School Personnel[a]

[a]Available in English and Spanish

blood glucose levels within a physiologic range requires the orchestration of several metabolic activities: pancreatic β cells must accurately sense glucose concentration and synthesize and release insulin, and insulin must bind to its receptors and facilitate the uptake of glucose by muscle, fat, and liver (Rosenbloom & Silverstein, 2003). In an insulin-resistant state, the usual amount of insulin does not produce the desired effect; therefore, the pancreas must secrete additional insulin to maintain blood glucose levels within a physiologic range. In the early phases of insulin resistance, normal glucose tolerance is maintained by release of greater than normal levels of insulin. However, β cell function gradually declines over time, resulting in inadequate insulin secretion to meet the demands of blood glucose regulation in an insulin-resistant state.

Puberty augments the problems imposed by insulin resistance for those predisposed to type 2 diabetes. Secretion of growth hormone as part of the pubertal growth spurt further increases resistance to insulin action. Adolescents with normally functioning pancreatic β cells secrete additional insulin to compensate for this puberty-related effect. However, when β cells do not function properly, metabolic decompensation begins and leads to a state of prediabetes (impaired fasting glucose and/or impaired glucose tolerance) with eventual progression to type 2 diabetes (American Diabetes Association, 2000). Table 18-2 identifies current American Diabetes Association definitions for prediabetes and diagnostic criteria for diabetes.

Epidemiology of Obesity and Type 2 Diabetes in Children
The phenomenon of type 2 diabetes in the pediatric population has emerged concurrent with the rising prevalence of overweight and obesity in U.S. youth. Data from the National Health and Nutrition Examination Survey (NHANES) indicate that approximately one third (31.9%) of U.S. children are either overweight or obese (BMI ≥ 85th percentile for age) (Ogden, Carroll, & Flegal, 2008). Among all age and gender categories, minority children have higher prevalence rates for overweight and obesity; for example, among teens, 44.5% of African American girls were overweight or obese compared to 31.7% of non-Hispanic white girls (Ogden et al., 2008).

The prevalence of type 2 diabetes has increased concurrent with the increase of pediatric overweight and obesity, with minority children disproportionately affected (Rosenbloom & Silverstein, 2003). In one large sample of Florida children cared for at pediatric diabetes centers, the percentage of children diagnosed with type 2 diabetes increased from 9.4% to 20% over a 5-year period (Macaluso

Table 18-2   American Diabetes Association Diagnostic Criteria for Prediabetes and Diabetes

Categorization	Diagnostic Criteria
Prediabetes	
Impaired fasting glucose	Fasting[a] plasma glucose between 100 and 125 mg/dL.
Impaired glucose tolerance	Plasma glucose between 140 and 199 mg/dL following a meal or glucose challenge as part of an oral glucose tolerance test.
Diabetes	Fasting[a] plasma glucose ≥ 126 mg/dL OR
	symptoms of hyperglycemia (e.g., polyuria, polydipsia, unexplained weight loss, enuresis) AND plasma glucose ≥ 200 mg/dL OR
	2-hour plasma glucose ≥ 200 mg/dL as part of an oral glucose tolerance test.

[a]Fasting defined as no calorie intake for a minimum of 8 hours

Source: Adapted from American Diabetes Association. (2008). Standards of medical care in diabetes–2008. *Diabetes Care, 31*(Suppl 1), S12–S54.

et al., 2002), although the total number of children diagnosed with diabetes remained stable during these years. Compared to children with type 1 diabetes, children with type 2 diabetes were more likely to be overweight or obese, of Hispanic ethnicity or African American race, female, and of older age.

Findings from the recent SEARCH for Diabetes in Youth Study (Liese et al., 2006), a large epidemiologic study, demonstrate that currently 154,000 children in the United States have diabetes; of these, approximately 39,000 (25%) have type 2 diabetes (Lipton, 2007). This study further suggests that the occurrence of type 2 diabetes in children less than 10 years of age is rare among U.S. children of all races and ethnicities. However, for children 10 years of age and older, race and ethnicity strongly influence the frequency of type 2 diabetes, with children of African American and Native American race most commonly affected. Therefore, it is important to consider type 2 diabetes in the differential diagnosis of older children who present with symptoms of diabetes. Although strongly linked to genetic predisposition, diet and lifestyle are also strongly implicated in the rise of type 2 diabetes in this age group. The combination of low physical activity with ingestion of high calorie, high fat foods of low nutritional quality creates an obesigenic environment leading to excess weight gain and obesity.

Obesity and Cardiovascular Disease Risk in Children
The Bogalusa Heart Study, a longitudinal epidemiologic study, was initiated in 1973 to study cardiovascular risk factors beginning in childhood. Several important relationships regarding obesity, insulin resistance, and cardiovascular risk have been identified using data from these participants. Investigators from the Bogalusa Heart Study (Svec et al., 1992) measured glucose and insulin levels in 377 children 7 to 11 years of age from a biracial community. Controlling for age, body weight, and pubertal stage, African American children had higher insulin levels compared to white children, placing African American children at higher risk for insulin resistance.

In another study (Freedman, Dietz, Srinivasan, & Berenson, 1999), researchers noted that children who were overweight were more likely to have elevations in a lipid profile component, blood pressure, and fasting insulin levels, thereby demonstrating a relationship between weight and cardio-metabolic risk. Importantly, more than half (58%) of the overweight children had at least one risk factor. Findings of this study demonstrate that, even among young children, presence of obesity is consistently related to cardiovascular risk factors. For example, among 5- to 6-year-old study participants, those who were overweight were 7.1 times more likely to have elevated triglyceride levels and 16 times more likely to have elevated systolic blood pressure compared to similar-age children of normal weight. In another study, autopsy reports of Bogalusa Heart study participants provided evidence of the presence of coronary and aortic atherosclerosis and its relationship to prior documented cardiovascular risk factors, and that severity of asymptomatic coronary artery disease increases with an increase in the number of cardiovascular risk factors (Berenson, Srinivasan, & Nicklas, 1998). Furthermore, childhood obesity results in a relative risk of about 1.5 for all-cause mortality and 2.0 for coronary heart disease mortality (Must & Strauss, 1999).

Pathophysiology of Type 1 Diabetes in Children

Type 1 diabetes, the second most common chronic disease in childhood, affects approximately 1 in 500 children in the United States, and is the more prevalent form of diabetes among children. Metabolic manifestations of both type 1 and type 2 diabetes are similar; however, the pathophysiology of type 1 diabetes differs from that of type 2 diabetes. Type 1 diabetes is an idiopathic and immune-mediated condition resulting in permanent loss of the body's ability to produce insulin due to progressive autoimmune destruction of the β cells of the pancreas (Asp, 2005). Approximately 75% of individuals with type 1 diabetes will test positive for the presence of autoantibodies at the time of diagnosis (Haller, Silverstein, & Rosenbloom, 2007). Prior to discovery of insulin in 1921, type 1 diabetes was a fatal disease.

Pancreatic β cell destruction occurs insidiously until the number of functioning pancreatic β cells is no longer sufficient to regulate blood glucose levels, and hyperglycemia occurs. When blood glucose concentrations exceed the kidney's ability to conserve glucose, glucose is excreted into the urine, leading to osmotic diuresis. Symptoms of diabetes, polydipsia and polyuria, are related to hyperglycemia. Type 1 diabetes has an abrupt clinical onset and generally occurs over a 2- to 3-week period (Roche, Menon, Gill, & Hoey, 2005). If diabetes is not recognized and treated, symptoms progress to weight loss, dehydration, and ketosis resulting from breakdown of body fat, and eventually progress to diabetic ketoacidosis, an absolute state of insulin deficiency (Haller et al., 2007). Approximately 20% to 40% of new cases of type 1 diabetes present in diabetic ketoacidosis, with young children and those with poor access to health care at particular risk (Mallare et al., 2003; Roche et al., 2005; Rosenbloom, 2007).

Epidemiology of Type 1 Diabetes in Children

The etiology of type 1 diabetes is multifactorial, combining a genetic predisposition with an environmental trigger (Rennert & Francis, 1999). The incidence of type 1 diabetes varies worldwide, ranging from Finland (greater than 40 per 100,000), where incidence is highest, to China (0.1 per 100,000), where incidence is lowest. In the United States the incidence of type 1 diabetes is estimated to be 16.1 per 100,000 per year (Soltesz, Patterson, & Dahlquist, 2007). Susceptibility to type 1 diabetes can be inherited; however, approximately 85% of cases occur sporadically. Siblings of an individual with type 1 diabetes have a 40-fold higher risk of developing diabetes; similarly, a child whose parent has type 1 diabetes has a 10-fold (if mother has diabetes) to 35-fold (if father has diabetes) increased risk (Winter, 2007). Researchers have studied the relationships between a variety of environmental agents such as cow's milk, vitamin D deficiency, and enteroviruses and development of type 1 diabetes (Eisenbarth, 2007). The TRIGR study, an international multi-site randomized controlled trial, is testing the hypothesis that compared to cow's milk–based formula, hydrolyzed infant formula decreases risk of developing type 1 diabetes in children with increased genetic susceptibility (TRIGR Study Group, 2007). However, to date, the factors responsible for activating autoimmune destruction of pancreatic β cells in children at risk for type 1 diabetes remain unknown.

In the 1980s, two international type 1 childhood population-based diabetes registries, Eurodiab and Diamond, were established to collect epidemiologic data (Soltesz et al., 2007) about type 1 diabetes in youth. These registries have provided important information regarding global incidence patterns, age and gender patterns, and trends over time. Incidence of type 1 diabetes increases with age, with children at highest risk during the pubertal years (10 to 14 years). Boys and girls are equally affected (Soltesz et al., 2007). The incidence of type 1 diabetes is rising globally, with the highest increase noted in children 5 years of age and younger (Dabelea et al., 2007; Gale, 2002). The SEARCH for Diabetes in Youth Study, a recent multi-center epidemiologic study of children in the United States (Dabelea et al.), demonstrates that the incidence of type 1 diabetes occurs among all racial/ethnic groups, with non-Hispanic white youth most commonly affected.

Treatment of type 1 diabetes in children has a strong evidence base. The Diabetes Control and Complications Trial (DCCT) (Diabetes Control and Complications Trial Research Group, 1993, 1994) clearly demonstrated that tight glycemic control achieved through intensive insulin therapy is critical in preventing or forestalling long-term complications of diabetes. The Epidemiology of Diabetes Interventions and Complications (EDIC) Study (White et al., 2001; Writing Team for the Diabetes Control and Complications Trial, 2002), a prospective epidemiologic study of DCCT participants, provides ongoing evidence that the improved metabolic control achieved for those in the intensively treated group remains protective against the long-term complications of diabetes. Application of DCCT findings to pediatric patients was initially cautious because of risk of hypoglycemia (DCCT Research Group, 1994) and safety of intensive insulin regimens when young children were away from parental supervision. Recent reports (Churchill, Ruppe, & Smaldone, 2009; DiMeglio et al., 2004; Fox, Buckloh, Smith, Wysocki, & Mauras, 2005; Jeha et al., 2005; Litton et al., 2002; Mack-Fogg, Orlowski, & Jospe, 2005; Wilson et al., 2005) provide evidence that intensive insulin regimens are both safe and efficacious, even when used in young children. Current American Diabetes Association standards of care for children with type 1 diabetes (Silverstein et al., 2005) reflect both lower glycemic targets and intensive insulin regimens using multiple daily injections or insulin pump therapy as the means to achieve them.

There is no diagnostic test to differentiate type 2 from type 1 diabetes; further, some features of diabetes formerly thought to be present only in type 1 diabetes (e.g., diabetic ketoacidosis and presence of autoantibodies) are now recognized as not being exclusive to one type of diabetes. Table 18-3 examines demographic, laboratory, and comorbidity factors and their frequency in type 1 and type 2 diabetes in childhood. The presence of a factor does not confirm or exclude one type of diabetes; however, a particular factor may occur more frequently in type 1 or type 2 diabetes (Dabelea et al., 2007).

Table 18-3   Differentiating Type 2 from Type 1 Diabetes

	Type 2 Diabetes	Type 1 Diabetes
Demographic/Physical Characteristics		
Age	≥ 10 years, particularly in minority children.	All ages.
Gender	More frequent in females.	Equal distribution by gender.
Race	More frequent in African Americans, Asian Americans, Native Americans, Hispanic Americans.	May occur in all racial ethnic groups, but most frequent in non-Hispanic whites.
Family history of diabetes	Common	Atypical
Overweight/obesity	Common	Not common but may be present.
Acanthosis nigricans	Common	Atypical
Clinical Presentation		
Diabetic ketoacidosis	Not common but does not exclude type 2 diabetes.	Occurs in approximately one third of new cases of diabetes.
Duration of symptoms	Insidious	Few weeks
Laboratory Evaluation		
Presence of autoantibodies	Uncommon	Common
C-peptide	Normal to elevated	Low
Presence of Comorbidities		
Hypertension	Common	Uncommon
Hyperlipidemia	Common	Uncommon
Polycystic ovarian syndrome	Common	Uncommon

Rethinking Mary's Diabetes Diagnosis

Hospital records document that Mary presented to the hospital emergency room with persistent vomiting, polyuria, and excessive thirst. She had been ill for the past 2 days. Her past medical history was uneventful and her prior health described as excellent. Although sluggish, she was oriented to time, person, and place. On physical examination her pulse was 108, respirations 30, temperature 37°C (98.6°F), blood pressure 130/90, and weight 142 lbs. Lungs were clear to auscultation, heart sounds were normal, and abdomen was soft without hepatosplenomegaly. Mary's initial laboratory evaluation included a basic metabolic panel, venous blood gas, complete blood count, and urinalysis. Subsequent laboratory evaluation included hemoglobin A1c and islet cell antibody (ICA) and glutamic acid decarboxylase (GAD) titers.

Notable among Mary's laboratory results, blood glucose was reported as 500 mg/dL (reference range 60–100 mg/dL), serum sodium 128 mEq/L (reference range 133–146 mEq/L), and blood urea nitrogen (BUN) 40 mg/dL (reference range 5–26 mg/dL). Venous blood gas results were indicative of a metabolic acidosis with pH 7.12 and pCO_2 10. Urinalysis results demonstrated specific gravity > 1.030, large glucose, and large ketones. Hemoglobin A1c was 12% (reference range < 6%) and ICA and GAD antibodies were reported as negative.

She was admitted to the intensive care unit for diabetic ketoacidosis (DKA) management, which included fluid resuscitation with normal saline to restore fluid balance, titration of blood glucose using an insulin infusion drip, and potassium replacement. No sodium bicarbonate was given. She remained in the intensive care unit for 36 hours, was discharged to a pediatric hospital unit for diabetes education, and was subsequently discharged to her aunt's home. The hospital discharge note indicated uncertainty regarding type of diabetes, a nonspecific plan for follow-up care in the child's community, and pending results of ICA and GAD antibody levels.

Making the Diagnosis

After thorough review of the pathophysiology and epidemiology of type 2 diabetes, the history and physical examination data, and Mary's hospital records, you begin to rethink Mary's initial diabetes diagnosis. Following review of Mary's family history and hospital laboratory data with your collaborating physician, you conclude that Mary has type 2 diabetes. Her laboratory results on hospital admission definitively document diabetes (blood glucose 500 mg/dL with symptoms of polyuria and polydipsia) (see Table 18-2) and presence of diabetic ketoacidosis (blood glucose 500 mg/dL, low serum pH, and low CO_2) (Frazier & Pruette, 2009; National High Blood Pressure Education Program, 2004). Her strong family history of type 2 diabetes, age, race, and negative ICA and GAD antibody status help to clarify her type of diabetes as type 2. Table 18-3 compares characteristics of children with type 1 and type 2 diabetes.

Management

Mary returns accompanied by her mother for her 2-week follow-up visit since her last visit with you. Mary has been well and brings blood glucose records with her today. She states that she has not had many low blood glucose readings and that she has been eating an apple for a snack instead of chips if she is hungry between meals. Her weight today is 147 pounds (3-pound weight loss) and blood pressure is 122/78 (90th percentile for age and height (Frazier & Pruette, 2009). Her blood glucose records show that most readings are in a range of 80–140, with occasional episodes of hypoglycemia after softball games.

Managing a teenager with diabetes is complex. Fortunately, a great deal of work has been done in this area that can help you develop a complete long-term healthcare plan.

Goals of Therapy

First, you need to establish goals for your care as well as goals for Mary and her family to achieve. Treatment goals for the adolescent diagnosed with type 2 diabetes are the following:

- Maintain blood glucose values as close to a normal range as possible while minimizing hypoglycemic episodes.
- Maintain hemoglobin A1c values at $\leq$ 7%.
- Prevent and/or identify comorbidities of diabetes and long-term microvascular complications of diabetes.
- Promote normal growth and development.
- Promote weight loss.
- Engage in healthy lifestyle behaviors.

Treatment Options

Although diabetes treatment and education approaches for children and adolescents with type 1 diabetes are well defined and supported by findings of the Diabetes Complications and Control Trial (DCCT) (DCCT Research Group, 1993, 1994), treatment of type 2 diabetes in youth remains in its infancy and currently lacks a strong evidence base. The TODAY Study, a multi-center randomized controlled trial presently in progress, was designed to identify the best "Treatment Options for Type 2 Diabetes in Adolescents and Youth." (Information about the TODAY Study may be accessed online at http://www.todaystudy.org/index.cgi.) The study is comparing the effectiveness of three treatment options for youth with type 2 diabetes: 1) metformin (currently the only oral diabetes agent approved for use in children), 2) metformin plus rosiglitazone, and 3) metformin plus an intensive behavioral intervention (Zeitler et al., 2007).

Medication Management

The hallmark of management of children and adolescents with type 2 diabetes is instituting a change from unhealthy to healthy nutritional and physical activity behaviors leading to weight loss. In the United States, fewer than 10% of individuals with type 2 diabetes are successful in achieving glycemic control with diet and exercise alone. Therefore, pharmacologic therapy is recommended in addition to diet and exercise.

Although a wide variety of medication choices are currently available for management of type 2 diabetes, metformin and insulin are the only medications currently approved by the Food and Drug Administration for use in the pediatric population (Atkinson & Radjenovic, 2007; Zeitler et al., 2007). However, because the pathophysiology of type 2 diabetes in children and adolescents is similar to that of adults, recent advances in different classes of medications for adults with type 2 diabetes have led to their off label use in children. Therefore, it is important that health professionals are well versed in the medications used in their particular setting.

Oral medications used in the treatment of type 2 diabetes lower blood glucose levels by increasing sensitivity to insulin (biguanides, thiazolidenediones, α-glucosidase inhibitors) or increasing insulin secretion (sulfonylureas, meglitinides) (Ludwig & Ebbeling, 2001). Over time, the natural course of type 2 diabetes will result in the body's inability to produce sufficient insulin and insulin replacement so that long- and/or short-acting insulin will be necessary.

Metformin, a biguanide, is recommended as the initial drug of choice in management of type 2 diabetes in adolescents. Metformin improves blood glucose levels without risk of hypoglycemia, and treatment is associated with a mild decrease in weight and decrease in low-density lipoprotein (LDL) and triglyceride levels. In girls with irregular menses or polycystic ovarian syndrome, treatment with metformin may also improve ovarian abnormalities and, therefore, increase the risk of unplanned pregnancy (American Diabetes Association, 2000). Metformin is contraindicated in patients with impaired renal function or hepatic disease, and treatment should be temporarily discontinued during any illness accompanied by dehydration or hypoxemia because of risk of lactic acidosis (American Diabetes Association). If monotherapy with metformin is unsuccessful in achieving glycemic targets, an agent from a different class or insulin may be added to the therapeutic regimen.

Medication may also be prescribed to control hypertension (National High Blood Pressure Education Program Working Group, 2004; Tan, 2009) and dyslipidemia, two frequent comorbidities of type 2 diabetes in youth. Guidelines for treatment of dyslipidemia in pediatric patients were recently amended to include children 8 years of age or older, particularly when accompanied by other cardiovascular risk factors such as obesity or diabetes (Daniels & Greer, 2008).

Children and families should receive both verbal and written instruction for each prescribed medication including purpose, dose, frequency, and potential side effects. It can be helpful to write medication changes in the blood glucose diary as an additional daily reminder. Medication adherence should not be assumed; it is important that adherence be assessed routinely at each patient encounter, particularly during adolescence.

Nutritional Changes
Healthful eating, in terms of both nutritional value and portion size, and improving physical activity are important components of the treatment plan for youth with type 2 diabetes. At diagnosis, the family should meet with a dietician experienced in nutritional management of children with diabetes to receive individualized, culturally appropriate medical nutrition therapy to achieve diabetes treatment goals, prevent cardiovascular disease, and promote behavior change (Gidding et al., 2005). Medical nutrition therapy recommendations should be reviewed with families at least yearly. Modest weight loss has been shown to decrease insulin resistance (American Diabetes Association, 2008). The Centers for Disease Control and Prevention (CDC) recently launched a "Healthy Weight" Web site (http://www.cdc.govhealthyweight/index.htm)

that provides nutrition information geared to parents and a site with interactive games specifically designed to promote healthy food choices and physical activity for children (http://www.smallstep.gov/kids/flash/index.html).

Physical Activity Changes

It is recommended that adolescents engage in 60 minutes of physical activity most days of the week (U.S. Department of Health and Human Services, 2005). Physical activity has multiple benefits for the child or adolescent with type 2 diabetes. In addition to lowering blood glucose levels, activity helps to burn fat, increase insulin sensitivity, and increase energy expenditure, and has beneficial effects on blood pressure and lipid levels. Because of their more sedentary lifestyle pattern, many children/adolescents with type 2 diabetes may need ongoing encouragement to initiate an exercise program and should be counseled to start slowly, gradually increase intensity, and build physical activity into lifetime habits. Overweight or obese adolescents may lack self-esteem or motivation to participate in school sports activities but may be willing to walk as a form of exercise. Use of pedometers has been effective in improving physical activity levels in adolescents, particularly when individualized behavioral goals are set (Butcher, Fairclough, Stratton, & Richardson, 2007; Schofield, Mummery, & Schofield, 2005).

Developmental Factors

Management of diabetes is complex and depends on daily performance of many behaviors and self-care tasks: taking medications for diabetes and possibly for blood pressure control and lipid reduction, monitoring blood glucose levels, and changing behaviors to incorporate healthy eating, weight control strategies, and physical activity into one's daily routine. Though it may appear to many as not much of a challenge, both research (Kaufman & Schantz, 2007; Zeitler et al., 2007) and common sense remind us that behavior change is difficult for virtually everyone. Adolescence is a period of profound physical, cognitive, and psychosocial change. During late childhood and early adolescence, children develop cognitive capacity for organized logical thought and begin to think abstractly (Child Development Institute, n.d.). Capacity for abstraction enables an adolescent to contemplate future possibilities or events. Despite their ability to think about the future, however, adolescents with chronic illness are primarily concerned with the present (Weinger, O'Donnell, & Ritholz, 2001) and are less influenced by what they perceive to be long-term health risks (Mulvaney et al., 2006; Sawyer & Aroni, 2005). Adolescence is also a time of seeking independence from parents. For adolescents with a chronic health condition, this means beginning to assume increasing responsibility for their diabetes self-management tasks, which often causes tension and conflict within the family (Anderson et al., 2002; Mulvaney et al.; Weinger et al., 2001). In a recent study, parents of adolescents with type 2 diabetes identified adolescents' food choices and failure to monitor blood glucose levels as common sources of family conflict (Mulvaney et al.).

The majority of research about transition of responsibility for diabetes self-management has been conducted with adolescents with type 1 diabetes. Although some issues may be similar, adolescents with type 2 diabetes have different physical, socioeconomic, and psychosocial issues compared to adolescents with type 1 diabetes. Because diagnosis of type 2 diabetes frequently occurs during mid-adolescence, these adolescents must adapt to the challenges imposed by a chronic health condition at the same time they are in the process of transitioning to greater autonomy.

Adolescents with type 2 diabetes need to deal with comorbid obesity within a family structure where obesity, type 2 diabetes, and poor lifestyle behaviors are prevalent (Pinhas-Hamiel et al., 1999); therefore, they may lack role models and/or emotional support needed to facilitate behavior change. Studies have shown that only a small minority of adolescents with type 2 diabetes exercised on a regular basis or followed their meal plan (Rothman et al., 2008). Obesity and its consequences may go unrecognized in these families (Skinner, Weinberger, Mulvaney, Schlundt, & Rothman, 2008).

Diabetes Comorbidities and Complications

Adolescents with type 2 diabetes are at risk for diabetes-related microvascular complications associated with poor glycemic control and psychosocial demands of living with a chronic health condition. In addition, similar to adults with type 2 diabetes, at diagnosis they are more likely to present with comorbidities, placing them at risk for future cardiovascular and renal disease: lipid disorders, hypertension, obesity, and insulin resistance.

Hypertension

Blood pressure should be measured at each visit. Hypertension is defined as a systolic and/or diastolic blood pressure that is ≥ 95th percentile for age, gender, and height using an appropriate-size cuff and confirmed on two or more repeated visits (National High Blood Pressure Education Program, 2004; Tan, 2009). If improved lifestyle behaviors are not sufficient in reducing blood pressure to target levels, first line therapy for treatment of hypertension is treatment using an angiotensin-converting enzyme (ACE) inhibitor. ACE inhibitors are contraindicated during pregnancy; therefore, sexually active girls treated with ACE inhibitors should be offered contraception counseling (Dean & Sellers, 2007).

Dyslipidemia

A fasting lipid profile should be measured at diagnosis and annually (Dean & Sellers, 2007) for all children with type 2 diabetes. Current guidelines (Dean & Sellers) support treatment of dyslipidemia (defined as LDL cholesterol ≥ 130 mg/dL) in children with diabetes age 8 years or older with either a bile acid–binding resin such as cholestyramine or a 3-hydroxy-3-methyl-glutaryl coenzyme A reductase inhibitor (statin) medication, and nutrition counseling. Fasting lipid levels, liver enzymes, and creatine kinase should be monitored semi-annually for those treated with statins to assess for therapy effectiveness and safety (Dean & Sellers).

Renal Disease
Children with type 2 diabetes should be screened at diagnosis for the presence of pre-existing renal disease with random urine microalbumin-to-creatinine ratio, and this screening should be repeated yearly (Dean & Sellers, 2007). First morning specimens are best to rule out the presence of orthostatic proteinuria.

Depression
Children with chronic illness are at higher risk to develop depression compared to healthy peers (Bennett, 1994; Grey, Whittemore, & Tamborlane, 2002; Hood et al., 2006). The combination of diabetes with comorbid depression places a child at further risk for poor glycemic control and poor medical outcomes (Dantzer, Swendsen, Maurice-Tison, & Salamon, 2003; Garrison, Katon, & Richardson, 2005; Grey et al., 2002; Stewart, Rao, Emslie, Klein, & White, 2005). In two recent cross-sectional studies (Hood et al.; Lawrence et al., 2006), 15–23% of youth with diabetes reported depressive symptoms. These findings highlight the importance of routine screening for depression in children and adolescents with diabetes, maintaining a high index of suspicion of depression in adolescents with poor diabetes control, and prompt initiation of treatment when depression is identified.

Microvascular Complications
Children with type 2 diabetes should be screened for the presence of retinopathy, nephropathy, and neuropathy at diagnosis with annual screening thereafter. A foot exam should be performed on an annual basis (Peterson, Silverstein, Kaufman, & Warren-Boulton, 2007).

Sociocultural Factors Affecting Diabetes Management
Cultural values are learned behaviors and influence how individuals receive and adopt health education messages. This section discusses how food, body weight perception, and spirituality may influence diabetes management in African Americans diagnosed with type 2 diabetes.

African Americans have retained some of their original culture through food, commonly referred to as "soul food." Preparation and consumption of foods high in fat reflect cultural practices (Airhihenbuwa et al., 1996). In one study (Maillet, D'Eramo Melkus, & Spollett, 1996), African American women with type 2 diabetes expressed concerns about their ability to include ethnic foods and participate in social occasions involving food while managing diabetes. Assisting families with modification of recipes, such as oven roasting rather than frying meat, for their preferred foods may improve dietary adherence (Kulkarni, 2004).

Accurate perception of body size is fundamental to the recognition of overweight/obesity and engagement in weight loss behaviors. In one sample of African Americans, caregivers of overweight children did not associate their child's body size with health risk (Young-Hyman, Schlundt, Herman-Wenderoth, & Bozylinski, 2003). Other studies found that African American girls perceived their female caregivers as role models for body size (Boyington et al., 2008; Katz et al., 2004) and were satisfied with their larger body size (Hesse-Biber, Howling, Leavy, & Lovejoy, 2004).

Religion and spirituality assume a central role in the lives of many African Americans (Quinn, Cook, Nash, & Chin, 2001). In one study, African American women associated the role of religion with health, life satisfaction, social support, coping, and stress management (Samuel-Hodge et al., 2000). On the other hand, religious beliefs and attitudes, such as beliefs that diabetes can be managed by prayer alone, may interfere with diabetes management.

What will you do to educate Mary and her mother about type 2 diabetes and its management? ■

Education Plan

Children and adolescents with type 2 diabetes and their families should receive age-appropriate, ongoing diabetes self-management education (Funnell et al., 2007). The goal of diabetes education is to provide the adolescent and family with the knowledge and skill required to perform daily self-care tasks, manage acute situations such as sick days and hypoglycemia episodes, and make lifestyle changes for effective disease management. Involving the family in lifestyle interventions to improve eating and exercise behaviors is an opportunity to improve health not only for the adolescent, but also for his or her family. The National Diabetes Education Program offers education materials specifically targeted to type 2 diabetes in youth (see Table 18-1). The diabetes management plan needs to emphasize lifetime behavior change as the key to successfully managing type 2 diabetes (Burnet, Plaut, Courtney, & Chin, 2002; Kaufman & Schantz, 2007).

Education content should be structured, age-appropriate, and include blood glucose monitoring, nutrition therapy, and physical activity with an emphasis on lifestyle changes and should be culturally sensitive and individualized to meet the needs of the family. Education may be delivered either individually or in group settings and should be based on assessment of attitudes, beliefs, learning style, baseline knowledge, and readiness to learn (Swift, 2007). Table 18-1 lists educational resources specifically geared to the needs of children and adolescents with type 2 diabetes.

Diabetes education and care is most successful when provided by a diabetes team. In the majority of situations, a child with diabetes will be co-managed by a primary care provider in conjunction with a pediatric endocrinologist and pediatric diabetes team. In cases where geographic access to specialty care is limited, telehealth services may be available through tertiary care centers; these have demonstrated some success with adolescents with diabetes (Batch & Smith, 2005; Heidgerken et al., 2006).

You review the laboratory results from her hospitalization with Mary and her mother and explain that Mary has type 2 diabetes. You discuss the option of initiating an oral antidiabetes agent, metformin, with gradual insulin reduction and the need for some baseline screening. You order the following laboratory tests to be completed prior to her next visit: fasting lipid panel, repeat hemoglobin A1c, and first morning urine for microalbumin, and refer Mary to an ophthalmologist for a dilated eye examination. You prescribe metformin 500 mg twice a day (before breakfast and before dinner) and explain the purpose, action, and possible side effects of the medication. In addition, you decrease Mary's insulin dose and ask Mary's mother to call in 1 week to review blood glucose records, sooner if hypoglycemia is present. You ask Mary's mom to supervise all medication administration and ask that she schedule Mary's 11-year-old brother for an office visit so that he may be screened for diabetes. You applaud Mary's efforts to make healthy food choices and to engage in physical activity and schedule Mary to return for follow up in a month.

In 1 month, Mary returns for follow-up. She is smiling and engages in conversation. Since her last visit, her insulin dose has been decreased on a weekly basis and her metformin titrated upward. Currently her metformin dose is 750 mg before breakfast and before dinner. She is monitoring blood glucose levels twice a day with occasional additional postprandial readings. Her blood glucose levels are recorded in her logbook and are all within her target range of 80-150. She is not experiencing hypoglycemia. Her last menstrual period occurred 1 week ago. The regional pediatric diabetes center has a satellite clinic located 50 miles from your community health center that meets quarterly. The diabetes center providers will follow Mary every 3 months.

Review of her laboratory results shows hemoglobin A1c level 6.5% (target $\leq$ 7%), fasting total cholesterol 165 mg/dL (normal < 170), LDL cholesterol 106 mg/dL (normal < 110), triglycerides 100 mg/dL (normal < 104), urine microalbumin 15 mcg/mg (normal 0-30), creatinine 0.6 mg/dL (normal 0.5-1 mg/dL). All are within normal ranges. The report from her screening eye exam is negative for retinopathy.

Mary reports that she is involved in an after-school program and is learning to swim. On weekends she is walking to the park with her family. She says her mom no longer purchases soda, and the family is drinking water as a beverage with meals. The family has decreased the amount of fried foods; they now eat fried chicken only once a week. She says that her brother has an appointment scheduled for next week and she thinks her mother is worried that he may have diabetes too.

On physical examination today, Mary's weight is 142 pounds (75-90th percentile for age) so she has lost 5 more pounds, and her blood pressure is 120/76 (90th percentile for age and height). Acanthosis nigricans is still present but less noticeable, and Mary mentions that she notices the difference and is pleased with the improvement. The remainder of her exam is negative.

You congratulate her on her excellent progress, noting her improved laboratory results, weight loss, and work to improve her diet and exercise habits. You also note that the family changes will be helpful to everyone. You tell Mary that you will continue to slowly reduce her insulin each week and titrate her metformin upward to the appropriate therapeutic dose.

When do you want this patient to return for follow-up? ■

Children and adolescents with type 2 diabetes should be evaluated every 3 months. In most cases, these children will receive diabetes follow-up from the diabetes care team with primary care services provided by the primary care provider. In cases where access to a pediatric diabetes team is geographically limited, primary care providers will assume a greater role in diabetes management. In either case, ongoing communication between primary and diabetes care providers is essential for achieving glycemic goals for adolescents with type 2 diabetes.

Today, you make no changes in Mary's metformin therapy, and encourage her to keep up the good work with her exercise and diet habits. You provide Mary's mother with a prescription for Mary's brother (fasting blood glucose) in preparation for his office visit next week. You schedule Mary for primary care follow-up in 3 months and send a note to the diabetes team regarding her progress.

Key Points from This Case

1. The incidence of type 2 diabetes is rising, particularly among African American teens. The presence of diabetic ketoacidosis at onset of disease does not exclude this diagnosis.

2. Screening for presence of diabetes comorbidities and complications should be initiated at diagnosis.

3. Type 2 diabetes is a family affair. Frequently, others in the family may have type 2 diabetes and may be either a positive or negative influence for the newly diagnosed adolescent. The diagnosis of type 2 diabetes in an adolescent may prompt screening in siblings or other family members for presence of the disease. The hallmark of management of type 2 diabetes is behavioral change leading to improvement in eating and physical activity behaviors for the entire family.

4. Diabetes management requires a team approach and coordination of services between primary care providers and the diabetes specialty team. In rural areas, this may require creative approaches for access to the diabetes team.

REFERENCES

Airhihenbuwa, C. O., Kumanyika, S., Agurs, T. D., Lowe, A., Saunders, D., & Morssink, C. B. (1996). Cultural aspects of African American eating patterns. *Ethnicity and Health, 1*(3), 245–260.

American Diabetes Association. (2000). Type 2 diabetes in children and adolescents. *Diabetes Care, 23*(3), 381–389.

American Diabetes Association. (2008). Standards of medical care in diabetes–2008. *Diabetes Care, 31*(Suppl 1), S12–S54.

Anderson, B. J., Vangsness, L., Connell, A., Butler, D., Goebel-Fabbri, A., & Laffel, L. M. (2002). Family conflict, adherence, and glycaemic control in youth with short duration Type 1 diabetes. *Diabetic Medicine, 19*(8), 635–642.

Asp, A. A. (2005). Diabetes mellitus. In L. C. Copstead & J. L. Banasik (Eds.), *Pathophysiology* (3rd ed., pp. 1000–1025). St. Louis: Elsevier Saunders.

Atkinson, A., & Radjenovic, D. (2007). Meeting quality standards for self-management education in pediatric type 2 diabetes. *Diabetes Spectrum, 20*(1), 40–46.

Batch, J., & Smith, A. C. (2005). Diabetes and telemedicine. In R. Wootton & J. Batch (Eds.), *Telepediatrics: telemedicine and child health* (pp. 89–104). London: Royal Society of Medicine Press.

Bennett, D. S. (1994). Depression among children with chronic medical problems: a meta-analysis. *Journal of Pediatric Psychology, 19*(2), 149–169.

Berenson, G. S., Srinivasan, S. R., & Nicklas, T. A. (1998). Atherosclerosis: a nutritional disease of childhood. *American Journal of Cardiology, 82*(10B), 22T–29T.

Boyington, J. E., Carter-Edwards, L., Piehl, M., Hutson, J., Langdon, D., & McManus, S. (2008). Cultural attitudes toward weight, diet, and physical activity among overweight African American girls. *Preventing Chronic Disease, 5*(2), A36.

Burnet, D., Plaut, A., Courtney, R., & Chin, M. H. (2002). A practical model for preventing type 2 diabetes in minority youth. *Diabetes Education, 28*(5), 779–795.

Butcher, Z., Fairclough, S., Stratton, G., & Richardson, D. (2007). The effect of feedback and information on children's pedometer step counts at school. *Pediatric Exercise Science, 19*(1), 29–38.

Child Development Institute. (n.d.). *Stages of intellectual development in children and teenagers*. Retrieved April 3, 2007, from http://www.childdevelopmentinfo.com/development/piaget.shtml

Churchill, J. N., Ruppe, R. L., & Smaldone, A. (2009). Use of continuous insulin infusion pumps in young children with type 1 diabetes: a systematic review. *Journal of Pediatric Health Care, 23*(3), 173–179.

Dabelea, D., Bell, R. A., D'Agostino, R. B., Jr., Imperatore, G., Johansen, J. M., Linder, B., et al. (2007). Incidence of diabetes in youth in the United States. *Journal of the American Medical Association, 297*(24), 2716–2724.

Daniels, S. R., & Greer, F. R. (2008). Lipid screening and cardiovascular health in childhood. *Pediatrics, 122*(1), 198–208.

Dantzer, C., Swendsen, J., Maurice-Tison, S., & Salamon, R. (2003). Anxiety and depression in juvenile diabetes: a critical review. *Clinical Psychology Review, 23*(6), 787–800.

Dean, H. J., & Sellers, E. A. (2007). Comorbidities and microvascular complications of type 2 diabetes in children and adolescents. *Pediatric Diabetes, 8*(Suppl 9), 35–41.

Diabetes Control and Complications Trial Research Group. (1993). The effect of intensive treatment of diabetes on the development and progression of long-term complications in insulin-dependent diabetes mellitus. *New England Journal of Medicine, 329*(14), 977–986.

Diabetes Control and Complications Trial Research Group. (1994). Effect of intensive diabetes treatment on the development and progression of long-term complications in adolescents with insulin-dependent diabetes mellitus: Diabetes Control and Complications Trial. *Journal of Pediatrics, 125*(2), 177–188.

DiMeglio, L. A., Pottorff, T. M., Boyd, S. R., France, L., Fineberg, N., & Eugster, E. A. (2004). A randomized, controlled study of insulin pump therapy in diabetic preschoolers. *Journal of Pediatrics, 145*(3), 380–384.

Eisenbarth, G. S. (2007). Update in type 1 diabetes. *Journal of Clinical Endocrinology and Metabolism, 92*(7), 2403–2407.

Fox, L. A., Buckloh, L. M., Smith, S. D., Wysocki, T., & Mauras, N. (2005). A randomized controlled trial of insulin pump therapy in young children with type 1 diabetes. *Diabetes Care, 28*(6), 1277–1281.

Frazier, A., & Pruette, C. S. (2009). Cardiology. In J. W. Custer & R. E. Rau (Eds.), *The Harriet Lane handbook: a manual for pediatric house officers* (18th ed., pp. 176–179). Philadelphia: Elsevier Mosby.

Freedman, D. S., Dietz, W. H., Srinivasan, S. R., & Berenson, G. S. (1999). The relation of overweight to cardiovascular risk factors among children and adolescents: the Bogalusa Heart Study. *Pediatrics, 103*(6 Pt 1), 1175–1182.

Funnell, M. M., Brown, T. L., Childs, B. P., Haas, L. B., Hosey, G. M., Jensen, B., et al. (2007). National standards for diabetes self-management education. *Diabetes Care, 30*(6), 1630–1637.

Gahagan, S., & Silverstein, J. (2003). Prevention and treatment of type 2 diabetes mellitus in children, with special emphasis on American Indian and Alaska Native children. American Academy of Pediatrics Committee on Native American Child Health. *Pediatrics, 112*(4), e328.

Gale, E. A. (2002). The rise of childhood type 1 diabetes in the 20th century. *Diabetes, 51*(12), 3353–3361.

Garrison, M. M., Katon, W. J., & Richardson, L. P. (2005). The impact of psychiatric comorbidities on readmissions for diabetes in youth. *Diabetes Care, 28*(9), 2150–2154.

Gidding, S. S., Dennison, B. A., Birch, L. L., Daniels, S. R., Gillman, M. W., Lichtenstein, A. H., et al. (2005). Dietary recommendations for children and adolescents: a guide for practitioners: consensus statement from the American Heart Association. *Circulation, 112*(13), 2061–2075.

Grey, M., Whittemore, R., & Tamborlane, W. (2002). Depression in type 1 diabetes in children: natural history and correlates. *Journal of Psychosomatic Research, 53*(4), 907–911.

Haller, M. J., Silverstein, J. H., & Rosenbloom, A. L. (2007). Type 1 diabetes in the child and adolescent. In F. Lifshitz (Ed.), *Pediatric endocrinology* (Vol. 1, pp. 63–81). New York: Informa Healthcare.

Heidgerken, A. D., Adkins, J., Storch, E. A., Williams, L., Lewin, A. B., Silverstein, J. H., et al. (2006). Telehealth intervention for adolescents with type 1 diabetes. *Journal of Pediatrics, 148*(5), 707–708.

Hesse-Biber, S. N., Howling, S. A., Leavy, P., & Lovejoy, M. (2004). Racial identity and the development of body image issues among African American adolescent girls. *The Qualitative Report, 9*(1), 49–79.

Hood, K. K., Huestis, S., Maher, A., Butler, D., Volkening, L., & Laffel, L. M. (2006). Depressive symptoms in children and adolescents with type 1 diabetes: association with diabetes-specific characteristics. *Diabetes Care, 29*(6), 1389–1391.

Jeha, G. S., Karaviti, L. P., Anderson, B., Smith, E. O., Donaldson, S., McGirk, T. S., et al. (2005). Insulin pump therapy in preschool children with type 1 diabetes mellitus improves glycemic control and decreases glucose excursions and the risk of hypoglycemia. *Diabetes Technology and Therapeutics, 7*(6), 876–884.

Katz, M. L., Gordon-Larsen, P., Bentley, M. E., Kelsey, K., Shields, K., & Ammerman, A. (2004). "Does skinny mean healthy?" Perceived ideal, current, and healthy body sizes among African-American girls and their female caregivers. *Ethnicity and Disease, 14*(4), 533–541.

Kaufman, F. R., & Schantz, S. (2007). Current clinical research on type 2 diabetes and its prevention in youth. *School Nurse News, 24*(3), 13–16.

Kulkarni, K. (2004). Food, culture, and diabetes in the United States. *Clinical Diabetes, 22*(4), 190–192.

Lawrence, J. M., Standiford, D. A., Loots, B., Klingensmith, G. J., Williams, D. E., Ruggiero, A., et al. (2006). Prevalence and correlates of depressed mood among youth with diabetes: the SEARCH for Diabetes in Youth study. *Pediatrics, 117*(4), 1348–1358.

Liese, A. D., D'Agostino, R. B., Jr., Hamman, R. F., Kilgo, P. D., Lawrence, J. M., Liu, L. L., et al. (2006). The burden of diabetes mellitus among US youth: prevalence estimates from the SEARCH for Diabetes in Youth Study. *Pediatrics, 118*(4), 1510–1518.

Lipton, R. B. (2007). Incidence of diabetes in children and youth—tracking a moving target. *Journal of the American Medical Association, 297*(24), 2760–2762.

Litton, J., Rice, A., Friedman, N., Oden, J., Lee, M. M., & Freemark, M. (2002). Insulin pump therapy in toddlers and preschool children with type 1 diabetes mellitus. *Journal of Pediatrics, 141*(4), 490–495.

Ludwig, D. S., & Ebbeling, C. B. (2001). Type 2 diabetes mellitus in children: primary care and public health considerations. *Journal of the American Medical Association, 286*(12), 1427–1430.

Macaluso, C. J., Bauer, U. E., Deeb, L. C., Malone, J. I., Chaudhari, M., Silverstein, J., et al. (2002). Type 2 diabetes mellitus among Florida children and adolescents, 1994 through 1998. *Public Health Reports, 117*(4), 373–379.

Mack-Fogg, J. E., Orlowski, C. C., & Jospe, N. (2005). Continuous subcutaneous insulin infusion in toddlers and children with type 1 diabetes mellitus is safe and effective. *Pediatric Diabetes, 6*(1), 17–21.

Maillet, N. A., D'Eramo Melkus, G., & Spollett, G. (1996). Using focus groups to characterize the health beliefs and practices of black women with non-insulin-dependent diabetes. *Diabetes Education, 22*(1), 39–46.

Mallare, J. T., Cordice, C. C., Ryan, B. A., Carey, D. E., Kreitzer, P. M., & Frank, G. R. (2003). Identifying risk factors for the development of diabetic ketoacidosis in new onset type 1 diabetes mellitus. *Clinical Pediatrics (Philadelphia), 42*(7), 591–597.

Mulvaney, S. A., Schlundt, D. G., Mudasiru, E., Fleming, M., Vander Woude, A. M., Russell, W. E., et al. (2006). Parent perceptions of caring for adolescents with type 2 diabetes. *Diabetes Care, 29*(5), 993–997.

Must, A., & Strauss, R. S. (1999). Risks and consequences of childhood and adolescent obesity. *International Journal of Obesity and Related Metabolic Disorders, 23*(Suppl 2), S2–S11.

National High Blood Pressure Education Program Working Group on High Blood Pressure in Children and Adolescents. (2004). The fourth report on the diagnosis, evaluation, and treatment of high blood pressure in children and adolescents. *Pediatrics, 114*(Suppl 2), 555–576.

Ogden, C. L., Carroll, M. D., & Flegal, K. M. (2008). High body mass index for age among US children and adolescents, 2003–2006. *Journal of the American Medical Association, 299*(20), 2401–2405.

Peterson, K., Silverstein, J., Kaufman, F., & Warren-Boulton, E. (2007). Management of type 2 diabetes in youth: an update. *American Family Physician, 76*(5), 658–664.

Pinhas-Hamiel, O., Standiford, D., Hamiel, D., Dolan, L. M., Cohen, R., & Zeitler, P. S. (1999). The type 2 family: a setting for development and treatment of adolescent type 2 diabetes mellitus. *Archives of Pediatric and Adolescent Medicine, 153*(10), 1063–1067.

Quinn, M. T., Cook, S., Nash, K., & Chin, M. H. (2001). Addressing religion and spirituality in African Americans with diabetes. *Diabetes Education, 27*(5), 643–644, 647–648, 655.

Rennert, O. M., & Francis, G. L. (1999). Update on the genetics and pathophysiology of type I diabetes mellitus. *Pediatric Annals, 28*(9), 570–575.

Roche, E. F., Menon, A., Gill, D., & Hoey, H. (2005). Clinical presentation of type 1 diabetes. *Pediatric Diabetes, 6*(2), 75–78.

Rosenbloom, A., & Silverstein, J. (2003). *Type 2 diabetes in children and adolescents: a guide to diagnosis, epidemiology, pathogenesis, prevention and treatment.* Alexandria, VA: American Diabetes Association.

Rosenbloom, A. L. (2007). Diabetes in the child and adolescent: diagnosis and classification. In F. Lifshitz (Ed.), *Pediatric endocrinology* (Vol. 1, pp. 57–62). New York: Informa Healthcare.

Rothman, R. L., Mulvaney, S., Elasy, T. A., VanderWoude, A., Gebretsadik, T., Shintani, A., et al. (2008). Self-management behaviors, racial disparities, and glycemic control among adolescents with type 2 diabetes. *Pediatrics, 121*(4), e912–e919.

Samuel-Hodge, C. D., Headen, S. W., Skelly, A. H., Ingram, A. F., Keyserling, T. C., Jackson, E. J., et al. (2000). Influences on day-to-day self-management of type 2 diabetes among African-American women: spirituality, the multi-caregiver role, and other social context factors. *Diabetes Care, 23*(7), 928–933.

Sawyer, S. M., & Aroni, R. A. (2005). Self-management in adolescents with chronic illness. What does it mean and how can it be achieved? *Medical Journal of Australia, 183*(8), 405–409.

Schofield, L., Mummery, W. K., & Schofield, G. (2005). Effects of a controlled pedometer-intervention trial for low-active adolescent girls. *Medicine and Science in Sports and Exercise, 37*(8), 1414–1420.

Silverstein, J., Klingensmith, G., Copeland, K., Plotnick, L., Kaufman, F., Laffel, L., et al. (2005). Care of children and adolescents with type 1 diabetes: a statement of the American Diabetes Association. *Diabetes Care, 28*(1), 186–212.

Skinner, A. C., Weinberger, M., Mulvaney, S., Schlundt, D., & Rothman, R. L. (2008). Accuracy of perceptions of overweight and relation to self-care behaviors among adolescents with type 2 diabetes and their parents. *Diabetes Care, 31*(2), 227–229.

Soltesz, G., Patterson, C. C., & Dahlquist, G. (2007). Worldwide childhood type 1 diabetes incidence—what can we learn from epidemiology? *Pediatric Diabetes, 8*(Suppl 6), 6–14.

Stewart, S. M., Rao, U., Emslie, G. J., Klein, D., & White, P. C. (2005). Depressive symptoms predict hospitalization for adolescents with type 1 diabetes mellitus. *Pediatrics, 115*(5), 1315–1319.

Svec, F., Nastasi, K., Hilton, C., Bao, W., Srinivasan, S. R., & Berenson, G. S. (1992). Black-white contrasts in insulin levels during pubertal development. The Bogalusa Heart Study. *Diabetes, 41*(3), 313–317.

Swift, P. G. (2007). Diabetes education. ISPAD clinical practice consensus guidelines 2006–2007. *Pediatric Diabetes, 8*(2), 103–109.

Tan, J. M. (2009). Nephrology. In J. W. Custer & R. E. Rau (Eds.), *The Harriet Lane handbook: a manual for pediatric house officers* (18th ed., pp. 507–536). Philadelphia: Elsevier Mosby.

TRIGR Study Group. (2007). Study design of the trial to reduce IDDM in the genetically at risk (TRIGR). *Pediatric Diabetes, 8*, 117–137.

U.S. Department of Health and Human Services. (2005). *Dietary guidelines for Americans.* Retrieved August 9, 2008, from http://www.health.gov/dietaryguidelines/dga2005/document/pdf/DGA2005.pdf

Weinger, K., O'Donnell, K. A., & Ritholz, M. D. (2001). Adolescent views of diabetes-related parent conflict and support: a focus group analysis. *Journal of Adolescent Health, 29*(5), 330–336.

White, N. H., Cleary, P. A., Dahms, W., Goldstein, D., Malone, J., & Tamborlane, W. V. (2001). Beneficial effects of intensive therapy of diabetes during adolescence: outcomes after the conclusion of the Diabetes Control and Complications Trial (DCCT). *Journal of Pediatrics, 139*(6), 804–812.

Wilson, D. M., Buckingham, B. A., Kunselman, E. L., Sullivan, M. M., Paguntalan, H. U., & Gitelman, S. E. (2005). A two-center randomized controlled feasibility trial of insulin pump therapy in young children with diabetes. *Diabetes Care, 28*(1), 15–19.

Winter, W. E. (2007). Diabetes autoimmunity. In F. Lifshitz (Ed.), *Pediatric endocrinology* (5th ed., Vol. 1, pp. 83–99). New York: Informa Healthcare.

Writing Team for the Diabetes Control and Complications Trial/Epidemiology of Diabetes Interventions and Complications Research Group. (2002). Effect of intensive therapy on the microvascular complications of type 1 diabetes mellitus. *Journal of the American Medical Association, 287*(19), 2563–2569.

Young-Hyman, D., Schlundt, D. G., Herman-Wenderoth, L., & Bozylinski, K. (2003). Obesity, appearance, and psychosocial adaptation in young African American children. *Journal of Pediatric Psychology, 28*(7), 463–472.

Zdravkovic, V., Daneman, D., & Hamilton, J. (2004). Presentation and course of
    type 2 diabetes in youth in a large multi-ethnic city. *Diabetic Medicine, 21*(10),
    1144–1148.
Zeitler, P., Epstein, L., Grey, M., Hirst, K., Kaufman, F., Tamborlane, W., et al.
    (2007). Treatment options for type 2 diabetes in adolescents and youth: a study
    of the comparative efficacy of metformin alone or in combination with rosigli-
    tazone or lifestyle intervention in adolescents with type 2 diabetes. *Pediatric
    Diabetes, 8*(2), 74–87.

Chapter 19

Migrant Farmworker's Toddler with Anemia

Veronica Kane

Sometimes a single cause may be the culprit when a child presents with multiple symptoms. However, there are those times when multiple symptoms stem from multiple causes, creating a diagnostic dilemma. To derive the most probable diagnoses and appropriate treatment plans, methodical synthesis of data about each of the multiple possible causes is imperative. Developing a schema for analyzing complex situations is essential for practitioners.

Educational Objectives
1. Develop a schema for approaching/evaluating the child who presents with multiple symptoms.
2. Integrate environmental histories into the data gathering for pediatric clients and their families.
3. Assess the child who presents with hematologic symptoms.
4. Analyze basic hematologic laboratory studies.
5. Differentiate among the causes and presentations of various anemias.
6. Integrate cultural information that might affect any aspect of the child's diagnosis, treatment, or compliance.
7. Integrate age-relevant information into the decision-making process.

Case Presentation and Discussion

Oswaldo Garcia, an 18-month-old, is here for his well-child visit. He is with his mother and the clinic's interpreter. Mrs. Garcia tells you that her family and friends in the housing area have expressed concern lately because the child is so pale and skinny. He recently has had a few nosebleeds and seems fussier than usual without any identifiable cause. You now look at Oswaldo for the first time and note blatant pallor in a quiet toddler sitting complacently on his mother's lap. He is wearing a diaper and tee shirt, with a holy medal around his neck and his thumb in his mouth.

Health History

What aspects of the history would be useful to help you refine the nature of Oswaldo's problem? ■

The following information would be helpful:

- History of present illness
- Past medical history
- Family medical history
- Social history
- Environmental history
- Complete review of systems

Oswaldo was last seen in the clinic 3 months ago for an ear infection and fever, and at that time he was given amoxicillin. Although he did not come in for follow-up, Mrs. Garcia reports that he got better very fast and has been fine. She states that she had an uncomplicated pregnancy except for hyperemesis and poor weight gain in the first 4 months of pregnancy. Her labor and delivery were uneventful, and he was discharged home at 2 days with mom and had no problems as a neonate. He has had no hospitalizations, surgeries, major illnesses, or visits to the emergency department.

Family medical history: The family consists of Mr. and Mrs. Garcia, Miguel (age 12 years, has mild asthma); Anna (age 10 years, in good health); Ignatio (age 9 years, recently diagnosed with ADHD), and Maria (age 5 years, with a seizure disorder for the past year). The parents are in good health, do not smoke or take medication, and have had no health problems. There is no family medical history of bleeding problems, G6PD, Fanconi anemia, chronic blood problems, autoimmune diseases, gall stone surgery, splenectomy, or heart disease.

Social history: The family moved to Yakima Valley, Washington, 6 months ago from California to work in the orchards. They had worked in California for a few years in the citrus industry before coming to Washington to be closer to family and to work at the same place year-round. Mrs. Garcia reports that the necklace that Oswaldo wears is a holy medal to keep him safe, which was given to him by his grandmother at his christening. Oswaldo's mom confides that since his change in activity and appetite, the ladies and parents have been praying to the Virgin for Oswaldo and light many candles. The curandera gave them tea to help Oswaldo, amulets of the Virgin for the Mal de Ojo, and oils to rub in for the "empacho" (Kemp, 2005). Box 19-1 discusses Mexican/Chicano health practices that may provide insight about their health belief system.

Environmental history: The family lives in a three-bedroom apartment in the company's housing complex, which was built just after World War II. The apple orchard and fruit farm where Oswaldo's father is employed utilizes pesticides, and the workers wear masks when they apply it. Dad does not change clothes before coming home and playing with the children. They recently have had problems with mice in the apartment so the parents put out some rat poison (super warfarin). There has not been any observed contact with the poison by any of the children, but Mrs. Garcia admits that she does not watch each of the children every second. The other children are all doing fine except as noted above.

Box 19-1   Mexican/Chicano Health Practices

- Mexican immigrants are typically Roman Catholic with a spiritualism that also harkens to their Aztec and Mayan predecessors.

- Healers, or *curanderas*, are usually females (mothers, grandmothers) who have learned their healing practices through an ages-old apprenticeship process.

- Prayer is commonly used to help with healing, especially prayer to important saints such as the Virgin of Guadalupe or Our Lady of San Juan.

- Families commonly have shrines in their homes where they lay amulets and light candles.

- When faced with illness, prayer, lighting of candles, wearing of holy medals and amulets, and even pilgrimages to shrines are common practices.

- Herbs, teas, and massage are also commonly employed as cures.

- Health is a matter of balance. The major balance is hot–cold. Belief in the fundamental nature of the hot–cold balance in health regulation may have an influence about what the sick person may eat, what medicine they will take, and when they do. An example of a "cold" illness is *empacho*, which literally translated means an impacted stomach. Anyone can have *empacho*, but it is commonly associated with gastrointestinal illnesses of children. This "cold" illness is said to be caused by soft or hard-to-digest foods adhering to the stomach wall.

- The *curandera* is an integral member of the immigrant's community with personal ties to the families she treats. Children and their families are not likely to reveal their interactions with these traditional healers until they feel very comfortable with the clinic and the provider.

Sources: Based on Spector, R. (1996). *Culture and diversity in health and illness* (4th ed.). Stamford, CT: Appleton & Lange; Kemp, C. (2005). *Mexicans and Mexican-Americans: health beliefs and practices.* Retrieved April 10, 2009, from http://bearspace.baylor.edu/Charles_Kemp/www/hispanic_health.htm

Review of systems: Because her son sometimes has "crampy stomachaches," Mrs. Garcia gives him Maltsupex 1 tsp, which she adds to his bottle once or twice per week to help him move his bowels when he seems to have a stomachache. Amoxicillin was completed 2 weeks ago; she denies using herbals or other complementary or alternative medicine (CAM) remedies. Mom has not noticed rashes or lesions except for increased bruising for about a month. When he fusses, which he does more and more lately, he shakes his head and closes his eyes. He seems to focus on objects; his eyes are clear with no redness or discharge. He has had several nosebleeds over the past couple of weeks, which seem to be more frequent the past few days. There is cracking at the corners of his mouth, and his tongue looks redder to his mother than usual but doesn't seem to hurt him.

There is no history of diarrhea or vomiting; he is still in diapers. Stools are dark clay-like about twice per week. No blood noted in his stools. He is a picky eater, preferring to drink cow's milk from the bottle, which he carries around with him. As he has gotten thinner and paler, mom has just been happy with whatever he eats. For breakfast he usually eats some oatmeal and fruit, lunch consists of some vegetables and rice, and dinner is rice and beans or casseroles. There is always fruit to eat at home, which mom washes as soon as she brings it home. Total cow's milk ingestion is between 32 and 40 ounces per day.

A review of his development reveals that he sat up at 6 months, stood alone at 11 months, is now walking, but lately prefers to crawl again. He said his first word at 12 months, now has 8–10 words in Spanish, puts everything in his mouth, and eats dirt when he plays outside. He plays quietly, preferring more and more to watch others play.

What should you know about the use of Maltsupex? ■

Maltsupex is commonly used in Mexican American populations for the treatment of constipation. You will address the use of laxatives with Oswaldo as part of your management plan.

Considering the child's age and developmental stage, what are the most common etiologies for pallor and anemia? ■

What possible causes for this presentation come immediately to mind? ■

Acquired pallor in a toddler is unusual and should cause one to think of problems of cutaneous blood flow, anemia, or some unknown mechanism. At 18 months of age, the likelihood of cutaneous blood flow issues is rare; anemia is much more likely. The recent onset of the pallor is more indicative of anemia. Anemia is diagnosed when the hemoglobin concentration (hematocrit) is more than two standard deviations below the mean. Pallor can also occur in association with bleeding, which expands diagnostic possibilities to include leukemia.

Based on the information at hand, what are your priorities for assessment during the physical examination? ■

There may have been exposure to several environmental toxins—rat poison (blood thinner), pesticides from the orchard transmitted on father's clothes (neurotoxin), and soil toxins such as lead or pesticides consumed via his pica behavior. The diet is inadequate in iron due to large quantities of milk ingestion and low ingestions of foods high in iron, and the milk ingestion could contribute to his constipation. Oswaldo's development has regressed slightly, as demonstrated by his now preferring crawling to walking. Oswaldo has become more sedentary and irritable over the past few weeks. Therefore, the neurological, skin and mucus membrane, abdominal, and cardiac examinations will be key areas to evaluate during the physical examination. A developmental assessment will also provide important information.

Likewise, the healthcare provider should review his growth chart (see Table 19-1), which reveals that his height to weight ratio has stayed around 10% from birth, but over the past 6 months a decline in his growth trajectory is evident by a flattened curve. Currently, height and weight are below the third percentile.

Table 19-1   Measurements from Oswaldo's Healthcare Visits

Age	Length	Weight	Weight for Length Percentiles[a]	Head Circumference (HC)	HC Percentile
Birth	19 in/ 48.4 cm	6 lbs 3 oz/ 2.7 kg	10%	33 cm	8%
2 months	21¾ in/ 55 cm	9 lbs 4 oz/ 4.27 kg	8%	37.5 cm	8%
4 months	23¾ in/ 60 cm	12 lbs 2 oz/ 5.6 kg	5–10%	40.4 cm	5–10%
6 months	25¼ in/ 64 cm	15 lbs/ 6.8 kg	10%	41.8 cm	5–10%
9 months	26¾ in/ 68 cm	17 lbs 5 oz/ 8.0 kg	5–10%	43.6 cm	5%
12 months	28½ in/ 71.5 cm	19 lbs 1 oz/ 8.6 kg [19 lbs 13 oz]	5%	44 cm [44.8 cm]	3%
15 months	29½ in/ 74.3 cm	20 lbs/ 9.1 kg [20½ lbs]	3%	44.6 cm [45.6 cm]	< 3% Just under line
18 months	29¾ in/ 76 cm [30¾ in]	20 lb 3oz/ 9.29 kg [22¼ lbs]	< 3%	44.8 cm [46 cm]	< 3%

[a]Numbers in brackets are *projected* values if growth were to be consistent.

Note. Center for Disease Control and Prevention information on Weight for Length Tables, Infants Selected Percentiles can be accessed at http://www.cdc.gov/nchs/about/major/nhanes/growthcharts/html_charts/wtleninf.htm

Physical Examination

Oswaldo presents as a quiet, attentive, subdued child sitting on mom's lap without moving around or reaching for toys or other objects. His vital signs are heart rate 112, respiratory rate 24, and height and weight below the third percentile. There are multiple 1 × 1 cm to 2 × 3 cm bruises of varying ages notable on extremities and forehead. Nails are without lesions with a capillary refill of 2 seconds. His anterior fontanel measures 1 × 1 cm and is flat. His ears and nose are within normal limits. The sclera have a bluish tint, and conjunctiva are pale; attempts to visualize fundi were futile. Irritation and cracking are noted at corners of mouth, and his tongue looks red but does not seem to hurt him. The oral mucosa is pale but no dark lines are noted along the gums. His neck, lungs, heart, and musculoskeletal exam are unremarkable. Abdominal exam is positive for palpable stool (left abdomen–midline and lower abdomen) and a palpable spleen 1 cm below the costal margin. His deep tendon reflexes are 2+ bilaterally, and cranial nerves are grossly intact.

The abnormal findings in the physical examination include:

- Decreased activity
- Central pallor
- Anterior fontanel borderline large for age
- Blue sclera
- Bruising
- Glossitis
- Angular stomatitis
- Splenomegaly
- Stool palpable in abdomen

Utilizing information from both the history and physical, what are the differential diagnoses to consider for Oswaldo? ■

The following are the possible differential diagnoses:

- Iron deficiency anemia
- Lead poisoning
- Leukemia/lymphoma
- Developmental delay, possibly secondary to neurotoxic effects of organophosphates
- Hypothyroidism
- Organophosphate toxicity
- Warfarin ingestion

Before refining the diagnosis by ordering any laboratory or radiologic tests, a review of each of the possible diagnoses will be useful.

Discussion of the Differential Diagnoses

What facts in the history indicate that Oswaldo is at high risk for environmental health hazards? ■

Oswaldo lives in a household where the parents are migrant workers in an agricultural environment known to use organophosphate pesticides; pesticides are used in his home to eradicate mice; crawling is his primary modality; and he spends much time on the floor playing.

Environmental Toxins and Children

Research conducted in the early 1990s revealed that approximately 75% of U.S. households used at least one pesticide product indoors (American Lung Association, n.d.). Such widespread use of pesticides makes the environmental history an integral aspect of data collection in pediatrics. Unique physical characteristics make children especially vulnerable to accumulating toxins in their bodies and exhibiting symptoms of both acute and chronic exposures. Children's bodies are less capable of detoxifying the toxins that get into their bodies due to immature levels of enzymes capable of accomplishing this task. Children spend much of their time close to the ground crawling and playing in the zones where pesticides accumulate. In this pesticide-rich environment, children breathe in fumes and ingest residue through hand-to-mouth activities, further increasing their ingestion of household pesticides.

Considering that the life expectancy of children from the time of toxic exposure is greater than if the exposure occurs in adulthood, there is more time for the development of diseases with long latency periods (Cohen, 2007). A child's respiratory rate is more than twice that of an adult's. Children consume seven times the amount of water as an adult in the first 6 months of life, and between ages 1 and 5 years children consume proportionally three times as much food as adults (Shea, n.d.). There are periods during development when certain systems are especially vulnerable, making them more susceptible to harm if exposed to toxins during these times, generally when organs such as the brain are rapidly growing. The timing of the ingestion of neurotoxic elements, such as lead, arsenic, mercury, PCBs, and alcohol, can have a more robust effect than the amount of the toxin itself.

Children's diets include large amounts of fresh fruits, vegetables, and juices. Breastmilk may also be contaminated. Other factors to consider are that children consume a greater volume of liquids and foods per kilogram than adults, therefore ingesting more toxins per body weight. Table 19-2 shows various fruits and vegetables and the relative amount of pesticide that is absorbed into the food and found by government testing. It is clear from viewing the list of fruits and vegetables that children are at greater risk for proportionally larger amounts of potential pesticides ingestion than adults.

Lower organophosphate metabolites are noted in the urine of children who ate organic foods, compared to children who did not. Children of agricultural workers repeatedly demonstrate higher organophosphate metabolites than children in other environments. Organophosphate metabolites are transmitted via aerial spraying or transmission from parents' clothing (Cohen, 2007; Curl et al., 2002; Thompson et al., 2008).

In the realm of acute effects, symptoms reflect the affected organ system: local irritation (skin, eyes, throat), respiratory system (respiratory distress), and the central nervous system (headache, seizure, coma, death). Chronic symptoms can range from birth defects, cancers, and asthma, to neurodevelopmental/ neurobehavioral symptoms. Many pesticides have been demonstrated to have disruptive effects on the endocrine systems.

Organophosphates (OP) are the most widely used pesticides in the United States, and those employed in agriculture experience the greatest levels of exposure. Data exist describing the health effects of both acute and chronic exposures. Repeated low-grade home spraying more often triggers acute toxic reactions than does agricultural exposure. The mechanism for these reactions is

Table 19-2 PESTnFOOD: Shoppers' Guide to Pesticide Residue in Produce	
High Levels	**Low Levels**
Apples	Asparagus
Bell peppers	Avocado
Celery	Banana
Imported grapes	Broccoli
Cherries	Sweet corn
Peaches	Onions
Potatoes	Peas
Pears	
Raspberries	
Spinach	
Strawberries	

Sources: Based on information from Cohen, M. (2007). Environmental toxins and health: the health impact of pesticides. *Australian Family Physician, 36*(12), 1002–1004; Karr, C. J., Solomon, G. M., & Brock-Utne, A. C. (2007). Health effects of common home, lawn, and garden pesticides. *Pediatric Clinical of North America, 54*, 63–80.

related to inhibition of cholinesterase activity, which results in accumulation of acetylcholine. These toxins target the central nervous system, and among the effects reported are verbal and visual attention problems, motor dexterity, confusion, cognitive deficits, and memory lapses, as well as muscle twitching, seizures, and coma (Fenske, Chensheng, Curl, Shirai, & Kissel, 2005; Karr, Solomon, & Brock-Utne, 2007). Organophosphates demonstrate a predilection for triggering hematologic and solid tumor cancers (Cohen, 2007; Lambert et al., 2005). Toxic symptomatologies can vary greatly between adults and children, with children's symptoms having a much broader presentation. This makes it imperative for healthcare providers to maintain a high index of suspicion. Other symptoms include anorexia, dyspnea, miosis, salivation, tearing, and sweating. Symptoms can persist long after exposure to organophosphates. The mnemonic I PREPARE can be employed to remember the aspects of an environmental history (see Table 19-3).

Oswaldo's environment is abundant in potential pesticide exposures: his father's work clothing, the types of foods he ingests, playing on the floor, hand-to-mouth behaviors, and home rat poison. The family history suggests that pesticide exposure may have had an impact on the siblings as well: Maria has a seizure disorder, Ignatio has ADHD, and Miguel has asthma. Further investigation should involve evaluation of the entire family's exposure level and urinary metabolites as well as other possible toxins. Although these conditions do not necessarily indicate toxicity, but are listed as possible complications, environmental toxins should be explored in Oswaldo's siblings.

Table 19-3   I PREPARE Mnemonic for Environmental History
Investigate potential exposures
Present work of child or parent
Residence (age and characteristics)
Environmental concerns
Past events
Activities (hobbies)
Referrals and resources
(http://www.epa.gov; http://www.atsdr.cdc.gov; http://www.aoec.org; http://www.hazard.com/msds; http://www.osha.gov)
Educate
Source: From Paranzino, G. K., Butterfield, P., Nastoff, T., & Ranger, C. (2005). I PREPARE: developmental and clinical utility of an environmental exposures history mnemonic. *American Association of Occupational Health Nursing, 53*(1) 37–42.

Specific tests would be based on history and symptomatology. Most urinary metabolite tests are nonspecific for the individual organophosphate. Treatment would be based on the agent and whether the poisoning was acute or chronic.

Decontamination of skin, nails, hair, and clothing is paramount because organophosphate absorption increases through breaks in the skin's integrity. Therefore, open areas should be cleansed first with the water flowing away from the wound.

Anemia

Because only 2% of 1 year olds are found to have iron deficiency anemia (IDA) during routine screening between 9 and 18 months of age, the U.S. Preventive Services Task Force does not find sufficient data to definitely recommend selective screening in the 6- to 12-month age group (U.S. Preventive Services Taskforce, 2006). However, general risk factors for anemia and the populations that should be screened for anemia have been identified.

- Premature infants (most hemoglobin accumulates in fetus during the last month of pregnancy)
- Cow's milk consumed before 1 year of age
- Low iron formula in infancy
- Children over 1 year who consume more than 24 ounces of cow's milk per day
- Menstruating adolescent females
- All children from low socioeconomic status families

In most of these situations there are cofactors of rapid growth and deficient nutritional states. These commonly occur together, making the child more susceptible to the depletion of iron at a time when the body has greater need for it. Some information regarding ethnic backgrounds can help point toward specific explanations for aberrant blood findings. Oswaldo's history reveals many of these risk factors.

Pathophysiology of Anemia

Anemia is defined as a low hemoglobin level in the blood. The physiologic impact of anemia on a growing child can be devastating. The human brain undergoes rapid and fundamental development during the first 2 years of life; therefore, lack of nutrition, as seen with decreased oxygen transportation in iron deficiency anemia (IDA), results in life-long cognitive sequelae when occurring during this critical period. Iron deficiency occurs gradually. Dietary requirements for iron are noted in Table 19-4.

In the *prelatent phase* the body's iron stores are depleted. During the *latent phase*, the serum iron and iron-binding capacity decrease below normal levels. Latency is also associated with reduced erythropoiesis that is reflected in a decreased mean corpuscular volume (MCV) and mean corpuscular hemoglobin (MCH) and an increase in the red cell distribution width (RDW) as iron deficiency alters red cell size unevenly. It is during the *frank phase* that anemia is evident through direct hematologic studies, noted through decreases in hemoglobin (Hgb) and hematocrit (Hct) (Berman, 2004; Lesperance, Wu, & Bernstein,

Age	Males (mg/day)	Females (mg/day)
0 to 6 months[a]	0.27	0.27
7 to 12 months	11	11
1 to 3 years	7	7
4 to 8 years	10	10
9 to 13 years	8	8
14 to 18 years	11	15
19 to 50 years	8	18
51+ years	8	8

Table 19-4   Recommended Dietary Allowances for Iron[a]

[a]A normal full-term infant is born with a supply of iron that lasts for 4 to 6 months. There is insufficient data to establish an RDA for iron for infants from birth through 6 months of age. Recommended iron intake for this age group is based on an Adequate Intake that reflects the average iron intake of healthy infants fed breastmilk.

Source: From National Institutes of Health, Office of Dietary Supplements. (n.d.). *Dietary supplement fact sheet: iron.* Accessed December 22, 2008, from http://ods.od.nih.gov/factsheets/iron.asp

2002). Early identification of anemias and intervention are essential for mitigating irreparable effects.

Anemia results from an imbalance between the destruction and production of red blood cells. In IDA, the iron stores are depleted to the extent that the hemoglobin essential to red cell production is no longer adequate for this to happen. Decreased red blood cell (RBC) production typically occurs gradually and causes chronic anemia. Any of several mechanisms may be responsible for this decreased production: bone marrow failure, impaired erythropoietin production, and defects in the maturation of red cells. Hemolysis, or increased RBC destruction, may be triggered by extracellular causes: mechanical injury (such as in hemolytic–uremic syndromes or cardiac valvular defects), antibodies (as from autoimmune disorders), infections, drugs, toxins, and thermal injury to RBCs (as in severe burns). Hereditary causes tend to decrease RBC production due to intracellular defects, including defects in cell membrane, enzyme defects, hemoglobinopathies, thalassemias, porphyrias, and paroxysmal nocturnal hemoglobinuria. Blood loss, either acute or chronic, represents the last category of decreased RBC production and can result from disease processes or trauma (Lesperance et al., 2002; Lee & Truman, 2007).

There are three kinetic categories of red blood cells used to describe anemias: *microcytic*, indicating undersized red blood cells; *normocytic*, indicating normal sized red blood cells; and *macrocytic*, referencing cells that are larger than normal. The second characteristic used to differentiate the types of anemia refers to the amount of hemoglobin contained in cells. When the hemoglobin is low, the anemia is referred to as *hypochromic*.

Oswaldo's history of acquired pallor, bluish sclera, lack of activity, and a diet of mostly cow's milk with no other significant iron source makes iron deficiency the most likely etiology of his anemia. His health history reveals many risk factors for iron deficiency anemia as well: low socioeconomic status, immigrant, age, diet, and appearance. This diagnosis is further suggested by the physical presence of glossitis and stomatitis.

Conditions with Anemia as a Symptom

IDA is classified as a *microcytic* and *hypochromic* anemia and is the most common of the anemias. Iron deficiency is the most common nutritional deficiency, and IDA is its most severe expression (Centers for Disease Control and Prevention [CDC], 2002). Children between 6 and 20 months, preterm infants, and menstruating adolescent females are at the greatest risk in general, but the incidence doubles in Mexican Americans and African Americans (Borgna-Pignatti & Marsella, 2008).

Thalassemia is another microcytic, hypochromic anemia, though it is most often encountered in its minor or trait variation. The thalassemias are genetically transmitted, with homozygous disease having the greatest health impact. Thalassemia minor is important to differentiate from iron deficiency anemia because thalassemia does not respond to iron therapy. It occurs with greater prevalence among certain racial and ethnic groups. Alpha-thalassemias are most prevalent in persons of Southeast Asian descent, whereas the beta-thalassemias are found among persons of Southeast Asian, Middle Eastern, or Mediterranean descent. Symptoms may appear between 3 and 6 months of age. Information gathered from the family medical history, such as anemia, miscarriage, jaundice, gallstones, or splenomegaly, should further raise the index of suspicion. Laboratory studies help to differentiate thalassemia minor from anemia. The Mentzer index is determined by dividing the MCV by the RBC count. A score greater than 13 suggests iron deficiency anemia, whereas less than 13 is indicative of thalassemia. The free erythrocyte protoporphyrin (FEP) test is another lab that is useful in differentiating the two anemias: a microcytic anemia with an elevated FEP rules out a diagnosis of thalassemia; however; it does not confirm the diagnosis of iron deficiency anemia. For a definitive diagnosis, hemoglobin electrophoresis is necessary, with a quantitative A2 and F hemoglobin. Beta-thalassemia trait will show elevations of either or both A2 and F hemoglobin (Garfunkel, Kaczorowski, & Christy, 2007).

Celiac disease is another common cause of iron deficiency (10–30% of cases) because it decreases the body's ability to absorb up to 46% of ingested iron. The only other disorder to equal this significant level of malabsorption is small bowel resection. Disorders that lead to decreased acid secretion, such as *H. pylori*, also impede iron absorption. Situations leading to blood loss (polyps, ulcers, hemorrhagic telangiectasia, and diverticulitis) also deplete iron stores, as do parasitic infestations (Irwin & Kirchner, 2001). After all other causes for a microcytic anemia have been ruled out, there is the possible explanation of anemia of chronic disease, which is only a diagnosis of exclusion.

It is interesting to note that in children with breath-holding spells there is a high incidence of iron deficiency anemia and that the rate of occurrence of these spells decreases following a therapeutic trial of elemental iron supplementation (Borgna-Pignatti & Marsella, 2008). Anemia in combination with leukopenia, neutropenia, or thrombocytopenia is more suggestive of failure of RBC production caused by conditions such as aplastic anemia, Fanconi anemia, or leukemia (Lee & Truman, 2007). This information underscores the need to seek the cause of anemia in order to provide the definitive treatment. Anemia is a symptom of an underlying disorder. As the anemia diagnosis narrows, the diagnosis of the underlying disorder then needs further treatment.

What physical findings in Oswaldo are suggestive of iron deficiency anemia? ▪

Relying solely on physical examination to make a diagnosis of iron deficiency anemia is not very reliable because the findings are nonspecific and often late manifestations, including pallor, fatigue, glossitis, edema (due to milk-induced protein-losing enteropathy with iron deficiency), spoon nails, angular stomatitis, bluish tint to sclera, irritability, frontal bossing, exercise intolerance, abnormal immune response, growth retardation, impaired collagen synthesis (blue sclera), epithelial abnormalities (gastrointestinal mucosal lesions, spoon-shaped nails), and chewing ice. Tachycardia is noted as a poor compensation for an acute process, such as blood loss. A normal heart rate is suggestive of a chronic process. Jaundice may be seen in the face of a hemolytic process as bilirubin accumulates. Splenomegaly occurs as a result of malignancies, acute infections, inherited hemolytic anemia, or the case of hypersplenism secondary to portal hypertension (Hermiston & Mentzer, 2002; Lesperance, Wu, & Bernstein, 2002).

What aspects of the history indicate risk factors for lead toxicity? ■

The following are aspects of Oswaldo's history that are risk factors for lead toxicity:

- Pica (eating non-nutritive substances)
- Crawling (increases amount of time on floor where residue accumulates)
- Mouthing behavior (young children explore their worlds)
- Age (toddlers are at increased risk due to floor play and hand–mouth exploration)
- Lower socioeconomic status
- Residing in an old building (lead paint was used until 1978 and still is utilized in some nonresidences and military installations [CDC, 2002])
- Wearing a medal on a chain–composition unknown

What physical findings would one look for in cases of suspected lead toxicity? ■

Lead Poisoning

Children with lead poisoning can be without symptoms until levels rise high enough to result in permanent neurologic damage. Lethargy may be noted in children with mild levels and perhaps a complaint of abdominal pain. As the severity of poisoning increases, diffuse abdominal, even colicky pain becomes evident. For serum lead levels > 300 mcg/dL, expected signs may include lethargy, nausea, vomiting, green or tarry stools, hypotension, rapid pulse, metabolic acidosis, shock, coma, hepatic necrosis, renal failure, and local gastrointestinal erosions. The nonspecific nature of these symptoms underscores the need for a high level of suspicion and an organized environmental history. Encephalopathies occur more commonly in children than in adults. These encephalopathies are characterized by seizures, mania, delirium, and even coma. A horizontal line across the nails or gumline may be evident, though such lines are in evidence so rarely as to have little clinical significance (Roberts & Reigart, 2002). As with other anemias, there may also be pallor. On radiograph, lead fragments may be visible in the gut, and uptake lines may appear on long bones, but these measures are indicated in a more severe presentation of toxicity.

Epidemiology of Lead Poisoning

Plumbism has long been recognized as having significant impact on the well-being of children, but lead is inescapably present throughout the environment.

The results of the National Health and Nutrition Examination Survey (NHANES) in 1994 and again in 1999–2002 indicate the occurrence of lead toxicity in the United States is on the decline as a result of increased public awareness and legislation. Rates in non-Hispanic African American children remain higher than in non-Hispanic white or Mexican American children (CDC, 2005; Roberts & Riegart, 2002).

Despite this improvement, lead toxicity remains a major health concern. A high index of suspicion and careful monitoring of children from at-risk populations is vital in order to provide early detection and treatment. The risk factors are the same as for iron deficiency, which itself facilitates lead absorption in children. Both pica and lead poisoning have been found to be associated findings in the presence of iron deficiency anemia.

Pathophysiology of Lead Poisoning
As in the discussion of environmental toxins, children absorb more lead and are more sensitive to its effects than are adults (Cohen, 2007). Children's bones store only 64% of the absorbed lead, whereas adults' bones sequester approximately 95%. That leaves 36% of the lead burden in the child's circulation and soft tissues where it results in acute toxic effects. Other deficiencies compound the rates at which iron is taken up into the body and the degree to which it is stored.

Lead competitively binds with many proteins: the sulfhydryl (SH) group of cysteine, the amino group of lysine, the carboxyl group of glutamic and aspartic acids, and the hydroxyl group of tyrosine (Piomelli, 2002). This widespread affinity for key proteins helps to explain the widespread effects within the body.

In blood, an elevated lead level interferes with heme synthesis by inhibiting essential mitochondrial membrane function and interfering with enzymatic functions. In lead toxicity, iron is blocked from being incorporated into protoporphyrin, despite the fact that it is available. However, in iron deficient states this lack of iron results in an accumulation of erythrocyte protoporphyrin in blood. Both situations result in elevated circulating levels of FEP (Piomelli, 2002). Therefore, an elevated FEP level with a microcytic RBC morphology could indicate either iron toxicity or iron deficiency.

The brain is very sensitive to exposure to heavy metals or other toxins, with children's brains being even more susceptible. The effect of these toxins is primarily reflected in neurobehavioral and neurodevelopmental disorders such as cognitive deficits, developmental delays, inattention problems, and psychosocial disorders, and in central nervous system dysfunctions such as ataxia, seizures, paresthesias, paralysis, coma, or death. The extent of sequelae is influenced by the level of intoxication.

Which of Oswaldo's physical findings would be suggestive of leukemia or another cancer? ■

The following findings could be suggestive of cancer:

- Pallor
- Fatigue
- Purpura
- Bleeding

Pathophysiology of Leukemia and Lymphoma

Although the specific cause of lymphoblastic leukemia is not known, in general cancers are known to stem from damage to DNA resulting in an uncontrolled overproduction of cells that overcrowd the bone marrow, crowding out normal cells. Because these abnormal cells are blood-borne, they can spread throughout the body and infiltrate organs and sites such as the liver, spleen, central nervous system, lymph nodes, and reproductive organs (Belson, Kingsley, & Holmes, 2007). These cells also develop abnormally long life spans. Leukemia may be the result of exposure to radiation or chemicals. Regarding chemical exposures, only benzene has been clearly demonstrated to cause cancer, but other agents, such as organophospates and other pesticides, have been noted as possible links (Belson et al., 2007).

Symptoms consistent with leukemias are typically present days to weeks before diagnosis. Disruption of hematopoiesis accounts for the most common presenting symptoms of anemia—infection, easy bruising, and bleeding. Other symptoms and signs of leukemia tend to be less specific (pallor, fatigue, fever, tachycardia, chest pain, malaise, and weight loss) and are attributable to anemia and a hypermetabolic state rather than to the direct effect of the cancer.

Multiple factors influence the outcomes for leukemia. Acute lymphoblastic leukemia (ALL) occurs most often in children and has a greater cure rate than acute myeloblastic leukemia (AML). Females tend to fare better than males. Whites tend to be diagnosed with ALL more often than African Americans, but Asian Americans and Hispanic Americans have survival rates higher than African Americans. Children between 1 and 10 years have greater survivability than older persons. Persons with Down syndrome have a greater likelihood of developing leukemia than do any other groups (Gamis et al., 2003; Robison et al., 1984). Overall survival rates drop off markedly if these cancerous cells are evident in the brain or central nervous system.

If suspicions of leukemia are strong, the initial evaluation would first include a complete blood count (CBC) and a peripheral blood smear (PBS). The red cell size may present as normocytic with decreased RBC production, and the MCV is occasionally increased. The presence of pancytopenia (thrombocytopenia/leucopenia/cytosis) and peripheral blasts suggest acute leukemia. The differential diagnosis of the finding of pancytopenia includes: aplastic anemia, viral infections such as infectious mononucleosis, and vitamin B_{12} and folate deficiency. The peripheral smear may also reveal tear-drop erythrocytes and leukocyte casts.

Blast cells in the blood smear may approach 90%, unless the WBC count is markedly decreased. Although the preliminary diagnosis can usually be made from the blood smear, bone marrow examination is the diagnostic gold standard. Blast cells in the bone marrow range between 30% and 95%. Immediate referral to a hematologist/oncologist is required.

A diagnosis of leukemia is unlikely in Oswaldo's case; however, you will do initial basic blood testing (CBC) that will assure you that leukemia is not the cause of his symptoms.

What physical findings are suggestive of warfarin (rat poison) ingestion? ■

The following symptoms are suggestive of warfarin ingestion:

- Nosebleeds
- Bruising and purpura
- Anemia secondary to acute blood loss

Pathophysiology of Warfarin Toxicity

The majority of accidental warfarin ingestions occur in children younger than 6 years of age and consist of ingestions of small amounts of warfarin. There are several long-acting coumarin derivatives, so-called Super warfarin anticoagulants (brodifacoum, diphenadione, chlorophacinone, bromodialone) commonly used as rodenticides. They produce profound effects and prolong anticoagulation. The mechanism of action of these common coumarin derivatives is to inhibit vitamin K_1-2,3 epoxide reductase, preventing vitamin K from being reduced to its active form (Olson, Trickey, Miller, & Yungmann-Hile, 2008). The degree of this effect is based on dose and duration of exposure to warfarin. The oral bioavailability is excellent. Once in the system, it is bound to plasma protein (albumin) and distributed to the kidneys, lungs, and spleen. Anticoagulant effects typically occur 5–7 days after a single dose; however, the Super warfarin effects may persist for weeks to months.

Minor bleeding complications are usually noted from mucosal surfaces, but also increase the ease of bruising, nosebleeds, and hematuria. As the ingested amount of Super warfarin increases, major complications become evident. Major bleeding commonly includes hemorrhages from gastrointestinal, intracranial, and retroperitoneal sites, but could progress to massive bleeding from any organ system.

What characteristics from the history and physical relate to the possible diagnosis of hypothyroidism? ■

The following could suggest hypothyroidism:

- Fatigue
- Loss of developmental skills
- Dullness

Pathophysiology of Hypothyroidism

Fatigue, constipation, poor feeding, delayed development, and the slow growth reported in Oswaldo's case are consistent with a diagnosis of hypothyroidism. In infants with congenital hypothyroidism, symptoms become evident within weeks to months of birth. Among the presenting symptoms are prolonged jaundice, poor feeding, constipation, cool mottled skin, excessive sleepiness, decreased crying, umbilical hernia, and large fontanel and tongue (Avery, 1994). A decrease in growth velocity in the presence of anemia suggests the possibility of hypothyroidism. This anemia tends to be normo- or macrocytic anemia. This finding should not be confused with the megaloblastic anemia associated with folate or cobalamin deficiency. Anemia associated with hypothyroidism responds when the primary hormone deficiency is treated (Irwin & Kirchner, 2001).

Of those neonates diagnosed with hypothyroidism, 10% will develop normal thyroid levels within days to months of birth. For the other 90% of affected neonates, if their hypothyroidism is left untreated, severe developmental delay and mental retardation as well as growth delays result (Kliegman, Greenbaum, & Lye, 2004).

Acquired hypothyroidism has an insidious onset, with slowing of growth being the most common initial symptom. Linear growth is very dependent on the amount of circulating thyroid hormone; in the absence of this hormone, growth will cease completely until it is replaced. A goiter often appears early and can be noted on routine examination even before growth slowing occurs. Hypothyroidism also impacts energy level and may produce a dull expression in children. Other findings include pale, thick, cool skin; constipation; delayed deep tendon reflexes; slow pulse and lowered blood pressure; and dulling of the child's cognitive ability, although these symptoms are reversible with hormone replacement therapy (Burchett, Hanna, & Steiner, 2009).

There are a few possible reasons for a young child to manifest signs and symptoms of hypothyroidism after the neonatal period. Delayed onset of congenital hypothyroidism occurs when the newborn has a vestigial or defective thyroid gland, which is incapable of meeting the demands of a growing child. Inhibition of thyroid hormone production within the gland itself is a more common explanation for the development of hypothyroidism. Inadequate dietary iodine is a cause that is common in less developed countries, but it is not a health concern in the United States (Kliegman et al., 2004). Some drugs may also block thyroid hormone production, and when prescribing lithium or iodine-containing drugs such as amiodarone, hormone level monitoring is essential (Taketomo, Hodding, & Kraus, 2008). Hypothyroidism from these causes can be reversed. Occasionally the body will have an autoimmune reaction to its own thyroid gland. In Hashmoto's thyroiditis, the antibodies attack and destroy thyroid cells.

Making the Diagnosis

Your diagnostic list now includes IDA, possible warfarin ingestion, and hypothyroidism as the most likely causes of Oswaldo's signs and symptoms. The next phase in determining Oswaldo's diagnosis and subsequent treatment is to perform laboratory diagnostic tests. For expediency and to minimize trauma to the toddler, several tests should be ordered simultaneously. Thus, you order the following tests:

- Complete blood count with white blood cell differential and peripheral blood smear (CBC with diff and PBS)
- Thyroid screen (T4, TSH, +/- T3)
- Lead level
- Prothrombin
- Urinary metabolites for organophosphates
- Stool guaiac

IDA: CBC with Differential

Specific tests to determine the type of anemia will be directed by the clinical presentation, history, and initial blood work. The causative factors of the anemia must be clarified. Information revealed in the complete blood count, peripheral blood smear, lead studies, thyroid studies, and hemoglobin electrophoresis would all help in refining the etiology of anemia. Findings in patient examination and history will further guide the diagnosis of anemia and the additional examinations needed to confirm the diagnosis. It is vital to remember that having the diagnosis of the type of anemia is not the end point. Bone marrow examination by itself is not a useful diagnostic tool in infants and toddlers because there is little or no iron stored in the marrow hemosiderin in these young children who do not have the marrow reserves that older children develop (Scott, 2006).

Warfarin Intoxication: Prothrombin Time

Serum measurements of warfarin are not readily available or useful in most ingestions because most labs are not able to provide timely reports of vitamin K–dependent clotting factors. Daily *prothrombin time (PT)* levels serve to quantify the anticoagulant effect of ingested rodenticide and to determine the necessary duration of vitamin K treatment. Some sources recommend repeating the PT test 24 and 48 hours post-ingestion (Olson et al., 2008). Mullins, Brands, and Daya's (2000) study, however, suggests that in normal pediatric exposures to Super warfarin the PT test is not necessary and does not affect outcome. Normalization of the PT level within 48–72 hours indicates the quantity of warfarin ingested was insignificant.

Lead Intoxication: Lead Level

An elevated lead level is diagnostic of plumbism. The sample may be from either a capillary or venous source, but preparation of the site is vital to getting an accurate result. The skin must be well-cleaned to prevent contamination from surface lead dust. Capillary samples are much more sensitive to surface contamination due to the small size of the sample. If a capillary sample yields a lead level greater than 10 mcg/dL, a venous sample must be obtained to provide diagnostic confirmation. Levels less than 10 mcg/dL are considered normal. Table 19-5 indicates the increments within elevated levels and how they are addressed therapeutically.

Hypothyroidism: Thyroxine and Thyroid Stimulating Hormone

A diagnosis of hypothyroidism would explain some but not all of Oswaldo's symptoms. The tests used to determine thyroid status are the thyroxine (T4) and thyroid stimulating hormone (TSH) levels. Eighty percent of circulating thyroid hormone is T4 and the remaining 20% is T3, so determining the T4 level is usually adequate, but one can also include the T3 level for a complete thyroid picture. TSH levels reveal the functioning and role of the pituitary gland in directing thyroid function. A normal TSH level with a low T4 level indicates that the pituitary gland is not sensing or responding to the low circulating level of thyroid hormone. An elevated TSH level indicates that the pituitary gland has detected the low serum thyroid levels and has attempted to spur the thyroid gland to greater activity to compensate. When the TSH is high and the T4 is low, the implication is that the thyroid gland is malfunctioning (Kliegman et al., 2004).

You review the results of your laboratory studies, which are found in Table 19-6. Based upon these findings you identify the following diagnoses:

Interpretation of CBC with differential and PBS:
- Microcytic, hypochromic anemia
- RDW is increased, consistent with iron deficiency anemia
- Normal white blood cell count
- Reticulocyte is increased, as is normally seen in IDA

Interpretation of iron studies:
- Serum iron and serum ferritin are very low, indicating inadequate iron stores.
- The FEP is elevated, consistent with IDA and/or elevated lead level.

  These results rule out thalassemia trait (diagnostic for thalassemia traits is microcytic anemia and normal FEP).

Lead level:
- A lead level of 42 constitutes a moderately high level, CDC classification III.

Table 19-5   Treatment Recommendations Based on Blood Lead Level

10–14 mcg/dL	15–19 mcg/dL	20–44 mcg/dL	45–69 mcg/dL	≥ 70 mcg/dL
Class II-A	Class II-B	Class III	Class IV	Class V Medical Emergency!
Lead education • Dietary • Environmental F/u blood lead monitoring	Community/environmental survey Remove lead source Lead education • Dietary • Environmental F/u blood lead monitoring Follow plan for 20–44 IF: • f/u BLL remains within this range at least 3 months after initial venous test • BLLs increase with retesting	Community/environmental survey Remove lead source Home visit: monitor Lead education • Dietary • Environmental F/u blood lead monitoring Complete history and physical exam Lab work: • Hemoglobin or hematocrit • Iron status Environmental investigation Lead hazard reduction Neurodevelopmental monitoring	Community/environmental survey Remove lead source Home visit: monitor Lead education • Dietary • Environmental F/u blood lead monitoring Complete history and physical exam Complete neurological exam Lab work: • Hemoglobin or hematocrit • Iron status • FEP or ZPP Environmental investigation	Community/environmental survey Remove lead source Home visit: monitor Hospitalize and begin chelation therapy at once Proceed according to actions for 45–69 mcg/dL

Table 19-5 Treatment Recommendations Based on Blood Lead Level (Continued)

10–14 mcg/dL	15–19 mcg/dL	20–44 mcg/dL	45–69 mcg/dL	≥ 70 mcg/dL
Class II-A	Class II-B	Class III	Class IV	Class V Medical Emergency!
		Abdominal X-ray with bowel decontamination if indicated Chelation challenge test	Lead hazard reduction Neurodevelopmental monitoring Abdominal X-ray with bowel decontamination if indicated Chelation therapy (DMSA)	

Notes. **The following actions are NOT recommended at any blood lead level:**

- Search for gingival lead lines
- Testing of neurophysiologic function
- Evaluation of renal function, except during chelation with EDTA
- X-ray fluorescence of long bones
- Testing of hair, teeth, or fingernails for lead
- Radiographic imaging of long bones

Abbreviations: BLL: blood lead level; f/u: follow-up; FEP: free erythrocyte protoporphyrin; ZPP: zinc protoporphyrin; DMSA: dimercaprol succinic acid.

Sources: Based on Roberts, J. R., & Reigart, J. R. (2007). *Managing elevated blood lead levels among young children: recommendations from the Advisory Committee on Childhood Lead Poisoning Prevention.* Retrieved July 30, 2008, from http://www.cdc.gov/nceh/lead/CaseManagement/chap3.pdf; Piomelli, S. (2002). Childhood lead poisoning. *Pediatric Clinics of North America, 49*, 1285–1304; Tietz, N. W. (1995). *Clinical guidelines to laboratory tests* (3rd ed.). Philadelphia: W.B. Saunders.

Table 19-6 Oswaldo's Laboratory Results with Norms for Children 6 Months to 3 Years

Test	Oswaldo's Values	Normal Range
Complete Blood Count (CBC)		
Hemoglobin (Hgb) *(g/dL)*	7	11–14
Hematocrit (Hct) *(%)*	20	33–41
Mean corpuscular volume (MCV)		70–84 fL/cell
Mean corpuscular Hgb		23–31 picograms/cell
Red cell distribution (RCD) width	19	11–16
White blood count *(× 1000 cells/mm³)*	10.0	6.0–16.0
Myelocytes	0	0
Neutrophils (segs) *(%)*	61	54–62
Neutrophils (bands) *(%)*	2	3-5
Lymphocytes *(%)*	30	25–33
Monocytes *(%)*	6	3–7
Eosinophils *(%)*	1	1–3
Basophils *(%)*	0	0.75
Reticulocyte count *(%)*	0.22	0–2
Serum iron *(mcg/dL)*	40	65–155
Serum ferritin (ng/mL)	24	40–160
Free erythrocyte protoporphyrin	elevated	
Lead level (mcg/dL)	42	0–10
Hemoglobin electrophoresis (with quantitative A2 and F)	pending	
Prothrombin time (sec)	13	< 12
Urinalysis	negative for heme	
Urinary metabolites	positive for OP	
Thyroid screen		
T4 (total) *(mcg/dL)*	6.8	4.9–9.5
TSH *(mIU/L)*	4.6	0.410–5.90
Stool guaiac	negative	

Thyroid screening:

- T4 and TSH are both within normal range, indicating there is no hypothyroidism.

    If hypothyroidism had been identified, primary treatment is by oral hormone replacement with levothyroxine. Because this medication can interact with many different drugs, it is important to review the child's medication history at each visit. Families should be instructed to limit ingestion of goitrogenic foods (asparagus, cabbage, peas, turnip greens, broccoli, spinach, brussel sprouts, lettuce, and soybeans), plus soybean-based formulas, cottonseed meal, walnuts, and dietary fiber, because these may decrease absorption (Takemoto, Hodding, & Kraus, 2008). The dosage varies by age, decreasing as the child ages. Laboratory monitoring of serum levels consists of annual TSH levels. Treatment is best accomplished in consultation with or referral to a pediatric endocrinologist.

Prothrombin time:
- The PT is elevated, which is consistent with ingestion of Super warfarin.

Developmental testing:
- The results of Oswaldo's developmental testing reveal he is delayed in gross and fine motor areas. There is a recommendation for close follow-up testing.

From these results, you arrive at your final list of diagnoses and determine their ICD codes. Table 19-7 lists the ICD-9 codes based upon your final diagnoses. These diagnoses are:

- Moderate-severe iron deficiency anemia
- Lead poisoning, moderate
- Organophosphate exposure and warfarin ingestion
- Poor growth and delayed development

Management

There are general guidelines to consider when managing the diagnostic problems that Oswaldo has.

Table 19-7 ICD-9 Codes for Oswaldo's Final Diagnoses	
Final Diagnosis	**ICD-9 Code**
Moderate-severe iron deficiency anemia	280.9
Lead poisoning, moderate	984.9
Organophosphate exposure	989.3
Warfarin ingestion (poison by agents affecting blood components)	964
Poor growth	253.2
Developmental delay	783.5

Iron Deficiency Anemia

Iron supplementation is necessary with laboratory monitoring of the child's response. Typically a trial of oral iron is started at 4 to 6 mg/kg/day of elemental iron in two to three divided doses per day. Reticulocytosis is typically seen after 4 days of therapy. Hemoglobin levels should be monitored. A return to normal Hgb level occurs within 4 to 6 weeks if iron supplementation is taken as prescribed. Because iron stores must be replenished, a course of iron supplementation is recommended for 2 to 3 months. Dietary counseling regarding iron-rich foods is an essential part of patient education. Blood monitoring of hemoglobin is typically done at 1 month. If there is an adequate response (an Hgb increase of at least 1 g/dL or a greater than 3% increase in hematocrit), the diagnosis of IDA is confirmed. A hemoglobin level is then drawn again approximately 6 months after iron supplementation is discontinued to confirm a full return to normal levels of Hgb (Schwartz, 2009). **Because Oswaldo does not simply have IDA but also has elevated lead levels and a hemoglobin of 7 gm/dL, you want to want to discuss his case with the hematologist.**

Plumbism

The CDC committee developed guidelines to direct treatment of plumbism in primary care practices (see Table 19-5). The primary step in treatment is to remove the lead source from the child's environment. Proper nutrition and the passage of time will generally serve to lower the levels of lead in mild to moderate intoxications. For symptomatic and severe intoxications by lead, it may be necessary to use chelation. Chelating agents are not without risks of their own and should be used by experienced healthcare providers in controlled situations.

Dimercaptosuccinic acid (DMSA) [Chemet] is a water-based oral agent approved in the treatment of heavy metals such as lead, cadmium, arsenic, and mercury toxicity by the Food and Drug Administration (FDA). DMSA is the safest of the chelating agents with a wide margin between the doses needed to be effective and the dosages that would be toxic. *British anti-lewit (BAL)* is oil-based and unpleasant to patients. Significantly, BAL forms a toxic substance when combined with iron, so it must *never* be given during iron therapy. *Edetate Calcium Disodium (Calcium EDTA)* is water-soluble and best given intravenously. It is possible to give intramuscularly, but is quite painful and should be drawn up with 2% procaine to minimize site discomfort. The primary risk associated with this chelating agent is that due to its actions within the body there is an increased likelihood of seizures.

Warfarin Intoxication

Vitamin K (phytonadione, AquaMEPHYTON) overcomes the coagulation, thereby blocking the effect of warfarin. It takes several hours for the liver to then produce clotting factors and release them into the circulation. Typical pediatric dosing is 1–5 mg orally; however, higher doses are necessary to reverse the Super warfarin coagulopathies, and these doses need to be titrated based on the results of daily prothrombin times (Taketomo, Hodding, & Kraus, 2008). Consultation with a hematologist is recommended.

> Although Oswaldo's PT level is only slightly above the normal range, you initiate a call to your hematologist consultant to determine whether vitamin K is needed at this point and to discuss the issue of his IDA, elevated lead levels, and positive urinary metabolite screen.

Plan of Care

You discuss your plan of care with Oswaldo's mother, which is as follows:

- Consult with hematologist regarding anemia, lead toxicity, and likely low level of warfarin ingestion.
- Department of Public Health involvement: Site visit and lead abatement.
- Visiting nurse to provide home monitoring, teaching, coaching, medication administration technique, and to promote success.
- Referral to early intervention program: for infant stimulation.
- Fer-in-sol (which comes in 75 mg/0.6 ml, in a 50 ml bottle) 6 mg/kg @ 9.2 kg = 0.2 ml orally bid, OR iron polysaccharide complex taken daily by mouth.
  - Take with orange juice or cranberry juice.
  - Wipe teeth clean after administering to minimize dark discoloration.
  - Put medicine toward back of mouth if possible.
- Consider iron chelation therapy with BAL or Calcium EDTA (doses) if lead levels do not drop as the environment becomes less toxic. This will necessitate a follow-up discussion with the hematologist.
- Nutritional consult: There will be much information for Mrs. Garcia to absorb, so an ongoing consult would be appropriate until Oswaldo's condition improves. Referral to address:
  - Decrease cow's milk to not greater than 16 ounces in a day.
  - Discontinue baby bottle.
  - Encourage iron-fortified foods and meats.
  - Discontinue the use of Maltsupex and encourage juices to help ease constipation, especially nectars, prune juice, and apple juice.
  - Increase caloric intake.
- Provide telephone follow-up in several days, not longer than 1 week, to determine how the family is doing with all the changes.
- Dental care: Iron may discolor teeth, but regular dental brushing and wiping teeth clean after administration of iron preparation will minimize this. This discoloration is temporary.
- Developmental assessment today, repeat in month, continue to monitor.
- Return to clinic in 2 weeks for repeat CBC and reticulocyte count.
- Provide telephone follow-up in several days, not longer than 1 week, to determine how the family is doing with all the changes.

With your written instructions, Oswaldo's mother seems to understand what will happen and how to manage his care at this point. She is happy to know that help is coming for his condition.

What long-term follow-up should be planned for Oswaldo? ▓

Long-Term Follow-up

Oswaldo should be followed closely for several months to ensure that his problems with anemia and lead poisoning are fully treated. Developmental assessments will be monitored regularly to determine if there has been a significant impact affecting Oswaldo's development. The primary care provider needs to contact the agencies that investigate toxic environments (Department of Public Health, Environmental Protection Agency, local Visiting Nurse Association, or other agencies) in order to ensure the environment is once again conducive for the health of children such as Oswaldo.

The follow-up reports indicate that Oswaldo's family now has been moved to one of the newer facilities at the orchard. There is no evidence of mice or lead. There is a functioning smoke detector. Mr. Garcia now showers at work and changes clothes before coming home, a change that the employer now encourages for all workers. The response from the employer has been very positive and several more safety measures have been instituted for these employees. The siblings have been screened but do not have toxic levels of organophosphates in their systems.

What information about the implications of IDA, even after treatment, could you give the concerned parents? ▓

There can be cognitive developmental implications, especially regarding reading scores and behavioral manifestations. The brain is undergoing significant development during the first 2 years of life. Lack of proper nutrition (oxygenation) results in irreparable damage and lost developmental opportunities. Oswaldo will need to be followed to help him maximize his development with early intervention programs.

For a toddler with an uncomplicated CBC indicative of a microcytic, hypochromic anemia, what further appropriate diagnostic process should you consider? ▓

Unlike the child with a complicated presentation, the average toddler with apparent IDA (microcytic, hypochromic) needs no further testing before initiating therapy. A therapeutic trial of oral iron is usually adequate in high-risk populations as a diagnostic measure for presumptive iron deficiency anemia (Hermiston & Mentzer, 2002). Fer-in-sol is prescribed at 6 mg elemental iron/kg, divided into two or three doses a day. It is important to follow up with a reticulocyte count in 2–4 weeks. An elevated reticulocyte count indicates that iron is adequate to promote RBC growth and reticulocytosis has begun. During the initial phase of therapy, the rate of RBC development is faster than normal and the reticulocytes are released early, with an extended lifespan of 2 days. Iron therapy needs to continue for 3–4 months to replenish the body's iron stores. Poor response to iron therapy necessitates further laboratory work-up of the anemia.

What evaluation should be pursued for the child with severe anemia, atypical hematological findings, or a history suspicious for iron deficiency, or who does not respond to an initial trial of iron therapy? ■

Specific tests will be directed by the clinical presentation, history, and initial blood work. The causative factors of the anemia must be clarified. Information revealed in the complete blood count, peripheral blood smear, lead studies, thyroid studies, and hemoglobin electrophoresis would all help in refining the etiology of anemia. Findings in patient examination and history will further guide the diagnosis of anemia and the examinations needed to confirm the diagnosis. It is vital to remember that having the diagnosis of the type of anemia is not the end point. Anemia is a symptom of an underlying disorder. The anemia diagnosis narrows the diagnosis of the underlying disorder that needs further treatment.

Key Points from the Case

1. Assessing the child with anemia is a complex process that necessitates careful data gathering to determine the ultimate etiology. Providers need to walk a fine line between making too narrow and too wide a focus.
2. Integrate information from all available sources to help formulate the final diagnosis. All variables must be considered, with a focus on the incidence at the child's stated age and health status. This necessitates a systematic and organized process of elimination.
3. A detailed history often reveals more useful data than the physical examination alone, so time is best spent obtaining as much relevant information as possible.
4. Keep in mind that the child is a product of his or her environment; explore environmental histories as a mainstay of healthcare visits.

REFERENCES

American Lung Association. (n.d.). *Pesticides.* Accessed November 9, 2008, from http://www.lungusa.org/site/c.dvLUK9OOE/b.35384/k.F5CC/Pesticides.htm

Avery, M. (1994). *Pediatric medicine.* Baltimore: Williams & Wilkins.

Belson, M., Kingsley, B., & Holmes, A. (2007). Risk factors for acute leukemia in children: a review. *Environmental Health Perspectives, 115*(1), 138–145.

Berman, B. W. (2004). Pallor and anemia. In R. M. Kliegman, L. A. Greenbaum, & P. S. Lye (Eds.), *Practical strategies in pediatric diagnosis and therapy* (2nd ed., pp. 873–894). Philadelphia, PA: Saunders.

Borgna-Pignatti, C., & Marsella, M. (2008). Iron deficiency in infancy and childhood. *Pediatric Annals, 37*(5), 329–337.

Burchett, M. L., Hanna, C. E., & Steiner, R. D. (2009). Endocrine and metabolic diseases. In C. E. Burns, A. M. Dunn, M. A. Brady, N. B. Starr, & C. G. Blosser (Eds.), *Pediatric primary care* (4th ed., pp. 584–611). St. Louis, MO: Saunders Elsevier.

Centers for Disease Control and Prevention. (2002). Iron deficiency—United States, 1999–2000. *Morbidity and Mortality Weekly Report.* Retrieved June 30, 2008, from http://www.cdc.gov/mmwr/preview/mmwrhtml/mm5140a1.htm

Centers for Disease Control and Prevention. (May 27, 2005). Blood lead levels—United States, 1999–2002. *Morbidity and Mortality Weekly Report, 54*(20), 513–516. Retrieved April 10, 2009, from http://www.cdc.gov/mmwr/PDF/wk/mm5420.pdf

Cohen, M. (2007). Environmental toxins and health: the health impact of pesticides. *Australian Family Physician, 36*(12), 1002–1004.

Curl, C. L., Fenske, R. A., Kissel, J. C., Shirai, J. H., Moate, T. F., Griffith, W., et al. (2002). Evaluation of take-home organophosphorous pesticide exposure among agricultural workers and their children. *Environmental Health Perspectives, 110*(12), A787–A792.

Fenske, R. A., Chensheng, L., Curl, C. L., Shirai, J. H., & Kissel, J. C. (2005). Biologic monitoring to characterize organophosphorus pesticide exposure among children and workers: an analysis of recent studies in Washington state. *Environmental Health Perspectives, 113*(11), 1651–1657.

Gamis, A. S., Woods, W. G., Alonzo, T. A., Buxton, A., Lange, B., Barnard, D. R., et al. (2003). Increased age at diagnosis has a significantly negative effect on outcome in children with Down syndrome and acute myeloid leukemia: a report from the Children's Cancer Group Study 2891. *Journal of Clinical Oncology, 21*(18), 3415–3422.

Garfunkel, L. C., Kaczorowski, J. M., & Christy, C. (2007). *Pediatric clinical advisor: instant diagnosis and treatment* (2nd ed.). Philadelphia: Mosby.

Hermiston, M. L., & Mentzer, W. C. (2002). A practical approach to the evaluation of the anemic child. *Pediatric Clinics of North America, 29*, 877–891.

Irwin, J. J., & Kirchner, J. T. (2001). Anemia in children. *American Family Physician, 64*(8), 1379–1386.

Karr, C. J., Solomon, G. M., & Brock-Utne, A. C. (2007). Health effects of common home, lawn, and garden pesticides. *Pediatric Clinical of North America, 54*, 63–80.

Kemp, C. (2005). *Mexicans and Mexican-Americans: health beliefs and practices.* Retrieved April 10, 2009, from http://bearspace.baylor.edu/Charles_Kemp/www/hispanic_health.htm

Kliegman, R. M., Greenbaum, L. A., & Lye, P. S. (Eds.). (2004). *Practical strategies in pediatric diagnosis and therapy* (2nd ed). Philadelphia: Saunders.

Lambert, W. E., Lasarev, M., Muniz, J., Scherer, J., Rothlein, J. Santana, J., et al. (2005). Variation in organophosphate pesticide metabolites in urine of children living in agricultural communities. *Environmental Health Perspectives, 113*(4), 504–508.

Lee, M. T., & Truman, J. T. (2007). Anemia, acute. *eMedicine from WebMD.* Retrieved June 30, 2008, from http://www.emedicine.com/ped/TOPIC98.HTM

Lesperance, L., Wu, A. C., & Bernstein, H. (2002). Putting a dent in iron deficiency. *Contemporary Pediatrics, 19*(7), 60–79.

Mullins, M. E., Brands, C. L., & Daya, M. R. (2000). Unintentional pediatric super-warfarin exposures: do we really need a prothrombin time? *Pediatrics, 105*(2), 402–404.

National Institutes of Health, Office of Dietary Supplements. (n.d.). *Dietary supplement fact sheet: iron.* Accessed December 22, 2008, from http://ods.od.nih.gov/factsheets/iron.asp

Olson, K. R., Trickey, D. N., Miller, M. A., & Yungmann-Hile, L. (2008). *Toxicity, warfarin and superwarfarins.* Retrieved June 30, 2008, from http://www.emedicine.com/emerg/topic872.htm

Paranzino, G. K., Butterfield, P., Nastoff, T., & Ranger, C. (2005). I PREPARE: developmental and clinical utility of an environmental exposures history mnemonic. *American Association of Occupational Health Nursing, 53*(1), 37–42.

Piomelli, S. (2002). Childhood lead poisoning. *Pediatric Clinics of North America, 49*, 1285–1304.

Roberts, J. R., & Reigart, J. R. (2002). *Managing elevated blood lead levels among young children: recommendations from the Advisory Committee on Childhood Lead Poisoning Prevention.* Retrieved July 30, 2008, from http://www.cdc.gov/nceh/lead/CaseManagement/chap3.pdf

Roberts, J. R., & Reigart, J. R. (2007). Managing elevated blood lead levels among young children: recommendations from the Advisory Committee on Childhood Lead Poisoning Prevention. Retrieved July 30, 2008, from http://www.cdc.gov/nceh/lead/CaseManagement/chap3.pdf

Robison, L. L., Nesbit, M. E. Jr, Sather, H. N., Level, C., Shahidi, N., Kennedy, A., et al. (1984). Down syndrome and acute leukemia in children: a 10-year retrospective survey from Children's Cancer Study Group. *Journal of Pediatrics, 105*(2), 235–242.

Schwartz, M. K. (2009). Hematologic disorders. In: C. E. Burns, A. M. Dunn, M. A. Brady, N. B. Starr, & C. G. Blosser (Eds.), *Pediatric primary care* (4th ed., pp. 612–633). St. Louis, MO: Saunders Elsevier.

Scott, J. P. (2006). Hematology. In: R. M. Kliegman, L. A. Greenbaum, & P. S. Lye (Eds.), *Practical strategies in pediatric diagnosis and therapy* (2nd ed., pp. 689–723). Philadelphia: Elsevier Saunders.

Shea, K. M. (n.d.). *Reducing low dose pesticide exposures in infants and children: a clinician's guide from Physicians for Social Responsibility* [pamphlet]. Washington, DC: Physicians for Social Responsibility. Retrieved April 10, 2009, from http://www.psr.org/site/DocServer/Reducing_Low-Dose_Pesticide_Exposures.pdf?docID=663

Spector, R. (1996). *Culture and diversity in health and illness* (4th ed.). Stamford, CT: Appleton & Lange.

Taketomo, C. K., Hodding, J. H., & Kraus, D. M. (2008). *Pediatric dosage handbook* (15th ed.). Hudson, Ohio: Lexi-comp.

Thompson, B., Coronado, G. D., Vigoren, E. M., Griffith, W. C., Fenske, R. A., Kissel, J. C., et al. (2008). *Para niños saludables:* a community intervention trial to reduce organophosphate pesticide exposure in children of farm-workers. *Environmental Health Perspectives, 116*(5), 687–694.

Tietz, N. W. (1995). *Clinical guidelines to laboratory tests* (3rd ed.). Philadelphia: W.B. Saunders.

U.S. Preventive Services Task Force. (2006). *Screening for Iron Deficiency Anemia.* Agency for Healthcare Research and Quality, Rockville, MD. Retrieved April 2, 2009, from http://www.ahrq.gov/clinic/uspstf/uspsiron.htm

Chapter 20

The Child with a Headache

Ritamarie John

Headache is a common problem in pediatric practice. Parents will bring children in for a headache complaint, concerned that their child has a brain tumor or infectious meningitis. The approach to the history and physical must be systematic and complete. Failing to do one part of the neurological exam can cause a delay in the correct diagnosis. In evaluating the chief complaint of headache, the provider needs to first determine whether the headache is a primary or secondary symptom.

Educational Objectives
1. Apply evidence-based guidelines to classify the presenting complaint of headache.
2. Apply shared decision making to develop the treatment plan.
3. Integrate knowledge of development, pharmacology, and complementary approaches to develop a treatment plan for the young child with primary headache.

Case Presentation and Discussion

John Brown is a 6-year-old who presents to a private practice with a complaint of headache. He has been having headaches for about 3 months and has seen two other providers without any relief. The child is accompanied by his father. The father explains that he is the primary parent since his 42-year-old wife died of lymphoma 3 years ago. He expresses concern that the child has missed 6 days of school over the past 3 months due to headaches and would like your opinion on the problem.

What questions will you ask John and his father about the "headache" problem? ■

Your symptom analysis reveals the following information: The child started with a headache 3 months ago and has been getting between two and three headaches per month. They are described as 5 of 6 on the Wong Pain Scale and are throbbing and bilateral over the top of the head or the forehead, lasting 5–8 hours. The headaches do not have any specific time that they commence; however, they do not wake the child up at night, and he has not had them in the morning. John generally feels nauseated with the headache but has vomited only once. During the headache episode, the child looks like he is sick. The father has not identified any precipitating factors or triggers. He reports that John's mother had migraines that would last for 2 days, and he does not want John to be as debilitated as his mother was. The headaches are not related to activity. He has been given acetaminophen (Tylenol) for the headaches by the other two providers without much relief. The father was not happy with the care of the other providers because they rushed through the exam and "made light" of his concerns.

What other questions do you need to ask John and his father? ■

Before answering this question, here is some information about headaches that you need to consider.

Headaches in Children

Headache is a common pediatric disorder that has become more common in adolescents (Lewis, 2007c). Overall, prevalence is between 37% and 51% in 7 year olds with an increase to as high as 82% in 15 year olds (Lewis, 2007a).

Pathophysiology of Migraine

The pathophysiology of migraine is not fully understood, but is now believed to be a neuronal process (Lewis, 2007b). The current thinking is that the cerebral cortex is hyperexcitable, with genetic influences causing disturbances in the neuronal ion channels (Lewis, 2007b; Lisi et al., 2005). This leads to a lowered threshold for a variety of external and internal factors to trigger episodes of excitation of the neuronal region. Subsequent to this, there is a cortical spreading depression that is likely responsible for the aura seen in migraine and for the activation of the trigeminovascular system (Lewis, 2007b). During the aura phase of migraine, there is regional neuronal depolarization as well as a decrease in blood supply or oligemia.

Because an aura is present in only about 30% of children, there are two mechanisms of pain generation (Lewis, 2007b). The first reason for pain is from the inflammation of the meningeal vessels, and the second reason is the sensitization of peripheral and trigeminal afferents (Lewis, 2007b). Some of the substances involved in the generation of the inflammation and sensitization of the vasculature in the brain include neurokinine, substance P, and calcitonin gene reactive peptide, which cause dilatation with subsequent pain. The vasoreactive neuropeptides act on blood vessels. Serotonin and glutamate may increase the sensitivity to pain in the blood vessel wall (Gunner, Smith, & Ferguson, 2008).

Migraine is now divided into three major subclassifications—migraine with aura, migraine without aura, and childhood periodic syndromes that are commonly precursors of migraine (Headache Classification Subcommittee of the International Headache Society [IHS], 2004). In children, a migraine headache must last between 1 and 72 hours with moderate to severe intensity, with aggravation by usual physical activities, and with behavioral signs of either photophobia or phonophobia (IHS, 2004). The diagnostic criteria for pediatric migraine without aura are not based on one attack. The patient must have five attacks that include the following criteria: 1) headache attacks last between 1 and 72 hours; 2) headaches minimally need two of the four characteristics—

unilateral or bilateral, frontotemporal but not occipital location; pulsing quality; moderate to severe pain; and physical activity limitations resulting from the headache; 3) headaches should have one of the following symptoms—nausea and/or vomiting, photophobia, or photophobia inferred from their behavior; and 4) cannot be attributed to another disease (IHS).

In migraine without aura, there may be autonomic symptoms such as nausea, anorexia, periumbical abdominal pain, diarrhea, pallor, photodysphoria, photophobia, a desire to sleep, cool extremities, goose flesh, increased or decreased blood pressure, or periorbital discoloration (Lewis, 2007b). In migraine with aura, the most common visual phenomena are binocular visual impairment with scotoma, with distortions or hallucinations, or monocular visual impairment occurring much less frequently (Lewis, 2007b).

Pathophysiology of Tension-Type Headache

Tension-type headaches (TTHs) are the most common type of headache and are now felt to have a neurobiological basis (IHS, 2004). Central pain mechanisms are felt to play a role in frequent tension headaches, whereas peripheral pain mechanisms play a role in infrequent episodic tension headaches (IHS). A TTH is described as a symmetrically distributed tightening "band-like" feeling around the head (Rubin, Suecoff, & Knupp, 2006). There may be associated photophobia or phonophobia, but without nausea, vomiting, or exacerbation with activity (IHS). The diagnostic criteria for tension-type headaches require at least 10 episodes of headache. The headaches must fulfill the following criteria: 1) last between 30 minutes and 7 days; and 2) need two of the four characteristics—bilateral location, pressing/tightening of a nonpulsating quality, mild to moderate intensity, and not be increased with routine activity such as walking or climbing stairs. In addition, there can be no associated nausea, vomiting, photophobia, and phonophobia. The headache cannot be the result of another disease process (IHS).

There are three subtypes of TTHs: infrequent episodic TTHs with headaches occurring less than 1 day a month, frequent episodic TTHs with headache episodes occurring 1 to 14 days a month, or chronic TTHs with headaches 15 or more days a month. In children, it may be difficult to distinguish between migraine and tension due to the developmental level of the child (Brna & Dooley, 2006).

Pathophysiology of Cluster Headache and Other Trigeminal Autonomic Cephalalgias

It is hypothesized that ipsilateral trigeminal nociceptive pathways are important in the etiology with the activation of the parasympathetic cranial system and ipsilateral parasympathetic nerves. An inflammation of the cavernous sinus and tributary veins is believed to be the main mechanism involved in cluster headaches (Lampl, 2002). A cluster headache is a unilateral burning pain that is most commonly found around the eye and orbits on the affected side, occurring from one to eight times during the course of the day (Lampl).

Epidemiology of Headaches

Migraine headaches can start at age 6 to 7 years and once puberty occurs, the female to male ratio is 2:1 (Lewis, 2007a). The headache is usually bilateral in children and usually frontotemporal, with occipital headaches being rare and needing immediate evaluation for structural lesions (IHS, 2004). Migraine with aura peaks at 5 to 6 years of age in boys and between ages 12 and 13 years in girls (Lewis, 2007a). Migraine prevalence estimates vary from 1–3% at 7 years of age with an increase to as high as 11% in the later school-age child and mid-adolescent (Brna & Dooly, 2006).

Cluster headaches are rare in the pediatric age group, with prevalence of 0.09% to 0.4% for male patients. From age 11–18, the prevalence of childhood-onset cluster headaches is 0.1% (Lampl, 2002).

Tension headache is more common in older girls. General prevalence is between 30% and 78% in the general population.

Social Factors

Mr. Brown is a single parent and has a full-time job. When questioned about his ethnicity, he denies belonging to any cultural group and feels he is a mixture of races. So in this case, it is important for you to explore what he believes about health care, medications, and complementary medications. Because the father has expressed concern about the management plan that was identified during prior healthcare visits related to John's headaches, you need to spend time explaining the diagnosis and evaluating Mr. Brown's acceptance of and desire to be involved in deciding on the management plan. Using the skills of motivational interviewing can be helpful in exploring parental expectations of the healthcare visit.

Further Assessment Data Required for the Differential Diagnosis?

The differential diagnosis is vast but needs to be approached systematically by first deciding whether the headache is a primary problem or a secondary symptom to another problem. A complete history and physical examination are the first steps in making the decision. Table 20-1 reviews possible differential diagnoses for headaches in children. The key to confirming the diagnosis is compliance with the treatment plan and good follow-up with the family.

From the above review, what additional questions should you ask? ■

History

- When did the headaches begin? If the problem has been going on for years, make sure there are no recent changes in the headache presentation.
- How often are the headaches, and has there been a change in frequency? What is the interval between the headaches? Migraines are not daily whereas TTHs can be daily or several times a week. Cluster

Table 20-1 Differential Diagnoses for Headache			
Acute	Acute Recurrent	Chronic Progressive	Chronic Nonprogressive or Daily Headache
Bacterial or viral infections: sinusitis, otitis media, dental abscess, infection of CNS	Migraine with aura	Neoplasm	Tension
	Migraine without aura	Pseudotumor cerebri	
	Complicated migraines	Hydrocephalus	
Vascular malformation		Brain abscess	
Acute stroke		Congenital malformation	
Other dental disease		Vascular malformation	
Toxins		Hypertension	
Carbon monoxide poisoning		Medication (oral contraceptives)	
Trauma			
Hypertension			
Congenital malformation			
Hydrocephalus			
Pseudotumor cerebri			
Posticteral after seizure			
Hypoxia			
Exertion			

Source: From Gunner, K. B., & Smith, H. D. (2007). Practice guidelines for diagnosis and management of migraine headaches in children and adolescents: part one. *Journal of Pediatric Healthcare, 21,* 327–332.

headaches occur in clusters of two to three per week over a few weeks and then do not occur for a period of time (Brna & Dooley, 2006).
- How did the headache begin? Asking about head trauma or recent changes in the child's social situation is an important part of this question.
- What is the time of onset of headache during the day? Ask about night waking due to headache, relationship to activity, or coughing causing the headache. Headache associated with coughing is an ominous sign (Gunner & Smith, 2007). Headaches that are predominantly nocturnal or early morning and associated with vomiting deserve neuroimaging (Brna & Dooley, 2006).

- How long does the headache episode last? Cluster headaches tend to be brief; migraines can last as short as 1 hour and as long as 72 hours; and TTHs can last the entire day (Brna & Dooley, 2006).
- Where is the headache located on the head? Bitemporal frontal headache is common in migraine whereas tension headache is around the head. Occipital headaches are an ominous sign and may indicate structural lesions (Gunner & Smith, 2007).
- What makes the headache better or worse?
- What are the characteristics of the pain? Younger children may describe migraine as pressing or heavy rather than throbbing (Brna & Dooley, 2006). The inability to locate the pain is more disturbing than not being able to describe it (Brna & Dooley).
- Are there any warning signs that the headache is coming? Auras that are persistently unilateral on the same side should have neuroimaging to rule out structural lesions (Brna & Dooley, 2006). Parents may be able to note changes in the child's appetite, mood, or thirst.
- What are the associated symptoms? Are there associated autonomic symptoms such as nausea, vomiting, numbness, or weakness? If the child complains of dizziness, you will need to ask more questions. Is the patient describing lightheadedness, unsteadiness, or vertigo? Lightheadedness suggests cerebral hypoperfusion or orthostasis (Lewis, 2007b). Unsteadiness or vertigo is associated with balance disorders, suggesting the need for neuroimaging to rule out vestibular or cerebellar pathology (Lewis, 2007b). Dizziness and vertigo at the onset of a throbbing headache suggest basilar-type migraine, which is a more complex type of migraine requiring referral (Lewis, 2007b).
- Do the headaches occur under any specific circumstances or after eating any particular food? Migraines may have a trigger.
- What makes the headache better or worse? Aggravating factors can include activities, light, noise, and smell. Headaches caused by increases in intracranial pressure will get worse when the child lies down (Brna & Dooley, 2006).
- What does the child do during the headache? Ask the child what he does if he gets the headache during playtime.
- What medications are taken for the headache? What other medications is the child taking? Asking specifically about alternative medications is also important. Headaches can be the side effects of other medications.
- Does the child have any other medical/psychiatric problems? Make sure there is no chronic health condition that may be causing headache or stress
- Would I as a healthcare provider know your child has a headache if I saw him?
- Has the child had a change in personality with the onset of the headache?

- Does anyone in the family have headaches? The genetics of migraine need to be explored.
- What does the parent think is causing the headaches?
- Is there any drug or alcohol use?
- What is the child's sleep pattern? Does the child snore? Is there day-time sleepiness? Children with migraine have increased sleep distur-bances (Heng & Wirrell, 2006; Isik et al., 2007).
- Are there any behavioral problems with the child? Children with headaches were initially thought to have psychopathology. However, recent reviews and studies have failed to show that a majority of chil-dren with headache have any psychopathology (Laurell, Larsson, & Eeg-Olofsson, 2005; Powers, Gilman, & Hershey, 2006; Vannetta et al., 2008)
- If the child is a female adolescent, does she use oral contraceptives?
- Does the child have a history of 2 weeks or more of purulent nasal discharge?
- When was the child's last visit to the dentist?

In addition to the data described earlier, you now learn on further questioning that with the first headache, there was no nausea reported but now Mr. Brown reports that John does not look well during the headache episodes. He does not feel the child has any aura. The headache is improved by lying down, but Tylenol provides only minimal relief. After sleeping, John is generally better. He has had about two to three headaches a month.

After the first headache, Mr. Brown took John to the doctor, and the child was diag-nosed with a tension headache. The father was advised to use Tylenol. After 6 weeks and three more headaches, John was seen by a second provider who did a CT scan, CBC, lead level, and thyroid screen. The results were all normal by the father's report and the family was given no further follow-up visits. Mr. Brown has not been able to identify a precipitat-ing cause but has not done a headache diary. John has had no associated head trauma or change in social situation. There are no other medical problems, and the father has not noted John to have purulent rhinitis. John's behavior and school performance is the same. He sees a dentist regularly. He generally sleeps 10 hours a night, but does report variability in sleep time. John eats three meals per day, and there has been no change in bowel or bladder habits. The maternal grandmother has babysat for the child for the past 3 years since the death of the mother. The previous medical record was not available at the time of the initial visit, but was later obtained and confirmed the father's history.

Physical Examination

John is at the 75th percentile in height and the 50th percentile in both head circumfer-ence and weight. His body mass index (BMI) is between the 50th and 75th percentile and his BP is normal. Developmentally, the child is able to answer questions and draw a diamond. He is able to read on grade level and do simple math and reading.

From the general physical examination, the following observations were made: There is one 1.5 cm café au lait spot on the right trunk but no other neurocutaneous manifestations. There is no tenderness over the maxillary sinus, and the nasal mucosa is pink with exudate. The mouth opens without clicking or popping of the temporomandibular joint. No caries are seen and there is no evidence of gingivitis. The cervical spine has full range of motion. Heart, lung, and abdomen examinations are normal.

A complete neurological exam was done. No cranial bruit was identified. Visual fields: grossly intact by confrontation. Visual acuity is 20/20, and extraocular movements are intact without nystagmus. The optic disc is sharp with normal disc to cup ratio. There is no blurring of the vessels along the disc margins. Pupils are equal, round, and reactive to light and accommodation. Fifth (trigeminal) nerve: intact bilateral masseter strength. Seventh (facial) nerve: face bilaterally symmetric; eighth (auditory) nerve: intact bilateral hearing; ninth (glossopharyngeal) nerve: normal gag; 11th (spinal accessory) nerve: full strength in bilateral trapezius and SCM; 12th (hypoglossal) nerve: tongue midline. Reflexes +2 symmetrical on all four extremities without clonus and with downgoing toes. Motor: right upper extremity muscle: normal; left upper extremity muscle: normal; right lower extremity muscle: normal; left lower extremity muscle: normal. Other: Able to walk on heels and hop three times on each foot. Right hand, right foot preference, able to do tandem gait. Sensory primary: Light touch: intact; Pinprick: intact. Secondary: Graphesthesia: able to perform; Stereognosis: able to perform. No neurological soft signs such as hyperactivity, poor attention span, or impulsivity demonstrated during exam. Coordination: dysdiadochokinesis (i.e., inability to quickly substitute antagonistic motor impulses) attempted. Gait: normal for age without ataxia.

In summary, no abnormal findings were identified in the physical examination.

Making the Diagnosis

The history and physical examination are consistent with the diagnosis of migraine headache. The need for neuroimaging should be considered when there are either historical features of recent onset of severe headache, changes in type of headache, or changes in neurological function (Lewis, 2007b). The need for neuroimaging should be considered if there are physical examination features of focal findings, increased intracranial pressure, or new onset of seizures. (See Table 20-2.) The child's history and physical have no worrisome characteristics and meet the criteria for pediatric migraine rather than tension-type headaches.

Management

How do you plan to treat his migraine headaches? ■

Do you need to do anything to confirm the diagnosis, such as laboratory studies? ■

No laboratory studies are recommended in the management of pediatric migraine (Guidetti & Galli, 2004; Gunner & Smith, 2007; Lewis, 2007a, b, c). Neuroimaging or lumbar puncture should be done if there are abnormalities during the history or physical examination that indicate the need for further testing.

Therapeutic plan: What will you do therapeutically? ■

Table 20-2	Worrisome History and Physical Examination Findings
History	Headache that increases on coughing or Valsalva maneuver
	Increasing frequency of or changes in type of headaches
	Changes in child's personality, behavior, or school performance
	Developmental delay
	Pubertal delay
	Headache with acute onset, associated with fever, neck stiffness, or vomiting
	Headache that gets worse when laying down
	Headache that wakes up the child at night, with morning headache
	Occipital headache
	Explosive onset of headache
	Epilepsy
	Changes in mental status including confusion or drowsiness
Physical examination	Signs of head trauma
	No increasing head circumference
	Normal level of consciousness
	Abnormalities of cranial nerves
	Anisocoria that varies in light and dark
	Abnormal growth parameters
	Cranial bruit
	Papilledema or optic pallor
	Visual disturbances
	Tenderness over maxillary or frontal sinuses
	Meningeal signs: neck stiffness, positive Brudzinski's sign or Kernig's sign
	Cervical spine with limitation of range of motion
	More than six café au lait spots on skin with axillary freckling
	No sensory or motor asymmetry
	Normal deep tendon reflexes: hyperreflexia indicates upper motor neuron lesion
	Weakness or paralysis on a side
	Ataxia
	No graphesthesia or stereognosis perceptions
	Gait disturbance

Sources: Adapted from Brna, P., & Doodley, J. (2006). Headache in the pediatric population. Seminars in Pediatric Neurology, 13, 222–230; Guidetti, V., & Galli, F. (2004). Headache in children: diagnostic and therapeutic issues. Seminars in Pain Medicine, 2(2), 106–114; Gunner, K. B., & Smith, H. D. (2007). Practice guidelines for diagnosis and management of migraine headaches in children an adolescents: part one. Journal of Pediatric Healthcare, 21, 327–332; Lewis, D. W. (2007b). Headaches in children and adolescents. Current Problems in Pediatric and Adolescent Health Care, 37, 207–246.

The plan is thoroughly discussed and decided with Mr. Brown's input. This is particularly important because the father had expressed his lack of satisfaction with the other two providers who did not schedule follow-up visits. The treatment plan you identify incorporates the goals outlined in the American Academy of Neurology Practice Parameters (Lewis et al., 2004) and the Guidelines of the National Association of Nurse Practitioners (Gunner et al., 2008) for the treatment of pediatric migraine. They include:

- Reduce the frequency, duration, severity, and disability from the headache.
- Reduce reliance on medication for acute migraine treatment that is ineffective or poorly tolerated.
- Improve the quality of life of migraine sufferers.
- Avoid overuse and escalating use of medication for acute migraine treatment.
- Educate patients to help them self-manage and self-control their migraine headache.
- Reduce headache-related distress and emotional symptoms in migraine sufferers.

Treatment Options

In order to develop a treatment plan, the options need to be explored with the father. First, it is important to assess the degree of headache disability. The PedMIDAS tool was developed at Cincinnati Children's Hospital and is available online at http://www.cincinnatichildrens.org/svc/alpha/h/headache/pedmidas. htm. The scoring information and PDF of the document are available at the Web site.

The next step would be to discuss nonpharmacological approaches because the family has not had a good experience with medication (see Table 20-3).

John's PedMIDAS score is 24, indicating a mild disability from the headache. A headache diary has not been done before, so you explain the reasons for the diary to Mr. Brown. Headache diaries can help identify triggers, allow for the child to express the headache symptoms, and help identify whether the treatment regimen is working. Headaches can be precipitated by different things including sleep, nutritional intake, physical activity changes, hormonal changes, lights, types of food, and stress. Minor stress can be missed by the parent, and a headache diary can help the child point out the problems to the father, who will share in the responsibility of keeping the diary.

Mr. Brown and John are interested in increasing John's amount of daily physical activity; however, it was more problematic for Mr. Brown because John is with a grandmother who is very protective of the child and does not allow playtime outside of the house. You ask Mr. Brown how he thinks he could increase John's daily exercise, and he decides that he will play catch with John after dinner.

Regular meal times, good hydration, and avoiding caffeine are discussed. Mr. Brown feels that John gets enough fluids in school, but he says he will talk with the teacher

Table 20-3	Biobehavioral Treatment in Pediatric Migraine
Sleep hygiene	Good sleep hygiene
	Going to bed and getting up at the same time, including on the weekend
	Avoidance of excess, inadequate, or irregular sleep patterns
Healthy lifestyle	Regular exercise
	Adequate amounts of fluids
	Avoiding caffeine
	Increasing fruits and vegetables
Progressive muscle relaxation	Involves tensing and relaxing a variety of muscles
	Teaching diaphragmatic and deep breathing
	Guided imagery by having the child visualize a pleasant scene
	More appropriate after 7 years, but can be used in younger children
Biofeedback	Needs to be done in a biofeedback lab
	Electromyographic activity or peripheral skin temperature is monitored and feedback given during a visual display.
Other techniques	There is no clinical evidence for the use of acupuncture, chiropractic treatment, hypnosis, osteopathic cervical adjustment, or hyperbaric oxygen in children.

Sources: Adapted from Gunner, K. B., Smith, H. D., & Ferguson, L. E. (2008). Practice guidelines for diagnosis and management of migraine headaches in children and adolescents: part two. *Journal of Pediatric Healthcare, 22,* 52–59; Lewis, D. W. (2007b). Headaches in children and adolescents. *Current Problems in Pediatric and Adolescent Health Care, 37,* 207–246; Powers, S. D., & Andrasik, F. (2005). Biobehavioral treatment, disability, and psychological effect of pediatric headache. *Pediatric Annals, 34,* 461–465.

about allowing extra fluids during the school day. You give Mr. Brown a list of caffeine-containing fluids, including sodas. After further discussion, Mr. Brown decides to try relaxation techniques because this is something he feels he could do with his son at home. The family is introduced to the technique in the office setting.

Pharmacological management of acute headache involves taking the medication as prescribed in the right dose at the onset of the headache.

Teaching Mr. Brown to identify and treat the pain early is a key point to abort the pain. John needs to have the medication with him so he can take it within 20–30 minutes of onset of the headache (Lewis, 2007b). You give Mr. Brown a note for the school. You discuss changing medication from Tylenol to ibuprofen at 10 mg/kg. Ibuprofen is an effective first line drug for migraine (Gunner et al., 2008; Lewis et al., 2004). Mr. Brown is happy about a change in medication.

Mr. Brown raises the issue of complementary medications such as feverfew, ginkgo, valerian root, or magnesium, so you discuss the lack of evidence of the efficacy of these medications. Mr. Brown also raises the issue of a multivitamin with a daily dose of magnesium as an alternative to a specific supplement. You agree to this as part of the treatment plan.

In addition, Mr. Brown has heard about medications to prevent migraines. It is important to explain that prevention medication would not be the first step in treatment. Medications for migraine prevention would be used only if the plan did not work. In addition, migraine prophylaxis does not have FDA approval (Eiland, 2007; Gunner et al., 2008; Lewis, 2007a, b, c).

When do you want to see this patient back again? ■

Generally, you would want to see this patient back in a month. You would want to review the diary, discuss the effectiveness of the treatment plan, and support the family in the new treatment management. As the family develops self-care skills, these appointments can be spread further apart.

John and his father agree on the treatment plan. You give them written instructions that go over the key points of the treatment plan. Mr. Brown is able to show you the dosage of ibuprofen to give the child, and a measurer is dispensed by the pharmacy. John likes the idea of doing imagery to help control his headaches. Mr. Brown schedules the 1-month follow-up appointment before leaving the office.

On the follow-up visit in one month, the family brings the diary. They have identified that lack of fluid was a trigger for the first migraine during the previous month. They increased fluid intake before school and at lunch because the teacher felt she could not allow fluids in the classroom. Ibuprofen was more effective than Tylenol in relief of migraine pain, and imagery seemed to help John relax. Mr. Brown wants to come back in a month and continue the diary.

Key Points from the Case

1. The management of pediatric migraine requires family education, use of biobehavioral measures, medications for acute treatments, and if needed, daily preventive medications.

2. The treatment requires a stepwise approach. This involves determining how much of an impact the headache has on the child's life, determining and then eliminating possible triggers, instituting a healthy lifestyle, teaching biobehavioral methods to control pain, and starting pain medication for acute headache early.

3. Offering treatment options and involving the family in the treatment decisions allows the patient and the family to practice self-care and manage the problem.

REFERENCES

Brna, P., & Doodley, J. (2006). Headache in the pediatric population. *Seminars in Pediatric Neurology, 13*, 222–230.

Eiland, L. S. (2007). Anticonvulsant use for prophylaxis of pediatric migraine. *Journal of Pediatric Healthcare, 21*, 392–395.

Guidetti, V., & Galli, F. (2004). Headache in children: diagnostic and therapeutic issues. *Seminars in Pain Medicine, 2*(2), 106–114.

Gunner, K. B., & Smith, H. D. (2007). Practice guidelines for diagnosis and management of migraine headaches in children and adolescents: part one. *Journal of Pediatric Healthcare, 21*, 327–332.

Gunner, K. B., Smith, H. D., & Ferguson, L. E. (2008). Practice guidelines for diagnosis and management of migraine headaches in children and adolescents: part two. *Journal of Pediatric Healthcare, 22*, 52–59.

Headache Classification Subcommittee of the International Headache Society. (2004). The International Classification of Headache Disorders. *Cephalagia, 24*(Suppl 1), S1–S160.

Heng, K., & Wirrell, E. (2006). Sleep disturbance in children with migraine. *Journal of Child Neurology, 21*, 761–766.

Isik, U., Ersu., R. H., Ay, P., Save, D., Arman, A. R., Karakoc, F., et al. (2007). Prevalence of headache and its association with sleep disorder in children. *Pediatric Neurology, 36*(3), 146–151.

Lampl, C. (2002). Childhood-onset cluster headaches. *Pediatric Neurology, 27*(2), 138–140.

Laurell, K., Larsson, B., & Eeg-Olofsson, O. (2004). Headache in schoolchildren: association with other pain, family history and psychosocial factors. *Pain, 119*, 150–158.

Lewis, D., Ashwal, S., Hershey, A., Hirtz, D., Yonker, M., & Silberstein, S. (2004). Practice parameter: pharmacological treatment of migraine headache in children and adolescents: report of the American Academy of Neurology Quality Society Standards Subcommittee and the Practice Committee of the Child Neurology Society. *Neurology, 63*, 2215–2224.

Lewis, D. W. (2007a). The epidemiology and treatment of pediatric migraine. *Current Medical Literature: Neurology, 22*(3), 65–74.

Lewis, D. W. (2007b). Headaches in children and adolescents. *Current Problems in Pediatric and Adolescent Health Care, 37*, 207–246.

Lewis, D. W. (2007c). Pediatric migraine. *Pediatrics in Review, 28*(2), 43–53.

Lisi, V., Garbo, G., Micchiche, F., Stecca, A., Terrazzino, S., Franzoi, M., et al. (2005). Genetic risk factors in primary paediatric versus adult headache: complexities and problematics. *Journal of Headache Pain, 6*, 179–181.

Powers, S. D., & Andrasik, F. (2005). Biobehavioral treatment, disability, and psychological effect of pediatric headache. *Pediatric Annals, 34*, 461–465.

Powers, S. W., Gilman, D. K., & Hershey, A. D. (2006). Headache and psychological functioning in children and adolescents. *Headache, 46*(9), 1404–1415.

Rubin, D. H., Suecoff, S. A., & Knupp, K. (2006). Headaches in children. *Pediatric Annals, 35*(5), 345–353.

Vannetta, K., Getzoff, E. A., Gilman, D. K., Noll, R. B., Gerhardt, C. A., Powers, S. W., et al. (2008). Friendships and social interactions of school-aged children with migraine. *Cephalalgia, 28*, 734–743.

Chapter 21

The Preschooler with a Red Eye

Michele Saysana

In many encounters in medicine, tests exist to confirm the diagnosis; however, the test results may not be readily available, thus leaving the practitioner to make a diagnosis as well as treatment recommendations based on the history and physical alone. By putting together the signs and symptoms based on the history and physical exam, the practitioner is able to make a diagnosis and treatment plan without the confirmatory test.

Educational Objectives

1. Identify the distinguishing signs and symptoms of bacterial, viral, and allergic conjunctivitis.
2. Discuss the different treatments of bacterial, viral, and allergic conjunctivitis.
3. Identify when patients need to be referred to an ophthalmologist for treatment of conjunctivitis.

Case Presentation and Discussion

Jack Cho is a 5-year-old Asian American boy who presents to your office because he was sent home from school today by the school nurse who said he had "pink eye." He is accompanied by his pregnant mother and his 19-month-old sister.

You talk with Jack and his mother about his symptoms and plan to complete a physical examination.

What questions will you ask Jack and his mother related to his "pink eye"? ■

Your symptom analysis reveals the following information: He woke up this morning with a crusted shut right eye. After his mother applied a warm washcloth to his face, the crusting disappeared. He had more yellow drainage out of his right eye while on the bus to school. He continued to have yellow drainage and a red eye at school, so his teacher sent him to the school nurse. He states his eye is not itchy or burning. Jack and his mother do not recall any trauma to the eye. Jack does not have any cough, rhinorrhea, fever, or ear or throat pain. He does not have any history of allergic rhinitis either. Upon further questioning, he tells you other children have been sent home from his class for "pink eye" this week, including the boy who sits next to him.

What other questions do you need to ask Jack? ■

Before answering this question, here is some more information about "pink eye" that you need to consider.

Information about "Pink Eye"

Epidemiology

Conjunctivitis is the most common pediatric eye disorder that primary care practitioners will encounter (Wald, 2004). In developed countries worldwide, acute bacterial or viral conjunctivitis has an annual incidence in adults and children of 1.5–2%, with one in eight school-age children affected each year (Rietveld, ter Riet, Bindels, Sloos, & van Weert, 2004; Rose et al., 2005). Bacterial pathogens account for 54–73% of conjunctivitis, with nontypable *Haemophilus influenzae* and *Streptococcus pneumoniae* as the most common bacterial pathogens (Buznach, Dugan, & Greenberg, 2005). Viral conjunctivitis can be caused by many different viruses, the most common being adenovirus (Langley, 2005). Enterovirus and influenza are also considered to be important causes of viral conjunctivitis (Pickering, Baker, Long, & McMillan, 2006).

Data for the Diagnosis

History

The differential diagnoses include bacterial, viral, and allergic conjunctivitis; hyperacute bacterial conjunctivitis; ophthalmia neonatorum; epidemic kerato-conjunctivitis; chemical conjunctivitis; ocular foreign body; periorbital and orbital cellulitis; keratitis; uveitis; glaucoma; or possible systemic disease processes such as Kawasaki disease, Stevens-Johnson syndrome, juvenile idio-pathic arthritis, inflammatory bowel disease, or lupus. (See Table 21-1.)

In this situation, the information that needs to be gathered includes the following:

- How old is the patient? (Certain causes for conjunctivitis are included and excluded based on age.)
- Is there drainage from the eye, what color, and how much? (Helps to distinguish among bacterial, viral, and allergic conjunctivitis, as well as hyperacute bacterial conjunctivitis and some of the systemic causes of red eye)
- Is the drainage persistent and yellow in color? (Bacterial conjunctivitis)
- Is the drainage watery in nature? (Viral conjunctivitis, allergic conjunctivitis)
- Does the patient wake up with the affected eye matted shut due to discharge? (Bacterial conjunctivitis)
- Is there associated itching of the eye? (Allergic conjunctivitis)
- Is the eye painful? (Keratitis, uveitis, orbital cellulitis, foreign body)
- Is there vision loss? (Uveitis, orbital cellulitis)
- Is there photophobia? (Bacterial conjunctivitis, viral conjunctivitis, epidemic keratoconjunctivitis, uveitis, keratitis)

Table 21-1   Distinguishing Causes of Red Eye

Condition	Etiology	Signs and Symptoms
Bacterial conjunctivitis	*H. influenzae,* *S. pneumoniae,* *M. catarrhalis,* *S. aureus*	Bilateral or unilateral purulent drainage, crusting of eyes upon awakening, normal vision, possible photophobia, conjunctival injection
Ophthalmia neonatorum	*N. gonorrhoeae,* *C. trachomatis*	Purulent drainage, swelling of eyelids, occurs in infants > 2 days of age
Lacrimal duct obstruction	Congenital stenosis of the lacrimal duct, inability to drain tears	Bilateral or unilateral yellow eye drainage, excessive tearing
Viral conjunctivitis	Adenovirus, enterovirus, influenza	Bilateral or unilateral watery drainage; conjunctival injection, burning sensation; may be hemorrhagic; normal vision; may have other symptoms such as fever, sore throat, myalgias, etc.
Allergic conjunctivitis	Allergen exposure	Bilateral involvement, chemosis, conjunctival injection, watery drainage, itching, normal vision
Ocular foreign body	Exposure	Unilateral, foreign body sensation, conjunctival injection, tearing
Chemical conjunctivitis	Exposure	Unilateral or bilateral, pain, conjunctival injection, possible corneal involvement
Periorbital cellulitis	*H. influenzae,* *S. pneumoniae,* group A *Streptococcus,* *M. catarrhalis,* *S. aureus*	Unilateral conjunctival injection, eyelid edema and erythema, normal vision, extraocular muscles intact without pain, fever
Orbital cellulitis	*H .influenzae,* *S. pneumoniae,* group A *Streptococcus,* *M. catarrhalis,* *S. aureus,* anaerobic bacteria of upper respiratory tract	Unilateral, conjunctival injection, proptosis, eyelid edema, eye pain, vision loss, impaired eye movement
Keratitis	Viral and bacterial pathogens, exposure	Unilateral, intense pain, photophobia, corneal clouding
Uveitis	Systemic illnesses	Bilateral or unilateral, photophobia, irregular pupil, ciliary flush, vision loss

- Does the patient wear contact lenses? (Keratitis)
- Has there been any trauma or toxin exposure to the eye? (Chemical conjunctivitis, foreign body)
- Does the patient have otitis media and conjunctivitis? (Nontypable *H. influenzae* conjunctivitis)
- Does the patient have associated symptoms such as sore throat and fever? (Viral conjunctivitis)
- Does the patient have significant swelling and erythema of the eyelids with or without proptosis? (Periorbital and orbital cellulitis, epidemic keratoconjunctivitis)
- Does the patient have clouding of the cornea? (Glaucoma, keratitis, epidemic keratoconjunctivitis)
- Does the patient have a nonpurulent conjunctivitis associated with fever for at least 5 days, perineal diaper rash, pharyngitis, strawberry tongue, or cervical lymphadenopathy? (Kawasaki disease)
- Does the patient have associated symptoms suggesting a systemic illness such as fever, weight loss, diarrhea, or arthritis? (Juvenile idiopathic arthritis, inflammatory bowel disease, lupus)
- Does the patient have associated symptoms such as bullae of skin and aphthous ulcers of oral mucosa? (Stevens-Johnson syndrome)

Physical Examination

Data from your physical examination will give you the remaining information that you need to make a reasonable diagnosis.

Upon physical examination, Jack is nontoxic in appearance and cooperative with your exam. His right eyelid margin and corners of his eye have purulent yellow discharge. His right eye has an injected, red conjunctiva. His left eye is normal without discharge or conjunctival injection. He has 20/20 vision in both eyes. His pupils are both equal and reactive to light and his extraocular muscles are intact without any pain upon movement of either eye. He does not have any photophobia. His ear exam is normal without any bulging or erythema of his tympanic membranes. Examination of his nose does not reveal any bogginess of the mucosa or nasal drainage. His oropharynx is normal without any erythema or cobblestoning. He does not have any lymphadenopathy.

Making the Diagnosis

This history and physical examination are consistent with a diagnosis of bacterial conjunctivitis. The combination of crusted eyelid in the morning, a red eye, and purulent discharge on physical exam are indicative of bacterial conjunctivitis (Patel, Diaz, Bennett, & Attia, 2007). Acute infectious conjunctivitis is defined as conjunctival injection with eye discharge (Wald, 2004); however, there are multiple causes of a red eye that must be included in the differential diagnosis of conjunctivitis.

Differential Diagnosis

Usually the diagnosis of conjunctivitis is not complicated and is based on the history and physical examination findings. The history and physical examination are important to help guide one down the right path on the differential diagnosis. When evaluating a patient with suspected conjunctivitis, the health-care provider needs to consider the following characteristic clinical findings to point to the causative agent.

Bacterial conjunctivitis is usually characterized by unilateral injected conjunctiva, purulent drainage, and matted eye upon awakening, and is most commonly caused by either nontypable *H. influenzae* or *S. pneumoniae* (Patel et al., 2007). Bacterial conjunctivitis due to *H. influenzae* may also be present with otitis media. Infants may also have lacrimal duct stenosis, which can present with unilateral or bilateral yellow drainage and is often confused with conjunctivitis. Usually the conjunctiva is not injected, and the drainage will often persist despite the use of topical ophthalmic antibiotic drops. Ophthalmia neonatorium occurs in infants less than 1 month of age and is usually due to *Neisseria gonorrhoeae* or *Chlamydia trachomatis*. It is acquired during vaginal delivery by a mother who is infected with *N. gonorrhoea* or *C. trachomatis* as a sexually transmitted infection. It is characterized by purulent drainage from the eye after 48 hours of life (Olitsky, Hug, & Smith, 2007). Older children, especially adolescents, may also develop an acute purulent conjunctivitis secondary to infection with *N. gonorrheae* or *C. trachomatis*.

Viral conjunctivitis is often characterized by watery discharge, burning, itching, and injection of the conjunctiva. Conjunctivitis due to adenovirus may also be associated with pharyngitis and fever called pharyngoconjunctival fever. Outbreaks have occurred in contaminated swimming pools and ponds. Adenovirus can also lead to epidemic keratoconjunctivitis, which usually is characterized by conjunctivitis with a foreign body sensation, discharge, photophobia, itching, burning, edema of the lid, and associated upper respiratory infection (URI) symptoms. Outbreaks have occurred in ophthalmology offices and neonatal intensive care units (Langley, 2005). Acute hemorrhagic conjunctivitis, caused by enterovirus, includes symptoms such as watery hemorrhagic discharge with painful eyes (Pickering et al., 2006; Olitsky et al., 2007). Influenza infection may also lead to conjunctivitis, which is often associated with sudden onset of fever, malaise, sore throat, myalgias, and cough and has a seasonal epidemic period in the winter months (Pickering et al.).

Bilateral conjunctival injection with watery discharge and itching rather than pain characterizes allergic conjunctivitis. It also may be associated with allergic rhinitis. Often there is a seasonal pattern, most commonly in the spring, summer, and fall with recurrence each year. Vernal conjunctivitis may develop due to severe allergic conjunctivitis. Patients will have cobblestoning on the upper tarsal plate due to giant papillae. This most commonly occurs in prepubertal children and boys more often than girls (Gigliotti, 1995).

Ocular foreign body is commonly characterized by unilateral conjunctival injection, watery discharge, and a foreign body sensation. Chemical conjunctivitis results when an irritating substance comes in contact with the conjunctiva. Common agents include silver nitrate used in newborns for prophylaxis of ophthalmia neonatorium, household cleaners, pesticides, and smoke (Olitsky et al., 2007).

Patients with periorbital and orbital cellulitis will have conjunctival injection as well. However, in both of these infections, patients will have significant unilateral eyelid edema, erythema, and chemosis or swelling of the bulbar conjunctiva. Often they are unable to open the eyelid due to swelling. They may have fever and will often appear ill with orbital cellulitis as well as have proptosis of the affected eye, pain with movement of the eye, impaired eye movement, and visual impairment (Wald, 2004).

Keratitis and uveitis are often associated with a red eye. Patients with keratitis may present with intense pain, photophobia, and corneal clouding. Patients may have a history of contact lens use. Herpes simplex virus can cause keratitis, as can *S. pneumoniae*, *S. aureus*, and *Pseudomonas*. Uveitis in children is often due to a systemic illness such as juvenile idiopathic arthritis, inflammatory bowel disease, lupus, Kawasaki disease, or Stevens-Johnson syndrome. Patients often complain of pain, vision loss, and photophobia in addition to conjunctival injection (Gigliotti, 1995). Kawasaki disease is characteristically associated with a bilateral bulbar, nonpurulent conjunctivitis, fever for 5 days or longer, rash, oral mucosal involvement, swelling of hands and feet, and lymphadenopathy (Pickering et al., 2006). In addition to widespread vesicles and bullae of the face, trunk, and extremities, patients with Stevens-Johnson syndrome often have eye involvement characterized by uveitis and corneal abrasion as well as oral mucosal involvement. Glaucoma may present with a red eye, corneal clouding, and pain; however, outside of the neonatal period, it is not a common disorder in children (Gigliotti).

Management

Do you need to do anything to confirm the diagnosis, such as laboratory studies? ■

Laboratory studies usually are not needed to confirm the diagnosis of bacterial conjunctivitis. Culture of the eye drainage may be obtained, but patients are usually treated presumptively based on the history and physical examination findings, which suggest bacterial conjunctivitis. In neonates, bacterial culture may be warranted because *N. gonorrhoea* or *C. trachomatis* require systemic treatment, not just topical treatment.

Therapeutic plan: What will you do therapeutically? ■

The plan is determined by the type of conjunctivitis the patient has. Different treatments exist for the various causes of conjunctivitis.

Treatment Options

Bacterial, viral, and allergic conjunctivitis are all generally self-limited illnesses. Treatment of bacterial conjunctivitis has some advantages because it will decrease the length of illness, possibly prevent the spread of the bacteria, and decrease the risk of complications. In addition, children are usually not allowed to return to the daycare or school setting unless treatment has been initiated. The mainstay of treatment of bacterial conjunctivitis is topical antibiotics. Because a culture is not usually obtained, a broad-spectrum topical antibiotic is usually the choice for treatment (Hwang, Schanzlin, Rotberg, Foulks, & Raizman, 2003). Topical antibiotics can be either drops or ointment, with ointment commonly used for infants. Typically older children do not tolerate ointment as well because it can cause distorted vision. Common antibiotics prescribed include erythromycin ointment, trimethoprim sulfate/polymyxin drops, or sulfacetamide drops. Fluoroquinolone drops and azithromycin drops are also used but may promote resistance and are generally more expensive than the other choices because they are relatively newer preparations. (See Table 21-2.) In cases of ophthalmia neonatorum, systemic treatment with intravenous antibiotics is required. In children who present with conjunctivitis with ipsilateral otitis media, oral antibiotics should be used such as amoxicillin/clavulanate. Patients who wear contact lenses need to be instructed to refrain from wearing their contacts until the conjunctivitis has resolved. If the lenses are disposable, they should be discarded along with the lens case (Olitsky et al., 2007).

Viral conjunctivitis does not generally require any treatment. The symptoms may last for up to 2 to 3 weeks. The emphasis should be placed on prevention of the spread of viral conjunctivitis. In cases of adenoviral conjunctivitis associated with swimming pools, adequate chlorination of the water will prevent the spread of adenovirus (Gigliotti, 1995).

Treatment of allergic conjunctivitis should include avoidance of the inciting allergen; however, this may be difficult to do because many allergens are pervasive and difficult for patients to avoid. Cold compresses and lubricating eye drops can also provide relief. Patients can use either topical or oral preparations to help manage allergic conjunctivitis. In cases when allergic conjunctivitis is present in combination with allergic rhinitis, patients will benefit from oral, nonsedating antihistamines such as cetirizine, loratadine, or fexofenadine. Topical ophthalmic medications include antihistamines, antihistamines and mast cell blockers, decongestants, and corticosteroids. Decongestants are not recommended because although they may reduce symptoms, they do not help stop the allergic reaction. Repeated use of these can cause a rebound conjunctival injection or conjunctivitis medicamentosa. The combination of an antihistamine and mast cell blocker

Table 21-2 Topical Antibiotics for Bacterial Conjunctivitis

Drug	Preparation	Dose	Notes
Erythromycin ophthalmic ointment	Ilotycin	½ inch inside the lower lid four times daily for 5 to 7 days	Use in infants, but generally not tolerated in children and adults Generic available
Polymyxin/ trimethoprim ophthalmic drops	Polytrim	1–2 drops four times daily for 5 to 7 days	Generic available
Sulfacetamide ophthalmic drops 10%	Sulf-10, Bleph-10, Sulamyd	1–2 drops four times daily for 5 to 7 days	Generic available
Azithromycin	AzaSite	1 drop twice daily for 2 days, then 1 drop daily for 5 days	Expensive No generic available at this time
Fluoroquinolone ophthalmic drops	Ciloxan, Ocuflox, Quixin, Zymar, Vigamox	Generally 1 to 2 drops four times daily for 5–7 days (may vary by medication)	Expensive Preferred drug for contact lenswearers Not approved for children < 1 year old

offers quick relief of the symptoms and helps stop the allergic reaction. Examples of this are epinastine hydrochloride 0.05%, ketotifen fumarate 0.025%, or olopatadine hydrochloride 0.1%. These medications are given twice daily, but sometimes cause burning. Refrigerating the medications can sometimes decrease the burning sensation. Corticosteroids should be used only in consultation with an ophthalmologist (Boguniewicz & Leung, 2007; Ono & Abelson, 2005).

Both chemical conjunctivitis and ocular foreign body require removal of the offending agent. Immediate irrigation of the eye with profuse amounts of water is necessary to help prevent the effects of chemical exposure of the eye. Conjunctival injection, edema, and irritation may persist even if the chemical or foreign body is removed. Consultation with an ophthalmologist may be necessary in certain cases of chemical exposure and foreign body.

Both periorbital and orbital cellulitis require treatment with systemic antibiotics and may require hospitalization. Orbital cellulitis requires intravenous antibiotics, and an ophthalmologist should be consulted to help manage the patient because surgery may be required (Wald, 2004). In patients with suspected uveitis and keratitis, referral to an ophthalmologist for evaluation and management is required.

The summary of treatments of different types of conjunctivitis is found in Table 21-3.

Table 21-3   Treatments for Allergic Conjunctivitis

Class	Medication	Route/Type	Dose	Notes
Antihistamine	Azelasine HCl 0.05% (Optivar)	Topical ophthalmic	1 drop twice daily	Children ≥ 3 yrs
	Emedastine difumarate 0.05% (Emadine)	Topical ophthalmic	1 drop four times daily	Children ≥ 3 yrs
	Levocabastine hydrochloride 0.05% (Livostin)	Topical ophthalmic	1 drop twice to four times daily for up to 2 weeks	Children ≥ 12 yrs. Not for use with contact lenses
	Cetirizine (Zyrtec)	Oral: tablets, liquid, chewable	2.5–10 mg daily depending on age	Useful in children with allergic rhinitis
	Fexofenadine (Allegra)	Oral: tablets, liquid, ODT (oral disintegrating tablets)	30–180 mg daily depending on age	Useful in children with allergic rhinitis
	Loratadine (Claritin)	Oral: tablets, liquid, quick-dissolving tablets	5–10 mg daily depending on age	Useful in children with allergic rhinitis
Antihistamine/ Vasoconstrictor	Naphazoline HCl/ pheniramine (Naphcon-A, Opcon-A)	Topical ophthalmic	1–2 drops four times daily	Children ≥ 6 yrs Not for use with contact lenses Limit use to 3–4 days to prevent rebound symptoms
Antihistamine/ Mast Cell Stabilizer	Epinastine HCl 0.05% (Elestat)	Topical ophthalmic	1 drop twice daily	Children ≥ 3 yrs
	Ketotifen fumarate 0.025% (Zaditor)	Topical ophthalmic	1 drop twice daily (8–12 hours apart)	Children ≥ 3 yrs
	Olopadatine HCl 0.1% (Patanol)	Topical ophthalmic	1 drop twice daily (8 hours apart)	Children ≥ 3 yrs
	Olopadatine HCl 0.2% (Pataday)	Topical ophthalmic	1 drop once daily	Children ≥ 3 yrs

In Jack's case, you decide to prescribe trimethoprim/polymyxin drops. His mother is instructed to instill two drops into the affected eye four times daily for 7 days.

Educational plan: What will you do to educate Jack and his mother about bacterial conjunctivitis and its management? ■

Points to make through discussion:

- Explain the diagnosis of bacterial conjunctivitis.
- Explain the use of the topical antibiotic drops and the benefit of treating bacterial conjunctivitis.
- Reassure them that his symptoms should decrease 1 to 2 days after treatment with complete resolution in about 7–10 days.
- Advise him to:
  - Either wash his hands with antibacterial soap or use hand sanitizer after touching his eyes, nose, or mouth to reduce the spread of the bacteria (Aronson & Shope, 2005).
  - Avoid sharing towels with other family members.
  - Stay out of school or daycare until antibiotics are initiated (Aronson & Shope, 2005). If his school is in the midst of an epidemic, he may be required to stay home until his conjunctivitis has resolved (Centers for Disease Control and Prevention, 2003).

When do you want to see this patient back again? ■

Usually patients are not seen in follow-up for bacterial or viral conjunctivitis unless symptoms do not resolve as expected. Patients should return if pain, vision changes, fever, or increased swelling of eyelids develop. If symptoms do not decrease as expected within 2 days of treatment, further evaluation is needed with possible referral to an ophthalmologist. In cases of allergic conjunctivitis and allergic rhinitis, patients should be instructed to return if the prescribed medications do not alleviate the symptoms or the symptoms worsen. These patients may need referral to an ophthalmologist for additional evaluation and treatment.

Key Points from the Case Study

1. Bacterial conjunctivitis is a diagnosis made based on clinical suspicion and exclusion of other causes of conjunctivitis.
2. Treatment of conjunctivitis varies based on the type of conjunctivitis the patient has.
3. The majority of cases of conjunctivitis can be managed by the primary care practitioner, but referral to an ophthalmologist may be required in certain cases.

REFERENCES

Aronson, S. S., & Shope, T. R. (2005). Pinkeye (conjunctivitis). In *Managing infectious diseases in childcare and schools* (pp. 97-98). Elk Grove Village, IL: American Academy of Pediatrics.

Boguniewicz, M., & Leung, D. Y. M. (2007). Ocular allergies. In R. M. Kliegman, K. J. Marcdante, H. B. Jensen, & R. E. Behrman (Eds.), *Nelson essentials of pediatrics* (pp. 978-979). Philadelphia: Elsevier Saunders.

Buznach, N., Dagan, R., & Greenberg, D. (2005). Clinical and bacterial characteristics of acute bacterial conjunctivitis in children in the antibiotic resistance era. *Pediatric Infectious Disease Journal, 24*, 823-828.

Centers for Disease Control and Prevention. (2003). Pneumococcal conjunctivitis at an elementary school—Maine, September 20-December 6, 2002. *Morbidity and Mortality Weekly Report, 52*, 64-66.

Giglotti, F. (1995). Acute conjunctivitis. *Pediatrics in Review, 16*, 203-207.

Hwang, D. G., Schanzlin, D. J., Rotberg, M. H., Foulks, G., & Raizman, M. (2003). A phase III, placebo controlled clinical trial of 0.5% levofloxacin ophthalmic solution for the treatment of bacterial conjunctivitis. *British Journal of Ophthalmology, 87*(8), 1004-1009.

Langley, J. M. (2005). Adenoviruses. *Pediatrics in Review, 26*, 244-249.

Olitsky, S. E, Hug, D., & Smith, L. P. (2007). Disorders of the conjunctiva. In R. M. Kliegman, K. J. Marcdante, H. B. Jensen, & R. E. Behrman (Eds.), *Nelson essentials of pediatrics* (pp. 978-979). Philadelphia: Elsevier Saunders.

Ono, S. J., & Abelson, M. B. (2005). Allergic conjunctivitis: update on the pathophysiology and prospects for future treatment. *Journal of Allergy and Clinical Immunology, 115*, 118-122.

Patel, P. B., Diaz, M. C., Bennett, J. E., & Attia, M. (2007). Clinical features of bacterial conjunctivitis in children. *Academic Emergency Medicine, 14*(1), 1-5.

Pickering, L. K., Baker, C. J., Long, S. S., & McMillan, J. A. (Eds.). (2006). *Red book: 2006 report of the Committee on Infectious Diseases* (27th ed., pp. 149, 202-203, 284, 401, 412-415). Elk Grove Village, IL: American Academy of Pediatrics.

Rietveld, R. P., ter Riet, G., Bindels, P. J., Sloos, J. H., & van Weert, H. C. (2004). Predicting bacterial cause in infectious conjunctivitis: cohort study on informativeness of combinations of signs and symptoms. *British Medical Journal, 329*(7459), 206-210.

Rose, P. W., Harden, A., Brueggemann, A. B., Perrera, R., Sheikh, A., Crook, D., et al. (2005). Chloramphenicol treatment for acute infective conjunctivitis in children in primary care: a randomized double-blind placebo-controlled trial. *Lancet, 366*(9479), 37-43.

Wald, E. R. (2004). Periorbital and orbital infections. *Pediatrics in Review, 25*, 312-320.

Chapter 22

The Toddler with Recurrent Ear Infections

Kathleen M. Boyd

In modern medicine, the primary care provider often relies heavily on advanced imaging technology and supportive laboratory evidence to clinch a diagnosis. On occasion, we are privileged to elucidate a clinical diagnosis based on just a thorough history and physical examination and provide treatment options based on that decision.

Educational Objectives

1. Identify the distinguishing signs and symptoms of acute otitis media (AOM) and otitis media with effusion (OME).
2. Apply the guidelines for management of acute otitis media and otitis media with effusion.
3. Recognize the risk factors associated with development of acute otitis media.
4. Identify when patients need to be referred to an otolaryngologist for treatment of otitis media.

Case Presentation and Discussion

Sam Burgess is a 16-month-old African American boy who presents to your office with a history of fever, rhinorrhea, and tugging at his ear. He is accompanied by his mother, who is 12 weeks pregnant, and his 3-year-old brother, who also seems to have cold symptoms.

You talk with Sam's mother about his presenting symptoms and past history and complete a detailed physical exam.

What questions will you ask Sam's mother related to his fever and ear pain? ■

Your symptom analysis reveals the following information: Sam started with a slight cough and runny nose 4 days ago. The rhinorrhea started with a small amount of clear discharge but has increased over the past 48 hours. Sam had been active and playful despite his symptoms until last night when his fever spiked to 102.2°F (39°C). His mother reports he was up most of the night crying and wanting to be held. He had one ear infection at 8 months of age and his mother is concerned that he may have another one because he is intermittently tugging at his right ear, acting as if it hurts. Ibuprofen has helped some with the fever and pain. Today Sam has been drinking well and has had several wet diapers, but he is not interested in eating. He has had no vomiting but his stools have been loose for the last 2 days.

What other questions do you need to ask Sam's mother? ■

Before answering this question, here is some more information about acute otitis media that you need to consider.

Epidemiology

Acute otitis media (AOM) is the most common bacterial infection in children, accounting for nearly 30 million clinic visits per year and costing over $5 billion in the United States yearly. It is the most frequent reason for childhood antibiotic consumption and outpatient surgery in developed countries (Rovers, Schidler, Zielhuis, & Rosenfeld, 2004). Fifty percent of U.S. infants have had at least one episode of AOM before 6 months of age, and 90% experience at least one episode by age 2 years (Siegel & Bien, 2004). There is an increased incidence in those younger than 2 years, with the peak age of incidence between 6 and 20 months. Males account for just over 50% of all cases.

Otitis media is especially prevalent and more severe among Native American, Inuit, and indigenous Australian children (Kerschner, 2007). Studies in the United States comparing otitis media rates among white and African American children have given conflicting results, but overall findings suggest that race-based difference rates seem most likely attributable to socioeconomic status, access to care, accuracy of diagnosis, and intensity of surveillance rather than race itself (Paradise et al., 1997).

Risk Factors

Age

The highest incidence for AOM is between 6 months and 2 years. Younger children are at increased risk for otitis media due to the relative immaturity of their immune systems. The developing immune systems of young children have less experience with common viruses than do those of adults. Viral infections likely are the direct or indirect cause of most middle ear infections (Kerschner, 2007).

More importantly, in infants and toddlers, the eustachian tube, responsible for draining middle ear secretions to the nasopharynx, is shorter, straighter, and floppier than an adult eustachian tube (Rovers et al., 2004). This straight, more easily closed design does not ventilate the middle ear as effectively, making it more susceptible to swelling, inflammation, and bacterial colonization (Maxson & Yamauchi, 1996).

Socioeconomic Status

Poverty has long been recognized as a major contributing factor in the development and the severity of OM. Recent studies strongly suggest that low socioeconomic status is one of the most important identifiable risk factors for the development of acute otitis media (Paradise et al., 2007). Crowded conditions, limited hygiene, suboptimal nutrition, limited access to health care, and limited resources for compliance with provider recommendations have all been suggested as playing a role in the relationship between poverty and the development of acute otitis media (Kerschner, 2007).

Secondhand Smoke Exposure

Passive smoke exposure increases the incidence of AOM and otitis media with effusion (OME), and the duration of the middle ear effusion. The precise mechanism remains unknown, but there is sufficient evidence to support a causal relationship between parental smoking and otitis media (U.S. Department of Health and Human Services, 2006). Recent studies suggest that nicotine and other toxins in secondhand smoke may enhance the invasion of bacteria into the middle ear and depress local immune function. Environmental tobacco smoke may cause toxic injury to the epithelium of the nasopharynx resulting in prolonged inflammation and congestion of the upper airways. It may also impair the mucociliary function of the eustachian tube and lead to impaired clearance of the nasopharyngeal airways (Kum-Nji, Meloy, & Herrod, 2006).

Etiology

Streptococcus pneumoniae, nontypeable *Haemophilus influenzae*, and *Moraxella catarrhalis* remain the leading bacterial pathogens responsible for acute otitis media (American Academy of Pediatrics [AAP], 2004). Viral infections, most commonly respiratory syncytial virus (RSV), influenza, and parainfluenza, are also common pathogens involved in AOM. It is uncertain whether viral infections alone can cause AOM, or whether their role is limited to setting the stage for secondary bacterial infection (Kerschner, 2007). It is suspected that viral co-infection amplifies the inflammatory process and contributes to delayed bacterial clearance (Rovers et al., 2004).

   S. pneumoniae accounts for 25–50% of AOM, *H. influenzae* accounts for approximately 40% of cases, and *M. catarrhalis* is responsible for one eighth of the recognized bacterial otitis media. There is some evidence to suggest that the microbiology of acute otitis media is changing due to the routine use of the heptavalent pneumococcal vaccine, with more cases now attributable to gram-negative and beta lactamase–producing organisms (Block et al., 2004).

Pathophysiology

Dysfunction of the eustachian tube and inflammation are the most important factors in the development of AOM. Commonly, viral upper respiratory infections precede or coincide with AOM. The viral infections induce inflammation and edema in the nasopharynx and eustachian tube, narrowing the eustachian tube lumen. Obstruction of the lumen causes negative pressure to build up, creating a relative vacuum within the middle ear space. This phenomenon reverses the flow of secretions, pulling fluid from the nasopharynx into the middle ear (Siegel & Bien, 2004). The resulting mucoid medium is ideal for bacterial colonization and overgrowth, stimulating an even greater inflammatory response.

Data for the Diagnosis

Often the diagnosis of acute otitis media is evident by the history and physical examination findings, but, as in all realms of medicine, it is important to generate a differential diagnosis to ensure proper management and counseling for the patients. Viral myringitis and otitis media with effusion (OME) may be mistaken for acute otitis media. In myringitis, characterized by otalgia and an erythematous ear drum, the tympanic membrane is inflamed; however, it is nonbulging and freely mobile on pneumatic otoscopy (Siegel & Bien, 2004). On the other hand, OME is characterized by a poorly mobile, nonbulging TM, indicating the presence of middle ear fluid. In OME, the tympanic membrane lacks the characteristic inflammation that is seen in AOM.

The differential diagnoses also include otitis externa, or swimmer's ear, which is an inflammation of the external auditory canal or auricle. Presence of a foreign body in the ear canal or impacted cerumen can also present as otalgia, but will typically lack the preceding upper respiratory infection (URI) symptoms and fever that accompany AOM, and will be evident on physical examination. Other diagnoses to consider when patients present with otalgia include local trauma, varicella zoster, herpes simplex, cellulitis or furunculosis of the ear canal, mastoiditis, and perichondritis. Referred pain from dental infections, stomatitis, pharyngitis, tonsillitis, and retropharyngeal abscesses must also be considered but are typically ruled out by physical examination (Sinai & Biggs, 2003).

From the above review, some other information you should obtain includes the following:

- Is there smoke exposure in the home? (Increased risk for development of AOM)
- Is the child breastfed? (Protective effect of breastmilk and breastfeeding if continued for at least 4 months)
- Does the child attend daycare? (Increased risk for development of AOM)
- Is there a family history of otitis media? (Increased risk for development of AOM with positive family history)
- Does the child have any speech delays or other developmental concerns? (Concern for conductive hearing loss due to AOM)
- Has the child been on antibiotics within the last month? (Increased risk for resistant organisms)
- Does the child have AOM and purulent conjunctivitis? (Nontypeable *H. influenzae*)
- Is there history of otorrhea? (TM perforation or myringotomy tubes)
- Is there increased pain with traction on pinna? (Otitis externa)

- Is the external auditory canal erythematous and/or edematous? (Otitis externa)
- Is there a vesicular exanthem involving the auricle or ear canal? (Varicella zoster, herpes simplex)

Physical Examination

Upon physical examination, Sam is ill appearing and quiet in his mother's lap. He has thick nasal discharge in both nares. Examination of the left tympanic membrane (TM) reveals a pearly gray tympanic membrane in neutral position. The light reflex and bony structures are clearly visible. Pneumatic otoscopy reveals movement of the left TM. The right tympanic membrane is cloudy, erythematous, and bulging. There are no visible landmarks. On pneumatic otoscopy of the right ear, there is no movement of the tympanic membrane. His oropharynx is moist and without erythema, ulceration, or exudates. Sam's neck is supple and without lymphadenopathy. His eye, heart, lung, and abdominal examinations are unremarkable.

Making the Diagnosis

The history and physical examination are consistent with the diagnosis of acute otitis media, right ear. Diagnostic criteria for AOM include 1) rapid onset of symptoms, 2) presence of middle ear effusion, and 3) signs and symptoms of middle ear inflammation (AAP, 2004). Fever, irritability, rhinitis, cough, decreased oral intake, trouble sleeping, and tugging at the ears are often associated with AOM but are nonspecific symptoms that can be seen in many childhood illnesses (Rothman, Owens, & Siemel, 2003). It is important to remember that acute otitis media cannot be differentiated from a common viral upper respiratory infection based on symptoms alone.

A bulging, cloudy, immobile tympanic membrane is the most helpful physical finding to clinch the diagnosis (Rothman et al., 2003). Color is not a defining feature of acute otitis media because the infected middle ear may appear red or yellow (Siegel & Bien, 2004). However, a tympanic membrane that is distinctly red, or "hemorrhagic, strongly red or moderately red," suggests AOM (Rothman et al.).

Detection of middle ear effusion by pneumatic otoscopy is a key element in the diagnosis of acute otitis media (AAP, 2004). Normally, the tympanic membrane is a convex, freely mobile, translucent barrier between the external ear canal and the inner ear. With insufflation, the healthy tympanic membrane moves easily in response to positive or negative pressure (Siegel & Bien, 2004). Normal mobility is evident when positive pressure is applied to the insufflator bulb and the eardrum moves rapidly inward; when the bulb is released, creating negative pressure, the TM moves out. The presence of a middle ear fluid, infectious or otherwise, significantly reduces the mobility of the TM. Evidence of middle ear effusion may also be demonstrated by the presence of purulent fluid in the external auditory canal, indicating a perforated tympanic membrane.

Management

How do you plan to treat Sam's acute otitis media? ■

Do you need to do anything to confirm the diagnosis, such as laboratory studies? ■

Typically, no laboratory studies are needed to confirm the diagnosis of acute otitis media. However, AOM can often be difficult to diagnose by exam alone. When the presence of middle ear fluid is difficult to detect clinically, tympanometry or acoustic reflexometry can be helpful in establishing the diagnosis (AAP, 2004). A tympanometer records compliance of the TM and provides information on the function of the middle ear and the presence of a middle ear effusion. Acoustic reflectometry detects middle ear fluid by analyzing a sound gradient reflected off of the tympanic membrane (Ramakrishnan, Sparks, & Berryhill, 2007).

Although not routinely done, the definitive diagnostic test for AOM is culture of the middle ear fluid via tympanocentesis. The indications for tympanocentesis include a severely ill or toxic child, AOM in a newborn or immunocompromised patient, or clinical suspicion of an unusual organism (Siegel & Bien, 2004). The clinician must have expertise in completing this procedure.

Therapeutic plan: What will you do therapeutically? ■

The goals of treatment for acute otitis media are twofold: pain management and reduction of recurrence. Nearly 80% of children with AOM will have spontaneous resolution within 2–14 days; therefore, it is not necessary that antibiotics be prescribed initially for all suspected cases of AOM (Rovers et al., 2004). Delaying antibiotics in select cases reduces antibiotic side effects, lowers treatment-related costs, and helps to minimize emergence of resistant bacterial strains (Ramakrishnan et al., 2007).

Children who will most likely benefit from antibiotic therapy are those younger than 2 years of age with severe AOM (defined as severe otalgia and fever > 39°C [102.2°F]), bilateral AOM, evidence of otorrhea on examination, and all children younger than 6 months of age (AAP, 2004). Children under 2 have a greater number of penicillin-resistant pneumococci isolated from the middle ear than older children; these infections are less likely to spontaneously resolve.

Antibiotics may be deferred in otherwise healthy children 6 months to 2 years of age in whom the disease is mild or the diagnosis is uncertain as long as there is a responsible, reliable caregiver and access to medical care if the symptoms worsen. Antibiotics may also be withheld in children older than 2 if the disease is mild or the practitioner is uncertain of the diagnosis, if in the presence of a reliable caregiver and ready access to medical follow-up (AAP, 2004).

Many practitioners have recently adopted a wait and see approach with regards to prescribing antibiotics because it allows for greater empowerment of the patient and family and enables shared decision making (Spiro & Arnold,

2008). It is a reasonable approach to give families a safety net antibiotic prescription (SNAP) with instructions not to fill the prescription unless symptoms worsen or fail to improve 48 hours after the initial visit (Spiro & Arnold). It is important to include an expiration date on the prescription within 5 days of the office visit.

The management of AOM should include a pain assessment and treatment of otalgia if present (AAP, 2004). Even with antibiotic therapy on board, significant otalgia may persist for up to 48 hours. A number of treatment options are available for pain management, including oral/rectal acetaminophen, ibuprofen, topical Auralgan (combination of antipyrine, benzocaine, and glycerin), and topical lidocaine. Antihistamines are not recommended and may prolong the middle ear effusion that often follows AOM. Decongestants may relieve nasal congestion but are not indicated in young children and do not improve healing or reduce complications of AOM (AAP, 2004).

When the decision is made to treat AOM with an antibiotic regimen, high dose amoxicillin is the preferred first line agent (AAP, 2004). Doubling the standard dose increases the drug concentration in the middle ear and provides activity against most intermediate strains of *S. pneumoniae* and many of the resistant strains. A 10-day antibiotic regimen is standard, but a 5- to 7-day regimen is adequate in older children with mild to moderate disease (AAP, 2004; Pickering, Baker, Long, & McMillan, 2006). In children who are vomiting and unable to tolerate an oral medication, an alternative for AOM management is a single dose of ceftriaxone, given intramuscularly or intravenously (Ramakrishnan et al., 2007).

Amoxicillin should not be first line therapy in patients who are at high risk for AOM caused by an amoxicillin-resistant organism. Those patients include children who have received antibiotics within the previous 30 days, patients with concurrent otitis and purulent conjunctivitis most likely due to nontypeable *H. influenzae*, and patients currently on amoxicillin prophylaxis (AAP, 2004; Pickering, Baker, Long, & McMillan, 2006). For children with penicillin allergy, please refer to Table 22-1 for antibiotic options. Table 22-2 outlines common agents used in the treatment of otitis media.

With appropriate antibiotic therapy and pain management, the signs and symptoms of systemic and local disease should begin to resolve within 24 to 72 hours. Lack of improvement in patients started on antibiotics suggests either

Table 22-1 Antibiotic Options in the Penicillin-Allergic Patient	
Type 1 Hypersensitivity (Presence of urticaria or anaphylaxis)	Non–Type 1 Hypersensitivity (No urticaria or anaphylaxis)
Azithromycin	Cefdinir
Erythromycin, sulfisoxazole	Cefuroxime
Clarithromycin	Ceftriaxone
Clindamycin	Cefpodoxime

bacterial resistance or the presence of another underlying disease process. High dose amoxicillin/clavulanate is the current recommended second line treatment option for persistent AOM. Cephalosporins such as cefdinir, cefpodoxime, cefuroxime, or a three-dose regimen of ceftriaxone are alternative regimens (AAP, 2004). Myringotomy or tympanocentesis to obtain cultures should be considered for cases that fail to respond to second line therapy (Pickering, Baker, Long, & McMillan, 2006).

When AOM is recurrent, despite appropriate antibiotic therapy, otolaryngology referral for possible surgical management with tympanostomy tubes is warranted. Recurrent AOM is defined as three episodes of AOM in 6 months or five to six episodes in 12 months (Kerschner, 2007).

In Sam's case, you decide to prescribe high dose amoxicillin. His mother is instructed to give him the antibiotic by mouth twice daily for 10 days. Since his pain improved with ibuprofen, you encourage his mother to continue to use it as needed every 6 hours for ear pain.

Educational plan: What will you do to educate Sam's mother about acute otitis media and its management? ■

Points to make through discussion:
· Explain the natural history of acute otitis media.
· Explain the benefits of treating the ear pain with analgesics.
· Explain the rationale of antibiotic use in the management of otitis media.
· Reassure Sam's mother that she should notice a decrease in his symptoms in 24–72 hours with the use of antibiotics and analgesics.
· Educate Sam's mother on the signs and symptoms of clinical deterioration.
· Educate Sam's mother on preventable risk factors.
  · Limit exposure to secondhand smoke.
  · Breastfeeding for at least 4 months (This may not help in Sam's case but may help with AOM prevention in future siblings.)
  · Limit pacifier use after 6 months to only when the child is falling asleep.
  · Avoid bottle propping; enure infants are given bottles while upright.
  · Receive all appropriate vaccines, especially influenza and pneumococcal.
  · Limit exposure to others with upper respiratory infections.

When do you want to see this patient back again? ■

Follow-up for AOM depends on the patient's age and history of underlying medical problems, particularly speech delay, hearing loss, or learning problems (AAP, 2004). Persistent middle ear effusion after resolution of AOM is typical and should not be seen as treatment failure or need for continued antibiotics. Seventy percent of children will have middle ear fluid at 2 weeks, 40% at 4 weeks, and 10–25% at 3 months (AAP, 2004). Current guidelines recommend follow-up ear checks for all children younger than 2 years. This is typically done at 6 to 8 weeks. It is also recommended that children over 2 years who have a history of speech or developmental delay also be seen for follow-up after AOM (AAP).

Sam's mother seems to understand the treatment regimen as explained and asks very appropriate questions. When she brings Sam back in 2 months for his previously scheduled 18-month well child visit, he seems to be doing well. On follow-up examination, the right ear is translucent and without erythema, but there is evidence of an air fluid level behind the TM. Pneumatic otoscopy reveals no movement of the TM when positive pressure is applied with the bulb. His left ear is completely normal, as is the remainder of his exam. Sam's mother reveals that he is doing well developmentally and has a vocabulary of 10 words. Sam's mother has no concerns with his hearing or speech.

Table 22-2   Agents Used in the Treatment of Acute Otitis Media

Drug	Preparation	Dosage	Notes
Amoxicillin		80–90 mg/kg/day orally in two divided doses	First line agent Inexpensive, safe, effective
Amoxicillin/ clavulanate	Augmentin	90 mg/kg/day (amoxicillin component) in two divided doses	Second line agent First line for patients on prophylactic amoxicillin, history of antibiotic use within the last 30 days and those with otitis-conjunctivitis Efficacious against beta-lactamase producers Diarrhea is common
Azithromycin		Single dose: 30 mg/kg × 1 day 3-day: 20 mg/kg/day × 3 days 5-day: 10 mg/kg day 1 and 5 mg/kg daily on days 2–5	Use in penicillin allergy (Type 1) Limited activity against nonsusceptible *S. pneumonaie* and beta-lactamase-producing *H. influenzae*
Cefdinir	Omnicef	14 mg/kg/day in one or two divided doses	Second line agent Warn patients it can turn stools red brick color
Cefuroxime	Ceftin	30 mg/kg/day in two divided doses	Second line agent Poor palatability
Cefpodoxime	Vantin	30 mg/kg/day	Poor palatability
Clarithromycin	Biaxin	30–40 mg/kg/day in four divided doses	Use in penicillin allergy (Type 1) Limited activity against nonsusceptible *S. pneumonaie* and beta-lactamase-producing *H. influenzae*

(continues)

Drug	Preparation	Dosage	Notes
Table 22-2 Agents Used in the Treatment of Acute Otitis Media (Continued)			
Ceftriaxone	Rocephin	Initial infection: 50 mg/kg × 1 IM/IV Treatment failure: 50 mg/kg/dose daily × 3 days	Useful for patient unable to tolerate oral medication due to vomiting Substantial cost
Clindamycin	Cleocin	30–40 mg/kg/day in three to four divided doses	Use in penicillin allergy (Type 1) Poor palatability
Erythromycin, sulfisoxazole	Pediazol	50–150 mg/kg/day of erythromycin in four divided doses	Use in penicillin allergy (Type 1) Poor palatability
Antipyrine/ benzocaine	Auralgan	Fill ear canal; moisten cotton pledget, place in external ear, repeat every 1–2 hours until pain and congestion are relieved	Used for pain management Not to be used if TM perforated

Otitis Media with Effusion

Otitis media with effusion, or serous otitis, is present in nearly all children after successful treatment of acute otitis media (Pickering, Baker, Long, & McMillan, 2006). In the majority of patients, OME resolves without medical intervention, but it may take weeks to months to do so. Prolonged OME increases the risk for language delay due to the associated conductive hearing loss. Current guidelines for the management of OME recommend watchful waiting if the patient has no underlying language delays or hearing loss. Hearing tests are recommended if OME persists longer than 3 months, or sooner if language delay, learning difficulties, or hearing loss are suspected. There is no evidence to support the use of antihistamines, decongestants, corticosteroids, or antibiotics in the treatment regimen of OME (American Academy of Family Physicians [AAFP] et al., 2004). Otolaryngology referral is indicated for patients with high risk of speech or learning problems, particularly children with permanent hearing loss, children with craniofacial anomalies or syndromes that affect hearing and eustachian tube function, children with uncorrectable vision loss, and those children with a cleft palate (AAFP et al., 2004).

You decide to bring Sam back for an ear recheck in 6 weeks to evaluate for resolution of the OME. On follow-up, the middle ear fluid has resolved. He continues to do well developmentally and his mother has no new concerns.

Key Points of the Case

1. Otitis media is a clinical diagnosis that requires both evidence of middle ear effusion and signs and symptoms of middle ear inflammation on physical examination.

2. Assessment of the child's pain and an appropriate plan for pain control should always be addressed in the management of acute otitis media.

3. Treatment of otitis media with antibiotics varies based on the child's age, risk factors, and the constellation of symptoms, but high dose amoxicillin is typically the first line antibiotic agent.

4. It is not uncommon to have evidence of middle ear effusion after successful treatment of AOM.

5. The majority of cases of AOM and OME can be managed by the primary care practitioner, but referral to an otolaryngologist may be required in cases of treatment failure.

REFERENCES

American Academy of Family Physicians, American Academy of Otolaryngology-Head and Neck Surgery, American Academy of Pediatrics, Subcommittee on Otitis Media with Effusion. (2004). Otitis media with effusion. *Pediatrics, 113*(5), 1412–1429.

American Academy of Pediatrics, American Academy of Family Physicians, Subcommittee on Management of Acute Otitis Media. (2004). Diagnosis and management of acute otitis media. *Pediatrics, 113*(5), 1451–1465.

Block, S. L., Hedrick, J., Harrison, C. L., Tyler, R., Smith, A., Findlay, R., et al. (2004). Community-wide vaccination with the heptavalent pneumococcal conjugate significantly alters the microbiology of acute otitis media. *Pediatric Infectious Disease Journal, 23*(9), 829–833.

Kerschner, J. E. (2007). Otitis media. In R. M. Kliegman, K. J. Marcdante, H. B. Jensen, & R. E. Behrman (Eds.), *Nelson essentials of pediatrics* (18th ed., pp. 2362–2646). Philadelphia: Elsevier Saunders.

Kum-Nji, P., Meloy, L., & Herrod, H. (2006). Environmental tobacco smoke exposure: prevalence and mechanisms of causation of infections in children. *Pediatrics, 117*(5), 1745–1754.

Maxson, S., & Yamauchi, T. (1996). Acute otitis media. *Pediatrics in Review, 17,* 191–195.

Paradise, J. L., Rockette, H. E., Colborn, K., Bernard, B. S., Smith, C. G., Kurs-Lasky, M., et al. (1997). Otitis media in 2253 Pittsburgh-area infants: prevalence and risk factors during the first two years of life. *Pediatrics, 99,* 318–333.

Pickering, L. K., Baker, C. J., Long, S. S., & McMillan, J. A. (Eds.). (2006). *Red book: 2006 report of the Committee on Infectious Diseases* (27th ed.). Elk Grove Village, IL: American Academy of Pediatrics.

Ramakrishnan, K., Sparks, R. A., & Berryhill, W. E. (2007). Diagnosis and treatment of otitis media. *American Family Physician, 76*(11), 1650–1658.

Rothman, R., Owens, T., & Simel, D. (2003). Does this child have acute otitis media? *Journal of the American Medical Association, 290*(12), 1633–1640.

Rovers, M. M., Schidler, A. G. M., Zielhuis, G. A., & Rosenfeld, R. M. (2004). Otitis media. *Lancet, 363*, 465–473.

Siegel, R. M., & Bien, J. P. (2004). Acute otitis media in children: a continuing story. *Pediatrics in Review, 25*, 187–193.

Sinai, L. N., & Biggs, L. M. (2003). Earache. In: M. W. Schwartz, L. M. Bell, P. M. Bingham, E. K. Chung, D. F. Friedman, & A. E. Mulberg (Eds.), *The 5-minute pediatric consult* (3rd ed., pp. 32–33). Philadelphia: Lippincott, Williams & Wilkins.

Spiro, D. M., & Arnold, D. H. (2008). The concept and practice of a wait-and-see approach to acute otitis media. *Current Opinion in Pediatrics, 20*(1), 72–78.

U.S. Department of Health and Human Services. (2006). *The health consequences of involuntary exposure to tobacco smoke: a report of the Surgeon General.* Atlanta, GA: U.S. Department of Health and Human Services, Centers for Disease Control and Prevention, Coordinating Center for Health Promotion, National Center for Chronic Disease Prevention and Health Promotion, Office on Smoking and Health.

Chapter 23

The Athlete Who Experienced Syncope

Patrick E. Killeen

An episode of syncope in a child or adolescent always merits careful investigation by the primary care provider (PCP). The clinical question that must be quickly answered when the child or teen is first seen is whether the syncopal event (or events) represents a serious underlying medical problem or a non-life-threatening, temporary annoyance. The PCP must obtain a detailed history to accurately identify the underlying cause of a particular child's syncope from the wide range of potential differential diagnoses associated with syncopal events. Omission of key questions may result in unnecessary and expensive diagnostic testing or failure to identify an underlying life-threatening medical problem. After having adequately explored essential historical questions and queried for significant associated symptoms with the child or teen and/or parent(s), a thorough physical examination is then performed. In addition to outlining history and physical findings that are critical elements of the assessment, this case study will also feature information about the often challenging issue of selecting diagnostic tests that should be ordered routinely or based on symptomatology and when to refer the child to a specialist for a definitive diagnosis or additional diagnostic work-up and management.

Educational Objectives
1. Identify key historical questions that need to be asked when a teen has experienced a syncopal episode.
2. Differentiate between signs and symptoms that point to a life-threatening syncopal condition versus a benign syncopal event.
3. Understand the underlying mechanisms of vasovagal-induced syncope.
4. Describe the key principles underlying the emergent evaluation of syncope in children and adolescents.
5. Identify the initial screening diagnostic work-up for a female teen who presents in the emergency department (ED) with a first-time episode of syncope.

Case Presentation and Discussion

> Emma Kaplan is a 14-year-old female who "fainted" after a field hockey game. Emma arrives with her field hockey coach to the ED via ambulance. She is alert and conscious. The coach states that immediately after the game while all the girls were in a huddle Emma "stood up and passed out." The coach states that Emma fell face down and was unresponsive for about 15–30 seconds or so. Emma states that she remembers playing the entire game while feeling hot, nauseated, sweaty, and short of breath. The last thing she remembers is suddenly feeling dizzy.

Before you proceed further, you need to review what you know about syncope episodes.

Overview of Syncope

Syncope is a sudden, brief loss of consciousness associated with loss of postural tone from which recovery is spontaneous (Kapoor, 2000). This abrupt loss of consciousness results from an interruption of energy sources to the brain, usually because of a sudden reduction of cerebral perfusion. Up to 15% of children experience a syncopal episode prior to the end of adolescence (Lewis & Dhala, 1999). Life-threatening causes of syncope can be identified by a detailed history and physical examination including family history and a few select diagnostic studies. There are multiple causes of syncope for the practitioner to consider, some of which may be life-threatening. (See Table 23-1.) Their origin can be:

- Neurologic
  - Seizure/migraine syndrome
  - Cerebral concussion
- Cardiac
  - Cardiac arrhythmias including long QT syndrome
  - Vasovagal
- Pregnancy
- Psychogenic
  - Hyperventilation or breath holding
  - Hysteria (somatization disorder) or a conversion disorder
- Medications or illicit drugs including antidepressant drugs
- Dehydration/volume depletion
- Toxins, e.g., carbon monoxide poisoning, inhalant/huffing

Etiology of Syncope

There are multiple causes of syncope that the healthcare provider must consider as part of the differential diagnoses of syncope. Some conditions are life-threatening whereas others are benign. Thus, the challenge for the primary care provider is to correctly distinguish a benign cause from a life-threatening problem, and to do so in a cost-effective manner without ordering unnecessary and costly diagnostic

Table 23-1   Causes of Syncope in Children[a]
Primary electrical disturbances: Long QT syndrome Brugada syndrome Familial catecholaminergic polymorphic ventricular tachycardia Short QT syndrome Preexcitation syndromes (such as Wolff-Parkinson-White) Bradyarrhythmias (complete atrioventricular block, sinus node dysfunction)
Structural abnormalities: Hypertrophic cardiomyopathy Coronary artery anomalies Arrhythmogenic right ventricular dysplasia/cardiomyopathy Valvar aortic stenosis Dilated cardiomyopathy Pulmonary hypertension Acute myocarditis Congenital heart disease
Other causes: *Vasovagal (neurocardiogenic) syndrome, including situational syncope (cough, micturation, hair combing)* *Breath-holding spell* *Orthostatic hypotension (hemorrhage, dehydration, pregnancy)* Toxic exposure Hypoglycemia
Conditions that may mimic syncope: Seizure Migraine syndromes Hysterical faint Hyperventilation
[a]Causes listed in **bold** are serious or life-threatening. Causes listed in *italic* are common. *Source:* © 2008 UpToDate.

tests. When life-threatening etiologies are identified, the responsibility of the primary care provider is to quickly refer the child or adolescent to the appropriate specialist. Table 23-1 lists causes of syncope in children from which to establish a list of differential diagnoses you will need to consider in Emma's situation.

Benign Causes of Syncope

The majority of causes of pediatric syncopal episodes are benign changes in vasomotor tone (Massin et al., 2004) such as breath holding and orthostatic hypotension. Other conditions that imitate syncope are overdose, drugs, seizures, migraine syndromes, hysteria, hyperventilation, and pregnancy.

Neurocardiogenic Syncope

Neurocardiogenic syncope (vasovagal) is a neurally mediated disorder and a common cause of syncope. Children with neurocardiogenic (vasovagal) syncope frequently report symptoms before the event that include dizziness, lightheadedness, sweating, nausea, weakness, and visual changes (blurred vision, tunnel vision, slow visual loss). Patients with orthostatic hypotension or vasovagal syncope may report that symptoms recurred when they tried to sit up immediately after the initial syncopal event. The duration of such activity is usually brief and recovery is rapid. In comparison, prolonged motor activity or postictal recovery time are consistent with a seizure (Reuter & Brownstein, 2002).

Children with a neurocardiogenic/vasovagal cause of syncope typically have been upright or changed position just prior to the event. A trigger such as pain or stress may be the precipitant in some cases. Syncope that occurs during physical exertion is very concerning for a cardiac etiology, whereas syncope after exertion may occur with neurocardiogenic/vasovagal syncope or cardiac conditions (Driscoll, Jacobsen, Porter, & Wollan, 1997; Massin et al., 2004). In a 2001 study reviewing recurrent syncope, neurocardiogenic/vasovagal syncope was considered the cause in 35% of such events (Mathias, Deguchi, & Schatz, 2001). However, neurocardiogenic/vasovagal syncope remains a diagnosis of exclusion.

The diagnosis can also be made by exclusion of other causes of syncope and by a characteristic response to upright tilt table testing, during which the patient may pass out from bradycardia and/or hypotension. These patients do not necessarily require treatment.

Seizure

Seizure refers to a transient occurrence of signs and/or symptoms due to excessive neuronal activity of the brain. Abnormal movement such as tonic clonic movement can occur. The duration of such activity is usually brief and recovery is rapid. Prolonged abnormal movements and/or prolonged recovery time are consistent with a seizure, as are loss of bowel or bladder control. In the patient with prolonged loss of consciousness, seizure activity, or a postictal phase, a routine outpatient electroencephalogram (EEG) or 24-hour video EEG should be considered. Neuroimaging may be indicated emergently for children with focal neurologic deficits, persistently altered mental status, or a significant head injury as a result of the syncopal episode. Syncope is distinguished from seizures by accompanying pallor, prodromal lightheadedness and visual changes, lack of postictal state, and no loss of bowel or bladder control.

Cardiac Causes

Cardiac issues that cause syncope can be life-threatening. Shortness of breath, chest pain, or palpitations prior to or during the event are concerning for a cardiac etiology. Sudden death in the young athlete occurs with an estimated prevalence of between 1:100,000 and 1:300,000 (Maron et al., 1996).

Cardiac issues that cause syncope are primary electrical disturbances and structural heart disease including exercise-related syncope. As stated earlier, syncope that occurs during physical exertion is very concerning for a cardiac etiology, whereas syncope after exertion may occur with vasovagal syncope or cardiac conditions (Driscoll et al., 1997; Massin et al., 2004). This is a major point that must always be considered.

One specific primary electrical disturbance that is worrisome is long QT syndrome. Triggers include a sudden startle or even auditory stimuli such as a fire alarm (Moss, 2003). An electrocardiogram (ECG) is considered a standard part of the syncope work-up. A patient with a normal ECG has a low likelihood of arrhythmia as a cause of syncope (Kapoor, 2000). ECG abnormalities may be variable and/or subtle, thus a cardiologist consult should be considered whenever there are incongruent clinical features, regardless of the ECG findings.

ECG findings consistent with life threatening causes of syncope that should be noted include:

- Bradycardia or atrioventricular block
- Prolonged QT interval/short QT interval (less than or equal to 0.30 seconds)
- Brugada pattern/pseudo right bundle branch block with ST elevation in leads V1 to V3
- Epsilon waves (arrhythmogenic right ventricular dysplasia)
- Preexcitation syndrome (Wolff-Parkinson-White)
- Nonsinus rhythm
- Signs of myocardial injury
- Ventricular hypertrophy or strain patterns

Recurrent syncope can be attributed to both psychogenic and cardiac etiologies. In a review of 433 patients, the cumulative incidence of recurrence of syncope at 3 years was 31% for patients with a cardiovascular etiology, 36% for those with a noncardiovascular cause, and 43% for those with syncope of unknown etiology (Kapoor et al., 1987).

What information do you need to evaluate Emma's fainting spell? ■

Historical Data Necessary for Syncope Analysis in Children

The first area to investigate relates to the specific facts about the situation immediately preceding the event. This includes a detailed description of the child's position and the activity the child was participating in prior to the syncopal episode. For example, if the child was in a seated position and then stood up and fainted, such syncope may be considered benign vasovagal or postural hypotension. In contrast, if the child was in full stride at a field hockey game and collapsed, this could indicate a life-threatening cardiac event. When asking for a description of the event, obtain the child's self-report of symptoms prior to the onset of syncope as well as witnesses' description of the syncopal event.

Here are a few suggested questions to ask:

- Did the child or adolescent feel dizzy or experience lightheadedness, sweating, nausea, weakness, numbness in hands or feet, and visual changes?
- Did the witness observe rapid breathing or emotional stress that may be indicative of hyperventilation or induced syncope?

Positive answers to these questions are consistent with a benign cause. Seek information about whether abnormal movements such as tonic clonic movements or focal movement of one extremity were noted, including the length of the time frame surrounding the abnormal activity, approximate length of loss of consciousness, and loss of bowel or bladder control with the syncopal episode. Positive findings would be consistent with a seizure.

For the child with a history of collapsing and being unresponsive, ask whether cardiopulmonary resuscitation was administered and/or whether an automated external defibrillator was used. If this is the case, obtain a detailed history of the sequence of basic life support interventions.

If a healthcare provider witnesses a syncopal event in a child or adolescent, there are a few additional assessment points to remember. During and immediately after the syncopal event, check for brady- or tachy- arrhythmias, check blood pressure for hypotension, and look for signs and symptoms of dehydration; all could be clinical symptoms and indicators of decreased perfusion. Observe for hyperventilation and ask about numbness of extremities or fingers or toes. If hyperventilation and numbness are consistent with the event, consider a diagnosis of hyperventilation-induced syncope or a conversion disorder.

Red flags that indicate a cardiac evaluation is needed include the following family issues: a family history of early cardiac death (less than 45 years of age), sudden deaths including unexplained accidents involving a single motor vehicle or drowning, known arrhythmia (long QT syndrome), and familial cardiomyopathy. If positive, any of these factors increases the concern for a cardiac etiology (Gillette & Garson, 1992). A family history may be present in up to 90% of children with vasovagal syncope (Reuter & Brownstein, 2002). A review of the past medical history of congenital heart disease or arrhythmia may focus attention on a potential cardiac etiology. Previous syncopal events suggest a vasovagal, psychogenic cause, or a cardiac etiology.

Other elements of the history should include questioning about the following:

- Presence of underlying medical problems (such as diabetes or cardiac history).
- Menstrual history—did the event occur while menstruating, cramping, or a heavy period with clotting?
- Access to and use of medications or illicit drugs.
- Prolonged loss of consciousness or unconscious for more than several seconds with a postictal period. If this occurs, the child should be evaluated for a neurologic disorder, such as a seizure or migraine syndrome.

- Transient loss of consciousness for less than several seconds in a child with a normal ECG and cardiac examination. This most likely represents noncardiac syncope.
- Typical characteristics of vasovagal-induced syncope. Vasovagal syncope is a neurocardiogenic incident that is usually diagnosed on clinical features. The absence of a significant prodrome, associated palpitations or chest pain, or a family history of syncope or sudden death may require further cardiac evaluation.
- Orthostatic hypotension. This is the likely etiology for syncope in patients with postural changes in heart rate and blood pressure and a normal ECG. The underlying cause of these changes such as dehydration/volume depletion should be identified and treated. Although orthostatic hypotension has also been associated with long QT syndrome, the ECG is abnormal in the vast majority of cases (Atkins, Hanusa, Sefcik, & Kapoor, 1991).
- A toxic exposure may be suggested by history such as the use of inhalants/huffing or identified by a urine toxicologic screen for medications or illicit drugs including antidepressant drugs or carbon monoxide poisoning.
- Hyperventilation-induced syncope. This demonstrates an abnormal respiratory pattern prior to the syncopal episode and is commonly seen in adolescents experiencing some type of emotional stress. They may describe additional symptoms such as chest pain, lightheadedness, paresthesias/numbness in hands or feet, and visual disturbances.
- Breath-holding spells occur in younger children (6 to 24 months). In this case, syncope develops in association with breath holding. A cardiac evaluation is indicated for children with a family history of syncope or sudden death or with episodes that are prolonged, frequent, or precipitated by startle or other nontraumatic stimuli.
- Somatization disorder/hysteria or a conversion disorder. This commonly occurs in adolescents. Expected physiologic signs of syncope such as sweating, pallor, or changes in heart rate and blood pressure are absent. In addition, patients may disclose details of the event that indicate no loss of consciousness and generally suffer no injury during collapse.
- Choking games in which an adolescent purposely attempts self-strangulation or allows strangulation by another person with the hands or a ligature. The goal of the game is to reach a euphoric state created by the hypoxia, and then release the pressure just before loss of consciousness. Failure to do so can result in death.
- Vasovagal (neurocardiogenic) syncope is a diagnosis of exclusion for patients with consistent clinical features.

Using the above information, what other history questions do you need to ask Emma and her mother? ■

Other questions that are an important consideration as part of your symptom analysis include:

- Did she have any posturing or shaking of her body or seizure-like activity?
- Did she experience flashing lights, stars, blind spots, or doubled or blurred vision?
- Is there a history of headaches, numbness, or tingling?
- Did anyone notice the color of her skin? Was it pink, blue, or mottled?
- Has she experienced any recent trauma?
- Were there palpitations or chest pain associated with the syncope?
- Did she have shortness of breath?
- Has she had fever or weight loss or complaints of tiredness or fatigue?
- What, if any, medication (or medications) is she taking including over-the-counter drugs, herbal or nutritional supplements, and antidepressant drugs?

Emma's mother, Mrs. Kaplan, has now arrived at the ED and together they provide you with the following information: Mrs. Kaplan reports that Emma has been very healthy. She has never been hospitalized or in the ED before. Her immunizations are up to date, and she has no food or medication allergies and takes no medication or nutritional supplements. She has never passed out before nor does she have a history of recent trauma, headaches, or a heart problem. She has not had a fever, weight loss, or complaints of tiredness or fatigue.

Emma has always been a "B" student and is now attending a new school after Mrs. Kaplan's recent divorce. Mrs. Kaplan states Emma has adjusted well to the recent divorce and she has made many new friends in a short time in her new school. She feels Emma's school performance continues to improve. Emma's last menstrual period was 2 weeks ago and described as a normal 5-day flow. She states she uses pads (not tampons) for her periods.

In the absence of her mother and coach, Emma denies any illicit drug, inhalant/huffing, and medication use. Emma states that it was a tough field hockey game against the Ridgefield Ravens. This was her first game playing with her new teammates, and she felt she had to prove to the other girls she was a great team player. She focused on making great passes and assists to make each team point. She denies chest pain or shortness of breath, and it seemed she was running more than usual and was very hot and sweaty. Emma recalls the events prior to her passing out and states when the team completed the huddle at the end of the game, she stood up and suddenly felt lightheaded, nauseous, and then things got blurry. The next thing she remembers is waking up, with one of her classmates holding her legs up and the coach asking her to tell him what happened.

You talk to Emma's coach. He states that there was no trauma during the game, and that at the end of the game, after the huddle, Emma "stood up and passed out." Emma fell face down and was unresponsive for about 15–30 seconds or so. Emma had no jerking movements, no color changes, and no loss of bowel or bladder control. When she came to, she seemed surprised she was on the ground and has seemed normal ever since.

In considering whether this syncopal episode could have resulted from an underlying life-threatening cardiac issue, you must quickly collect information from Emma and her mother and document their answers about the following key issues:

- Did the syncope occur during activity/exertion?
- Is there a family history of early cardiac death?
- Does Emma have a history of congenital heart disease?
- Is her past medical history significant for cardiac disease or risk factors (e.g., elevated blood pressure, supraventricular tachycardia, anorexia nervosa)?

From your interviews with Emma, her mother, and her coach, you know that Emma's syncope took place after the game, and you have also been given assurance that there is no family history of early cardiac death nor does Emma have congenital heart disease or arrhythmias or a history of anorexia or blood pressure problems.

What would be your next plan of action? ■

Based on Emma's presenting symptoms, you ask the ED nurse to draw a standard blood panel including complete blood count, chemistry, toxicology, and pregnancy test. You look up at the cardiac monitor and note that she is in normal sinus rhythm. You are now ready to begin your physical examination of Emma.

Physical Examination

The healthcare provider should perform a complete physical exam that includes full vital signs including orthostatic pulse and blood pressure measurements and cardiac and neurologic examinations.

Abnormal blood pressures include a decrease in systolic blood pressure by 20 mm Hg or an increase in heart rate by 20 beats per minute from sitting to standing. More significant than changes in blood pressure is the recurrence of symptoms such as lightheadedness or syncope on standing. However, the presence of orthostatic hypotension does not rule out other causes of syncope, particularly long QT syndrome (Atkins et al., 1991). An age-appropriate neurologic exam should be performed to identify focal deficits or seizures.

Emma's vital signs reveal blood pressure (BP) 110/60, temperature 97.9°F, pulse 70, respirations 18, and pulse oximetry 98%. Orthostatic BPs are as follows: sitting 110/60 and standing 102/55. Heart rate: sitting 70 and standing 78. Her four-point BPs lying down are: right arm 110/60; left arm 118/64; right leg 100/55; left leg 100/56. General appearance is that of an alert, oriented, well-developed, and well-nourished 14-year-old who is holding her mother's hand. You perform a thorough cardiac and neurologic examination of Emma. The cardiovascular exam reveals a regular rate and rhythm, normal S1 and S2, and no cardiac gallop, rub, or murmur including with a Valsalva maneuver and squatting. There is no carotid bruit, jugular venous distention, or peripheral edema.

She has strong distal pulses with warm extremities and her capillary refill is less than 2 seconds. Her liver is at the right costal margin without hepatomegaly. The neurologic exam reveals full recall of all incidents before and after her syncopal event. She is alert and oriented to person, place, and time. Her cranial nerves II–XII are intact; she has symmetric bilateral deep tendon reflexes, with good muscle tone and strength, and has a normal gait and stance. The remaining findings of her physical exam are likewise unremarkable.

Children and adolescents, like Emma, with a normal ECG and cardiac examination are unlikely to have a cardiac etiology. However, a change in cardiac exam with evidence of new heart sounds, including gallops, rubs, and murmurs, may suggest the following structural lesions:

- Aortic stenosis is associated with a systolic ejection murmur and ejection click.
- Valvar stenosis may be associated with coarctation of the aorta. Four extremity blood pressures should be recorded. A difference in the systolic measurement of 20 mm Hg in the arm greater than in the legs is significant.
- Hypertrophic cardiomyopathy causes a murmur that is heard best during a Valsalva maneuver or squatting.
- New onset congestive heart failure may be diagnosed if findings such as rales, a gallop, and hepatomegaly, not noted before, are now evident on examination.

What laboratory tests did you need to order and what were the results? ■

Here are the initial laboratory studies and data that are important to help you determine the probability of potential differential diagnoses related to the cause of Emma's syncopal episode and to assist you in developing a management plan.
Blood studies with normal values indicated in parentheses:

- Na (sodium): 145 (136–146) mmol/L; K (potassium): 5 (3.5–5.0) mmol/L; Cl (chloride): 110 (95–108) mmol/L; BUN (blood urea nitrogen): 5 (7–18) mg/dL; HCO_3 (bicarbonate): 28 (22–30) mmol/L; CR (creatinine): 0.79 (0.8–1.2) mg/dL; glucose: 69 (70–99) mg/dL
- WBC (white blood cell count): 13.3 (4.0–14.0) × 1,000 cells/mm³; hemoglobin: 15 (12.0–16.0) g/dL; hematocrit: 42 (36.0–46.0) %; PLT: 223 (150–400) × 10³/mm³
- Opiate screen: Negative
- ETOH (alcohol): Nondetected
- Serum pregnancy: Negative
- UA (urinalysis): Negative

The results of these laboratory studies and your complete physical exam allow you to rule out dehydration, hypoglycemia, anemia, pregnancy, and drug and alcohol use as the etiology of Emma's syncopal episode.

At this point, what are the differential diagnoses you should consider in this case? ■

Upon review of your differential diagnosis you note the following:

Neurologic: Both seizure and cerebral concussion diagnoses are unlikely due to lack of history or physician findings that indicate trauma, headaches, or seizure activity.

Cardiac: A cardiac problem is an unlikely diagnosis with a normal ECG. You know that syncope that occurs during physical exertion is very concerning for a cardiac etiology, whereas syncope after exertion may occur with vasovagal syncope or cardiac conditions (Driscoll et al., 1997).

- *Cardiac arrhythmias including long QT syndrome:* Unlikely diagnosis due to a physical examination with normal cardiac sounds and normal ECG without prolonged QT or other cardiac arrhythmias or structural abnormalities and no family history of sudden death.
- *Neurocardiogenic/vasovagal:* This is your most likely diagnosis due to a history of syncope after physical exertion associated with change of posture, dizziness, blurred vision, and short recovery. Finally, there is no evidence by history of seizure activity or a prolonged postictal period associated with loss of bowel or bladder control.

Pregnancy: This is not supported by history, physician exam, and/or laboratory testing.

Psychogenic: There is no presyncopal report of hyperventilation or breath holding. There is a remote possibility that an added benign cause of syncope could be due to recent school change, family stressors, and divorce; however, this is not supported by report and family history from Emma, Mrs. Kaplan, or her coach.

- *Hyperventilation or breath holding:* Not supported by history.
- *Hysteria (somatization disorder) or a conversion disorder:* Not supported by Emma's report, coach's report, and mother's history.

Medications or illicit drugs including antidepressant drugs or toxins: *carbon monoxide poisoning, inhalant/huffing:* Not supported by history and laboratory testing.

Dehydration/volume depletion: Not supported by physical exam, weight loss, vital signs, and laboratory findings.

What other tests do you need to make your diagnosis and then decide on a plan of care? ■

Laboratory Blood Work

In the asymptomatic patient, laboratory blood work is rarely helpful; however, specific laboratory tests may be useful.

- Bedside blood glucose for children who present immediately after the episode
- Hematocrit for children who are at risk for anemia
- Urine pregnancy test in postmenarchal females
- Urine toxicology screen in patients with altered metal status

Electrocardiogram, Echocardiogram, and Imaging Studies

Cost Effectiveness of Testing

In a study of 480 pediatric patients, an abnormal history, physical examination, or electrocardiogram identified 21 of the 22 patients with a cardiac cause of syncope. Electrocardiography provides a screening protocol that allows the identification of a cardiac cause of syncope in the overwhelming majority of pediatric patients. In the absence of ECG changes, the echocardiogram does not contribute to the evaluation of syncope in children (Ritter et al., 2000).

In a retrospective review of 169 pediatric patients with new onset syncope, the results revealed the cost based on testing for fiscal year 1999. A total of 663 tests were performed at a cost of $180,128. Only 26 tests (3.9%) were diagnostic in 24 patients (14.2%). The average cost per patient was $1,055, and the cost per diagnostic result was $6,928. Echocardiograms, chest radiographs, cardiac catheterizations, electrophysiology studies, and serum evaluations were not diagnostic. Thus, the evaluation of pediatric syncope remains expensive and the above testing has a low diagnostic yield. An approach that focuses on the use of testing to verify findings from the history and physical examination or exclude life-threatening causes is justified (Steinberg & Knilans, 2005).

> Given your list of possible diagnoses and the information regarding the value of various tests, you decide that you need to order a 12-lead ECG, which reveals a normal sinus rhythm. In Emma's case, the results for all of the listed studies conducted on her were normal.

Making the Diagnosis

What is the most likely diagnosis regarding Emma's syncopal episode? ∎

You have arrived at your diagnosis of neurocardiogenic syncope/vasovagal-related syncope using an algorithmic approach to the emergent evaluation of syncope in children and adolescents, as outlined in Figure 23-1. This algorithm provides a systematic method to assess the etiology of a syncope episode in a child or adolescent and serves as a practice guide that the healthcare provider can quickly use in either the ED or primary care setting.

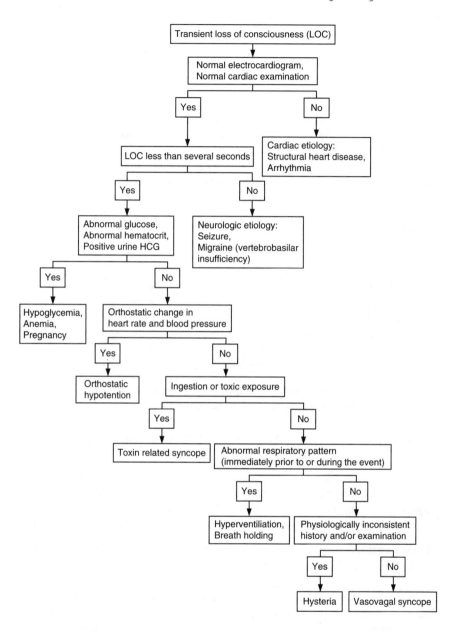

Figure 23-1   Emergent evaluation of syncope in children and adolescents.

Source: © 2008 UpToDate.

Management

Does Emma need further specialty referrals or admission to the hospital? ■

Indications for Referral or Admission

The majority of children, like Emma, who have had syncope with a negative evaluation can be followed as outpatients. Concerning features such as absence of a significant prodrome, palpitations or chest pain, a family history of syncope or sudden death, and recurrent episodes should be referred for further cardiac evaluation. Follow-up consultation with a neurologist should be considered for children with prolonged loss of consciousness and/or a history of focal neurologic findings.

Admission to the hospital for further evaluation and observation should be considered under the following circumstances:

- Evidence of cardiovascular disease
- An abnormal ECG
- Chest pain
- Cyanosis
- Apnea or bradycardic spells that resolve only with vigorous stimulation
- Abnormal neurologic findings
- Orthostatic hypotension that does not resolve with fluid therapy

Emma's clinical presentation and subsequent findings meet none of the criteria for admission to the hospital for additional observation or testing.

Best Practice Evidence for Managing Emma's Syncopal Event

Now that you have thoroughly evaluated Emma's syncopal event using data obtained from her history, physical examination, and first line diagnostic studies using a systematic approach to data collection, and having come to your diagnosis of neurocardiogenic syncope (vasovagal), you are ready to discuss this event and its likely etiology with Emma and her mother.

Emma's mother is very upset after all the questions and many tests, which seem to her to indicate that Emma might have a "heart condition." What will you tell her? ■

It is important that Mrs. Kaplan, Emma, and her coach understand that Emma does not have a heart problem. There are no family risk factors such as a family history of early cardiac death (less than 45 years of age), sudden deaths including unexplained accidents involving a single motor vehicle or drowning, known arrhythmia (long QT syndrome), and familial cardiomyopathy. In addition, syncope that occurs during physical exertion is very concerning for a cardiac etiology, whereas syncope after exertion may occur with vasovagal syncope or cardiac conditions (Driscoll et al., 1997). Emma passed out *after* physical activity, which is more consistent with a noncardiac etiology. A normal ECG is one of the most important tests to evaluate syncope. Emma's ECG is normal, indicating the unlikelihood that Emma has a heart condition.

It is documented that up to 15% of children experience a syncopal episode prior to the end of adolescence (Lewis & Dhala, 1999), and that fainting is a transient loss of consciousness, which typically occurs after activity. Similarly, Emma's symptoms match patients who have had vasovagal syncope. Prior to the event and her loss of consciousness, Emma changed position, going from the huddle to standing. She reported feeling dizziness, lightheadedness, sweating, nausea, and weakness, and had blurred vision. Her loss of consciousness was short with no postictal state/prolonged unconsciousness, and she did not have seizure activity or loss of bladder or bowel control. These are Emma's exact symptoms and are due to vasovagal syncope.

Emma wants to know if she can return to sports tomorrow. What will you tell her? ■

Emma may return to sports tomorrow. She should take the following precautions:

- Increase fluids intake and avoid dehydration.
- Increase salt in diet.
- Assume sitting/supine position at onset of symptoms.
- Avoid noxious stimuli (i.e., avoid hot environment or prolonged standing/kneeling).
- Address anxiety/stress/emotional concerns.

Other potentially helpful management interventions that might be considered in select cases include:

- Use of physical exercise/training to increase muscular tone. Exercise prompts fitness, which counteracts neurocardiogenic syncope but can make symptoms worse initially. Therefore, it should be done cautiously at first.
- Use of waist-high support hose to prevent pooling (knee-high hose may not work well).

The coach was also worried about Emma and asked that you send him a note or call him regarding her condition.

What will you tell the coach? ■

With the family's approval, the healthcare provider can tell the coach and also write him a note stating Emma's ECG findings are normal and that she does not have a cardiac etiology to this fainting spell. By Emma taking the precautions listed previously, she will decrease the possibility of a similar event. However, if Emma and the coach do not follow the precautions, it is remotely possible that she may have another syncopal event.

Suggest that the coach and athletic trainers consider administering the 2004 American Academy of Pediatrics Pre-sports Participation Form as a part of their screening procedure for students applying for school sports.

Key Points from This Case

1. Syncope is a sudden, brief loss of consciousness associated with loss of postural tone from which recovery is spontaneous.
2. Syncope in children is most often benign. However, syncope can also occur as the result of more serious cardiac disease with the potential for sudden death.
3. A complete history and physical examination and ECG findings typically identify children with a life-threatening cause of syncope.
4. A patient with a normal ECG has a low likelihood of arrhythmia as a cause of syncope (Kapoor, 2000).
5. The use of additional testing, beyond history, physical examination, and ECG, can be avoided in many patients with transient loss of consciousness (van Dijk et al., 2008).
6. Syncope that occurs during physical exertion is very concerning for a cardiac etiology, whereas syncope after exertion may occur with vasovagal syncope or cardiac conditions (Driscoll et al., 1997).
7. In some studies, echocardiograms, chest radiographs, cardiac catheterizations, electrophysiology studies, tilt table test, and serum evaluations were found to be neither cost-effective nor diagnostic.
8. The responsibility of the primary care provider is to quickly identify the child or adolescent who needs a referral to the appropriate specialist. For example, when a cardiac etiology is identified, such as a structural heart disease or arrhythmias, a cardiology consult should be made for further evaluation and management. Similarly, when a neurologic etiology is identified, such as a seizure or head trauma, a neurologic consult should be made for further evaluation and management.
9. An algorithmic approach to syncope is recommended.

REFERENCES

Atkins, D., Hanusa, B., Sefcik, T., & Kapoor, W. (1991). Syncope and orthostatic hypotension. *American Journal of Medicine, 91*, 179–185.

Driscoll, D. J., Jacobsen, S. J., Porter, C. J., & Wollan, P. C. (1997). Syncope in children and adolescents. *Journal of the American College of Cardiology, 29*, 1039–1045.

Gillette, P. C., & Garson, A. Jr. (1992). Sudden cardiac death in the pediatric population. *Circulation, 85*, (1 Suppl): 164–169. Review.

Kapoor, W. N. (2000). Syncope. *New England Journal of Medicine, 343*, 1856–1862.

Kapoor, W. N., Peterson, J. R., Wieand, H. S., & Karpf, M. (1987). Diagnostic and prognostic implications of recurrences in patients with syncope. *American Journal of Medicine, 83*, 700–708.

Lewis, D. A., & Dhala, A. (1999). Syncope in the pediatric patient. The cardiologist's perspective. *Pediatric Clinics of North America, 46*, 205–219.

Maron, B. J., Shirani, J., Poliac, L. C., Mathenge, R., Roberts, W. C., & Meuller, F. O. (1996). Sudden death in young competitive athletes. Clinical, demographic, and pathological profiles. *Journal of the American Medical Association, 276*, 199–204.

Massin, M. M., Bourguignont, A., Coremans, C., Comte, L. Lepage, P., & Gerard, P. (2004). Syncope in pediatric patients presenting to an emergency department. *Journal of Pediatrics, 145*, 223–228.

Mathias, C. J., Deguchi, K., & Schatz, I. (2001). Observations on recurrent syncope and presyncope in 641 patients. *Lancet, 357*, 348–353.

Moss, A. J. (2003). Long QT syndrome. *Journal of the American Medical Association, 289*, 2041–2044.

Reuter, D., & Brownstein, D. (2002). Common emergent pediatric neurologic problems. *Emergency Medicine Clinics of North America, 20*, 155–176.

Ritter, S., Tani, L. Y., Etheridge, S. P., Williams, R. V., Craig, J. E., Minich, L. L. (2000). What is the yield of screening echocardiography in pediatric syncope? *Pediatrics, 105*, E58.

Steinberg, L. A., & Knilans, T. K. (2005). Syncope in children: diagnostic tests have a high cost and low yield. *Journal of Pediatrics, 146*(3), 335–338.

van Dijk N., Boer, K. R., Colman, N., Bakker, A., Stam, J., van Grieken, J. J., et al. (2008). High diagnostic yield and accuracy of history, physical examination, and ECG in patients with transient loss of consciousness in FAST: the Fainting Assessment Study. *Journal of Cardiovascular Electrophysiology, 19*, 48–55.

Chapter 24

The Child Presenting with Cough

Jennifer Newcombe

Respiratory problems are the leading cause of illness in children. Viral infections are the primary causative agents and seasonal variations are noted. Children with respiratory infections are commonly seen in the primary care setting and are brought in by parents who are concerned about relieving their child's associated respiratory symptoms. Children typically do well with outpatient treatment. However, it is important to recognize circumstances that warrant hospitalization.

Educational Objectives

1. Explain the findings of pneumonia typically found upon physical examination.
2. List differential diagnoses for pneumonia.
3. Outline the antibiotics used to treat *Mycoplasma pneumoniae* in an outpatient setting.
4. Describe circumstances that warrant hospitalization for an infant or child with pneumonia.

Case Presentation and Discussion

Mary Dixon, a previously healthy 5-year-old white female, is brought to your clinic by her father because of difficulty breathing for 1 day. Two days prior she developed a runny nose, cough, and low grade fever; her maximum temperature was 101°F (38.3°C) yesterday. Her temperature this morning was 103°F (39.4°C) and she was breathing fast, working hard to breathe. Her mother was concerned and had Mary's father bring her in to be seen because she had to go to work. Mary's appetite is fair. She takes liquids well, but her solid intake has decreased. Mary's father denies that his daughter has had any nausea, vomiting, or diarrhea. Her activity level is good. She has had no recent contact with others with respiratory or other illnesses and does not attend daycare or preschool. Her past medical history is negative for allergies or asthma. She is not taking medications other than Tylenol (acetaminophen). Her last dose of Tylenol was yesterday evening before bedtime. Her immunizations are up to date by record review, and she has no known drug allergies, hospitalizations, or surgeries.

What other questions will you ask her father related to her illness? ■

The main symptoms of pneumonia are fever and cough; although children with these two symptoms don't necessarily have pneumonia, clinicians should always consider the possibility of pneumonia if these symptoms are present (Durbin & Stille, 2008). A typical history should focus on the duration of illness, respiratory symptoms (i.e., quality of cough, wheezing, difficulty with breathing), and extra respiratory symptoms such as fever, headache, sore throat, lethargy, or rash (Durbin & Stille).

> Her father states her cough is wet sounding, productive, and is persistent throughout the day. He describes the sputum as yellowish in color. Her father said Mary complained of a mild headache earlier this morning but said she didn't have a sore throat or lethargy.

Pathophysiology of Pneumonia

Pneumonia is a lower respiratory tract infection that is associated with consolidation of the alveolar space and lung parenchyma involvement. It usually follows an upper respiratory tract infection that permits invasion of the lower respiratory tract by bacteria, viruses, or other pathogens. This invasion triggers the immune response to produce inflammation (Jenson & Baltimore, 2006). Agents that cause lower respiratory tract infections are usually transmitted by droplets spread directly from close personal contact or indirectly by contaminated fomites (Durbin & Stille, 2008). *S. pneumoniae* is responsible for 90% of childhood bacterial pneumonias and is common in all age groups. Mycoplasma pneumonia is common after 5 years of age (Brady, 2009). The incubation period after exposure for mycoplasma pneumonia averages 3 weeks (Pickering, Baker, Long, & McMillan, 2006). If the normal host defense mechanisms does not function properly and effectively, pneumonia can occur. The normal respiratory defense functions include: nasopharyngeal air filtration; laryngeal protection of the airway to prevent aspiration of oral and gastric fluid; mucociliary clearing of particles and pathogens from the upper and lower airways; a strong defensive cough reflex; anatomically correct and unobstructed airway drainage; normal immune function at both the humoral and cellular levels; and normal innate biochemical and redox-based host defense mechanism (Gaston, 2002). However, defects in the host defenses increase the risk of pneumonia.

The infectious agents that commonly cause pneumonia vary by age of the child and setting in which the infection is acquired (community or nosocomial), along with the presence of any underlying disease. (See Table 24-1.) The most common infecting agents by age are respiratory syncytial virus (RSV) in infants; RSV, parainfluenza viruses, influenza viruses, adenoviruses in children younger than 5 years old; and *M. pneumonia* and *S. pneumoniae* in children older than five (Jensen & Baltimore, 2006).

Complications that may result from acute bacterial pneumonia include pleuritis (inflammation of the pleura), pleural effusion, pyothorax (pus in the pleural cavity), empyema (organized pyothorax with fibrous walls), and bacteremia (Jenson & Baltimore, 2006).

Epidemiology of Pneumonia

According to the World Health Organization, there are 150.7 million cases of pneumonia every year in children younger than 5 years (Rudan et al., 2004). In the United States, the annual incidence of pneumonia in children younger than 5 years is estimated to be 34 to 40 cases per 1,000, while the incidence decreases to 7 cases per 1,000 in adolescents 12 to 15 years of age. The mortality rate in developed countries remains low, at less than 1 per 1,000 per year; however, in third world countries, respiratory tract infections are more prevalent and severe. Pneumonia in these countries accounts for more than 4 million deaths annually (Durbin & Stille, 2008).

Viral and bacterial pneumonia occur throughout the year; however, they are more prevalent in fall and winter. Many speculate that during cooler months there is enhanced person-to-person droplet spread of respiratory pathogens due to crowding, along with diminished host resistance due to impaired mucociliary clearance from dry indoor air (Durbin & Stille, 2008).

Children who have underlying cardiopulmonary disorders and other medical conditions are at higher risk for pneumonia and its complications.

Table 24-1 Childhood Community-Acquired Pneumonia: Common Pathogens	
Age	**Pathogen**
3 weeks to 3 months	*Chlamydia trachomatis*
	Respiratory syncytial virus
	Parainfluenza
	Streptococcus pneumoniae
	Bordetella pertussis
3 months to 4 years	Respiratory syncytial virus
	Parainfluenza
	Human metapneumovirus
	Influenza
	Rhinovirus
	S. pneumoniae
	Mycoplasma pneumoniae
5 years through adolescence	*Mycoplasma pneumoniae*
	Chlamydophila pneumoniae
	S. pneumoniae
	Mycobacterium tuberculosis

These conditions include congenital heart disease, bronchopulmonary dysplasia, asthma, sickle cell disease, gastroesophageal reflux, and acquired immunodeficiency disorders. Also, children exposed to cigarette smoke are at higher risk for acquiring pneumonia as a result of impaired mucociliary clearance and increased risk of aspiration. In addition, the use of alcohol has been associated with increased colonization of the oropharynx with aerobic gram-negative bacilli (Durbin & Stille, 2008).

Clinical Manifestations

Typical clinical findings of pneumonia depend somewhat on the infecting agents. Bacterial and viral pneumonias occur at all ages and can have an acute or gradual onset with mild URI symptoms a few days beforehand. In contrast, mycoplasmal pneumonia typically occurs after 5 years of age and tends to have a slow onset. A temperature of $\geq$ 102°F ($\geq$ 39°C), chills, cough and dyspnea are suggestive of bacterial pneumonia. Viral pneumonias commonly have a slower onset and a less prominent fever compared to what occurs with bacterial pneumonia. Cough, wheezing, and stridor may also be found in viral pneumonia. A dry persistent cough, a prodrome of chills, headache, sore throat, gastrointestinal complaints, and malaise are characteristic of mycoplasmal pneumonia (Brady, 2009).

What diagnoses would you consider with this history and physical examination? ■

Differential Diagnosis

You consider the following diagnoses:

- Bronchiolitis
- Foreign body aspiration
- Cystic fibrosis
- Asthma
- Tuberculosis

These are the typical conditions to consider. Other possibilities, although remote in this case, include congestive heart failure, acute bronchiectasis, and pulmonary abscess.

Given those diagnostic possibilities, what other information would help you make the diagnosis? ■

From the above review, some other information you should obtain includes the following:

- History of previous episodes of respiratory illness (immuncompromised)
- History of travel
- History of contacts with confirmed or suspected infectious tuberculosis

- History of choking (foreign body aspiration)
- History of foul smelling stools (cystic fibrosis)
- Results of prior purified protein derivative (PPD) skin testing (tuberculosis)
- History of animal exposure/insect bites

Mr. Dixon reports that Mary has no previous history of pneumonia or significant respiratory illness—just the usual colds. The family has no history of recent travel nor a history of contacts with confirmed or suspected TB infections. Her PPD skin test was negative at 12 months of age. Mary has not experienced any episodes of choking, and her stools are not foul smelling. The family does not have pets, and she has not had contact with animals and has had no recent insect bites.

Physical Examination

Vital signs: Temperature 103°F, pulse 130, respiratory rate 32, O_2 saturation 96% on room air. Her weight is 23 kg (75th percentile) and length is 115 cm (95th percentile). Body mass index is at the 85th percentile for age.

General: She is awake and alert, in mild respiratory distress. Head/eyes/ears/throat: Her conjunctiva and tympanic membranes (TMs) are normal. Her nasal mucosa is erythematous with yellowish discharge. There is mild maxillary sinus tenderness. Her lips and mucous membranes are moist. Tonsils are 1+, pharynx with mild erythema, no exudates noted. Tachycardia is present with regular rhythm and no murmurs noted.

Mild intercostal retractions are noted with decreased air entry over left lower lobe with fine crackles. No expiratory wheezes are auscultated. There is increased vocal fremitus over the left base with dullness to percussion. Exam of the abdomen reveals bowel sounds present; it is soft and nontender to palpation.

Her skin and neurologic examinations are unremarkable.

The physical exam should focus on the respiratory system. The clinician should assess for tachypnea, retractions (intercostal, subcostal, suprasternal), wheezing, nasal flaring, or grunting. Tachypnea is a significant, although at times subtle, clinical finding associated with lower airway illness. Durbin and Stille (2008) use the following criteria as key indicators of the presence of pneumonia in a pediatric patient: > 50 breaths/min at 2 to 12 months of age, > 40 breaths/min at 1 to 5 years, > 20 breaths/min for those older than 5 years, subtracting 10 if the child is febrile. They emphasize that tachypnea is the most sensitive and specific sign of pneumonia, found twice as frequently in children who have evidence of pneumonia on chest radiography as in those who have no such findings (Durbin & Stille, 2008).

"The most common signs of pneumonia detected by office-based clinicians are dullness to percussion, crackles, decreased breath sounds and bronchial breath sounds (louder than normal tubular breath sounds often accompanied by egophony)" (Durbin & Stille, 2008, p. 150). New onset wheezing is not typically associated with bacterial pneumonias (Durbin & Stille).

Making the Diagnosis

This history and physical examination are consistent with a diagnosis of pneumonia. There are three child and adolescent pneumonia syndromes: bacterial, atypical, and viral. (See Table 24-2.) Viruses are the most common etiology of pneumonia in older infants and children younger than 5 years of age. However, bacterial pathogens including *M. pneumoniae* and *C. pneumoniae* are most prevalent in school-age children (Gaston, 2002). Determination of the precise etiology of pneumonia is difficult due to a lack of sensitive and specific tests. Many clinicians treat pneumonia empirically with minimal laboratory or radiographic evaluation.

Do you need to do anything to confirm the diagnosis, such as a chest X-ray or laboratory studies? ■

In most instances, blood tests such as a complete blood count with differential (CBC), chemistries, or serology will not help to identify the cause of pneumonia or aid in the treatment. However, in a highly febrile child or infant

Table 24-2 Common Clinical Pneumonia Syndromes			
Syndrome	Typical Cause	Age Group	Clinical Features
Bacterial	*S. Pneumoniae*; others including *Staphylococcus aureus*	All ages; younger children (< 6) more common	Abrupt onset, high fever, ill appearance, chest and abdominal pain, focal infiltrate if chest X-ray is obtained, white blood count often elevated > 15 ($\times$ 1000 cells/mm^3)
Atypical: infancy	*Chlamydia trachomatis*	< 3 months	Tachypnea, mild hypoxemia, lack of fever, wheezing, interstitial infiltrates on chest X-ray
Atypical: older children	Mycoplasma	> 5 years	Gradual onset, low-grade fever, diffuse infiltrates if chest X-ray obtained
Viral	Multiple viruses (e.g., respiratory syncytial virus, influenza, parainfluenza, adenoviruses, human metapneumovins, and, rhinovirus)	All ages; 3 months to 5 years more common	Prominent upper respiratory infection symptoms, low grade or absent fever, wheezes on examination, possible diffuse interstitial infiltrates if chest X-ray is obtained, normal or slightly elevated white blood count

less than 3 months, a blood culture and CBC may be warranted (Brady, 2009). The white blood cell count is usually normal or mildly elevated with neutrophil predominance (Brady). When a more precise diagnosis is necessary, more invasive techniques are required. Bacteria found in blood, pleural fluid (thoracentesis), or lung tissue are considered diagnostic in a patient presumed to have pneumonia (Nohynek, Valkeila, Leinonen, & Eskola, 1995). Chest radiograph can be used to verify the clinical suspicion of pneumonia and characterize the disease process, but is not necessary for every patient.

This child's history and symptoms are typical of mycoplasmal pneumonia. Therefore, you decide that a chest radiograph is not needed at this time.

Management

Treatment must first be directed at whether the child needs to be admitted to the hospital or remain at home. The decision to hospitalize a child with pneumonia must be individualized and based upon age and several clinical factors. Typically, children who are less than 3 months old are hospitalized because they can deteriorate rapidly and are prone to hypoxemia and bacteremia (Durbin & Stille, 2008). A child of any age whose family cannot provide appropriate care and assure compliance with the therapeutic plan needs to be hospitalized. Other indications for hospitalization include:

- *Hypoxemia:* Oxygen saturation consistently less than 92% on room air
- *Dehydration* or inability to maintain oral hydration
- *Moderate to severe respiratory distress:* Respiratory rate > 70 breaths/min in infants less than 12 months or > 50 breaths/min in older children, difficulty breathing, apnea, or grunting
- *Toxic appearance*
- *Failure of outpatient therapy:* Worsening or no response in 24 to 72 hours

Children who have none of these features can be treated as outpatients.

How do you plan to treat this patient's pneumonia? ▇

Based on the patient's age, history, and physical exam, the most likely organism for her pneumonia is *Mycoplasma*. A macrolide is the drug of choice. Azithromycin is recommended most often because of its ease of administration, with once daily dosing for 5 days (Durbin & Stille, 2008). Usual dosage for azithromycin is 10 mg/kg QD day 1, then 5 mg/kg QD days 2–5. A more cost-effective alternative is erythromycin 50 mg/kg per day divided Q 6 hours for 10 days; maximum dose 2 g/day. For children who are older than 8 years, doxycycline is an alternative. The dose for doxycycline is 4 mg/kg per day in two divided doses for 10 days; maximum 200 mg/day.

You write a prescription for azithromycin 230 mg PO day 1, then 115 mg PO days 2–5 for pneumonia and instruct the father to follow up with you in 24 hours either by phone or office visit if either parent has concerns.

Most children have an uneventful recovery, but it is important to inform parents that their child's cough can last for several weeks (Brady, 2009).

Educational plan: What will you do to educate the father about pneumonia and its management? ■

You discuss the following with Mr. Dixon:

- Explain the diagnosis and pathophysiology of pneumonia.
- Inform the father of the name, dose, frequency, and duration of the antibiotic. Review the dosage of acetaminophen and frequency of its administration.
- Discuss that over-the-counter decongestants should not be given to the child because of dangerous side effects
- Emphasize the need to finish all antibiotics, even if the child is feeling better and fever subsides. Alert Mr. Dixon to the fact that with azithromycin exposure to sunlight (photosensitivity) may cause severe sunburn and skin rashes. Protection from the sun is advisable (e.g., use of sunscreen and wearing of protective clothing).
- Advise the father that uncomplicated bacterial pneumonia should improve within 48 hours.
- Teach the father how to monitor for signs of increased respiratory distress.
- Educate the father that cough can last several weeks.
- Discuss the need to keep Mary hydrated, and emphasize that he should not be worried about her appetite, which should return in 2 to 3 days when she is feeling better.

When do you want to see this patient back again? ■

Tell Mrs. Smith to call and ask for a same-day appointment if Mary is not better in 48 hours or to return sooner (or at any time) if her symptoms worsen. It is important to provide an immediate recheck if there is no improvement within 48 hours because this generally indicates the need to rethink the diagnosis and management plan. If her condition has worsened at follow-up, she should be evaluated for potential complications and the need for a chest X-ray, complete blood count, and/or hospitalization. If improved, schedule a recheck at the completion of antibiotic therapy.

Is this child infectious to others and what is the typical progression of recovery? ■

Transmission of *Mycoplasma pneumoniae* is by person-to-person contact with respiratory secretion. Its incubation period is 1 to 4 weeks. Typically, within 24 to 48 hours of antibiotic coverage the child will no longer be considered contagious (Centers for Disease Control and Prevention, 2005).

Overall outcomes in children with pneumonia are excellent. A change in respiratory sounds is typically noted by the second or third day with consolidation of the infection. Resolution occurs around the seventh day (Brady, 2009). The majority of children recover without complications. Radiographs may be abnormal for 6 weeks; therefore, serial X-rays are not recommended in uncomplicated pneumonia (Durbin & Stille, 2008). Follow-up radiographs 2 to 3 weeks after completion of therapy may be helpful in assessing alternate diagnoses or coincident conditions in children with recurrent pneumonia, persistent symptoms, severe atelectasis, or unusually located infiltrates.

Key Points from this Case

1. A macrolide is the drug of choice for the treatment of *Mycoplasma pneumoniae*.
2. The decision to hospitalize a child with pneumonia must be individualized and is based on age, underlying conditions, and severity of illness.
3. Children who are treated for pneumonia as outpatients should have follow-up within 24 hours. Those whose complications have worsened at follow-up should be evaluated for potential complications and hospitalization.

REFERENCES

Brady, M. A. (2009). Respiratory disorders. In: C. E. Burns, A. M. Dunn, M. A. Brady, N. B. Starr, & C. G. Blosser (Eds.), *Pediatric primary care* (4th ed., pp. 767–794). St. Louis, MO: Saunders Elsevier.

Centers for Disease Control and Prevention. (2005). *Mycoplasma pneumoniae.* Retrieved May 11, 2009, from http://www.cdc.gov/ncidod/dbmd/diseaseinfo/mycoplasmapneum_t.htm

Durbin, J. W., & Stille, C. (2008). Pneumonia. *Pediatrics in Review, 2,* 147–160.

Gaston, B. (2002). Pneumonia. *Pediatrics in Review, 23,* 132–140.

Jenson, H. B. & Baltimore, H. J. (2006). Pneumonia. In: R. M. Kliegan, K. J. Marcdante, H. B. Jenson, R. E. Behrman (Eds.), *Nelson essentials of pediatrics* (5th ed., pp. 503–509). Philadelphia: Elsevier Saunders.

Nohynek, H., Valkeila, E., Leinonen, M., & Eskola, J. (1995). Erythrocyte sedimentation rate, white blood cell count and serum C-reactive protein in assessing etiologic diagnosis of acute lower respiratory infections in children. *Pediatric Infectious Disease Journal, 14*(6), 484–490.

Pickering, L. K., Baker, C. J., Long, S. S., & McMillan, J. A. (Eds.). (2006). *Red book: 2006 report of the Committee on Infectious Diseases* (27th ed.). Elk Grove Village, IL: American Academy of Pediatrics.

Rudan, I., Tomaskovic, L., Boschi-Pinto, C., & Campbell, H. (2004). Global estimate of the incidence of clinical pneumonia among children under five years of age. *Bulletin of the World Health Organization, 82,* 895–903.

Chapter 25

The Child with Vomiting and Diarrhea

Ardys M. Dunn
Victoria Winter

Vomiting and diarrhea are common phenomena in children. They often occur simultaneously, especially in the young child, and are most often associated with gastroenteritis. This case study focuses on the question of when the child with diarrhea can be managed with a telephone consultation and when he or she needs to be seen by the healthcare provider. In answering this question, we will examine the presentation of gastroenteritis in children, its epidemiology, etiology, differential diagnosis, diagnostic criteria, and treatment.

A case of gastroenteritis can be short-lived and managed with minimal intervention, or it can be the initial manifestation of a wide spectrum of acute and chronic disorders requiring more intensive therapy. The history and physical examination are essential for accurate assessment and diagnosis, and in conjunction with occasional laboratory tests, should guide care. Patient and family education on preventive measures can be effective in limiting the number of episodes of gastroenteritis in the home and the community.

Educational Objectives
1. Identify the major etiologies of gastroenteritis in the United States.
2. Explain the pathophysiology of the different types of diarrhea.
3. State the factors that place the child at increased risk for hospitalization or death due to diarrhea.
4. Determine when a healthcare provider can use telephone assessment versus in-person office assessment of the child.
5. Describe treatment plans for acute, self-limited gastroenteritis and for severe gastroenteritis with dehydration.

Case Presentation and Discussion

Sara's mother is on the phone, calling about her 4-year-old daughter, who is sick with vomiting and diarrhea. "I feel ridiculous calling again, but Sara is sick. She started out with vomiting and then diarrhea, and now she is running a fever. I've tried everything I can think of to keep her well but this is the third time this year she has been sick. I think I need to bring her into the office. Do you think there is something seriously wrong with her that is causing all of this?"

Your office assistant informs you about this phone call. She asks what you want her to tell Sara's mother. Do you want her to bring Sara into the office? Or is this something that can be handled on the phone?

Before you answer, the following provides some important information about gastroenteritis.

Epidemiology of Gastroenteritis

Diarrhea results in over 1 billion episodes of illness and 3–5 million deaths annually worldwide, placing it with upper respiratory tract infections as the most common infectious disease syndromes of humans. In the United States, gastroenteritis is a leading cause of morbidity and the second most common disease seen in children (Jenson & Baltimore, 2006; Lopez, Mathers, Ezzati, Jamison, & Murray, 2006; Pickering & Snyder, 2004). Most cases in this country are self-limited and require only minimal intervention aimed at dietary and fluid management. However, occasional episodes of severe, life-threatening gastroenteritis may occur, necessitating aggressive therapeutic intervention.

By definition, acute gastroenteritis is an illness of rapid onset that includes diarrhea with possible nausea, vomiting, lethargy, fever, abdominal pain, or dehydration (common in young children). Liquidity and frequency of stool are characteristic features (Jenson & Baltimore, 2006; Pickering & Snyder, 2004). Caring for a child with gastroenteritis can present a challenge to parents who must make judgments about how to keep their child hydrated during this illness, when to call or have their child seen by the pediatric primary care provider, and how to prevent this illness from occurring again or spreading to other members of the family or close contacts of the child.

Etiology of Gastroenteritis

The most common causative agents of gastroenteritis in the United States include (Pickering, Baker, Long, & McMillan, 2006):

- *Viral agents:* Rotavirus, adenovirus, Norwalk, and calicivirus
- *Bacterial agents:* Shigella, Salmonella, and *Campylobacter jejuni*
- *Parasitic agents: Giardia lamblia, Entamoeba histolytica,* and Cryptosporidium
- *Agents that produce enterotoxins: S. aureus, E. coli* (0157:H7), and *C. difficile*

Acute viral infectious gastroenteritis accounts for 70–80% of the cases of diarrhea in developed countries and results in more than 1.5 million outpatient visits and 200,000 hospitalizations in the United States each year (King, Glass, Bresee, Duggan, & Centers for Disease Control and Prevention, 2003).

Diarrhea in children can also be due to a systemic, nongastrointestinal infection; antibiotics; feeding patterns; and enzyme deficiency.

Important studies on the etiology of gastroenteritis reveal the following pattern:

- A common disorder seen in the pediatric population in the emergency department (ED) is viral gastroenteritis. Rotavirus and norovirus play key roles in such viral illnesses. It is estimated that four out of five children in the United States will develop a symptomatic rotavirus gastroenteritis by age 5 years. One in seven will be seen in an ambulatory health setting, with an additional 205,000 to 272,000 ED visits due to this virus (Payne, Stockman, Gentsch, & Parashar, 2008). It is estimated that the noroviruses may be responsible for more than 235,000 clinic visits and 91,000 ED visits in children under 5 years of age living in the United States (Patel et al., 2008). With the use of the rotavirus vaccine, their numbers should decrease.
- Extra-intestinal infections, such as otitis media, urinary tract infections, and pneumonia, can cause acute diarrhea that is mild and self-limited in nature (Berkun et al., 2008; Defilippi et al., 2008).
- Antibiotic-associated diarrhea (AAD) occurs commonly (Turck et al., 2003) and is thought to be associated with a disruption in normal flora (Surawicz, 2003).
- Overfeeding, especially with hyperosmolar fluids (i.e., soft drinks, apple juice, and broth) can cause diarrhea (Dennison, 1996). Limiting intake of solid foods can cause a thin, watery, green stool.
- Lactase deficiency in the form of hypolactasia or lactase nonpersistence can cause diarrhea (Heyman & AAP Committee on Nutrition, 2006).

Pathophysiology of Vomiting and Diarrhea

Vomiting is the forceful expulsion of stomach (and sometimes duodenal) contents, often preceded by nausea. It should not be confused with regurgitation, which is the flow of undigested material from the lower esophagus and stomach without the associated forceful muscle contractions. Vomiting is a function of neuronal activity in the brainstem, specifically in the medulla oblongata of the hindbrain. The hypothalamus, stimulated by the same neuronal activity, also plays a role in vomiting. Two dynamics appear to occur leading to vomiting seen in conjunction with diarrhea: Chemosensitive receptors detect emetic agents in the bloodstream and transmit a message to the nucleus tractus solitarius (NTS) in the medulla, and vagal afferent nerves detect changes in intestinal contents and tone and send messages to the same site. The NTS is a complex of subnucleii related to gastric, laryngeal, and pharyngeal sensation; swallowing; baroreceptor function; and respiration. Neurostimulation of this center leads to the autonomic changes seen in vomiting (Hornby, 2001).

Vomiting with secretory and cytotoxic diarrhea may be due to a functional ileus seen in these conditions. As a result of the decreased intestinal tone and slowed peristalsis of a functional ileus, the intestinal lumen dilates causing abdominal pain and vomiting; gastric emptying is delayed, causing vomiting; and the patient experiences cramping due to peristaltic rushes.

Common causative factors for vomiting in infancy that are included in a differential diagnosis are congenital obstructive lesions (neonatal period), allergic reactions to formula (the first 2 months of life), pyloric stenosis, and metabolic disorders. For older children, viral or bacterial gastroenteritis or food poisoning are the more common causes of vomiting. Urinary tract infections, streptococcal pharyngitis, and otitis also are associated with vomiting. Central nervous system problems, migraine headaches, and other gastrointestinal anomalies must also be considered (Bishop, 2006).

The major pathophysiologic dynamic in diarrhea is an alteration in the balance of fluid exchange across the intestinal wall, resulting in excess fluid elimination. It is a function of a relative increase in secretion of fluid into the bowel and decrease in absorption of fluid from the small bowel. There are four main types of diarrhea commonly seen in infants and children:

1. *Osmotic diarrhea:* Occurs when the concentration of nutrients and electrolytes in the intestine is high enough to be osmotically active. As a result, fluid is drawn into the intestine to dilute these particles. Intestinal tissue is not typically damaged in osmotic diarrhea. Malabsorption syndromes, lactose intolerance, overfeeding, and excessive ingestion of hypertonic juices are examples of causes of osmotic diarrhea.

2. *Secretory diarrhea:* Occurs when bacterial enterotoxins stimulate secretion of fluids and electrolytes from small intestinal crypt cells into the intestine. Absorption by the small intestine villous cells is also inhibited. The excess fluids result in diarrhea. Common agents leading to secretory diarrhea include *Aeromonas, Clostridium, E. coli, Salmonella, Shigella, Yersinia, Vibrio,* and *Giardia.*

3. *Cytotoxic diarrhea:* Occurs when an agent (usually viral) destroys mucosal villous cells of the small intestine. Secretory cells tend to be spared, but shortened villi lead to decreased absorption of fluids and electrolytes. Rotavirus, Norwalk virus, *Cryptosporidium,* and *E. coli* bacteria are major causes of cytotoxic diarrhea.

4. *Dysenteric diarrhea:* Occurs when the bowel is inflamed, damaging the mucosa and submucosa. Subsequent edema, infiltration, and bleeding compromise the ability of the intestine to absorb water, nutrients, and electrolytes. This inflammatory process can occur with bacterial infections, celiac disease, and irritable bowel syndrome, affecting the functional ability of the bowel.

Acute versus Chronic Diarrhea

Acute diarrhea is typically defined as duration of diarrheal symptoms for 5 days or less. Chronic (or persistent) diarrhea is the presence of loose or more frequent stools for more than 2 weeks (Ghishan, 2004; Pickering & Snyder, 2004). Dehydration is a major cause of morbidity and mortality in acute diarrhea, less so in chronic diarrhea. Growth retardation, both physical and cognitive, is more commonly seen with chronic diarrhea, though this is more of a problem in developing countries than in the United States (Bhutta et al., 2008).

The etiology of chronic diarrhea may be age-related, with cow's milk protein intolerance being the most common cause in infants. However, the causes of chronic diarrhea in young children are largely uncertain and probably multiple. Mucosa damaged by an episode of acute diarrhea may be slow to heal, limiting absorption from the gut and resulting in a persistent osmotic diarrhea. Allergies or food sensitivities, dietary or nutritional deficiencies, unknown pathogens, or underlying conditions (such as enzyme deficiency, celiac disease, or an autoimmunity) may cause chronic diarrhea (Bhutta et al., 2008). One study of children with persistent diarrhea in the United States found that 59% of the stool samples sufficient for analysis contained no pathogens, and another 17.9% contained only *C. difficile* and *E. coli* that appeared unrelated to the diarrhea (Vernacchio et al., 2006). This same study found that viruses most typically associated with persistent diarrhea were rotavirus, norovirus, and sapovirus; it remains unclear what role these viruses play in chronic diarrhea in developing countries where malnutrition and other diseases complicate the presentation (Bhutta et al.; Vernacchio et al.). Protracted diarrhea also can be caused if vomiting and gastroenteritis are managed by a high-carbohydrate, low-fat, and low-protein diet (Petersen-Smith & McKenzie, 2009).

In the United States, chronic nonspecific diarrhea of childhood (CNDC), also called toddler's diarrhea or irritable colon of infancy, is usually a benign condition, but it often leads to an outpatient medical visit and must be evaluated to determine if treatment is necessary. CNDC is a diagnosis of exclusion. The term has been in the medical literature for over 50 years, and the characteristics of the condition specified in 1966 remain valid (Kleinman, 2005). These characteristics include (Davidson & Wasserman, 1966):

- Diarrhea typically begins between 6 and 20 months of age (> 75%); 12% of infants presented with diarrhea before 6 months of age.
- The child is growing and developing well.
- The first stool of the day is large and semi-formed; subsequent stools are smaller and looser.
- Most (87%) children have diarrhea with mucous.
- A family history of functional bowel disorders is common.

Clearly, the history and physical examination are critical to identify the condition and possible underlying causes. Laboratory and diagnostic studies are ordered as indicated. Key factors to consider in assessing and managing chronic diarrhea are:

- In CNDC, the best treatment is reassurance and returning the child to a full, normal diet for age. In Davidson and Wasserman's study (1966), 88% of children with CNDC cleared by 39 months of age; another 10% by 48 months of age, without growth delay.
- Treat underlying causes if known.
- Treat the effects of diarrhea as indicated (e.g., oral or parenteral rehydration).
- Refer to a gastroenterologist if:
  - Newborns present with diarrhea in the first hours of life.
  - The child has abnormal or delayed growth patterns.
  - Severe illness is present.

What additional information do you need to help you make the determination about a telephone consultation versus having Sara come in for an office visit? ■

Risk Factors for Hospitalization and Death Due to Gastroenteritis

Before the initiation of treatment either by telephone or in person, one must review risk factors that place a child with gastroenteritis at increased risk for hospitalization or death (Fischer et al., 2007; Ho et al., 1988). These include:

- Age < 12 months
- Malnutrition
- Immunodeficiency
- Underlying disease
- Low socioeconomic status of the family
- Race
- Maternal factors:
  - Little prenatal care
  - Low level of education
  - Young
- Poor capability of the parents to monitor and care for their child
- Winter season

If the child in question has one or more of these risk factors, there is concern for dehydration, especially during the first 6 hours of a primary infection such as rotavirus. For a telephone assessment, the provider's knowledge of the patient's family is crucial in assessing the validity of the information.

In addition to family data, the following information related to the specific illness is essential in assessing the child's condition and determining if he or she should be seen in the office:

- Age of child
- Onset and duration of the illness

- Number of diarrhea and vomiting episodes
- Presence of blood or mucus in the stool
- Intake of fluids—what and how much over the past 24 hours
- Moisture on the mucus membranes
- Fever
- Urine frequency, amount, color, and last void
- Activity of the child

Assessing fever and bloody stool, two features that can be present in gastroenteritis, is particularly helpful in determining the differential diagnosis and guiding the provider to make appropriate decisions regarding care (see Table 25-1).

The above information, along with the season of the year, can help guide the provider in diagnosing and treating the child. However, in order to distinguish an acute self-limited episode of gastroenteritis from a more serious disorder, additional historical information must be obtained, including:

- Contacts with ill individuals
- Exposures to illness or environmental contaminants such as in daycare, travel, water source, or foods
- Previous episodes of gastroenteritis or dehydration (how many and time of last episode)
- Medications being taken, including over-the-counter or prescription, and any complementary or alternative medications or herbal remedies
- Prior history of other significant infections

Table 25-1   Differential Diagnosis of Gastroenteritis by Fever and Bloody Stool

	Febrile	Afebrile
Bloody stool	Infectious enteritis	Intussusception
	Pseudomembranous colitis (if child recently treated with antibiotics)	Hemolytic uremic syndrome (HUS)
		Pseudomembranous colitis
	Amoebiasis (recent travel overseas)	Acute gastroenteritis (only after above have been excluded)
	Inflammatory bowel disease (occasionally presents with fever)	
Nonbloody stool	Viral infection	Viral enteritis
		Antibiotic-associated diarrhea
		Overfeeding
		Excessive fluid or juice intake

- Presence of concurrent infections
- Underlying diseases
- History of allergies
- Family history of gastrointestinal conditions

For the child who is seen in person, the provider needs to assess and evaluate the following:

- The infant's or child's level of consciousness; activity and energy level
- Vital signs
- Signs of dehydration
- A careful abdominal exam looking for the presence of any localizing and/or meningeal signs

What additional questions will you need to ask when you return Sara's mother's phone call? ▪

With the information from the office triage nurse and a review of Sara's records that indicate she is up-to-date on her immunizations, has no known allergies to medications or food, no family history of gastrointestinal conditions, and no history of recent hospitalization or serious illness, you telephone Sara's mother. You ask her the following questions:

· *How long has Sara been sick? What started first, the vomiting or the diarrhea?* She had been fine until just a few days ago. Two days ago, she threw up twice and then she had the loose stools. She had four loose stools today.

· *What do the stools look like? Any blood or mucus?* They are loose greenish stools. There doesn't seem to be any blood in them.

· *When did her fever start, what has it been, and how have you dealt with her fever?* I first noticed she felt hot last night about 9 p.m. Her temperature was 100°F. I gave her some Tylenol, and it came down to normal within an hour. Her temperature this morning was 99.8°F. I haven't given her anything for fever today, and she really doesn't feel very warm now.

· *Is anybody in the family sick? Have you traveled anywhere recently? Has Sara eaten any new foods? Is Sara in daycare?* Nobody in the family is ill. We have not gone anywhere lately. Sara's been eating her normal diet, but we did change daycare about 2 weeks ago to a center nearer to home.

· *Has Sara been eating and drinking? How many times has Sara voided today including the time of her last urination?* She had some dry cereal and milk today and some peaches for lunch, and she didn't vomit after eating this time. She has gone to the bathroom at least three times to void, with her last voiding about 2 hours ago.

· *Has she been playing or lying around napping?* She has been playing with her dolls this morning and watched one of her videos this afternoon. Do you think something else is wrong with her since she has been sick so much this year? What am I doing wrong?

You reassure Sara's mom that she isn't doing anything wrong, though you understand how anxious she is because Sara is sick again.

What are the possible differential diagnoses? ■

Do you need to see this child, and are diagnostic tests needed at this point? ■

Differential Diagnosis

Watery and/or frequent stools may be the initial manifestation of a wide spectrum of acute and chronic disorders, some of which may be life threatening in children. Of particular concern are intussusception, hemolytic uremic syndrome (HUS), pseudomembranous colitis, appendicitis, and toxic megacolon.

Intussusception is most common in infants 6–12 months of age, but can occur later in life; the majority of cases are seen in children less than 2 years of age. Without treatment, it can be life threatening. Most children experience sudden onset of severe, intermittent, crampy abdominal pain accompanied by inconsolable crying. These episodes typically occur at 15- to 20-minute intervals. As the obstruction progresses, the attacks become more frequent and there can be bilious gastric emesis, passage of "currant jelly" stool, and a sausage-shaped mass in the right side of the abdomen. The classic triad of symptoms of pain, palpable sausage-shaped abdominal mass, and currant jelly stools are seen in less than 15% of patients with intussusception. Between episodes, the infant behaves normally, and initial symptoms can be confused with gastroenteritis.

Hemolytic uremic syndrome (HUS) should be a consideration for any child with bloody diarrhea. This illness begins 5 to 10 days after the onset of diarrhea, is sudden in onset, and is characterized by the triad of microangiopathic hemolytic anemia, thrombocytopenia, and acute renal failure (Amiriak & Amiriak, 2006). The prodromal symptoms of abdominal pain, vomiting, and diarrhea that are experienced can mimic those of ulcerative colitis, other enteric infections, and appendicitis.

Pseudomembranous colitis is a rare but serious disorder that results almost exclusively from an overgrowth of toxin-producing *Clostridium difficile* organisms in the bowel. It is commonly associated with antibiotic therapy and prior hospitalization of the child. The typical presentation is lower abdominal pain accompanied by watery diarrhea, low-grade fever, and leukocytosis that start during or shortly after antibiotic administration. This infection can progress to toxic megacolon and shock (Brook, 2005).

Appendicitis typically begins with diffuse abdominal pain with the following three predominant clinical features: pain in the right lower quadrant, abdominal wall rigidity, and migration of periumbilical pain to the right lower quadrant (Paulson, Kalady, & Pappas, 2003). Predictive indicators of appendicitis in preadolescent children include lower right quadrant tenderness, nausea, inability to walk, and elevated white blood cell and neutrophil counts. Diarrhea may be present in children with appendicitis but is not a useful diagnostic indicator (Colvin, Bachur, & Kharbanda, 2007).

Toxic megacolon can occur as a complication of a Shigella infection, pseudomembranous colitis, Hirschsprung disease, or inflammatory bowel disease. It is a life-threatening complication. Its clinical manifestations are fever, massively dilated colon, painful abdominal distention, and anemia with a low serum albumin level (Bishop, 2006).

In addition to these life-threatening conditions, what other conditions should you include in the differential diagnoses when a child has vomiting and diarrhea? ◼

The following diagnoses should also be considered:

- Urinary tract infection
- Other infections: otitis media, strep pharyngitis
- Inflammatory bowel disease
- Malabsorption: lactose intolerance, celiac disease, cystic fibrosis
- Milk protein allergy
- Chronic diarrhea
- Viral gastroenteritis
- Overfeeding
- Excessive fluid or juice intake
- Amoebiasis

Diagnostic Testing

Laboratory testing is not necessary in acute gastroenteritis unless one of the following is present:

- Blood or mucus in the stools.
- No improvement in signs and symptoms after 5–6 days.
- Signs and symptoms of severe dehydration. Specific blood work should be done to check blood urea nitrogen (BUN), white blood cell count and differential, and electrolytes. Urine should be checked for specific gravity.

Testing for a specific virus is rarely necessary because the disease is self-limited. However, if a specific organism is suspected, the following stool tests can be performed:

- *Bacterial infection:* Stool can be sent for culture (e.g., *E. coli* 0157:H7 if child has bloody stools).
- *Giardia:* Send stool for Giardia antigen.
- *Cryptosporidium:* Send stool for ova and parasite test.
- *C. difficile:* Send stool for *C. difficile* toxins text.

Making the Diagnosis

You continue your phone conversation, telling Sara's mom that you think Sara just has a viral infection that is causing the vomiting and diarrhea, also known as acute gastroenteritis. Some of this may be related to changing day-care centers—especially if other children are sick.

Management

The goals of treatment in diarrhea are to restore and maintain hydration and resume full bowel function as soon as possible. At the least, acute gastroenteritis is a self-limited disease that requires no intervention other than administration of oral fluids and resumption of an age-appropriate diet, as is the case with Sara. Management of more severe illness in children who present with fever and dehydration should include the following steps:

1. *Restore and maintain hydration.* With a diagnosis of acute gastroenteritis, initial therapy is directed at correcting any fluid deficit and electrolyte imbalance. The American Academy of Pediatrics (AAP), Centers for Disease Control and Prevention (CDC), and World Health Organization (WHO) have established fluid replacement guidelines for children with diarrhea (AAP, 2004; King et al., 2003). All are based on the degree of dehydration or volume depletion. Severe dehydration requires immediate intervention with rapid intravenous fluid resuscitation. With mild to moderate hypovolemia, oral rehydration is preferred, and can be accomplished with oral rehydration solution (ORS) or with the use of a number of prepared commercial solutions. Inappropriate liquids are Kool-Aid, fruit juices (e.g., apple juice), sports drinks, and sodas; gelatin should also be avoided. See Table 25-2 for recommendations regarding treatment of various degrees of dehydration.

2. *Resume feedings.* Both the AAP and the CDC recommend the resumption of feedings of an age-appropriate diet as soon as rehydration is complete. A relatively unrestricted diet reduces the stool output and the duration of the illness (King et al., 2003). For the infant, on-demand breastfeeding should be continued without disruption when a child has diarrhea. If the infant is receiving formula, feedings should continue unchanged as tolerated. In older children, full strength cow's milk or other nonhuman milks are usually tolerated without problems. Use of probiotics or lactose-free formulas appear to be generally unnecessary (Salazar-Lindo, Miranda-Langschwager, Campos-Sanchez, Chea-Woo, & Sack, 2004), but in a study of Thai and Asian children with genetic lactase deficiency, acute diarrhea resolved more quickly with a lactose-free formula (Simakachorn, Tongpenyai, Tongtan, & Varavithya, 2004). Foods that have high levels of fat and simple sugars are less well

Table 25-2   Rehydration Therapy

Severity of Diarrhea	Replacement Fluid	Amount	Comments
Mild	ORS	40–50 mL/kg over 4 hours (10 mL/kg/hr)	Resume normal diet as soon as possible. Avoid fatty foods and sugary foods. Continue breastfeeding or formula feeding.
Moderate	ORS	60–100 mL/kg over 4–6 hours (20 mL/kg/hr)	Resume normal diet as above.
Severe	IV fluids: Ringer's lactate or normal saline Once the child has voided, follow with D5W with NaCl and KCl for maintenance fluids and to replace fluid following continued severe diarrhea.	20 mL/kg bolus over 1 hr See below for 24-hour amount of maintenance fluids and replacement fluids in the event of continued severe diarrhea. Give one-half amount over 8 hours, the other half over the next 16 hours. Include bolus in 24-hour total amount.	May repeat bolus if needed until pulse, perfusion, and mental status are normal. Begin ORS as soon as possible.

Maintenance Fluids	Weight of Child	Amount	Comments
Total fluid volume	0–10 kg	100 mL/kg/24 hr	Once replacement fluids have been completed, continue with maintenance fluids.
	10–20 kg	1,000 mL + 50 mL/kg for each kg over 10 kg/24 hr	
	> 20 kg	1,500 mL + 20 mL/kg for each kg over 20 kg/24 hr	
If severe diarrhea continues		10 mL/kg or 4–8 oz ORS for each diarrhea stool (1–1.5 times the amount of stool)	

Notes. hr, hours; IV, intravenous; ORS, oral rehydration solution; D5W, Dextrose 5% in water; NaCL, sodium chloride; KCL, potassium chloride

Source: Adapted from Petersen-Smith, A. M., & McKenzie, S. B. (2009). Gastrointestinal disorders. In C. E. Burns, A. M. Dunn, M. A. Brady, N. B. Starr, & C. Blosser (Eds.). *Pediatric primary care* (4th ed., pp. 795–844). St. Louis, MO: Elsevier Saunders.

tolerated than complex carbohydrates, lean meats, yogurt, fruits, and vegetables (King et al., 2003). Contrary to practices from years past, fasting or "letting the bowel rest," and exclusive use of the BRAT diet (bananas, rice, applesauce, toast) or a diet of clear liquids (like apple juice) are unusually restrictive measures and provide suboptimal nutrition for the child. The child should not fast, and the foods in the BRAT diet can be included in a normal diet as tolerated, but should not be the dietary mainstay. Toddlers and older children should eat a wide variety of healthful foods, fruits, vegetables, grains, protein, and carbohydrates as tolerated. Smaller portions, given more frequently, may be better tolerated. High-carbohydrate (especially sugared drinks and sugary foods), high-fat, and spicy foods should be avoided. Boiled milk should *never* be given (AAP, 2008).

3. *Prescribe appropriate antibiotics (only if an identified bacterial agent is the cause of the diarrhea) and other medications only if indicated.* Do not prescribe diphenoxylate-atropine (Lomotil) because it slows intestinal motility, can contribute to paralytic ileus, and can complicate the clinical outcome if the diarrhea is due to antibiotic administration, pseudomembranous colitis, or an enterotoxin-producing bacteria. Repetitive or incorrect dosing of diphenoxylate-atropine has also been associated with mortality in toddlers (Thomas, Pauze, & Love, 2008). Avoid use of Pepto-Bismol because it can mask symptoms of nausea and upset stomach and may interact with prescription drugs, making diagnosis and resolution of the underlying problem more difficult. Also, the active ingredient in adult preparation Pepto-Bismol, bismuth subsalicylate, has been associated with toxicity in infants (Lewis, Badillo, Schaeffer, Hagemann, & McGoodwin, 2006); the active ingredient in children's Pepto-Bismol is calcium carbonate, which can be used cautiously in older children.

4. *Administer zinc.* Some studies have shown the administration of zinc to children in developing countries with diarrhea decreases the duration of the illness (King et al., 2003; Strand et al., 2002).

5. *Administer parenteral fluids if signs of severe dehydration are present or if the child is at high risk for rapid dehydration.* See Table 25-2 for parenteral treatment of severe dehydration. Intravenous therapy may be administered in an urgent care center or emergency department, where the child can be carefully observed. Hospitalization may be required.

6. *When giving a telephone consultation, always tell the child's care provider when to follow up with the healthcare provider.* They should also be advised to seek care if severe symptoms develop or if the child's symptoms become worse or do not resolve in a projected length of time. Identify what signs and symptoms are worrisome and require evaluation. In addition, provide a specified time frame in which the child should show signs of improvement. Tell the child's care provider to seek assistance in an emergency department on weekends or after the clinic or office is closed if necessary.

7. *Follow up.* Follow up with a telephone call to check on the child's progress.

Sara's mom asks what she can do about her being sick. You tell her that one of the most important measures she, Sara, and the other members of her family can do is simple handwashing with soap and water. Everyone needs to do this after using the bathroom and before eating any food. You recommend that she also check with the head of the daycare to see how they are cleaning the toys and equipment at the center. Proper cleaning of supplies and equipment will help keep all of the children healthy.

You tell her to make sure Sara continues to eat and drink as much as she is comfortable with. She shouldn't give her juice, soda, or any sweetened drinks, and she should avoid fatty foods like chips, french fries, or ice cream; fried foods like chicken nuggets; or any sweets like candy or cookies. She may want to eat smaller portions, more frequently, rather than three meals a day. Her mother should try giving her foods like fresh fruits, cooked vegetables, cereal, bread, rice, pasta, yogurt, and some lean meats like chicken. The foods she has eaten today are the right ones and should help her recover quicker.

The diarrhea should stop in a day or so. If it continues for a total of 6 days, she should call you back because you will want to see Sara. She should also call back if her fever is higher than 101 degrees or if she is acting unusual, more "tired" or "weird." If she seems worse, won't eat or drink, or only voids once or twice a day, she should call right away so that you can see her as an urgent visit.

Sara's mother asks how she can keep her from getting sick all the time. What will you tell her? ■

You tell her that children Sara's age often have minor illnesses, especially if they are around other children. Once she is back to her normal self, the best way to keep Sara healthy is to make sure she gets the rest she needs and that she eats a variety of healthy foods—fruits, vegetables, breads, grains, and protein like milk, cheese, yogurt, nuts, and meat. She doesn't have to eat all of these every day, but she should provide her with good foods. Sara should avoid fried foods and fatty foods like french fries and chips, and avoid sugary drinks and soda. She should also limit the amount of juice Sara drinks to about 8 ounces a day. She should limit sweets too, but it's fine if she has a cookie, ice cream, or sweet once every day or two. Finally, she should make sure Sara and everyone else in the family washes their hands often.

Key Points from This Case

1. History is essential for accurate diagnosis of gastroenteritis.
2. Viral enteritis is the most common cause of gastroenteritis in children.
3. Telephone consultation may be appropriate for the management of many cases of acute, self-limited gastroenteritis, but close follow-up is critical to assess outcome.
4. Risk factors for dehydration must be considered in making decisions about assessment and treatment.

5. Oral rehydration following diarrhea and vomiting promotes more rapid healing than parenteral therapy alone.

6. Parenteral therapy may be appropriate for children at high risk for dehydration and/or children with severe dehydration; resume oral rehydration as soon as possible.

7. A normal diet should be resumed as soon as possible after replacement fluids have been administered.

8. Handwashing and healthful diets are key factors in preventing gastroenteritis in children. Patient, parent, and community education should emphasize these factors.

REFERENCES

American Academy of Pediatrics. (2004). Statement of endorsement: managing acute gastroenteritis among children: oral rehydration, maintenance, and nutritional therapy. *Pediatrics, 114*(2), 507.

American Academy of Pediatrics. (2008). *Diarrhea, vomiting, and water loss (dehydration)*. Retrieved December 12, 2008, from http://patiented.aap.org/AtoZIndex.aspx?letter=D

Amiriak, I., & Amiriak, B. (2006). Haemolytic uraemic syndrome: an overview. *Nephrology, 11*(3), 213–218.

Berkun, Y., Nir-Paz, R., Ami, A. B., Klar, A., Deutsch, E., & Hurvitz, H. (2008). Acute otitis media in the first two months of life: characteristics and diagnostic difficulties. *Archives of Disease in Childhood, 93*(8), 690–694.

Bhutta, Z. A., Nelson, E. A., Lee, W. S., Tarr, P. I., Zablah, R., Phua, K. B., et al. (2008). Recent advances and evidence gaps in persistent diarrhea. *Journal of Pediatric Gastroenterology and Nutrition, 47*(2), 260–265.

Bishop, W. P. (2006). The digestive system. In R. M. Kliegman, K. J. Marcdante, H. B. Jenson, & R. E. Behrman (Eds.), *Nelson essentials of pediatrics* (5th ed., pp. 579–624). Philadelphia: Elsevier Saunders.

Brook, I. (2005). Pseudomembranous colitis in children. *Journal of Gastroenterology and Hepatology, 20*(2), 182–186.

Colvin, J. M., Bachur, R., & Kharbanda, A. (2007). The presentation of appendicitis in preadolescent children. *Pediatric Emergency Care, 23*, 849–855.

Davidson, M., & Wasserman, R. (1966). The irritable colon of childhood (chronic nonspecific diarrhea syndrome). *Journal of Pediatrics, 69*, 1027–1038.

Defilippi, A., Silvestri, M., Tacchella, A., Giacchino, R., Melioli, G., Di Marco, E., et al. (2008). Epidemiology and clinical features of *Mycoplasma pneumoniae* infection in children. *Respiratory Medicine, 102*(12), 1762–1768.

Dennison, B. A. (1996). Fruit juice consumption by infants and children: a review. *Journal of the American College of Nutrition, 15*(5 Suppl), 4S–11S.

Fischer, T. K., Viboud, C., Parashar, U., Malek, M., Steiner, C., Glass, R., et al. (2007). Hospitalizations and deaths from diarrhea and rotavirus among children <5 years of age in the United States, 1993–2003. *Journal of Infectious Diseases, 195*, 1117–1125.

Ghishan, F. K. (2004). Chronic diarrhea. In: R. Behrman, H. B. Jenson, & R. M. Kliegman (Eds.), *Nelson textbook of pediatrics* (17th ed., pp. 1276–1281). St. Louis, MO: WB Saunders.

Heyman, M. B., & AAP Committee on Nutrition. (2006). Lactose intolerance in infants, children, and adolescents. *Pediatrics, 118*(3), 1279–1286.

Ho, M. S., Glass, R. I., Pinsky, P. F., Young-Okoh, N. C., Sappenfield, W. M., Buehler, J. W., et al. (1988). Diarrheal deaths in American children. Are they preventable? *Journal of the American Medical Association, 206*(22), 3281–3285.

Hornby, P. J. (2001). Central neurocircuitry associated with emesis. *American Journal of Medicine, 111*, 106S–112S.

Jenson, H. B., & Baltimore, R. S. (2006). Infectious diseases. In R. M. Kliegman, K. J. Marcdante, H. B. Jenson, & R. E. Behrman (Eds.), *Nelson essentials of pediatrics* (5th ed., pp. 445–577). Philadelphia: Elsevier Saunders.

King, C. K., Glass, R., Bresee, J. S., Duggan, C., & Centers for Disease Control and Prevention. (2003). Managing acute gastroenteritis among children: oral rehydration, maintenance, and nutritional therapy. *Morbidity and Mortality Weekly Report, 52*(RR-16), 1–16.

Kleinman, R. E. (2005). Chronic nonspecific diarrhea of childhood. *Nestlé Nutrition Workshop Series, Paediatric Programme, 58*, 73–84.

Lewis, T. V., Badillo, R., Schaeffer, S., Hagemann, T. M., & McGoodwin, L. (2006). Salicylate toxicity associated with administration of Percy medicine in an infant. *Pharmacotherapy, 26*(3), 403–409.

Lopez, A. D., Mathers, C. D., Ezzati, M., Jamison, D. T., & Murray, C. J. L. (2006). Global and regional burden of disease and risk factors, 2001: systematic analysis of population health data. *Lancet, 367*, 1747–1757.

Patel, M. M., Widdowson, M.-A., Glass, R. I., Akazawa, K., Vinje, J., & Parashar, U. D. (2008). Systematic literature review of role of norovirus in sporadic gastroenteritis. *Emerging and Infectious Diseases.* Retrieved December 27, 2008, from http://www.cdc.gov/EID/content/14/8/1224.htm

Paulson, E. K., Kalady, M. R., & Pappas, T. N. (2003). Clinical practice. Suspected appendicitis. *New England Journal of Medicine, 348*(3), 236–242.

Payne, D. C., Stockman, L. J., Gentsch, J. R., & Parashar, U. D. (2008). Rotavirus. In: Centers for Disease Control and Prevention, *VPD Surveillance Manual* (4th ed., chap. 9). Retrieved December 27, 2008, from http://www.cdc.gov/vaccines/pubs/surv-manual/chpt13-rotavirus.htm

Petersen-Smith, A. M., & McKenzie, S. B. (2009). Gastrointestinal disorders. In C. E. Burns, A. M. Dunn, M. A. Brady, N. B. Starr, & C. G. Blosser (Eds.), *Pediatric primary care* (4th ed., pp. 795–844). St. Louis, MO: WB Saunders.

Pickering, L. K., Baker, C. J., Long, S. S., & McMillan, J. A. (Eds.). (2006). *Red book: 2006 report of the Committee on Infectious Diseases* (27th ed.). Elk Grove Village, IL: American Academy of Pediatrics.

Pickering, L. K., & Snyder, J. D. (2004). Gastroenteritis. In R. Behrman, H. G. Jenson, & R. M. Kliegman (Eds.), *Nelson textbook of pediatrics* (17th ed., pp. 1272–1276). St. Louis, MO: WB Saunders.

Salazar-Lindo, E., Miranda-Langschwager, P., Campos-Sanchez, M., Chea-Woo, E., & Sack, R. B. (2004). Lactobacillus casei strain GG in the treatment of infants with acute watery diarrhea: a randomized, double-blind, placebo controlled clinical trial. *BMC Pediatrics, 4*, 18.

Simakachorn, N., Tongpenyai, Y., Tongtan, O., & Varavithya, W. (2004). Randomized, double-blind clinical trial of a lactose-free and a lactose-containing formula in dietary management of acute childhood diarrhea. *Journal of the Medical Association of Thailand, 87*(6), 641–649.

Strand, T. A., Chandyo, R. K., Bahl, R., Sharma, P. R., Adhikari, R. K., Bhandari, N., et al. (2002). Effectiveness and efficacy of zinc for the treatment of acute diarrhea in young children. *Pediatrics, 109*(5), 898–903.

Surawicz, C. M. (2003). Probiotics, antibiotic-associated diarrhoea and *Clostridium difficile* diarrhoea in humans. *Best Practice and Research: Clinical Gastroenterology, 17*(5), 775–783.

Thomas, T. J., Pauze, D., & Love, J. N. (2008). Are one or two dangerous? Diphenoxylate-atropine exposure in toddlers. *Journal of Emergency Medicine, 34*(1), 71–75.

Turck, D., Bernet, J. P., Marx, J., Kempf, H., Biard, P., Walbaum, O., et al. (2003). Incidence and risk factors of oral antibiotic-associated diarrhea in an outpatient pediatric population. *Journal of Pediatric Gastroenterology and Nutrition, 37*(1), 22–26.

Vernacchio, L., Vezina, R. M., Mitchell, A. A., Lesko, S. M., Plant, A. G., & Acheson, D. W. K. (2006). Characteristics of persistent diarrhea in a community-based cohort of young US children. *Journal of Pediatric Gastroenterology and Nutrition, 43*(1), 52.

Chapter 26

Three Cases of Oral Trauma

Prashant Gagneja
John Peterson

Oral trauma frequently occurs during the life of a young child and adolescent. Often, the consequences of this trauma are minor and may even go unnoticed. However, many injuries to the teeth can have long-lasting significance. It is the purpose of this chapter to present three common dental trauma scenarios and their management.

Educational Objectives

1. Understand the diagnosis and management of the following types of dental trauma:
   - Avulsion of primary incisors
   - Avulsion of permanent incisors
   - Crown fracture of a permanent incisor with no pulp exposure
   - Crown fracture of a permanent incisor with pulp exposure
2. Describe the primary care provider's role in management of dental trauma.

Case Presentations and Discussion

Child #1

Maria Lopez is a 3-year-old Latino female who avulsed the maxillary right primary central incisor 3 hours ago. Her mother reports that Maria was running through the living room when she tripped on the carpet and fell face first into the coffee table. She was not reported to have lost consciousness. After wiping away some of the tears and blood, mom saw that Maria's upper front tooth was missing. She found it on the floor and called her primary healthcare provider. However, due to logistical complications, she was not able to get to the office for approximately 3 hours. When she does arrive, Maria seems calm and cooperative.

Child #2

Prashant Kumar is a 10-year-old Indian American male who avulsed his maxillary left permanent incisor about 15 minutes ago. Prashant and his family are visiting his cousin's house where there is a swimming pool. While running around the pool, he slipped and hit his mouth on the concrete. The avulsed tooth fell into the pool, but his sister found it moments later. Since they were vacationing far away from their dentist, his father chose to go to a nearby urgent care center.

Child #3

Johnny Smith is a 12-year-old white male who, upon leaving school, fell off his bicycle. It was a rather minor crash but, after dusting himself off, he realized he had hit the handlebars with his mouth. He felt his maxillary incisors with his tongue and realized that two of them were broken. He quickly went to the school's healthcare office. The school nurse noticed that, although two teeth were fractured, only one of them showed any blood from the broken area. Mom was called and immediately came to the school.

What questions would you like to ask all three children and parents to help in the development of a diagnosis and treatment plan? ■

As with all head injuries, you will want to know the following information:

- Time of injury
- Where and how the injury occurred
- History of neurologic signs or symptoms before arriving at your clinic
  - Loss of consciousness
  - Headache
  - Nausea or vomiting
  - Disorientation, dizziness, or confusion
  - Unexplained sleepiness
  - Bleeding or fluid from ears, eyes, or nose
- General medical history
- History of other traumatic injuries

What physical examination data will you collect for all these cases in addition to the observed dental trauma? ■

Physical examination for head injuries should include the following assessments:

- Vital signs.
- Sign and symptoms of child abuse or possible abuse.
- Neurological examination:
  - Begin by noting any signs or symptoms of neurological trauma as reported by the caregiver.
    - Loss of consciousness
    - Headache
    - Nausea or vomiting
    - Disorientation, dizziness, or confusion
    - Unexplained sleepiness
    - Bleeding or fluid from ears, eyes, or nose
  - Evaluate functions controlled by the cranial nerves.

- Evaluate pupils for equality, roundness, reaction to light, and accommodation (PERRLA).
- Range of motion for the head and neck.
- Pain in the head and neck that cannot be attributed to the dental trauma.

How would the results from the histories and physical examinations above affect your triage of the children? ■

Before we go further, here is some information about various types of oral/dental trauma.

Dental Trauma Background Information

Unfortunately, dental injuries are all-too-frequent events in the life of some children. Dental trauma may happen at home, during sports, in motor vehicles, or as a result of abuse. When dental injuries affect the primary or young permanent dentition, the child may not always report directly to the dentist. Instead, they may first arrive at the emergency department or other primary healthcare facility. Thus, it is important for primary care healthcare providers to be prepared to manage these injuries prior to the child being sent on to the dentist.

Epidemiology

In the primary dentition, the frequency for dental injuries seems to be about equally distributed between females and males. However, later on, in the permanent dentition, boys appear to injure their teeth more often than girls (Bastone, Freer, & McNamara, 2000). In both the primary and permanent dentition, the teeth most commonly traumatized are the maxillary incisors.

Children with a variety of dental injures may present themselves to primary healthcare facilities. Typical injuries include avulsions, intrusions, luxations, fractures of the root, and crown fractures. It is not the purpose of this case study to discuss all of these various types of dental trauma. Instead, three commonly occurring injuries are used to illustrate how the primary healthcare provider can be of help not only to the child, but also to the dentist to whom the case will ultimately be referred.

Avulsion of a Primary Incisor

The avulsion of a primary incisor is an event that is traumatic not only to the child, but also to the parent. When a beautiful upper front baby tooth is lost suddenly and unexpectedly, it is not hard to imagine that the first thing a parent would like is for the tooth to be replaced in the socket. However, this is not the recommended treatment. In fact, the most appropriate treatment is to leave the tooth out (Andreasen & Andreasen, 1994; Andreasen, Andreasen, Bakland, & Flores, 2003) and manage the other components of the injury, including the emotional one. This advice to not replant the primary tooth can be disconcerting to parents because the popular press may have led them to think that all avulsed teeth should be replanted. It is important for the primary care provider to help the parents understand the differences in treating an avulsed primary incisor versus a permanent incisor. In most cases, only a permanent incisor should be replanted as soon as possible. Of great importance when considering the appropriate management for an avulsed primary incisor is the effect that the initial trauma, and any subsequent treatment, may have on the underlying permanent incisor. (See Figure 26-1.) The initial displacement of the primary incisor or an attempt at replantation may damage the developing permanent tooth lying underneath it in the jaw (Christophersen, Freund, & Harild, 2005; Zamon & Kenny, 2001). In addition, consideration should also be given to the long-term health of a replanted primary incisor. The possible negative sequelae of replantation include, but are not limited to, an abscess of the primary tooth itself (Zamon & Kenny). Thus, in review, the recommended treatment for an avulsed primary incisor is to not replant it.

Avulsion of a Permanent Incisor
The avulsion of a *permanent* incisor is also a very traumatic event in the life of an adolescent and parent. (See Figure 26-2.) However, the dental management for an avulsed permanent incisor is entirely different from that of a primary incisor. The goal here is to replant the tooth and have it physiologically reattach to the dental socket. The two parts of an avulsed tooth that are most susceptible to damage are the cells and tissues of the dental pulp and those in the periodontal ligament. Thus, to maintain viability of these cells and enhance the possibility for successful replantation, time is of the essence. In fact, if more than 1 hour of extra-alveolar time passes, there is considerable damage to the periodontal ligament tissues and the chance for successful replantation is significantly

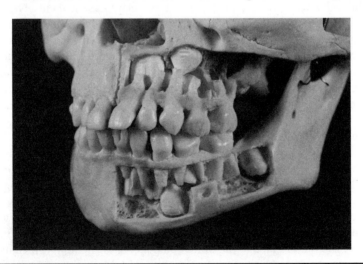

Figure 26-1   Skull of 4 year old showing proximity of primary teeth roots to developing primary incisors.

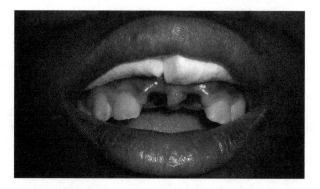

Figure 26-2   Avulsion of permanent central molars.

reduced. The best way to decrease the extra-oral time is to replant the tooth immediately after the injury. To do this, the child or an adult first washes off any contaminates with cold tap water and then replants it into the tooth socket (Andreasen et al., 2003). If this is not possible, the tooth should be placed in an appropriate storage medium and taken as quickly as possible to the primary healthcare provider or dentist. A variety of storage media have been suggested to help maintain the viability of periodontal ligament cells until the tooth can be replanted, including Viaspan, Hank's balanced salt solution, cold milk, saliva, physiologic saline, and water (American Academy of Pediatric Dentistry, 2008). Of these, milk is usually the most available to a layperson and thus is probably the liquid of choice in which to transport the tooth to the primary healthcare provider. Once the tooth has been replanted, it should be stabilized with a splint attached to the adjacent teeth. (See Figure 26-3.) In addition, it is suggested by some to start the child on a regimen of oral antibiotics at the time of replantation (Andreasen et al., 2003). Subsequently, the pediatric dentist or endodontist will usually begin root canal therapy within the first week after the avulsion and continue to follow the child for an extended time thereafter.

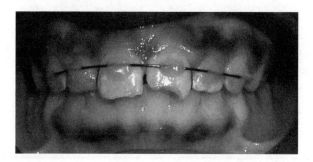

Figure 26-3   Same patient as Figure 26-2 with teeth reimplanted and splinted.

Fractured Permanent Incisor

When a permanent incisor is injured, it can also take the form of a fractured crown. In this case, the traumatic forces may be dissipated by breaking part of the crown rather than displacing the entire tooth. The least damaging fracture is that involving just the enamel; however, more severe fractures will include the enamel and dentin, with the most harmful of these involving the dental pulp. (See Figure 26-4.) The immediate and long-term consequences become increasingly significant when the pulp is involved (Cavalleri & Zerman, 1995). The tooth with a crown fracture can be restored in a variety of ways including esthetic crowns, composite restorations, or the reattachment of the broken crown fragment. Fortunately, in most cases, bonding on a composite resin or reattaching the broken fragment provides a very functional and esthetic restoration. If the broken crown fragment is used, it should be kept moist until it arrives at the dentist. Usually the pulp will respond well, without complication, when it is not exposed; however, when the pulp is exposed, there is an entirely different treatment protocol and potential outcome.

Treatment of the exposed pulp will range from sealing it with various medications to performing a root canal. The dentist will make these treatment decisions based on how long the pulp has been exposed, how extensive the pulp exposure is, and whether the tooth has an incompletely or completely formed root apex. Although all crown fractures should be referred to the dentist, the most urgent referral is for fractures that involve the pulp. The role of the primary healthcare provider is, unfortunately, limited and, in most cases, consists of calling the dental care provider to the emergency department or immediately referring the child to the dental clinic.

Other Dental Trauma

In addition to the dental trauma presented here, the primary healthcare provider may encounter other types of injuries to the primary and young permanent

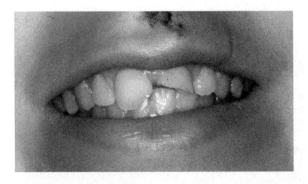

Figure 26-4   Tooth fracture of permanent central incisors.

dentition. The most common of these is the displacement or luxation of an incisor. The initial injury may or may not be noticeable enough to the parent to bring the child to the primary healthcare provider. However, traumatic luxation of a primary incisor may lead to a variety of consequences including changes in the color of the crown, gingival recession around the tooth, necrotic pulp tissue, and resorption of the root and early loss of the tooth that is not attributable to regular exfoliation (Borum & Andreasen, 1998). If signs or symptoms such as color change, pain, inflammation, or abscess formation are recognized by a primary healthcare provider, the child should be referred to a dentist.

Continuing on with the three children, how would you diagnose and manage each case? ■

Child #1: Avulsion of a Primary Incisor

Summary of trauma findings:
  - No signs or symptoms of nondental trauma or child abuse.
  - Complete avulsion of the maxillary right primary central incisor.
  - No other hard or soft tissue trauma except minor damage to the gingival tissue immediately surrounding the tooth socket.

Making the Diagnosis

Maria has an avulsed primary incisor. The extra-oral time has been about 3 hours. There are no other hard or soft tissue injuries and no medical contraindications to treatment.

Management

Recommended dental treatment for an avulsed primary incisor is as follows:

- If the avulsed tooth was not retrieved, obtain a dental radiograph to confirm that the missing tooth has not been intruded, out of sight, into the gingiva and alveolar bone.
- Do not replant. Avulsed primary teeth are *not* replanted, in contrast to avulsed permanent incisors.
- Confirm that tetanus immunizations are up to date.
- Immediately refer the child for dental care.

After explaining the plan, you proceed. Immunizations are not needed. The family has a dentist that they can take her to. They feel badly that she has lost a tooth but are glad it was a "baby tooth."

Prognosis
The prognosis is good for Maria. Generally, the premature loss of a maxillary anterior primary incisor will not have long-term adverse effects on speech

(Gable et al., 1995) or the ability to chew. The effect the initial trauma has on the developing permanent incisors is unknown until these teeth develop further.

Child #2: Avulsion of a Permanent Incisor

Summary of trauma findings:
- · No signs or symptoms of nondental trauma or child abuse.
- · Complete avulsion of maxillary left permanent central incisor.
- · No other hard or soft tissue trauma except minor damage to the gingival tissue immediately surrounding the tooth socket.

Making the Diagnosis

Prashant has an avulsed permanent incisor with an extra-oral time of only 15 minutes. There are no other hard or soft tissue injuries and no medical contraindications to treatment.

Management

Recommended dental treatment: Despite Prashant's pain, you go ahead and put the tooth back into the socket after first rinsing it off carefully with tap water to remove a bit of debris and being careful to hold the tooth by the crown, without touching the root. You then have him hold the tooth in place. You confirm with his father that his tetanus immunization is up to date.

If you hadn't been able to get Prashant's cooperation or, due to other problems, you couldn't replant the tooth, you would have stored the tooth in milk (or Hank's balanced salt solution) and sent him to the dentist immediately. Note: if the tooth is left to dry for an extended time, it may be contraindicated to attempt replantation.

You next call a nearby dentist with the family's permission and send them to that dental office immediately for stabilization, pulp therapy, and management of any other complications. If the tooth hadn't been retrieved, you would have obtained a dental radiograph to confirm that the missing tooth has not been intruded, out of sight, into the gingiva and alveolar bone.

Prognosis

The prognosis for replanted permanent teeth is very dependent on the amount of extra-alveolar time. This is especially true if the root is left to dry during this time. With extended extra-oral time, the possibility for the root to ankylose directly to the alveolar bone is significantly increased.

Complications

At least two significant complications may occur with replanted permanent teeth (American Academy of Pediatric Dentistry, 2008). First, if the tooth becomes ankylosed, the root usually begins to resorb over a period of time. In addition, a tooth that is ankylosed and cannot be moved orthodontically might necessitate a compromise to the orthodontic treatment plan. Secondly, the tooth will need root canal treatment. If this is not done, the pulp will usually abscess. **You tell the father that when he returns home, he will need periodic dental follow-up to be sure the replanted tooth is not developing complications.**

Child #3: Crown Fracture of a Permanent Incisor

Summary of trauma findings:
- No signs or symptoms of nondental trauma or child abuse.
- Fracture of the enamel and dentin of the maxillary right permanent central incisor.
- Fracture of the enamel and dentin of the maxillary left permanent central incisor; however, on the left incisor, the fracture is large enough to expose the dental pulp.
- No other hard or soft tissue trauma.

Making the Diagnosis

Johnny clearly has a crown fracture without pulp exposure of the maxillary right incisor. He also has a crown fracture with pulp exposure of the maxillary left incisor. There do not appear to be other hard or soft tissue injures. Neither are there any medical contraindications to the proposed treatment.

Management

Recommended dental treatment: You send an aide to the school to get Johnny's bicycle and try to find the broken tooth fragment. If she finds it, you will send it to the dentist in a glass of water. You ask the mother to give you the name of Johnny's dentist so that you can call ahead and arrange for him to be seen immediately. In the interest of time, and because of your school setting, you will not try to obtain a dental radiograph to confirm the extent of the crown fracture and to rule out additional fractures to the roots and surrounding bone.

The school health aide was not able to find any tooth fragments and Johnny's mom takes him to the dental office. Before leaving, you alert her that the pediatric dentist will treat each tooth differently in light of the fact that one tooth has the complication of a pulp exposure. Dental treatment will consist of managing the dental pulp conditions and restoring the fractured tooth.

You also confirm with her that his tetanus immunizations are up to date.

Prognosis

The prognosis for this type of trauma is usually good. However, the possible complications are presented in the next section.

Complications

There are two areas for complications. First, the dental pulp may have been irreversible damaged. It is often unknown until some time after this initial period if the pulp will suffer necrosis. If it does, usually it can be treated with root canal therapy. Secondly, the crown of the tooth may need additional repair from time to time because even the best of dental restorations may not last a lifetime.

How would you follow up with these children as a primary care provider? ■

The follow-up plan and the educational plan are the same for all three children: Confirm with the child/caregiver that follow-up dental care was obtained and confirm with the dentist that appropriate follow-up care was given.

Educational Plan

- Counsel the child and caregiver about the appropriate age-related trauma prevention strategies.
- Encourage the child/caregiver to become proactively established with a pediatric dentist for regular dental care.

Key Points from These Cases

1. The assessment of dental trauma should also consider head trauma findings.
2. The immediate reimplantation of an avulsed tooth depends upon whether it was a primary or permanent tooth.
3. Preservation of an avulsed permanent tooth requires a physiologic medium for transport to the dentist.
4. Fractured teeth are also important to assess; evidence that the pulp has been exposed makes the case more emergent.

REFERENCES

American Academy of Pediatric Dentistry Council on Clinical Affairs. (2008). American Academy of Pediatric Dentistry reference manual: guideline on management of acute dental trauma. *Pediatric Dentistry, 29*(7),168–172.

Andreasen, J. O., & Andreasen, F. M. (1994). *Textbook and color atlas of traumatic injuries to the teeth* (3rd ed.). Munksgaard-Copenhagen, Denmark: Mosby.

Andreasen, J. O., Andreasen, F. M., Bakland, L. K., & Flores, M. T. (2003). *Traumatic dental injuries* (2nd ed.). Munksgaard, Denmark: Blackwell.

Bastone, E. B., Freer, T. J., & McNamara, J. R. (2000). Epidemiology of dental trauma: a review of the literature. *Australian Dental Journal, 4*, 2–9.

Borum, M. K., & Andreasen, J. O. (1998). Sequelae of trauma to primary maxillary incisors. I. Complications in the primary dentition. *Dental Traumatology, 1*, 31–44.

Cavalleri, G., & Zerman, N. (1995). Traumatic crown fractures in permanent incisors with immature roots: a follow-up study. *Dental Traumatology, 1*, 294–296.

Christophersen, P., Freund, M., & Harild, L. (2005). Avulsion of primary teeth and sequelae on the permanent successors. *Dental Traumatology, 21*, 320–323.

Gable, T. O., Kumner, A. W., Lee, L., Creaghead, N. A., & Moore, L. J. (1995). Premature loss of the maxillary primary incisors: effect on speech production. *Journal of Dentistry for Children, 62*, 173–179.

Zamon, E. L., & Kenny, D. J. (2001). Replantation of avulsed primary incisors: a risk-benefit assessment. *Journal of the Canadian Dental Association, 67*, 386.

Chapter 27

The Preschooler with Urinary Urgency and Urinary Incontinence

Shelly J. King

Children may not present with the typical complaints for a urinary tract infection (UTI), making them a challenge to diagnose and treat. In this case study the child has no complaints, but the parents state the child has urinary urgency and incontinence. As you further investigate, you find the child has infrequent urination and hard stools. She also has a prior visit to the emergency room for similar symptoms and fever.

A UTI is a bacterial infection of the kidneys, bladder, or a combination of both. It is a common cause of febrile illness in children. It can be challenging to diagnose because young children cannot communicate symptoms well. Prompt diagnosis and treatment are essential to minimize acute morbidity and decrease the risk of progressive renal dysfunction. The origin of a urinary tract infection is often unclear. Detailed history, complete data collection, and a physical examination are necessary to provide an individualized plan of care.

Educational Objectives

1. Apply the guidelines for urinary tract infection management.
2. Determine appropriate interview questions for gathering pertinent data.
3. Discuss variables affecting management, including age, sex, presentation of illness, compliance, and cultural and socioeconomic factors.
4. Identify appropriate testing.

Case Presentation and Discussion

Ashley Jones is a 4-year-old white female who presents in the pediatric clinic for complaints of urinary urgency and foul-smelling urine. Mom describes symptoms of rushing to the bathroom and minor urine leakage during the day over the last 48 hours. She also wet the bed the last two nights. She does not complain of pain with urination and there has been no fever.

Mom reports her concern regarding multiple urinary tract infections over the last year. One infection was associated with fever, flank pain, and vomiting. Mom is very frustrated that this continues to be a problem.

What aspects of the physical examination will be most important? ■

Physical Examination

Upon physical examination, you find Ashley has no specific abnormalities. Her abdomen is soft and nontender; there is no evidence of a mass. Stool is palpable in the right lower quadrant. She denies costal-vertebral angle (CVA) tenderness. You palpate her lower spine and it is normal. There is no visual evidence of any abnormality, no sacral dimple, discolorations, asymmetry, or hair patch. Her feet are not high-arched and her toes are straight. She has no complaints of back pain, lower extremity pain, or weakness. She has full range of motion and ambulates with a normal gait. The external genitalia yield separate urethral and vaginal openings; the perineum is normal aside from some minor irritation. (In males who present with UTI, the scrotal examination is important to rule out epididymitis.) Her vital signs are within normal limits. She is afebrile.

Pathophysiology of Urinary Tract Infection

The majority of urinary tract infections have an ascending route of origin. Despite good perineal hygiene, the perineum and urethral meatus are colonized by intestinal flora that can ascend the urethra into the bladder. Bacterial virulence factors and host susceptibility contribute to development and severity of infection. *Escherichia coli* accounts for approximately 75–95% of urinary tract infections (Gaylord & Starr, 2009).

Disturbances of bowel and bladder function (dysfunctional elimination syndrome) are common in children with urinary tract infections. A detailed elimination history is important to determine and treat this disorder. Successful management of urinary tract infections will not occur if the elimination pattern is not addressed (Koff, Wagner, & Jayanthni, 1998). Symptoms associated with dysfunctional elimination syndrome (DES) include urinary incontinence, fecal incontinence, constipation, dysuria, urinary frequency and urgency, posturing (such as squatting or crossing legs tightly) to avoid accidents, and infrequent or delayed voiding.

Obstruction and other anomalies of the urinary tract can present with UTI; these infections can be difficult to manage. Vesicoureteral reflux (VUR) is a condition of retrograde flow of urine from the bladder to the kidney. It is graded in order of severity I through V. Children with VUR may be at higher risk for significant infection and resultant renal scarring. Decreased renal function and hypertension can result from renal scarring. Approximately one third of siblings of children with reflux also have reflux, and 50% of offspring of mothers with reflux also have reflux (Elder, 2007).

Epidemiology of Urinary Tract Infection

Bacteriuria can occur in all age groups; in the first year of life it is more common in males, especially if uncircumcised (1:47 compared to circumcised 1:445) (Schöen, Colby, & Ray, 2000). After the first year, it is more likely in females (10:1) (Elder, 2007). The short urethra is an accepted explanation for the increased incidence of UTI in girls. By age 11, it is estimated that 1% of males and 3% of females will be affected by UTIs (Alon, 2006).

Social and Economic Factors

Urinary tract infections are common in children. Parents often do not understand the importance of antibiotic use and follow-up. Some believe that home remedies such as cranberry juice effectively treat urinary tract infections. Lack of insurance and difficulties with transportation also often preclude follow-up. These issues need to be respectfully addressed.

Are there lab tests you want to order? ■

With the symptoms Ashley presents with, a clean-catch, midstream urine specimen would be appropriate to obtain now.

Her urinalysis is leukocyte and nitrite positive today.

What other questions do you want to ask the parents and child to help make the diagnosis? ■

You want to ask the following questions:

- How often does the child void? (Elimination disturbances)
- Does your child have any stool incontinence or constipation? (Elimination disturbance)
- Does the child have posturing behaviors, or attempts to delay voiding? (Elimination disturbance)
- What symptoms has the child experienced previously?

You need to differentiate between upper tract infection (pyelonephritis) and lower tract bladder infections:

- How were previous urine specimens obtained? Did the child urinate in a cup or was she catheterized? Where were the specimens obtained? (Rule out specimen contamination; the provider needs to determine if the specimens show true infection or a contaminate.)
- Is there any family history of renal anomalies? (Determine genetic risk for renal anomalies.)
- Does the child have any lower extremity pain or weakness? Are there any gait problems? (Neurologic disorders)
- Have you tried any home remedies to help your child? (Homeopathic approach)

Mom responds that Ashley voids infrequently; she sometimes goes up to 2 hours after awakening in the morning before she urinates. During the day, she holds it until the last minute and sometimes they see her squatting or crossing her legs to avoid going to the bathroom. She has occasional damp spots in her underwear during the day, but is typically dry at night; during infections she has accidents both day and night.

The first infection was approximately 9 to 10 months ago. A clean-catch midstream specimen grew 100,000 *Escherichia coli*. She did not have a fever, flank pain, nausea, or vomiting. Mom had taken her to a clinic because of the incontinence. She was treated with amoxicillin and her symptoms resolved. Six weeks later, mom noticed she had an episode of nocturnal enuresis. At that time, a repeat culture was done, which grew less than 50,000 *Escherichia coli*. She was treated again, but still had occasional day accidents.

Mom reports Ashley's bowel movements are infrequent and hard to pass. She has stool streaks in her underwear.

Approximately 2 months prior to this clinic visit, Ashley was seen in the local emergency department with a fever of 102°F. She was complaining of generalized abdominal pain, nausea, and a headache. She vomited several times. She was started on antibiotics and treated as an outpatient. Her urine culture grew greater than 100,000 *Klebsiella pneumoniae*.

Mom had a history of urinary tract infections as a child, but does not recall being evaluated.

Making the Diagnosis

The differential diagnoses for urinary tract infection include differentiating among upper urinary tract infections (pyelonephritis), lower urinary tract infections, external perineal irritation, foreign body insertion, vaginitis, pin worms, renal calculi, hypercalcuria, constipation, and structural anomalies of the urinary tract such as obstruction or vesicoureteral reflux.

History and physical findings are consistent with the diagnoses of 1) a urinary tract infection, and 2) dysfunctional elimination syndrome. The urinalysis is both leukocyte and nitrite positive and should be sent to the laboratory for culture and sensitivity.

How a specimen is collected directly correlates to its validity: most valid is suprapubic bladder aspirate, second is sterile urethral catheterization, and third is clean-catch midstream. The least reliable is the bagged specimen (Gaylord & Starr, 2009).

Ashley has no known allergies. She has delayed voiding, posturing to prevent enuresis, and constipation, which are symptoms consistent with dysfunctional elimination syndrome. There is one documented upper tract infection with fever, nausea, and vomiting. Pyelonephritis may be indicative of structural abnormality and warrants additional evaluation. Structural abnormalities such as VUR, obstruction, or other anatomical defects may present as urinary tract infection (Gaylord & Starr, 2009).

Management

The treatment plan is determined by the findings of urinary tract infection, dysfunctional elimination syndrome, and any complications such as vesicoureteral reflux. It will be customized to the child's age.

The goals are to:

- Protect the kidneys from damage.
- Prevent urinary tract infections.
- Resolve dysfunctional elimination syndrome.
- Monitor vesicoureteral reflux.
- Educate the family on how to achieve the above goals.

What additional studies are necessary to confirm the diagnosis? ■

Urine culture and sensitivity are indicated to identify the causative organism and specific antibiotic management. Febrile infection and more than one infection in a child less than 5 years of age require evaluation by a renal and bladder ultrasound and voiding cystourethrogram (Shortliffe, 2007).

What is the first thing you need to do to manage her UTI? ■

Medications

Ashley should be started on antibiotics empirically. Two months ago she was seen in the ED, at which time her urine specimen grew greater than 100,000 colonies of *Klebsiella pneumoniae*. She was treated in the ED with a single dose of ceftriaxone and discharged on oral cephalexin. The culture was sensitive to the prescribed treatment and sulfamethoxazole. Today's clinical symptoms are consistent with a lower tract bladder infection; she does not have fever, flank pain, nausea, or vomiting, which are symptoms of pyelonephritis. **She is started on trimethoprim-sulfa; when she finishes the treatment dose, she will be started on prophylaxis.** Trimethoprim-sulfa is a good choice; it is inexpensive, does not need to be refrigerated, has a relatively long shelf life, and is unlikely to cause gastrointestinal upset. The side effect profile overall is low.

Antibiotic prophylaxis is appropriate for a child with a history of a febrile infection, until she has been evaluated fully. She is at risk for anatomical abnormalities and should be maintained on prophylaxis until her X-ray evaluation is complete (Gaylord & Starr, 2009).

Further Diagnostic Studies

A renal and bladder ultrasound is used to rule out kidney abnormalities, and a voiding cystourethrogram is obtained to rule out vesicoureteral reflux or bladder abnormalities. In children, it is important to discover anatomical sources for bacterial persistence that may necessitate surgical intervention (Shortliffe, 2007). A renal and bladder ultrasound and voiding cystourethrogram should be obtained in any child with a febrile urinary tract infection, any male child, and any infant or child under age 5 (Shortliffe). Patients with hydronephrosis or grade IV–V VUR should be referred to a pediatric urologist.

An X-ray evaluation was obtained. An ultrasound shows normal kidneys, with a significant postvoid residual. A voiding cystourethrogram (VCUG) shows grade II vesicoureteral reflux into the right renal pelvis. She did not empty her bladder on VCUG and has a spinning-top urethra, the classic finding of detrusor sphincter dyssynergia. Detrusor sphincter dyssynergia is a lack of coordination between the bladder contraction and relaxation of the external sphincter. This discoordination leads to incomplete evacuation of the bladder. A KUB (kidneys, ureters, and bladder) X-ray typically precedes the VCUG, and in Ashley's case reveals a moderate stool burden. Constipation may provoke detrusor-sphincter activity. The bony structure of the spine appears normal. The X-ray evaluation is consistent with dysfunctional elimination and vesicoureteral reflux.

How do you plan to manage her dysfunctional elimination syndrome? ◾

Dysfunctional Elimination Syndrome

Dysfunctional elimination must be addressed regardless of the results of her X-ray evaluation. She needs to be placed on a timed voiding regimen during the day. She is in the habit of holding her urine to the point of having urge incontinence. Often these children have difficulty relaxing the external sphincter and do not take time to void to completion. This is complicated by constipation, which increases colonization of the intestinal flora and may create difficulty with voiding to completion.

You explain to the mother that Ashley's dysfunctional elimination will be managed by placing her on a strict timed voiding schedule during the day, every 2 hours by the clock, whether she has the urge to urinate or not. You suggest using a simple behavioral modification chart with days of the week and times of the day for scheduled voiding, which can be created with stickers to recognize her cooperation with the plan.

During today's visit, Ashley is trained in the proper toileting posture to facilitate relaxation of the external sphincter and voiding to completion (Yeung, Sihoe, & Bauer, 2007). She is instructed to sit on the toilet with her legs widely separated. She should be sitting comfortably on the toilet with her feet supported. In small children this requires a seat adapter.

For constipation, she will be given a cleanout regimen, a pediatric Fleet enema given once a day for 2 to 3 days. A stool softener is also started and can be tapered as the stools become normal. There are many effective bowel management programs. The family is instructed on a high-fiber diet and increasing fluids during the day.

Urinary Tract Infection and Vesicoureteral Reflux

Ashley is started on trimethoprim-sulfamethoxazole treatment dose and then will be maintained on prophylaxis. Trimethoprim-sulfamethoxazole can be used in children older than 2 months of age. The treatment dose is based on trimethoprim 6–12 mg/kg/day given BID for 10 days. The prophylaxis dose is also based on trimethoprim, but at 1–2 mg/kg/day. Trimethorprim-sulfamethoxzzole diffuses into vaginal fluid and decreases bacterial colonization.

Macrodantin or furadantin elixir is another effective treatment and/or prophylactic agent. It does not achieve high blood levels and should not be used for systemic or febrile infections. The most common side effect is gastrointestinal upset. To help prevent this problem, the medication should be given with food. The liquid form is not tolerated well by children. The capsules can be opened and sprinkled on applesauce, yogurt, or pudding. It can be given to children older than 2 months of age, and the treatment dose is 5–7 mg/kg/day given QID. Prophylaxis is 1–2 mg/kg/day in a single dose.

Amoxicillin is also used to treat urinary tract infections and is often used for prophylaxis in children under 3 months of age. It is tolerated well and has a low side effect profile, but can cause candidiasis in high doses. The suspension has to be refilled every 14 days, which makes it less convenient for families to use. Prophylaxis is 20 mg/kg/day in a single dose. Treatment dosing of amoxicillin is variable, based on age and severity of infection. Cephalosporins can also be used for treatment and/or prophylaxis.

Antibiotic management of pediatric UTIs is always done with caution. Age-related dosing restrictions, comorbid conditions, and severity of infection must be considered before treatment is recommended. These issues also affect the decision of whether to utilize inpatient intravenous therapy versus outpatient oral management. Children who appear toxic and those under 2 months of age who have suspected pyelonephritis should receive intravenous treatment. Ampicillin and aminoglycoside (if no known drug allergy) are started until culture and sensitivity results are final (Brown, Burns, & Cummings, 2002). Fluoroquinolones have been approved by the Food and Drug Administration (FDA) for the treatment of complicated UTIs in children. In children who present with a febrile UTI but do not appear toxic, 1 to 2 days of intramuscular ceftriaxone can provide coverage until culture results are final and appropriate oral therapy is determined

The family should be educated on the signs and symptoms of a UTI at this appointment. They should be able to differentiate between a significant upper tract or kidney infection and lower tract symptoms or bladder infection. With a history of vesicoureteral reflux, at the first sign of infection the child should be evaluated. The signs and symptoms of UTI should be revisited when discussing the X-ray evaluation with the family. If a urinalysis is positive, treatment should be started before culture results have been received to prevent the development of pyelonephritis. Vesicoureteral reflux should be evaluated by ultrasound and VCUG every 12 to 18 months. As long as the child has good overall renal growth, no evidence of scarring, no infections while on prophylaxis, and no worsening reflux, the child can be managed conservatively. If they have breakthrough infections or upper tract changes, alternate management would need to be considered. This would warrant a referral to a pediatric urologist. Other variables that might lead to surgical management are allergies to multiple antibiotics and poor compliance with medical management.

Parent Education

You provide patient education as follows:

- Explain the diagnosis, pathophysiology, and typical progression of the disorder.
- Explain that antibiotics are necessary to hopefully prevent urinary tract infection. They do not treat or resolve vesicoureteral reflux.
- Discuss the use of oral antibiotics, the importance of giving them on a routine basis, and completing any treatment antibiotics that are prescribed.
- Discuss potential side effects of antibiotics and any evaluation that is necessary.
- Reassure the family that with urinary tract infection prevention, the child will likely do well. It does require patience, however, to work with children this young to modify behavior.
- Provide positive reinforcement to the child for practicing the toileting habits that improve bladder and bowel emptying.
- Instruct parents to bring the child to the clinic for prompt evaluation of urine if there are any signs or symptoms of urinary tract infection.
- Discuss the importance of dysfunctional elimination management to prevent infection and promote VUR resolution.

Ashley is only 4 years old, but you tell her in simple terms about:

- the specific toilet posture to facilitate emptying (have the child demonstrate in the office)
- the importance of not delaying urination or stooling
- the use of a chart and stickers to reward her efforts
- the importance of an appropriate diet and fluid intake to decrease symptoms of constipation

When do you want to see this patient back again? ■

Renal ultrasound and voiding cystourethrogram should be obtained about 10 days after beginning treatment of a UTI. A time should be scheduled to review results with family, recheck the urine, and determine compliance with dysfunctional elimination management and antibiotic prophylaxis. An abdominal examination should be performed to assess for constipation. The bladder should not be percussible after voiding if the child is emptying well.

At the next visit 2 weeks later, Ashley is taking her antibiotics on a daily basis. She has been working hard on voiding every 2 hours and has been practicing the voiding techniques to help empty her bladder. Her abdomen is soft and nontender, and there is no evidence of a mass indicating constipation. The parents report that she is having a daily bowel movement that is soft and not painful. Her bladder is not percussible, and her urinalysis today is negative. Renal ultrasound and VCUG results are normal.

The plan will be to see her back in 6 to 8 weeks. If she continues to do well, then surveillance could be spread out to 6 months and then a year. At that point, her ultrasound and VCUG should be repeated.

Complications

There are rare cases in which children with dysfunctional elimination, UTI, and reflux have symptoms that persist or worsen, even with appropriate management. This outcome could indicate a neurologic abnormality, so evaluation of the lower spine by MRI may need to be done. Other symptoms that can be associated with neurologic issues are chronic back and lower extremity pain, gait abnormalities, and stool incontinence. Physical evidence of bony abnormalities can sometimes be seen on plain radiographs, or as sacral dimples, gluteal asymmetry, lower spine discolorations, or a sacral hair patch.

Key Points from the Case

1. Guidelines simplify the care of recurrent urinary tract infections, vesicoureteral reflux, and dysfunctional elimination syndrome.
2. Treatment of dysfunctional elimination syndrome, reflux, and urinary tract infection requires an understanding of the pathophysiology and development of the patient and a family care plan.
3. Urinary tract infections will not improve unless dysfunctional elimination is addressed.
4. Significant abnormalities of the urinary tract can present with urinary tract infection and must be kept in mind when evaluating a patient.
5. Antimicrobial management is dependent on age, comorbid conditions, and severity of infection.

REFERENCES

Alon, U. S. (2006). Urinary tract infection and perinephric/intranephric abscess. In F. D. Burg, J. R Ingelfinger, R. A. Polin, & A. A. Gershon (Eds.), *Current pediatric therapy* (18th ed., pp. 594–596). Philadelphia: Saunders.

Brown, J., Burns, J., & Cummings, P. (2002). Ampicillin use in infant fever: a systematic review. *Archives of Pediatric and Adolescent Medicine, 156*, 27–32.

Elder, J. S. (2007). Urologic disorders in infants and children. In R. E. Behrman, R. M. Kliegman, & H. B. Jensen (Eds.), *Nelson's textbook of pediatrics* (18th ed., pp. 2221–2272). Philadelphia: Saunders.

Gaylord, N. M., & Starr, N. B. (2009). Genitourinary disorders. In C. Burns, M. A. Brady, A. M. Dunn, & N. Starr (Eds.), *Pediatric primary care* (4th ed., pp. 866–905). Philadelphia: Elsevier.

Koff, S. A., Wagner, T. T., & Jayanthni, V. R. (1998). The relationship among dysfunction elimination syndromes, primary vesicoureteral reflux and urinary tract infections in children. *Journal of Urology, 160*, 1019–1022.

Schöen, E. J., Colby, C. J., & Ray, G. T. (2000). Newborn circumcision decreases incidence and costs of urinary tract infections during the first year of life. *Pediatrics, 105*(4), 789–793.

Shortliffe, L. D. (2007). Infection and inflammation of the pediatric genitourinary tract. In A. J. Wein, L. R. Kavoussi, A. C. Novick, A. W. Partin, & C. A. Peters (Eds.), *Campbell-Walsh urology* (pp. 3252–3254). Philadelphia: Saunders.

Yeung, C. K., Sihoe, J. D., & Bauer, S. B. (2007). Voiding dysfunction in children: non-neurogenic and neurogenic. In A. J. Wein, L. R. Kavoussi, A. C. Novick, A. W. Partin, & C. A. Peters (Eds.), *Campbell-Walsh urology* (pp. 3604–3655). Philadelphia: Saunders.

Chapter 28

The 15-Year-Old Girl Who Wants Birth Control

Deborah Stiffler

Prescribing contraception to adolescent females can be a difficult and time-consuming task. Assisting the adolescent to choose a contraceptive that is right for her, and also finding one that she can use consistently and correctly to prevent pregnancy and help her to prevent any sexually transmitted infections, can be challenging.

Educational Objectives

1. Differentiate among the types of contraceptives currently available.
2. Compare the risks and benefits of each contraceptive.
3. Choose a safe and effective contraceptive method for a patient.
4. Formulate an individualized management plan for a patient.

Case Presentation and Discussion

Jaime Hoskins, a 15-year-old African American young woman, presents to your office requesting birth control. Jaime relates to you that she has been sexually active for about a year. She has had two different partners in that year, but she was only having sex with one at a time. She has been with her current boyfriend, Blair, for almost 3 months. Blair is 18 years old. As far as she knows, he is only having sex with her. She does not know how many partners he has had previously. They usually use a condom when they have sex, but sometimes Blair isn't in the mood, so they don't use one. Jaime tells you the reason she has come in today is that she and Blair recently had a scare. They were using a condom, but it slipped off during sex. When her period was a few days late, she was sure she was pregnant. Jaime's mom is waiting for her in the waiting room; she brought Jaime in today thinking that Jaime had a yeast infection. Jaime does not want her mom to know that she is here for birth control because "she would just freak" if she knew that Jaime was sexually active.

What questions would you ask Jaime to expand on the above information? ■

Jaime's immunizations are current, she has had no surgeries, has no allergies, and is taking no medications.

Jaime's family is fairly healthy. Her mother is 33 years old and somewhat overweight, but otherwise, she is healthy. Her maternal grandmother is deceased from a stroke at age 61. Jaime's maternal grandfather is currently 68 years old and has adult onset diabetes. Her sisters are healthy. Jaime does not know anything about her father's side of the family.

Jaime started her periods at age 11. They have always been regular, about 26–28 days apart, and they last for 5 days. Jaime relates moderate to heavy flow for the first 3 days, saturating three or four maxi pads each day. She also has moderate cramping with her periods. The cramping does not cause her to stay home from school, but she is "not worth much" on those days. Other than occasional condom use, she has never used any methods of birth control nor has she had a pap smear. Her last menstrual period was 2 weeks ago, and she and Blair have had unprotected intercourse since then.

Social history: Jaime is a sophomore at the local high school. She is on the cheerleading squad and plays volleyball on the school team. She lives at home with her mother and two younger sisters, ages 14 and 11. Her parents are divorced. She sees her father occasionally. She denies using street drugs and occasionally drinks alcohol, mostly beer on the weekends. She admits to being drunk twice, and doesn't smoke.

What findings are important on the physical examination? ■

You chart her examination as follows: Vital signs: temperature 98.2°F, oral; blood pressure 110/58; pulse 82; respirations 16; height 64 inches; weight 137 pounds; body mass index (BMI) 23.5.

Physical examination: EENT WNL; thyroid not enlarged; heart RRR without murmurs; lungs clear to P&A; back no CVA tenderness; abdomen soft, nontender, no splenohepatomegaly. She has a negative Homan's sign, bilaterally. Pelvic: escutcheon, normal female; vulva without lesions; vagina moist, normal leukorrhea; cervix small, nulliparous; uterus anteverted, small, no tenderness on palpation; adnexa without cysts or masses, no tenderness to palpation.

What testing should be done? ■

In this case, the following laboratory testing should be done:

- *Urine human chorionic gonadotropin:* An easy test for pregnancy that can be done quickly in the office.
- *Pap smear:* The newest guidelines from the American Cancer Society (ACS) state the first pap smear should be done by 3 years of initiation of intercourse or by the age of 21, whichever comes first (ACS, 2008).
- *Gonorrhea/chlamydia cultures:* Jaime is already sexually active and does not always use condoms, so she is at risk for currently having or acquiring a sexually transmitted infection in the future.
- *Hemoglobin/hematocrit count (H&H):* This will check for anemia due to Jaime's heavy menstrual periods.

You collect the specimens and send them off for laboratory studies.

After completing the history and physical, what information should you consider? ■

Jaime is in her adolescent years. This is a period of time when adolescents start to take risks. Risk-taking is a way for an adolescent to define and develop his or her identity. Healthy risk-taking, such as playing sports, seeking out new friends, or starting a job is a valuable experience (Ponton, 1997); however, adolescents frequently make unhealthy choices. Adolescents are at risk for behaviors such as drinking, smoking, drug use, reckless driving, unsafe sexual activity, disordered eating, self-mutilation, running away, stealing, and gang activity. Jaime does engage in occasional binge drinking. Alcohol decreases inhibitions, and this could put Jaime at risk for unintended sexual activity, decrease the potential for using a condom, or affect her use of other contraceptives. Adolescents under the influence of alcohol or drugs may take chances with their personal safety (U.S. Department of Health and Human Services, 2008). Currently, Jaime is engaging in another unhealthy behavior: unprotected sexual activity. This is an important area to discuss with Jaime.

It is important to have Jaime start some method of contraception. However, adolescents tend to be inconsistent users of contraception (Frost, Singh, & Finer, 2007). They can be forgetful, not taking their oral contraceptive pills or not keeping a condom with them when there is the potential for intercourse (Frost et al., 2007). Adolescents who have initiated sexual activity early in their teen years have the potential for multiple sexual partners. Jaime has stated that she is only having intercourse with Blair right now, but she has been sexually active with someone previously. Plus, there is no way to know how many partners Blair has had. When Jaime has sexual intercourse with Blair, she is essentially having intercourse with every other person he has had sex with (Stiffler, Sims, & Stern, 2007). She is at risk for HIV/AIDS along with other sexually transmitted infections (STIs). Adolescent females are biologically more at risk for STIs than adolescent males (Chambers & Rew, 2003). During the adolescent years, the transformation zone of the cervix is lower in the cervical canal. This is the area where the cells are changing from squamous epithelium to columnar epithelium, and it is especially vulnerable to infection and disease (Moore et al., 2005).

Jaime is very active, playing on her school volleyball and cheer teams. She travels with her teams frequently, which could cause her schedule to be erratic. Any contraceptive that would need a strict schedule could be affected.

Another risk that you must consider for Jaime is that of partner violence. Blair refuses to use condoms at times; this could potentially cause discord in the relationship. Women who do not feel that they have power in their relationships are less likely to use condoms with each sexual act (Harvey, Bird, Galavotti, Duncan, & Greenberg, 2002). Although Jaime has not said anything today that warrants concern, it would be advisable to consider this possibility for her.

Jaime is not communicating with her mother throughout this situation. Although this is not unusual for adolescents, Jaime might find her mother's insights helpful because Jaime's mother was an adolescent when Jaime was born. When adolescents do talk with their parents about contraceptive use, they are more likely to consistently use contraceptives (Manlove, Ryan, & Franzetta, 2003).

Jaime suffers from menorrhagia and dysmenorrhea with her monthly menses. Some contraceptive methods could potentially decrease her symptoms. It would be important to discuss these with Jaime and assist her to choose a contraceptive that could decrease her flow of blood and alleviate some, if not all, of her cramping.

Jaime would like to prevent a pregnancy without jeopardizing her future ability to have children. Her contraceptive needs should be effective, reversible, not linked to coitus, and assist in preventing sexually transmitted infections. Adolescents at this stage have the cognitive ability to make good decisions; however, they do not always make the most appropriate decisions in light of future consequences (Commendador, 2003). When adolescents have higher self-esteem, they tend to make decisions that are better for them (Commendador). Jaime, however, tends to allow Blair to decide whether or not he wants to use a condom when they have sex. This is not uncommon because Blair is older than Jaime; however, this means the chances that they will use contraception with intercourse decreases. Older partners tend to have a greater influence on the adolescent (Manlove et al., 2003).

What contraceptive options should you consider? What are the advantages and disadvantages of each option? Which would be reasonable options for Jaime? ◼

A list of possible contraceptives is provided in Table 28-1, and discussed here:

- Abstinence
  - *Advantages:* Nonhormonal, no need to remember to take a pill every day.
  - *Disadvantages:* There are no risks to abstinence. except that it requires self control under all circumstances. This is the only 100% effective and safe method of contraception, if followed (Caufield, 2004; Kowal, 2007). Once an adolescent has become sexually active, it is unlikely that he or she will cease having intercourse, especially if he or she continues in the same relationship (Chambers & Rew, 2003).
  - Option for Jaime: Although a good option for any adolescent, this is not likely an option Jaime will choose.
- Combined estrogen/progesterone (oral, transdermal, transvaginal)
  - *Advantages:* Highly effective in preventing pregnancy when taken correctly; not related to coitus; rapid return to fertility after discontinuation; very safe when prescribed for appropriate users; can be

Table 28-1   Types of Contraception
• Abstinence
• Combined estrogen/progesterone
○ Combined oral contraceptive pills (oral)
○ Ortho Evra patch (transdermal)
○ Vaginal ring (transvaginal)
• Progesterone only
○ Depo-Provera (injectable)
○ Progestin-only pills (oral)
• Barrier methods/spermicidal
○ Condoms (male or female)
○ Diaphragm
○ Sponge
○ Various spermicides
• Intrauterine devices
○ Paraguard (nonhormonal)
○ Mirena (progestin)
• Fertility awareness/natural family planning
○ Sympto-Thermal
○ Calendar
• Permanent contraception
○ Bilateral tubal ligation
• Emergency contraception

used throughout the reproductive years; decreased maternal deaths; reduction in risk of ectopic pregnancy; decrease in dysmenorrhea; decrease in menorrhagia; reduction in premenstrual syndrome (PMS) symptoms; reduction in endometrial and ovarian cancer risks; decrease in benign breast conditions; improvement of androgen-sensitivity or androgen-excess conditions (such as PCOS).

- *Disadvantages:* Must be taken consistently and correctly to be effective; storage, access, lack of privacy; no protection against STIs. Common side effects include nausea, vomiting, weight gain, decrease in libido, headaches, breast tenderness, and skin hyperpigmentation. The transdermal form may be linked to an increased risk of thromboembolic disease because of higher concentrations of estrogen in the system.

- *Contraindications:* Personal history of thrombosis, known clotting disorder, personal history of stroke or MI, labile hypertension, estrogen-sensitive malignancy, active liver disease, migraines with focal neurologic symptoms.

- *Complications:* Venous thromboembolism, myocardial infarction, stroke, hypertension, liver disease (Caufield, 2004; Nelson, 2007).
- Option for Jaime: Any one of these methods could be an option for Jaime, but not alone. These methods do not protect against STIs, so it would be essential for Jaime to also use condoms to decrease transmission of STIs.

- Progesterone only
  - *Advantages:* No estrogen; reversible; amenorrhea or scanty bleeding after prolonged use; improvement in dysmenorrhea, menorrhagia, premenstrual dysphoric disorder (PMDD), premenstrual symptoms, and endometriosis symptoms; decreased risk of endometrial or ovarian cancer; decreased risk of PID; compatible with breastfeeding. Depo Provera–specific: highly effective, discreet and private, not linked to coitus, requires user to remember only four times a year.
  - *Disadvantages:* Menstrual cycle irregularities; weight gain; depression; headaches; no protection against STIs. When taking progestin-only pills, they must be taken at almost the exact same time every day. Progestin-only pills are not as effective as combined oral contraceptive pills. Depo-Provera–specific: weight gain, prolonged return to fertility, adverse effect on lipids, decreased bone mineral density with prolonged use (Caufield, 2004; Raymond, 2007).
  - Option for Jaime: The progestin-only pills need to be taken precisely on time. Being an adolescent, this might not be the best option, plus Jaime is looking for an effective means of birth control. Depo-Provera, in contrast, is very effective; however, with decreased calcium absorption at the time when the most bone mass is being laid down, and the recommendation of not being on this method for more than 2 years, this might not be the optimal method for Jaime.

- Barrier methods/spermicides
  - *Advantages:* Male participation, no prescription needed, very inexpensive, effective in preventing pregnancy if used correctly with every intercourse, minimal side effects, provides some STI protection, no hormones.
  - *Disadvantages:* Reduces sensitivity, reduces spontaneity, male erection problems, lack of cooperation from the male, embarrassment about purchasing, not very effective with "typical use," latex allergy, some methods (diaphragm) need professional fitting (Cates & Raymond, 2007; Caufield, 2004; Warner & Steiner, 2007).
  - Option for Jaime: This is certainly an option for Jaime, along with another method. At the very least, she would need to use a condom with spermicide with every act of intercourse. Blair has been resistant to this at times. With whatever method Jaime chooses, she needs to use condoms in addition to help prevent STIs.

- Intrauterine device (Paraguard and Mirena)
  - *Advantages:* Highly effective, no user error, convenient, long-lasting (10 years for Paraguard, 5 years for Mirena), reversible, discreet, cost-effective with prolonged use, low incidence of side effects, independent of coitus.
    - *Paraguard:* Can remain in place for up to 10 years, nonhormonal, normal menstrual pattern continues.
    - *Mirena:* Can remain in place for up to 5 years, protective against endometrial cancer, reduces menstrual bleeding by 90%, 20% of users become amenorrheic, low incidence of progestin side effects.
  - *Disadvantages:* Menstrual problems, discomfort with insertion, expulsion of the device, perforation of the uterus, requires office visit with trained professional, high initial cost, no protection against STIs.
    - *Paraguard:* Can cause heavier menses with more severe cramping, especially the first few cycles.
    - *Mirena:* Irregular bleeding, especially during the first 6 months (Grimes, 2007; Caufield, 2004).
  - Option for Jaime: Although not necessary, most providers would prefer to place an IUD in someone who has previously borne a child because the uterus has been stretched. The Paraguard can cause increased bleeding and cramping. This is something that Jaime is already concerned with, so the Paraguard would not be recommended. The Mirena, which decreases bleeding, could possibly be an option, but the irregular bleeding early in use might be a deterrent.
- Fertility awareness/natural family planning
  - *Advantages:* No hormones, no side effects, enables a woman to understand her body's cycles, promotes cooperation between partners, can also be used to achieve pregnancy or to identify fertility problems, only method approved by the Catholic church.
  - *Disadvantages:* Methods require varying amounts of training and cost, which detracts from spontaneity; causes friction between partners if not in agreement; difficult to use if recent childbirth, breastfeeding, recent menarche, approaching menopause, recent discontinuation of a hormonal method, irregular cycles, or unable to interpret fertility signs (Caufield, 2004; Jennings & Arevalo, 2007).
  - Option for Jaime: This method takes training, enthusiasm for the method, and support from the partner. At Jaime's time of life, this is probably not a good method for her.
- Permanent sterilization
  - *Advantages:* Permanent, highly effective, safe, quick recovery, lack of significant long-term side effects, cost-effective, partner cooperation not required, not coitus linked.

- *Disadvantages:* Possibility of patient regret, difficult to reverse in the future, achieving pregnancy could require assistive reproductive techniques (Caufield, 2004).
- Option for Jaime: This is a permanent method, so it would not be an option for a 15-year-old girl.
- Emergency contraception
  - *Advantages:* To be used for contraceptive failure, error in withdrawal or periodic abstinence, rape, any unintended sperm exposure.
  - *Disadvantages:* Not to be considered ongoing contraception (Caufield, 2004; Stewart, Trussel, & Van Look, 2007).
  - Option for Jaime: In the incidence of method failure, emergency contraception could be an option, but not as an ongoing method of contraception.

Making the Diagnosis

Given her history and physical information, it is helpful to identify Jaime's risk factors. In this case, Jaime is at risk for unhealthy lifestyle choices such as unprotected sexual intercourse, STIs, partner violence, and binge drinking. These risks must be addressed. Also, due to her menorrhagia, Jaime is at risk of becoming anemic. Jaime should be encouraged to discuss these issues with her mother. Her mother could be a tremendous help for her in dealing with them.

Although her maternal grandmother had a stroke and her maternal grandfather has adult onset diabetes, these do not significantly alter Jaime's choices of contraception.

Management

After much discussion, Jaime decides she would like to try combined oral contraceptive pills (COCs).

You explain to Jaime what she needs to know regarding taking COCs, including how to take the pills, when to start the pills, risks and benefits, and warning signs of problems (Box 28-1). Providing accurate and understandable information relating to using the method of choice increases the chance that the contraception will be used properly and consistently, thus decreasing unwanted pregnancies (Frost et al., 2007). Explain that Jaime may also experience less bleeding during her period and less cramping. You could give her a nonsteroidal anti-inflammatory medication (such as Anaprox DS or ibuprofen) to decrease her pain from the cramping. A prescription for no more than 3 months of COCs should be given at this visit.

You explain to Jaime that her partner must also use a condom every time she has intercourse, even though she is taking COCs. This is to help prevent the transmission of STIs. You explain that using condoms every time does not prevent the transmission of all

Box 28-1   Instructions for Taking Combined Oral Contraceptive (COC) Pills

When you get home after having your prescription filled, make sure you read the package insert. There is a lot of information in there that is very helpful. It has directions for how to take the pills, what to do if you miss a pill, and warning signs of problems. Always keep a copy of the package insert tucked away in a drawer.

Most combined oral contraceptive pills come in a package with 28 pills in them. The first 21–24 pills are "active" pills, which means they have the estrogen and progesterone in them that prevent pregnancy. The 4–7 pills at the end of the package are "inert," meaning there is no medicine in them. They are there to remind you to keep taking a pill once every day. The last 4–7 pills are a different color from the "active" pills.

Starting Your Pills

There are three different ways to start taking COCs:

- *Sunday start method:* This means you take the very first pill in the package on the Sunday *following* the start of your period. If your period starts on Sunday, take your first pill that same day. Most pill packages are set up for a Sunday start. The theory behind this is that you will always start your pill packages on a Sunday and finish taking the last pill on a Saturday. You will probably start your period on the Tuesday or Wednesday following the last "active" pill in the pack. For most women, their period will finish before the weekend. If you choose this start method, you should use a back-up method of contraception (condom and/or spermicide) until you have taken at least seven consecutive active pills. I encourage my patients to use a back-up method for the entire first month they are taking their pills.

- *First day start:* This method has you start your first active pill on the first day of your menstrual period no matter what day of the week it is. Even though the majority of pill packages are set up for a Sunday start, they will usually have stickers with the days of the week on them that you can place on the package to remind you what day you are on. Start with the very first pill in the package. When using the first day start, you should not need a back-up method, but I still encourage my patients to use condoms for the first month they are on the pills.

- *Today start.* Take your first pill in the package today, no matter where you are in your cycle. You can only use this method if you are *ABSOLUTELY POSITIVE* that you are not pregnant. Start with the very first day of the package and take each one of the pills. Because you are starting your pills in the middle of your cycle, it is very common to have some break through bleeding for a while until your body matches the hormone cycle of the pills. If there is any way that you could possibly be pregnant, I do not recommend starting your pills this way.

Always remember: COCs prevent pregnancy. They do *NOT* protect against sexually transmitted infections. If there is any possibility that your partner has an infection, always use a condom along with your pills. Always using a condom is just a smart thing to do, anyway.

(continues)

Box 28-1   Instructions for Taking Combined Oral Contraceptive (COC) Pills (Continued)

Taking Your Pills

You need to take one pill every day at about the same time every day. You need to take it at a time when you will easily remember to take it. For some women, that is first thing in the morning. For others, it is the last thing at night. Try to take them when you can consistently take them at the same time (or close) every day. If you usually get up at the same time every day, that may be good. If you go to bed at the same time every night, that may work. You need to find a time that works for you and stick with it. Keep taking one pill each day until the end of your pack. When you start taking the "inert" pills, you know that your period should start in the next day or two. When you have taken the last pill in that package, start the next package the very next day.

Benefits

The nice thing about taking COCs is that your period will become very regular. You may be able to set your watch by it. You should be able to know what day, and maybe even what time it will start. That way you can always be prepared for it. You should notice less bleeding and less cramping with your periods. Depending on what pill you are taking, some women notice that they do not get as much acne as they had before. Others may not have as many PMS symptoms, like bloating, moodiness, and so on. Taking COCs helps to decrease your chances of some types of female cancer like ovarian and endometrial cancer (inside of the uterus). The research on whether COCs play any role in breast cancer is inconclusive.

Side Effects

It sometimes takes our bodies a few months to get used to being on COCs. It would not be unusual for you to feel some mild *nausea* or have some *breast tenderness*. If you take your pills at night or with a meal, the nausea should go away. If you keep taking your pills, the nausea and breast tenderness should go away on their own. Some women may have some *spotting* between their periods. Others may notice *mood changes* or *headaches*. If you get a headache that doesn't go away with a mild pain reliever and rest, call the office. If the headache is severe and won't go away, go to the emergency room. Most side effects resolve by themselves within 3 months. You need to keep taking your pills for at least 3 months. If you continue to have problems, you need to call the office and come in to see me.

Warning Signs

A warning sign is one that says something may really be wrong. If you have any of these signs, we want you to call the office right away or go to the emergency room. To help you remember them, we use the mnemonic ACHES:

   A: Abdominal pain (severe)

   C: Chest pain (severe), cough, shortness of breath

   H: Headache (severe), dizziness, weakness, or numbness

   E: Eye problems (vision loss or blurring, speech problems)

   S: Severe leg pain (calf or thigh)

   So remember ACHES!

Box 28-1   Instructions for Taking Combined Oral Contraceptive (COC) Pills (Continued)

Other Questions

If you forget to take an "active" pill, take it as soon as you remember it. Take your next pill at its usual time. That may mean that you are taking two pills at the same time. If you forget to take an "inert" pill, that is OK as long as you start your "active" pills at the normal time.

If you forget to take two pills in a row, take two pills as soon as you remember and then take two pills at the next scheduled time. That should catch you back up. It would not be unusual to have some spotting when you miss pills. You should also use a back-up method of contraception for 7 days.

If you miss more than two pills, take one "active" pill each day until you can talk to me. You should use a back-up method of contraception for the rest of the cycle.

Remember: COCs are only effective if you take them! If you forget pills, you put yourself at risk for pregnancy.

If you miss a period and have taken every pill on time on the right day, there is little chance that you could be pregnant. Go ahead and start your new package of pills when it is time. If you are concerned, or you miss a second period, call the office and come in for a pregnancy test, just to make sure you are not pregnant. If you have forgotten one or more pills and then miss a period, keep taking one pill each day and come in for a pregnancy test.

There are many different types of COCs, just like there are many different types of women. Not all pills work well for all women. Keep taking the pills that were prescribed for you for at least 3 months. If you are not feeling "right" or you are having side effects that are unpleasant, call and come in for an appointment. Sometimes we need to adjust the dosages. We are almost always able to find a pill that works well.

STIs, but it does decrease her risk. The only way to be 100% sure of no risk of STIs is with abstinence.

You also caution Jaime about the potential for partner violence, explaining that it is important that she should *never* feel pressured to do something that she doesn't want to do. Blair should *always* respect her right to say no to anything that doesn't feel right. She needs to talk to Blair ahead of time about what she will and will not do (U.S. Department of Health and Human Services, 2008). Some tips for healthy and safe relationships that you give her include getting to know a person by talking on the phone or at school before going out with him for the first time, going out with a group of friends to a public place, planning fun activities other than being alone, talking to her parents about the person and giving them the specifics on where she is going and when she will be home, and always carrying her cell phone or change to make a call, if necessary (U.S. Department of Health and Human Services).

Jaime has become drunk a couple of times, so you let her know that not everyone drinks. There are many teens who do not drink. It does not make a person cool to drink alcohol. She does not need to drink to have fun, be popular, or be comfortable with other people. In fact, alcohol can cause her to lose control over what happens to her and her body. She could end up in potentially dangerous situations. You also warn Jaime about the potential of people spiking her drink with a date rape drug (U.S. Department of Health and Human Services, 2008). You encourage Jaime to talk to her mother or another safe adult about what is going on in her life.

Research has shown that adolescent girls who talk and have meaningful communication with their parents are less likely to experiment with high risk behaviors (Stiffler et al., 2007).

What other issues would you like to discuss with Jaime? ■

You want to discuss the following with Jaime:

- *Healthy lifestyle habits:* Jaime should be encouraged to eat a nutritious diet following the U.S. government's food pyramid (U.S. Department of Agriculture, 2008). She should exercise 60 minutes on most days (U.S. Department of Health and Human Services, 2008). She should take a multivitamin every day that contains at least 400 micrograms of folic acid. Folic acid helps to prevent neural tube defects in children, and all women of childbearing age should make sure they get enough folic acid. She should be encouraged to keep a menstrual diary or keep track of her menses to note improvement after initiation of COCs or continued problems.
- *Healthy sexuality decisions:* Throughout the history, physical, and discussion of findings, Jaime should be counseled on knowing whether she is ready for intercourse. Healthy relationships should be discussed as well as signs of potential partner violence.
- *Immunizations:* Jaime should keep current on her usual childhood vaccinations. She should be encouraged to receive the human papillomavirus (HPV) vaccine, if she has not already done so. The HPV vaccine is a series of three injections that help protect against the strains of HPV that are most likely to cause external genital warts and internal cervical, precancerous changes. She should also be encouraged to receive the meningococcal vaccine (U.S. Department of Health and Human Services, 2008).

Jaime says that she understands what you have told her. She has had concerns for a while now and would like to change some of her behaviors, especially drinking alcohol. She is still hesitant about talking with her mother, but she promises you that she will think about it.

When would you like to see Jaime again? ■

Since Jaime is just starting COCs for the first time, she should return to the office within 1–2 months. At this visit, her blood pressure can be taken to rule out any hypertension as a result of starting the COCs. Information on how to take COCs can be reviewed and further instructions can be given if Jaime is having any problems. If Jaime is doing well at that time and does not have any questions or concerns, she should receive a prescription for up to 9 months (1 year total).

Jaime returns to your office a little more than a month after her first visit. Her blood pressure is 116/54, pulse 78, and respirations 12. She tells you that she is doing well remembering to take her pills every day. She has had some slight nausea and breast tenderness, but this seems to be improving. She has had one period since beginning her COCs. She was very happy that her cramping wasn't bad, and she didn't seem to flood as much. She relates that she still hasn't talked to her mother, but she does want to. She and Blair are doing well together and he is doing better about wearing condoms, though he still doesn't like it much. Jaime has thought about the HPV vaccine and would like to start it today. You review with Jaime how to take COCs and the warning signs to watch for, and give her a prescription for 9 months of COCs. You administer her first HPV immunization injection and remind her to return at 2 and 6 months for the other shots. Jaime states that she doesn't have any other questions and that she will come back for the rest of the injections.

Other than for the vaccinations, she should return to the office in 1 year unless she has any concerns prior to that time.

Key Points from the Case

1. It is important to look at the whole person when providing contraceptive counseling and prescribing. Assisting the patient to choose the appropriate type of contraception will increase her ability to take/use it effectively.

2. The hormones estrogen and progesterone, although safe, do have side effects associated with their use. Careful explanation of the potential risks is crucial along with warning signs to watch for.

3. Although in this case Jaime came to the office for contraception, there were other very important issues that needed to be addressed. Be watchful for these other issues.

4. Try to help the adolescent to feel comfortable with the care being provided. Make the office a safe place where she feels comfortable discussing anything with you.

REFERENCES

American Cancer Society. (2008). Cervical cancer: prevention and early detection. Retrieved December 18, 2009, from http://www.cancer.org/docroot/CRI/content/CRI_2_6x_cervical_cancer_prevention_and_early_detection_8.asp?sitearea=PED

Cates, Jr., W., & Raymond, E. G. (2007). Vaginal barriers and spermicides. In R. A. Hatcher, J. Trussel, T. L. Nelson, W. Cates Jr., & F. Stewart (Eds.), *Contraceptive technology* (19th ed., pp. 317–336). New York: Ardent Media.

Caufield, K. A. (2004). Controlling fertility. In E. Q. Youngkin & M. S. Davis (Eds.), *Women's Health: A Primary Care Clinical Guide* (3rd ed., pp. 165–226). Upper Saddle River, NJ: Pearson/Prentice Hall.

Chambers, K. B., & Rew, L. (2003). Safer sexual decision making in adolescent women: perspectives from the conflict theory of decision-making. *Issues in Comprehensive Pediatric Nursing, 26*(3), 129–143.

Commendador, K. A. (2003). Concept analysis of adolescent decision making and contraception. *Nursing Forum, 38*(4), 27–35.

Frost, J. J., Singh, S., & Finer, L. B. (2007). Factors associated with contraceptive use and nonuse. *Perspectives on Sexual and Reproductive Health, 39*(2), 90–99.

Grimes, D. A. (2007). Intrauterine devices (IUDs). In R. A. Hatcher, J. Trussel, T. L. Nelson, W. Cates Jr., & F. Stewart (Eds.), *Contraceptive technology* (19th ed., pp. 117–146). New York: Ardent Media.

Harvey, S. M., Bird, S. T., Galavotti, C., Duncan, E. A., & Greenberg, D. (2002). Relationship power, sexual decision making and condom use among women at risk for HIV/AIDS. *Women and Health, 36*(4), 69–84.

Jennings, V. H., & Arevalo, M. (2007). Fertility awareness-based methods. In R. A. Hatcher, J. Trussel, T. L. Nelson, W. Cates Jr., & F. Stewart (Eds.), *Contraceptive technology* (19th ed., pp. 343–360). New York: Ardent Media.

Kowal, D. (2007). Abstinence and the range of sexual expression. In R. A. Hatcher, J. Trussel, T. L. Nelson, W. Cates Jr., & F. Stewart (Eds.), *Contraceptive technology* (19th ed., pp. 81–86). New York: Ardent Media.

Manlove, J., Ryan, S., & Franzetta, K. (2003). Patterns of contraceptive use within teenagers' first sexual relationships. *Perspectives on Sexual and Reproductive Health, 35*(6), 246–255.

Moore, A., Cofer, L., Elliot, G., Lanneau, J., Walker, M., & Gold, M. (2005). Adolescent cervical dysplasia: histologic evaluation, treatment, and outcomes. *American Journal of Obstetrics and Gynecology, 197*(2), 141.e1–141.e6.

Nelson, A. (2007). Combined oral contraceptives. In R. A. Hatcher, J. Trussel, T. L. Nelson, W. Cates Jr., & F. Stewart (Eds.), *Contraceptive technology* (19th ed., pp. 193–270). New York: Ardent Media.

Ponton, L. E. (1997). Ten tips for parents: understanding your adolescent's behavior. *The Romance of Risk: Why Teenagers Do the Things They Do*. Jacksonville, TN: Basic Books.

Raymond, E. G. (2007). Progestin-only pills. In R. A. Hatcher, J. Trussel, T. L. Nelson, W. Cates Jr., & F. Stewart (Eds.), *Contraceptive technology* (19th ed., pp. 181–192). New York: Ardent Media.

Stewart, F., Trussel, J., & Van Look, P. F. A. (2007). Emergency contraception. In R. A. Hatcher, J. Trussel, T. L. Nelson, W. Cates Jr., & F. Stewart (Eds.), *Contraceptive technology* (19th ed., pp. 87–116). New York: Ardent Media.

Stiffler, D., Sims, S. L., & Stern, P. N. (2007). Changing women: mothers and their adolescent daughters. *Health Care for Women International, 28*, 638–653.

United States Department of Agriculture (USDA). (2009). *MyPyramid.gov*. Retrieved June 3, 2009, from http://www.mypyramid.gov/?gclid=CJuj8NDm7poCFRJ4xgod9lsnkg

U.S. Department of Health and Human Services, Office of Women's Health. (2008). *Be healthy, be happy, be you, beautiful*. Retrieved October 15, 2008, from http://www.girlshealth.gov.

Warner, L., & Steiner, M. J. (2007). Male condoms. In R. A. Hatcher, J. Trussel, T. L. Nelson, W. Cates Jr., & F. Stewart (Eds.), *Contraceptive technology* (19th ed., pp. 297–316). New York: Ardent Media.

Chapter 29

The 16-Year-Old Girl with a Vaginal Discharge

Teral Gerlt

Working with adolescents is both challenging and rewarding. Adolescent healthcare encounters are often situations in which the provider's agenda may be quite different from that of the teen. There is so much that healthcare providers need to teach teens about healthy life behaviors and practices, and the reception is frequently lukewarm at best. Time, patience, and mutual respect are essentials for open communication.

Educational Objectives
1. Identify the developmental influences impacting adolescent behaviors and learning.
2. Describe important components when communicating with adolescents.
3. Identify factors that increase the risk for sexually transmitted infections (STIs).
4. Apply the Centers for Disease Control and Prevention (CDC) guidelines concerning management and treatment of STIs.

Case Presentation and Discussion

Leslie Montgomery, a 16-year-old white female, comes to your clinic today because she wants to start birth control pills. She has been in a new relationship for the past 2 months and wants to use something to keep her from getting pregnant "besides condoms." She is very concerned about having to have a pelvic exam because she has never had one before. She was told by one of her girlfriends that she didn't have to have one to start the pill. She also mentions that perhaps she should have an examination because she has a discharge that is new and she doesn't like it.

How will you approach this teen? ■

Approach to Taking a Sexual History from an Adolescent

Generally, adolescents, especially females, are reluctant to seek health care about sexuality concerns or issues unless they can depend upon a confidential environment in which to do so (Reddy, Fleming, & Swain, 2002). Therefore, it is important to establish confidentiality at the start. Also, keep in mind that an open, respectful, and nonjudgmental attitude is essential when working with adolescents in order to obtain a thorough sexual history and deliver prevention messages effectively.

Taking a sexual history should be integrated into the general health history. The clinician should reassure the individual that asking sexual questions is a normal part of clinical practice: "I'm going to ask you a few questions that I ask all my young-adult patients about their health and relationships" (Rakel, 2002, p. 14). Giving appropriate, factual information that uses medical-sexual terminology rather than slang is helpful to the extent that the teen understands what is being said.

One also needs to ask open-ended, broad, nonjudgmental questions that will allow the teen to discuss his or her ideas and sexual activities. For example, asking the question, "Have you ever had a romantic relationship with a boy or a girl?" allows for a more inclusive description of sexual activity than asking the traditional, "Are you sexually active?" question. Phrases such as "Explain how that happened," "What happened next," or "Tell me about a typical date" elicit more complete information than do close-ended questions. "When you think of people to whom you are sexually attracted, are they males, females, both, neither, or are you not sure yet?" is a useful question that opens up a conversation for youth struggling with their sexual orientation (Murphy & Elias, 2006). Questions that contain "why" can require a level of analysis beyond the capabilities of young people operating at a concrete level of cognition.

Phrase questions that may be emotionally laden in a way that lets clients know that their experience may not be exceptional (e.g., "Many people have been sexually abused or molested as children; did this happen to you?" [Rakel, 2002] or "How often do you masturbate?" rather than "Do you masturbate?" [Rakel]).

Begin the interview using open-ended questions, setting the tone to be accepting as much as possible. It is essential that you assure the teen that the information from the visit will be kept confidential unless the provider believes the teen may do harm to him- or herself or someone else.

The Centers for Disease Control and Prevention (CDC) has a practical set of questions to incorporate into the sexual history (see Box 29-1).

Further sexual history reveals that she and her partner do not always use condoms because her partner does not like them. Their last vaginal intercourse was this past weekend but she says, "we did use condoms that time." Her current partner is an 18-year-old who dropped out of high school his junior year but is working. Age at first coitus for Leslie was 15 years and consensual. She has had two other sexual partners in the past. She states that she has never had anal intercourse but does have both oral and vaginal intercourse with her current partner. She has only had sex with males and has only used condoms as a birth control method.

Box 29-1   The CDC's Five Ps

1. Partners
   - "Do you have sex with men, women, or both?"
   - "In the past 2 months, how many partners have you had sex with?"
   - "In the past 12 months, how many partners have you had sex with?"
2. Prevention of pregnancy
   - "Are you or your partner trying to get pregnant?"
     - If no, "What are you doing to prevent pregnancy?"
3. Protection from STIs
   - "What do you do to protect yourself from STIs and HIV?"
4. Practices
   - "To understand your risks for STIs, I need to understand the kind of sex you have had recently."
   - "Have you had vaginal sex, meaning 'penis in vagina sex'?"
     - If yes, "Do you use condoms: never, sometimes, or always?"
   - "Have you had anal sex, meaning 'penis in rectum/anus sex'?"
     - If yes, "Do you use condoms: never, sometimes, or always?"
   - "Have you had oral sex, meaning 'mouth on penis/vagina'?"

   For condom answers:
   - If never: "Why don't you use condoms?"
   - If sometimes: "In what situations, or with whom, do you not use condoms?"
5. Past history of STIs
   - "Have you ever had an STI?"
   - "Have any of your partners had an STI?"

   Additional questions to identify HIV and hepatitis risk:
   - "Have you or any of your partners ever injected drugs?"
   - "Have any of your partners exchanged money or drugs for sex?"
   - "Is there anything else about your sexual practices that I need to know about?"

Source: From Centers for Disease Control and Prevention. (2006b). *Sexually transmitted diseases: treatment guidelines, clinical prevention guidance.* Atlanta, GA: U.S. Department of Health and Human Services. Retrieved September 17, 2008, from http://www.cdc.gov/std/treatment/2006/clinical.htm#clinical2

Menarche was at age 12; her cycles are usually regular every 28 to 30 days and last about 4 days. She complains of severe cramping for the first 2 days with medium flow. Her last menstrual period (LMP) was approximately 2 weeks ago, although she does not really keep track of dates for her cycles.

She denies a history of any skin lesions or rash, dysuria, abdominal pain, dyspareunia, or a sexually transmitted infection. She has noticed a little spotting a couple of times this last month, especially after having sex, and a little white vaginal discharge for the past few weeks.

She has a negative personal medical history. Her family history is positive for hypertension (father) and type 2 diabetes (maternal grandmother).

Leslie's social history is positive for "occasional" alcohol at parties, which she describes as three to four drinks once a month. She admits to smoking socially when at parties, but denies any other drug use. She describes herself as a "good" student with a B average. She plans to go to college but is unsure what she wants to major in.

What are your concerns after getting this history? ■

See the STI risk factors listed in Box 29-2.

Leslie is at risk for both pregnancy and STIs due to irregular condom use and having three sexual partners in the last year. She is having some vaginal spotting, which could be related to a STI. She is also using both alcohol and tobacco.

What are your working diagnoses prior to your physical examination? ■

You start with the following working diagnoses:

- Contraceptive need
- Rule out pregnancy
- Rule out STIs
- Bloody vaginal spotting and discharge of unknown etiology
- Alcohol and tobacco use

What type of physical examination would you do? ■

In accordance with current recommendations of the American Cancer Society's "Guidelines for Early Detection of Cervical Cancer," which states that screening should begin approximately 3 years after first sexual intercourse (Saslow et al., 2002), she does not need a pap screening today. However, she does need a pelvic and STI examination.

What clinical findings are you looking for? ■

The three most common sexually transmitted infections in teenage women are chlamydia, gonorrhea, and syphilis. Chlamydia is the most common of these. In 30–70% of women chlamydia is asymptomatic, but the usual symptoms, if they appear, include vaginal discharge that may be clear to white or yellow; bloody vaginal spotting; dysuria and/or pyuria; mucopurulent cervicitis with edema, erythema, and hypertrophy; mild abdominal pain;

Box 29-2   Risk Factors for Sexually Transmitted Infections

- Adolescent younger than 15 years of age
- Sexually active adolescent, especially with two or more partners in 6 months, high frequency of intercourse, or high rate of new partners
- Use of drugs or alcohol, or other high-risk behaviors
- Pregnancy or abortion
- Homosexual
- Victim of abuse, rape, or incest
- Incarcerated, runaway, homeless, or in a group shelter or detention home
- Clients in sexually transmitted infection (STI) clinics or with any other STI or previous history of STI
- Lack of family availability; low level of parental support and monitoring
- Beliefs about normative behaviors among peers
- Inappropriate healthcare behaviors (e.g., not seeking medical care, not adhering to treatment regimen, failure to recognize symptoms, delay in notifying partners, nonuse of barrier contraceptive)

Sources: In Gerlt, T. J., Kollar, L. M., & Starr, N. B. (2009). Gynecologic conditions. In C. E. Burns, A. M. Dunn, M. A. Brady, N. B. Starr, & C. Blosser (Eds.), *Pediatric primary care* (4th ed., p. 933). Philadelphia, WB Saunders; data from Biro, F. M., & Rosenthal, S. L. (1995). Adolescent STDs: diagnosis, developmental issues, and prevention. *Journal of Pediatric Health Care, 9,* 256–262; Bonny, A. E., & Biro, F. M. (1998). Recognizing and treating STDs in adolescent girls. *Contemporary Pediatrics, 15,* 119–143; Shrier, L. A. (2005). Bacterial sexually transmitted infections: gonorrhea, chlamydia, pelvic inflammatory disease, and syphilis. In S. J. Emans, M. R. Laufer, & D. P. Goldstein (Eds.), *Pediatric and adolescent gynecology* (5th ed., pp. 565–614). Philadelphia: Lippincott Williams & Wilkins.

Fitz-Hugh-Curtis syndrome (right upper quadrant pain); or foreign body sensation in eyes with conjunctivitis.

Gonorrhea (GC) is also usually asymptomatic in women. The typical signs and symptoms of GC infection include dysuria; urethritis; thick, green, profuse vaginal discharge; cervicitis; bleeding; dyspareunia; Skene's or Bartholin's gland abscess; or exudative pharyngitis.

Syphilis is less common. The primary form usually presents with a single painless papule with serous discharge on a smooth base with raised edges. The location of the chancre may be vaginal, anal, or oral. In secondary syphilis, the classic copper-penny rash presents, generally on the palms of the hands and soles of the feet. There also may be mucocutaneous lesions and painless regional lymphadenopathy.

Height and weight, body mass index (BMI), blood pressure, thyroid, heart, lungs, breast, abdominal, and pelvic examinations are all parts of the assessment needed before beginning hormonal contraception and to rule out STIs.

Leslie's general physical examination reveals: height 5' 3"; weight 112 pounds; BMI 19.8 (25%); blood pressure 116/68. Her thyroid is smooth, without enlargement. Her heart rate is regular with no murmurs, rubs, or clicks. Lungs are clear to auscultation. Breasts are nontender, Tanner stage 4, without masses. Her abdomen is soft, nontender, with no masses, and without organomegaly.

Pelvic examination: Your examination reveals external genitalia without lesions, negative Bartholin's, urethra, and Skene's; Tanner stage 4. Her vagina is pink with normal ruga and minimal clear to white discharge. Her cervix appears nulliparous and pink with thick clear mucous at the os.

Bimanual examination: You perform a bimanual examination and find her uterus to be anteverted, firm, smooth, nontender, and nonenlarged; her adnexa is without masses or tenderness; and the cervix is firm, without cervical motion tenderness.

What laboratory studies would you order? ■

In deciding which studies to order, the provider needs to know what organisms to look for and the difference in and accuracy of tests.

Epidemiology

Sexually transmitted infections are considered an epidemic in the United States at this time. Their highest rates are among adolescents; almost half of the 19 million new cases yearly occur in teens (CDC, 2007). Young adults ages 15–24 years and young women between the ages of 15 and 19 have the highest rates of *N. gonorrhoeae* and *C. trachomatis* (CDC, 2006a). Youth in detention facilities; male homosexuals; injection drug users; and minorities, especially African Americans, are all at high risk.

Some factors that contribute to this epidemic in teenagers include the increasingly early age and frequency of sexual activity, inconsistent use of contraceptive and protective devices, physiologic characteristics that predispose adolescents to infection, adolescents' lack of access to and use of health care, and societal influences. The increased use and availability of accurate screening tests for diseases, especially chlamydia, is another factor that may be contributing to the higher reported numbers of STIs.

Chlamydia Trachomatis and Testing

Chlamydia infection is the most frequently reported bacterial STI, with a rate of 347.8 cases per 100,000 reported in 2006, up 5.6% from 2005 (CDC, 2007). Adolescent females have the highest percentage of these cases. Young women ages 15 to 19 years old account for 37% of the chlamydia infections, and 20- to 24-year-olds represent 36%. Because of the increased incidence in female adolescents, all sexually active young women in this age group should be screened at least annually because chlamydia is frequently asymptomatic. Untreated chlamydia can progress to pelvic inflammatory disease (PID); as many as 40% of women with untreated infections develop PID, and 20% of those may lose their fertility (CDC, 2007).

For sexually active adolescents with possible chlamydia, many family planning clinics use direct immunofluorescent smears. Nucleic acid hybridization tests (DNA probes) and nucleic acid amplification testing (NAAT) are acceptable alternatives for teens, especially in high-prevalence populations. Only NAATs can be done using either a cervical swab or urine and, thus, are the preferable testing method for adolescents (CDC, 2006a). It is important to note, however, that if chlamydia is suspected in younger children, a culture is the only acceptable method to diagnose this agent. Chlamydia in young children may be associated with sexual abuse and must be correctly identified. Therefore, culture results, not DNA detection, must be used.

Gonorrhea and Testing

Gonorrhea is caused by *Neisseria gonorrhoeae*, a nonmotile, gram-negative diplococcus. It is often found along with chlamydia or other STIs. The gonorrhea rate for 2006 was 120.9 cases per 100,000, which is up 5.5% from 2005 and an increase for the second year in a row (CDC, 2007). The highest rate for adolescents occurs in the 15- to 19-year-old group. There are more reported cases of GC in African Americans than whites (18:1). The infection is often asymptomatic, with as many as 80% of young women infected with GC reporting no symptoms (Stamm & McGregor, 2001). Untreated GC can also progress to PID, with the issue of infertility as a possible outcome.

The definitive test for gonorrhea in women is a culture on selective media with determination of penicillin resistance. DNA probes and NAATs are also available for GC testing (Spigarelli & Biro, 2004). NAATs are more reliable with cervical swab testing than urine testing for GC (Shrier, 2005); gram stains of vaginal discharge or cervical secretions are not recommended (CDC, 2006a).

Syphilis and Testing

Syphilis, caused by *Treponema pallidum*, is a motile spirochete with a prevalence rate of 3.3 cases per 100,000 in 2006, an increase of 13.8% from 2005. Although the majority of this increase (11.8%) was in males and primarily in men having sex with men (MSM), the rate for women increased for the second year in a row (from 0.9 per 100,000 to 1.0 in 2006). Furthermore, the rate of congenital syphilis, after being down 12% from 2004 to 2005 to 8.2 per 100,000 live births, went up to 8.5 in 2006 (CDC, 2007).

To test for syphilis, direct visualization with dark-field microscopy or direct immunofluorescent antibody (DFA) provides definitive results. Several serologic nontreponemal tests including the Venereal Disease Research Laboratories (VDRL), rapid plasma reagin (RPR), and the automated reagin test correlate with disease activity. Because they decline after treatment, they are used to monitor disease progression. Treponemal tests such as the fluorescent treponemal antibody absorption (FTA-ABS) and the microhemagglutination test for *Treponema pallidum* (MHA-TP) are confirmatory, but once positive, they usually remain so for years (CDC, 2006a).

HIV and Testing

HIV is another sexually transmitted infection that can occur in persons who engage in unprotected sexual intercourse. Adolescents in the United States are often at risk due to their sexual behaviors. Although the Youth Risk Behavior Survey for 2007 indicated a decrease in those who have ever had sexual intercourse, the decreases have leveled off. Condom use has also leveled off at about 61.5% (CDC, 2008). Thus, adolescents are still at risk for this serious disease.

Usually HIV is diagnosed by tests for antibodies against HIV-1, although some combination tests also detect antibodies against HIV-2. The first step in diagnosing this condition is the use of a sensitive screening test, either the enzyme immunoassay (EIA) or the newer rapid test. The latter test has allowed clinicians to make a significantly accurate presumptive diagnosis of HIV-1 infection within half an hour. Reactive screening tests must then be confirmed by a supplemental test such as the Western blot (WB) or an immunofluorescence assay (IFA) (CDC, 2006a).

All 50 states require most STIs to be reported; however, mandated reporting rules vary from state to state. All 50 states allow adolescents to be evaluated and to receive confidential treatment for STIs, but management of children younger than 13 years old requires coordination between the pediatric provider and child protective authorities.

Laboratory Tests for Leslie

The wet mount of vaginal secretions was checked immediately after the pelvic examination was completed. The results, which included saline for microscopic examination to look for white blood cells (WBCs), clue cells, trichomonads, and bacteria and the 10% potassium hydroxide (KOH) for whiff test and microscopic examination to look for yeast (branching hyphae and spores), were all negative. You also checked a urine specimen for pregnancy and the result was negative.

Specimens were also sent to the laboratory.

- Chlamydia: NAAT on cervical swab
- Gonorrhea: NAAT on cervical swab

Recommended blood work for rapid plasma reagin (RPR) for syphilis and an enzyme immunoassay (EIA) for HIV were declined by Leslie.

Making the Diagnosis

What is your assessment? ■

First, Leslie has a contraceptive need, which she has expressed and is evident from her sexual history. Second, she also has a possible sexually transmitted infection that, if diagnosed, needs treatment.

Management

What will be your plan, given the two diagnoses you have made? ▦

You mentally outline your plan as follows:

- Contraceptive need.
- Patient education about oral contraceptive pills (OCPs).
- Patient education about condom use.
- Provide an Rx for OCPs.
- Rule out a sexually transmitted infection: chlamydia, gonorrhea, syphilis, or HIV.
- Await lab results.
- Patient education and counseling about safer sex.

Counseling of the Adolescent

The adolescent's perspectives about sexual activities that are appropriate for them may not match those of the primary care clinician. Teens and young adults are faced with media portrayal of sexuality at a time when they are using role models for their own behaviors. Family and community cultural norms as well as peer group pressures can affect the attitudes and beliefs about sexuality and sexual behaviors that they are developing (American Academy of Pediatrics [AAP], 2001; Brown & Brown, 2006). All these influences need to be considered and addressed when counseling the teen.

Using the answers given by the adolescent in the sexual history will help guide the counseling and education provided to the individual teen. Trust, honesty, mutual respect, an open nonjudgmental attitude, and confidentiality are extremely important to the adolescent (Burgis & Bacon, 2003). It may take several visits for the trust relationship to grow before the adolescent is willing to divulge more private thoughts and behaviors. The clinician's job is to assure the adolescent of the confidential nature of the relationship and provide opportunities for trust to develop.

Adolescents need to know that they have choices about sexual behaviors that have different outcomes. Adolescents should be counseled that abstinence is the most effective strategy for the prevention of pregnancy, STIs, and HIV/AIDS (American Academy of Family Physicians [AAFP], 2006; AAP, 2001; American College of Obstetricians and Gynecologists [ACOG], 2005). It is a choice to remain abstinent and a choice to become sexually active, not just something that happens, and with that choice comes responsibilities. Open communication and respect for self and partner will lead to choices that include protection from STIs and pregnancy.

Counseling and Development

Counseling adolescents requires that the clinician make adjustments based on the teen's stage of psychosocial developmental (Burgis & Bacon, 2003; Clark, 2003) because not all teens are developmentally at the same level. Piaget demonstrated that early adolescents, ages 12–14 years, are concrete thinkers and lack the ability to comprehend the abstract thought of "what if." When counseling youth at this age, the healthcare provider needs to use language that is characterized by simple concrete terms. Pictures, direct questions, and statements will help facilitate their understanding. Middle adolescents such as Leslie, ages 15–17 years, are starting to understand abstract concepts but often regress to concrete thinking in stressful situations. The clinician needs to adjust the approach to the middle adolescent accordingly, helping him or her to identify inconsistencies in reasoning and guide the teen's thought processing through to logical consequences of choices and behaviors. Late adolescents, ages 18–21 years, generally have abstract thought more firmly established and are future oriented. However, this ability will vary, as with the general adult population.

Contraceptive and Safer Sex Counseling

Clinicians who provide contraceptive and safer sex counseling to adolescents should understand that the successful use of any method requires a complex process of knowledge, decision-making skills, and public behaviors. It is also important to use gender-neutral phrasing when discussing safer sex and contraception and not assume heterosexuality. To use contraceptives/protective barriers successfully, an individual must master the following (Gerlt, Blosser, & Dunn, 2009):

- *Knowledge for contraception:* Most adolescents need to learn about a barrier method for contraception, such as male or female condoms, to prevent an STI as well as about a variety of hormonal methods for contraceptive purposes.
- *Ability to plan for the future:* Adolescents need to admit to themselves that they will have sex in the future and that they have the ability and resources necessary to use a contraceptive method consistently and correctly. Further, they must be willing to use the chosen method of protection consistently, not just when it is convenient to do so.
- *Willingness to acquire needed contraceptive/barrier methods publicly:* Adolescents wanting to be successful in using contraceptive/barrier methods successfully will need to be public with requests for contraceptive and/or protective devices; for example, to purchase condoms at a local pharmacy or to seek services at the local clinic, school-based health facility, or private practice. This is not an easy step for many teens and may need rehearsal.
- *Communication skills:* Adolescents must be able to communicate with another person or persons such as their partner, healthcare provider,

pharmacist, or salesperson about their individual contraceptive/ protective barrier needs. The ability to express their feelings about sexual activity, how it affects them, and the thinking behind their decisions to be sexually active is also a needed communication skill.

The next afternoon you receive a faxed lab report: Leslie's NAAT is positive for chlamydia but negative for GC.

What is your plan now? ▮

You need to consider how to contact Leslie to assure her confidentiality. Will you treat her partner too? If not, who will you refer him to? Do you need to report to the public health officials, or will your lab do that? Many healthcare systems have guidelines or protocols to help you answer these questions.

Per CDC guidelines (CDC, 2006a), treatment of an uncomplicated chlamydial infection includes:

- Azithromycin 1 g orally in a single dose *OR* doxycycline 100 mg orally twice a day for 7 days.
- Refer partners for treatment. It is recommended to treat the last partner and any partner exposed within the 60 days before the onset of symptoms.
- Recommend that the client abstain from intercourse for 1 week after single dose treatment or until completion of a 7-day course. The client also needs to abstain until after her partner has completed treatment.
- Rescreen 3 to 4 months after the positive test because a high prevalence of *C. trachomatis* infection is found in women with a chlamydial infection in the preceding several months. Reinfection is usually the cause of infection and elevates the risk for PID.

For general STI treatment measures, see Box 29-3.

After contacting Leslie, she wants to come into the clinic to take her one-time dose of azithromycin and talk further about this new issue. When you see her the next day, she is very upset about having an STI and does not know how to talk with her boyfriend about this. How did this happen? Did he give it to her or her him? Was he cheating on her? Will this make her unable to have babies?

How will you answer her questions? ▮

You answer Leslie's many questions and reassure her that with treatment her risk of long-term sequelae is minimal; however, with reinfection the risk would increase. You help her problem solve talking with her partner about the chlamydial infection and plan for his evaluation and treatment. Once again you review with Leslie the guidelines for practicing safer sex in the future and role play negotiating skills that she can use with her partner.

Box 29-3   General Treatment Measures for Sexually Transmitted Infections

- Have patient abstain from sexual intercourse until patient and partner are cured (treatment complete and symptoms resolved). The consequences of untreated sexually transmitted infections (STIs) should be explained.
- Test for other STIs, including hepatitis B, human immunodeficiency virus, bacterial vaginosis, and trichomonas.
- Notify, examine, and treat all partners of patient for any identified or suspected STI.
- Report STIs to the state health department. Reporting to appropriate authorities is important to identify those at risk, recognize new strains, and assess the extent of infection in the community and the effect of prevention efforts.
- Provide regular sex health assessment including Papanicolaou (pap) testing, vaginal examination, and testing for STIs.
- Give hepatitis B and HPV vaccines if not done already.
- Discuss safer sex practices, including abstinence and use of condoms.
- Educate and counsel about complications and transmission of STIs, as well as perinatal consequences.

Source: From Gerlt, T. J., Kollar, L. M., & Starr, N. B. (2009). Gynecologic conditions. In C. E. Burns, A. M. Dunn, M. A. Brady, N. B. Starr, & C. Blosser (Eds.), *Pediatric primary care* (4th ed., p. 936). Philadelphia: WB Saunders.

When will you see Leslie again? ■

You plan to see her again in 3 to 4 months for a repeat NAAT, to see how she is doing with her OCPs, and to generally check in. Keeping frequent contact with the adolescent helps build rapport and your education and counseling can be reinforced.

Key Points from the Case

1. Understanding the developmental level of your patient is essential for excellent care.
2. Open, honest, and nonjudgmental communication is crucial when working with adolescents.
3. Understanding the risk factors for STIs and why adolescents are inherently at risk by nature is important to their care.
4. Knowing where to find information, guidelines, and evidence-based resources (e.g., CDC, AAP, your healthcare system, etc.) will simplify your work.

REFERENCES

American Academy of Family Physicians. (2006). *Adolescent health care, sexuality and contraception.* Retrieved September 20, 2008, from http://www.aafp.org/online/en/home/policy/policies/a/adol3.html

American Academy of Pediatrics, Committee on Psychosocial Aspects of Child and Family Health and Committee on Adolescence. (2001). Sexuality education for children and adolescents. *Pediatrics, 108,* 498–501.

American College of Obstetricians and Gynecologists. (2005). *Committee on Adolescent Health Care Resource Guide: Adolescent sexuality and sex education.* Retrieved September 20, 2008, from http://www.acog.org/departments/dept_notice.cfm?recno=7&bulletin=3271

Biro, F. M., & Rosenthal, S. L. (1995). Adolescent STDs: diagnosis, developmental issues, and prevention. *Journal of Pediatric Health Care, 9,* 256–262.

Bonny, A. E., & Biro, F. M. (1998). Recognizing and treating STDs in adolescent girls. *Contemporary Pediatrics, 15,* 119–143.

Brown, R. T., & Brown, J. D. (2006). Adolescent sexuality. *Primary Care, 33,* 373–390.

Burgis, J. T., & Bacon, J. L. (2003). Communicating with the adolescent gynecology patient. *Obstetrics and Gynecology Clinics of North America, 30,* 251–260.

Centers for Disease Control and Prevention. (2006a). Sexually transmitted diseases: treatment guidelines. *Morbidity and Mortality Weekly Report, 55*(RR-11), 1–94.

Centers for Disease Control and Prevention. (2006b). *Sexually transmitted diseases: treatment guidelines 2006, clinical prevention guidance.* Atlanta, GA: U.S. Department of Health and Human Services. Retrieved September 17, 2008, from http://www.cdc.gov/std/treatment/2006/clinical.htm#clinical2

Centers for Disease Control and Prevention. (2007). *Trends in reportable sexually transmitted infections in the United States, 2007.* Atlanta, GA: U.S. Department of Health and Human Services. Retrieved April 15, 2009, from http://www.cdc.gov/std/stats07/main.htm

Centers for Disease Control and Prevention. (2008). Trends in HIV- and STD-related risk behaviors among high school students—United States, 1991–2007. *Morbidity and Mortality Weekly Report, 57*(30), 817–822.

Clark, L. R. (2003). Tips for clinicians: approaching the adolescent patient from a psychodevelopmental framework. *Journal of Pediatric and Adolescent Gynecology, 1,* 327–330.

Gerlt, T. J., Blosser, C. G., & Dunn, A. M. (2009). Sexuality. In C. E. Burns, A. M. Dunn, M. A. Brady, N. B. Starr, & C. Blosser (Eds.), *Pediatric primary care* (4th ed., pp. 395–410). Philadelphia: Elsevier.

Gerlt, T. J., Kollar, L. M., & Starr, N. B. (2009). Gynecologic conditions. In C. E. Burns, A. M. Dunn, M. A. Brady, N. B. Starr, & C. Blosser (Eds.), *Pediatric primary care* (4th ed., pp. 906–941). Philadelphia: Elsevier.

Murphy, N. A., & Elias, E. R. (2006). Sexuality of children and adolescents with developmental disabilities. *Pediatrics, 118,* 398–403. Retrieved September 20, 2008, from http://aappolicy.aappublications.org/cgi/content/full/pediatrics;118/1/398

Rakel, R. E. (2002). *Textbook of family practice* (6th ed.). Philadelphia: WB Saunders.

Reddy, D. M., Fleming, R., & Swain, C. (2002). Effect of mandatory parental notification on adolescent girls' use of sexual health care services. *Journal of the American Medical Association, 288,* 710–714.

Saslow, D., Runowicz, C. D., Solomon, D., Moscicki, A. B., Smith, R. A., Eyre, H. J., et al. (2002). American Cancer Society guideline for the early detection of cervical neoplasia and cancer. *CA: A Cancer Journal for Clinicians, 52,* 342–362.

Shrier, L. A. (2005). Bacterial sexually transmitted infections: gonorrhea, chlamydia, pelvic inflammatory disease, and syphilis. In S. J. Emans, M. R. Laufer, & D. P. Goldstein (Eds), *Pediatric and adolescent gynecology* (5th ed., pp. 565–614). Philadelphia: Lippincott Williams & Wilkins.

Spigarelli, M. G., & Biro, F. M. (2004). Sexually transmitted disease testing: evaluation of diagnostic tests and methods. *Adolescent Medicine Clinics, 15,* 287–299.

Stamm, C. A., & McGregor, J. A. (2001). Diagnosing and treating STDs in young women. *Contemporary Pediatrics, 18,* 53–67.

Chapter 30

The Child with an Itchy Rash

Donald W. Kennerley

The child who presents in a clinic with an itchy rash is usually miserable and the parents are anxious for a quick fix to the problem. The dilemma for the healthcare provider is to quickly identify the problem and find a treatment plan that provides immediate relief as well as a long-term cure, or amelioration in the chronic case that won't be cured. The source of the problem may be an infection, infestation, environmental toxin/irritant, or allergy/immunologic problem. This scenario will help the clinician sort through those issues.

Educational Objectives
1. Develop a multimodal approach for the treatment of atopic dermatitis.
2. Understand the complex role that the environment and aeroallergens have in the development of atopic dermatitis.
3. Review and understand new therapies for compromised barrier function.
4. Understand the effects that atopic dermatitis has on the social, financial, and psychological well-being of a family with a child affected with this disorder.

Case Presentation and Discussion

Anna Logan is a 3-year-old white female who comes into the office accompanied by her mother. She has come today because of a persisting rash that the mother indicates comes and goes and was first noted when her daughter was 1 year old. Though the rash does at times get better, it has never left her daughter. In fact, as her daughter gets older the intensity of the rash worsens and is spreading to other areas of her body. Originally the rash started on Anna's face but is now on her neck, arms, and legs. Mrs. Logan indicates that her daughter is scratching more now than in the past and is often awake at night due to the scratching. Further questioning of the mother reveals that, apart from the rash, her daughter also has trouble with chronic sneezing and a constant running nose. The child does not have a history of asthma. The mother is concerned about the spreading rash and is worried about the possibility of her daughter causing further damage to her skin as a result of her constant scratching. The mother comes with her daughter to find out what the rash is and how to get rid of it.

Physical Examination

Upon general physical examination you notice that Anna appears healthy with a slight paleness in her color and darkness beneath her eyes. She scratches during the entire examination. She has a red, dry, inflamed rash on her face, neck, wrists, and antecubital and popliteal fossae. Some of the areas show scratch marks and are lichenified. There are no areas of weeping. She has signs of chronic rhinitis with redness of the nasal turbinates. The rest of her physical examination is unremarkable.

What questions do you feel would help you to make a diagnosis? ■

Before proceeding with those questions, let us now look at atopic dermatitis in more detail.

Atopic Dermatitis

Epidemiology

Atopic dermatitis (AD) is a common skin condition in children, often beginning in early childhood. Its presentation can be quite severe. Approximately 15–20% of school-age children are affected, with 1–2% having severe involvement. About 1–3% of adults are affected by this condition (Barclay, 2008; Krakowski, Eichenfield, & Dohil, 2008). Approximately 60–65% of patients with atopic dermatitis develop their disease before age 1 year, and by age 5 years, 85–90% of patients have developed signs of their disease (Krakowski et al., 2008; Lewin Group, 2005). The prevalence of atopic dermatitis, asthma, and allergic rhinitis has been rising in industrialized countries (Spergel & Paller, 2003).

Atopic dermatitis is a chronic and relapsing disease and persists from an average of 4.4 years in children to 18.2 years in adults (Lewin Group, 2005). Most forms of this childhood disease improve with the onset of puberty, but up to 40% of cases do not and can recur even into adulthood. AD is often associated with other atopic predispositions; many patients suffering with atopic dermatitis will go on to develop asthma or allergic rhinitis in what is known as the "atopic march" (Spergel & Paller, 2003). Up to 30–60% of patients with atopic dermatitis will go on to develop asthma and 35–66% will go on to develop allergic rhinitis (Lewin Group).

This condition has a significant impact on the quality of life of the individual and his or her family. Cost estimates for the United States range from $364 million to $3.8 billion annually, depending upon the study parameters (Carroll et al., 2005; Mancini, Kaulback, & Chamlin, 2008). The condition accounts for an estimated 7.4 million office visits in the United States alone (Krakowski et al., 2008). Studies have shown that AD can affect sleep, negatively affect school performance, cause low self-esteem, decrease participation in sports and other social activities, and induce stress and anxiety (Krakowski et al.).

Pathophysiology

Although the pathogenesis of atopic dermatitis is not completely understood, in the simplest terms it is believed to be due to a combination of T-cell downregulation and skin barrier dysfunction (Gilliam & Frieden, 2006). The underlying immunologic abnormality for acute disease appears to be related to the overexpression of T-helper-cell type 2 hypersensitivity, whereas chronic disease is related to augmented T-helper-cell type 1 activity (Novark, Bieber, & Leung, 2003). Genetic studies have found that AD has a complex genetic pattern. Some studies have shown that a primary defect in the skin barrier may be one central factor in the condition. Other factors are still being studied (Spergel, 2008).

The permeability barrier, which relies on the functional integrity of the stratum corneum, is altered in patients with atopic dermatitis, leading to accelerated transepidermal water loss and skin dryness. Improving that functional permeability barrier is a cornerstone of AD treatment.

The immune system response in atopic dermatitis involves both intrinsic (nonallergic) and extrinsic (allergic) components. Approximately 70–85% of cases of atopic dermatitis involve the extrinsic system whereas 15–30% of cases are intrinsic. Extrinsic atopic dermatitis is associated with high serum IgE levels and exhibits allergen-specific IgE to aeroallergens and foods, positive skin prick reactions, and a cytokine profile of high interleukin-4 (IL-4) and IL-13 levels (Bardana, 2004). Intrinsic atopic dermatitis is associated with normal IgE levels, negative skin prick reactions, and low IL-4 and IL-13 levels, and the individual does not have allergen-specific IgE to aeroallergens and foods (Bardana). Patients with intrinsic disease are characterized by an absence of other atopic diseases, asthma, and allergic rhinitis (Schmid-Grendelmeier, Simon, Simon, Akdis, & Wirthrich, 2001).

Presentation

There are three distinct phases, related to stages of growth, in which atopic dermatitis can present. They include an infantile phase, a childhood phase, and an adult phase. In the infantile phase, which occurs from birth up to age 2, the disease presents with pruritic, erythematous papules, patches, and vesicles on cheeks and extensor surfaces of the extremities (Peterson & Chen, 2006). Other areas of involvement may include the scalp, forehead, chin, and trunk, but not in the diaper area in the majority of cases (Spergel & Paller, 2003). In the childhood phase, from age 2 to puberty, lichenification and scarring appear as a result of chronic rubbing and scratching. Distribution of the lesions changes to the flexor surfaces, particularly the antecubital and popliteal fossae as well as the neck, periorbital, perioral, hands, feet, wrists, and ankles (Spergel & Paller). The adult phase begins at puberty and may follow a continuous course. Areas of involvement include the flexor folds, face, hands, upper arms, back, wrists, and the dorsa of the hands, fingers, feet, and toes (Spergel & Paller). Large lichenified plaques; scaly, erythematous papules and plaques; and pruritic papules are featured in the adult phase (Leung & Bieber, 2003).

A diagnostic formula was established in 1996 to aid in the diagnosis of atopic dermatitis. A patient has to have a history of itchy skin and three or more of the following presentations: a history of rash in skin folds, a personal history of asthma or hay fever, a history of dry skin, onset before age 2 years, and visible flexural dermatitis (Williams et al., 1996).

Triggers

Allergies play a major role in triggering atopic dermatitis. Approximately 20–40% of young children and infants with atopic dermatitis have clinically relevant food allergies that worsen their disease (Leung & Bieber, 2003). The most common food allergies include cow's milk, eggs, fish, peanuts, soy, tree nuts, and wheat (Rudikoff & Lebwohl, 1998). Aeroallergens include animal dander, cockroaches, dust mites, human dander, molds, and pollens (Schmid-Grendelmeier et al., 2001). Tests for allergies are not necessary in most children with mild eczema. Radioallergosorbent/skin prick (RAST/SPT) testing has only a 20% positive predictive accuracy (Rowlands, Tofte, & Hanifin, 2006). A double blind placebo-controlled food challenge is considered the gold standard for diagnosing food allergies; however, if there is a history of anaphylaxis, a food challenge should be used with caution and only if the patient is closely monitored (Peterson & Chen, 2006).

Other triggers such as climate, irritants, and micro-organisms are also factors that have a pronounced effect on the severity of atopic dermatitis. Decreased humidity in winter allows the skin to dry out easier through increased transdermal water loss. Irritants such as hot water, soaps, cigarette smoke exposure, laundry detergents, household disinfectants, solvents, synthetic clothing fibers, and juice from fresh fruits are commonly implicated in atopic dermatitis (Abramovits, Goldstein, & Stevenson, 2003).

Bacteria, viruses, fungi, and yeast aggravate atopic dermatitis. Approximately 90% of atopic dermatitis lesions are colonized by *Staphylococcus aureus*, as opposed to only a 5% rate of colonization in skin of healthy controls (Abramovits, 2005; Chung, Jeon, Sung, Kim, & Hong, 2008). Community-acquired methicillin-resistant *S. aureus* (MRSA) accounted for 18.3% of those isolates in the Chung et al. study (2008).

Other information that should be ascertained includes the following:

- Does this child have food or other types of allergies?
- What type of clothing does the child wear?
- Is there a family history of asthma or hay fever?
- Has the rash ever been weeping or covered in an exudate?
- What type of soap is used in bathing and in laundry care?
- Has the mother been trying any home remedies on the rash?
- Has the child been seen by a physician in the past and treated for skin problems?
- How much sleep does the child get at night?

The mother responds that Anna is one of three children in the family. Her eldest daughter is on medication for asthma while the other child has intermittent seasonal allergies. Anna has had a history of some early childhood milk allergies that she seems to have outgrown. The mother indicates that she changed her daughter's clothes from wool to cotton fiber when she discovered that her daughter's scratching became worse in the wool clothing. During bathing, the mother uses Dove soap and has been applying Lubriderm cream after her daughter gets out of the bath. The rash persists despite the lotion treatment, and her daughter is getting only about 4–5 hours of sleep at night. The mother and her husband are getting less sleep also because they have to get up with their daughter in the night when she cannot sleep. This is beginning to cause some stress in the family. There have been no other medical visits or treatments.

Making the Diagnosis

The common conditions that should be considered in the differential diagnosis for atopic dermatitis are as follows:

- Classic atopic dermatitis
  - Infantile seborrheic dermatitis
  - Irritant or allergic contact dermatitis
  - Nutritional dermatitis; immunodeficiency
- Nummular dermatitis
  - *Dry form:* Tinea corporis, psoriasis, pityriasis rosea
  - *Wet form:* Impetigo, burns, allergic contact
- Dyshidrotic eczema
- Bullous impetigo
- Allergic bullous tinea
- Contact dermatitis

Reviewing the facts gained from the history and the correlating physical findings, you are assured that this child has atopic dermatitis. The patient has chronic scratching as well as a red erythematous rash on the flexor folds of her arms and knees with early lichenification. There is a history of asthma in the family and allergic rhinitis. The rash first appeared at age 1 year, and Anna has a mild to moderate case of atopic dermatitis.

Diagnostic tests are not indicated at this time because the child has mild involvement and the family is aware of the triggers for this disease and have already made changes to her clothing, bathing, and allergy exposure.

Management

Management of atopic dermatitis in children should follow a stepped approach, with treatment steps tailored to the severity of the eczema. Even when the eczema clears, emollients should always be used and should form the basis of the management. Parents should be counseled on symptoms of atopic dermatitis flares, which include increased dryness, itching, redness, swelling, and general irritability, as well as how to treat the flares through a step-wise care plan (Barclay, 2008; Krakowski et al., 2008).

General Measures

All patients with atopic dermatitis, including children, have hyper-irritable skin. It is important to avoid irritants such as soaps, cleaning agents, detergents, heat, and wool clothing. Over-the-counter preparations such as Aquaphor, CeraVe, Eucerin, or Vaseline are helpful. Newer prescription emollients such as Epiceram or Hylira are also available. Barrier repair formulations have recently come on the market and include ceramide-based creams such as TriCeram, Impruv, TriXera, Nouriva Repair, and Stelatopia. Their drawback is expense, particularly when the medication is used to cover large areas of the body. Emollients should be applied twice daily and immediately after bathing (Darsow et al., 2005).

Bathing remains somewhat controversial. On the one hand, bathing promotes skin hydration, cleansing, and absorption of topical therapies. On the other hand, bathing can dry the skin and disrupt the stratum corneum barrier during evaporation if emollients are not immediately used to maximize moisture retention (Krakowski et al., 2008). Soaps such as Eucerin, Dove, Aveeno, and Alpha Keri may provide benefit.

Treatment of the pruritis in children is also extremely important because sleep deprivation becomes a factor parents have to deal with frequently. General measures may include cooling the skin with cool wraps or cool baths. Moisturizing and minimizing itching are essential. Oral antihistamines have not been shown to be very effective at reducing itch, but sedating antihistamines may promote night-time sleep.

Topical Corticosteroids

Topical corticosteroids are divided into classes based on their potency. Class 1 is the most potent of steroids whereas class 7 is the least potent (Table 30-1). Class 1–5 steroids are not to be used in areas of thinner skin including the eyelids, face, mucous membranes, genitalia, and intertriginous areas because those areas have increased likelihood of transepidermal corticosteroid absorption (Leung et al., 2004). Higher potency steroids should be avoided in children (Paller et al., 2005).

Topical steroids should be used for only a few weeks in a continuous fashion and then tapered as soon as symptoms improve. It is preferable to use low-potency steroids for maintenance therapy and mid- to high-potency steroids for flares (Leung et al., 2004). Traditional vehicle choices are ointments for dry skin, creams or lotions for moist skin, lotions or foams for hair-bearing areas, and lotions for facial skin in teens. Local side effects of steroids include striae, telangiectasis, skin atrophy, dyspigmentation, and acneiform eruptions.

Table 30-1   Common Topical Corticosteroids by Potency

Class/ Potency	Generic Name	Dosage Form	Trade Name
I. Super-high and II. High	*Should not be used in children.*		
III. Medium-high	Betamethasone dipropionate	Cream	Diprosone cream 0.05%
	Betamethasone valerate 0.1%	Ointment, cream, lotion	Valisone, Betatrex
	Desoximetasone 0.05%	Cream	Topicort LP
IV. Medium	Betamethasone valerate 0.12%	Foam	Luxiq
	Flucosinolone acetonide 0.025%	Ointment	Synalar
	Flurandrenolide	Cream, ointment, lotion	Cordran
	Hydrocortisone valerate 0.2%	Ointment	Westcort
	Mometasone furoate 0.1%	Cream, lotion, solution	Elocon
	Triamcinolone acetonide 0.1%	Cream	Kenalog, Aristocort A
V. Medium-low[a]	Betamethasone dipropionate 0.05%	Lotion	Diprosone
	Flucosinolone acetonide 0.025%	Cream	Synalar
	Triamcinolone acetonide 0.025%	Ointment	Kenalog, Aristocort
VI. Low[a]	Alclometasone dipropionate 0.05%	Cream, ointment	Aclovate
	Betamethasone valerate 0.1%	Lotion	Beta-Val, Valisone
	Desonide 0.05%	Foam	Verdeso
	Flucosinolone acetonide 0.01%	Cream	Synalar
	Flucosinolone acetonide 0.01%	Oil, body and scalp aerosol spray, cream, lotion	Derma-Smoothe/FS
VII. Very low[a]	Fluocinolone acetonide 0.01%	Solution	Synalar
	Hydrocortisone base or acetate 1%,	Cream, ointment	Cortisporin
	Hydrocortisone base or acetate 2.5%	Cream, lotion, ointment	Cortisporin, Hytone, U-cort, Vytone
	Hydrocortisone base or acetate 0.5%	Cream	Cortaid cream

[a] Only low-potency or medium-to-low potency steroids should be used on the face, diaper area, axilla, and in young children, and only for short periods of time.

Sources: Adapted from Cohen, B. A. (2005). *Pediatric dermatology* (p. 11). Philadelphia: Mosby; Nurse Practitioners' Prescribing Reference. (2007, Fall). Haymarket Media, Inc. (p. 117); Lehne, R. (2007). *Pharmacology for nursing care* (p. 1203). St. Louis, MO: Saunders/Elsevier.

Topical Calcineurin Inhibitor (TCIs)

This class of medications exhibits a potent anti-inflammatory effect without the immune suppression caused by corticosteroids. Pimecrolimus (Elidel) and tacrolimus (Protopic) are safe products in children after the age of 2 years. Pimecrolimus is effective in treating mild to moderate atopic dermatitis whereas tacrolimus is more often used to treat moderate to severe atopic dermatitis. Both are applied two times a day and can be used concomitantly with topical steroids. In addition, both can be used in areas of thinner skin without the risk of skin atrophy and striae (Peterson & Chen, 2006). These agents inhibit the phosphatase activity of calcineurin, thereby preventing the expression of a number of proinflammatory cytokines (interleukin [IL]-2, IL-3, IL-4, IL-5, granulocyte-macrophage colony-stimulating factor, tumor necrosis factor-alpha, and interferon-gamma), which play significant roles in the pathophysiology of atopic dermatitis (Nghiem, Peterson, & Langley, 2002). These agents have decided advantages over topical corticosteroids because they can be used safely on the face and in intertriginous areas without causing skin atrophy, striae, hypopigmentation, or hypothalamic-pituitary-adrenal (HPA) axis suppression.

Topical calcineurin inhibitors can be used safely around the eyes of atopic dermatitis patients without concern for increasing intraocular pressure or contributing to cataract formation (Tharp, 2005).

Systemic Therapy

Systemic steroids may be employed for a short period of time to treat severe atopic dermatitis. However, concerns over side effects and a rebound effect that may occur after discontinuation limit their use (Abramovits, 2005). In severe recalcitrant atopic dermatitis immunomodulators (cyclosporine, azathioprine, mycophenolate mofetil) may also be needed, but it is imperative that these patients be followed closely to detect any side effects. These types of medications should not be used long term (Paller et al., 2005).

Other Treatments

Some other treatments that may be used include:

- *Ultraviolet (UV) light therapy:* Psoralen plus ultraviolet A light (PUVA) therapy should only be used in patients with severe, widespread, recalcitrant atopic dermatitis (Leung & Bieber, 2003). Referral to a dermatologist would be indicated for such a condition.
- *Antibiotics:* These are recommended for patients with an active infection or heavy colonization of *S. aureus* (Darsow et al., 2005). If a flare-up of atopic dermatitis occurs with evidence of skin infection, a course of oral antibiotics is recommended.

- *Antivirals:* Acyclovir should be used in herpeticum eczema because this infection can be life threatening in patients with atopic dermatitis.
- *Atopiclair:* This is a new steroid-sparing prescription cream whose safety and efficacy have been previously demonstrated in adults with atopic dermatitis. It is also reported to be effective and safe in children and infants. The most frequent side effects are stinging, burning, fever, urinary tract infection, and the common cold (Louden, 2007). Its main drawback is its price. Again, a dermatologist probably should prescribe this medication if more common, less expensive medications are ineffective.
- *MimyX:* This product is indicated for relief of burning and itching associated with atopic dermatitis, allergic contact dermatitis, and radiation dermatitis. It contains olive and vegetable oils, glycerin, squalene, lecithin, and palmitoylethanolamide (PEA). PEA is thought to be missing in atopic skin. Its main action seems to be downregulating mast cell activation. When applied two times a day, studies have shown a decrease of 80% in itching, a 63% reduction in steroid use, and a 65% improvement in sleep quality in children (Smith, 2008).

How would you proceed to treat this patient with mild to moderate atopic dermatitis? ▮

Parental education is key to the successful treatment of AD in a child. Bathing is first addressed by instructing the mother to use only tepid bath water and Dove soap. After patting her daughter dry, she is to apply Aquaphor cream two times a day. On the affected areas she is to apply triamcinolone 0.1% ointment three times a day for 4–5 days. At night the child is to be given Benadryl liquid to help her sleep until the eczema improves and the itching subsides. You ask the mother to follow this initial treatment plan for 5 days and then return for re-evaluation. You are expecting improvement in that time.

The child is rechecked in 5 days and the areas of involvement are already healing well. The mother is instructed to use a step-up/step-down approach to her daughter's eczema, and hydrocortisone 2.5% ointment is prescribed for application to the affected areas until the inflammatory reaction has cleared. Once the inflammation has resolved, emollients alone are recommended for daily application to the skin of her body and face.

Patient Education

Patient and family education is an integral part of managing atopic dermatitis (Chisolm, Taylor, Balkrishnan, & Feldman, 2008). Education should include information on causes and triggers of atopic dermatitis, prognosis, treatment, and its prevention. Written instructions facilitate understanding and adherence (Chisolm et al., 2008). The healthcare provider must also address the patient's quality of life. **In this particular case, you instruct the mother to avoid the triggers that contributed to her daughter's condition, especially clothing and bathing,** and tell her that the routine use of emollients on a daily basis is foremost in the care of a child with atopic dermatitis. You may address food allergens later if Anna's condition remains problematic after treatment is started.

The use of midpotency corticosteroids with emollients during periods of flare-up and how to taper to less potent steroids over the course of the treatment needs to be understood by the family. Educate that there will be flare-ups and exacerbations, but provide reassurance that with a step-up/step-down treatment approach by the family these conditions can be brought under quick control. A significant percentage of children will outgrow atopic dermatitis in time, so constant reassurance to the family is extremely important and helps the family to adjust to the difficult times they may often have.

When do you wish to see this patient again? ■

Anna and her mother were to follow up in 3 weeks to reassess the treatment program and address any new questions the family may have.

When the patient and her mother return in 3 weeks, you notice a happier child with improved color and no dark lines under her eyes. The mother says her daughter is sleeping much better and her scratching has almost cleared. Reexamination of the patient's skin shows only a faint redness in the affected areas, and the lichenified areas are almost clear now. The mother is advised to continue with the emollients daily and to return if her daughter has a new flare-up that does not respond to step care by the family.

Key Points from the Case

1. Atopic dermatitis is treated through a multimodal approach.
2. In mild to moderate disease, the use of emollients and mild potency corticosteroids should be initiated.
3. In moderate to severe cases, the primary care provider may need to use emollients, moderate potency topical steroids, and topical calcineurin inhibitors in a step-wise approach.
4. In extreme cases, one would use all of the above as well as phototherapy and even systemic therapy. Care would be transferred to a dermatologist at this level.
5. Therapy for barrier dysfunction, inflammation, infection, and pruritus as well as the identification of possible trigger factors are all necessary in the management of atopic dermatitis.
6. Sometimes bacterial superinfection also needs to be treated.

REFERENCES

Abramovits, W. (2005). A clinician's paradigm in the treatment of atopic dermatitis. *Journal of the American Academy of Dermatology, 53*(Suppl 1), S70–S77.

Abramovits W., Goldstein, A. M., & Stevenson, L. C. (2003). Changing paradigms in dermatology: topical immunomodulators within a permetational paradigm for the treatment of atopic dermatitis and eczematous dermatitis. *Clinics in Dermatology, 21*(5), 383–391.

Barclay, L. (2008). Atopic dermatitis. *National Institute for Health and Clinical Excellence (NICE).* Retrieved July 2, 2008, from http://www.medscape.com/viewarticle/573546

Bardana, E. J. (2004). Immunoglobulin E (IgE) and non-IgE mediated reactions in the pathogenesis of atopic eczema/dermatitis syndrome (AEDS). *Allergy, 59*(S78), 25–29.

Carroll, C. L., Balkrishnan, R., Feldman, S. R., Fleischner, A. B., & Manuel, J. C. (2005). The burden of atopic dermatitis: impact on the family and society. *Pediatric Dermatology, 22*, 192–199.

Chisolm, S., Taylor, S., Balkrishnan, R., & Feldman, S. (2008). Written action plans: potential for improving outcomes in children with atopic dermatitis. *American Journal of Dermatology, 59*, 677–683.

Chung, H., Jeon, H., Sung, H., Kim, M., & Hong, S. (2008). Epidemiological characteristics of methicillin-resistant *Staphylococcus aureus* isolates from children with eczematous atopic dermatitis lesions. *Journal of Clinical Microbiology, 46*, 991–995.

Cohen, B. A. (2005). *Pediatric Dermatology.* Philadelphia: Mosby.

Darsow, U., Lubbe, J., Taieb, A., Seidenari, S., Wollenberg, A., Calza, A. M., et al. (2005). Position paper on diagnosis and treatment of atopic dermatitis. *Journal of the European Academy of Dermatology and Venereology, 19*(3), 286–295.

Gilliam, A., & Frieden, I. (2006). Treatment of atopic dermatitis: optimizing management and implications of the new labeling for topical calcineurin inhibitors (CME/CE). *Medscape.* Retrieved July 2, 2008, from http://www.medscape.com/viewarticle/535793

Krakowski, A., Eichenfield, L. F., & Dohil, M. A. (2008). Management of atopic dermatitis in the pediatric population. *Pediatrics, 122*, 812–824.

Lehne, R. (2007). *Pharmacology for Nursing Care.* St. Louis, MO: Saunders/Elsevier.

Leung, D. Y., & Bieber, T. (2003). Atopic dermatitis. *Lancet, 361*, 151–160.

Leung, D. Y., Nicklas, R. A., Li, J. T., Bernstein, I. L., Blessing-Moore, J., Boguniewicz, M., et al. (2004). Disease management of atopic dermatitis: an updated practice parameter. *Annals of Allergy, Asthma, and Immunology, 93*(3 Suppl.2), S1–S21.

Lewin Group. (2005). *The burden of skin diseases 2005. Executive summary prepared by the Society for Investigative Dermatology and the American Academy of Dermatology.* Falls Church, VA: Author.

Louden, K. (2007). New nonsteroidal cream for atopic dermatitis is effective, safe in infants and children. *Medscape Medical News.* Retrieved July 2, 2008, from http://www.medscape.com/viewarticle/560266

Mancini, A. J., Kaulback, K., & Chamlin, S. L. (2008). The socioeconomic impact of atopic dermatitis in the United States: a systematic review. *Pediatric Dermatology, 25*, 1–6.

Nghiem, P., Peterson, G., & Langley, R. G. (2002). Tacrolimus and pimecrolimus: from clever prokaryotes to inhibiting calcineurin and treating atopic dermatitis. *Journal of the American Academy of Dermatology, 46*, 228–241.

Novark, N., Bieber, T., & Leung, D. Y. (2003). Immune mechanisms leading to atopic dermatitis. *Journal of Allergy and Clinical Immunology, 112*, S128–S139.

Nurse Practitioners' Prescribing Reference. (2007, Fall). Haymarket Media, Inc.

Paller, A. S., Lebwohl, M., Fleischer, Jr., A. B., Antaya, R., Langley, R. G., Kirsner, R. S., et al. (2005). Tacrolimus ointment is more effective than pimecrolimus cream with a similar safety profile in the treatment of atopic dermatitis: results from 3 randomized, comparative studies. *Journal of the American Academy of Dermatology, 52*(5), 810–822.

Peterson, J., & Chen, L. (2006). A comprehensive management guide for atopic dermatitis. *Dermatology Nursing, 18*(6), 531–542.

Rowlands, D., Tofte, S., & Hanifin, J. (2006). Does food allergy cause atopic dermatitis? Food challenge testing to dissociate eczematous from immediate reactions. *Dermatologic Therapy, 19*, 97–103.

Rudikoff, D., & Lebwohl, M. (1998). Atopic dermatitis. *Lancet, 351*, 1715–1721.

Schmid-Grendelmeier, P., Simon, D., Simon, H. U., Akdis, C. A., & Wirthrich, B. (2001). Epidemiology, clinical features, and immunology of the intrinsic (non-IgE-mediated) type of atopic dermatitis (constitutional dermatitis). *Allergy, 56*(9), 841–849.

Spergel, J. (2008). Immunology and treatment of atopic dermatitis. *American Journal of Clinical Dermatology, 9*, 233–244.

Spergel, J. M., & Paller, A. S. (2003). Atopic dermatitis and the atopic march. *Journal of Clinical Immunology, 112*(6 Suppl), S118–S127.

Tharp, M. D. (2005). A multifaceted approach to the treatment of atopic dermatitis. *Medscape Dermatology, 6*(1). Retrieved July 2, 2008, from http://www.medscape.com/viewarticle/506964

Williams, H. C., Burney, P. G., Pembroke, A. C., & Hay, R. J. (1996). Validation of the U.K. diagnostic criteria for atopic dermatitis in a population setting. U.K. Diagnostic Criteria for Atopic Dermatitis Working Party. *British Journal of Dermatology, 135*, 12–17.

Chapter 31

The Teen Boy with Acne

Catherine E. Burns
Danielle J. Poulin

Sometimes a diagnosis seems to be quite apparent from the onset of the visit. Still, the provider needs to do the appropriate data collection via history and physical examination, consider alternative diagnoses, and plan care that is individualized to the patient—the "art of medicine."

Educational Objectives
1. Apply the guidelines for management of acne to a teenage patient.
2. Discuss the impact of age upon the management plan.
3. Identify lifestyle factors that might affect the condition.
4. Discuss the cultural factors that might affect the management plan and the family's understanding and compliance with the plan of care.

Case Presentation and Discussion

José Gutierrez is a 16-year-old Mexican American male who comes to your migrant clinic for a sports physical. He has recently joined the wrestling team at his high school. He is accompanied by his mother, who speaks mostly Spanish. She explains via his interpreting that she wants you to help José with his acne, which has been getting worse over the past year and he agrees, hesitantly, though in excellent English, that he doesn't like the lesions on his face, chest, and back and would like help with this problem.

You ask Mrs. Gutierrez to wait in the waiting room while you talk with José about his health and complete the physical examination, assuring her that you will address the acne problem.

What questions will you ask José related to the acne problem? ■

Your symptom analysis reveals the following information: The lesions first appeared a year or two ago on his forehead. They seem to be getting worse and now are there all the time and have been appearing on his chest for the past 6 months. He has been showering daily, using Dial soap, but this doesn't seem to help. He has also bought some acne medicine at a local pharmacy and has been using that but sees little improvement. He can't remember what the name of the product is. His mother advises him to stop eating fries and chips but he hasn't done that. She also wants him to use an ointment that she got from her sister in Mexico but it stings and makes his skin red and sore so he doesn't use it.

What other questions do you need to ask José? ■

Before answering this question, here is some more information about acne that you need to consider.

Pathophysiology of Acne

Acne is a disorder of the pilosebaceous unit (PSU). Most often the PSUs of the face, chest, back, shoulders, and upper arms are affected. The unit is made up of a wide, stratified squamous epithelium-lined follicle, a rudimentary hair, and large, multi-lobulated sebaceous glands.

The pathogenesis involves androgen stimulation, which causes an enlargement of the sebaceous glands and an increase of sebum production. The androgens also stimulate hyperkeratosis of the follicle causing increased density of keratin and abnormal shedding of the epithelial cells lining the follicle. The combination of sebum and epithelial cell proliferation creates a microcomedone, a precursor to the visible acne lesion. As the microcomedone enlarges, it becomes a noninflammatory or inflammatory lesion.

The noninflammatory lesions are open or closed. *Propionibacterium acnes* (*P. acnes*) are anaerobic bacteria normally present on the skin. The closed comedones create the anaerobic environment with the sebum substrate that supports bacterial proliferation. The bacteria stimulate inflammation and weaken the follicular walls. When the walls break, the sebum spills out into the dermis where it causes additional inflammation and formation of a papule, pustule, or nodule. Multiple nodules and cysts can merge to form sinus tracts in the most severe cases (Gollnick, 2003; Kerkemeyer, 2005).

Scars occur in up to 95% of acne cases (Gollnick, 2003). Postinflammatory hyperpigmentation occurs with patients who are darker in skin color such as Hispanics.

Epidemiology

Acne is the most common dermatologic problem affecting adolescents, with 80% affected at some point between 11 and 30 years (Paller & Mancini, 2006). It is also the most common dermatologic diagnosis among Hispanics (20.4%) (Halder & Nootheti, 2003). Acne occurs more frequently in adolescents, coinciding with puberty and the increases in androgen hormones. Some health problems associated with acne include XYY (Klinefeller Syndrome), hyperinsulinemia, insulin resistance, adrenal tumor, and pituitary tumor (Leonard et al., 2009; Paller & Mancini, 2006). Many medications can also trigger or exacerbate acne, including androgens, topical and systemic glucocorticosteroids, anabolic steroids, isoniazid, lithium, hydantoin, and gold (Cohen, 2005; Paller & Mancini, 2006). Other contributing factors include lotions, creams, or oils applied to the skin, which can be physically occlusive. Sports gear such as helmets or shoulder pads can also promote acne.

Use of anabolic steroids is relatively common among adolescents involved in sports (Vandenberg, Neumark-Sztainer, Cafri, & Wall, 2007). Anabolic steroid use may also cause weight gain, seborrhea, deepening voice, gynecomastia, and depression. There is an increased risk of acne when there are first-degree relatives with the condition. Environmental conditions can also contribute to acne. Working at a gas station or in a restaurant cooking fried foods are examples of risky environments.

Cultural/Ethnic Factors

Mexicans usually bathe or shower daily and may apply lotions to their skin (Guarnero, 2005); Hispanic males may use pomade when grooming their hair, a predisposing factor for pomade acne (Halder & Nootheti, 2003).

The Mexican American patient may seek the services of a curandera instead of or in addition to the services of Western healthcare providers. This may be true especially if the client lacks health insurance or access to Western health care (Guarnero, 2005). Lack of insurance, illegal status, and/or healthcare beliefs may lead the patient to self-treat acne with folk remedies (Guarnero) such as oregano (Howell et al., 2006).

Differential Diagnosis

The differential diagnoses for acne include cosmetic, mechanical, environmental, or drug-induced acne; rosacea; flat wart; milia; perioral dermatitis; and folliculitis. Other skin conditions common to wrestlers on sports teams include *herpes gladiatorum, tinea corporis gladiatorum,* and methicillin-resistant *Staphylococcus aureus* (MRSA) infections.

From the above review, some other information you should obtain from José includes the following:

- How much has he been wrestling recently? (Exposure to infectious agents)
- What head gear does he wear for wrestling? (Mechanical acne)
- Is he using any steroids to build muscle for his wrestling? (Steroid use)
- Is he taking any medications? (Drug-induced acne or drugs from Mexico)
- Is he working at a gas station, fast food restaurant, or elsewhere where oils are present? (Environmental factors)
- Does he use pomades to groom his hair (Halder & Nootheti, 2003) or other special soaps or cleansing products? (Cosmetic acne)

- Has he had any boils, other rashes, painful blisters, itching, or dryness? (MRSA, tinea, herpes)
- Have there been any other changes in his health—changes in weight, polydipsia, polyuria, polyphagia (Diabetes mellitus, adrenal tumor, insulin resistance), or hypertension? (Anabolic steroid use)
- Have they seen a curandera for this problem and, if so, what was recommended (Howell et al., 2006)? (Integrative medicine approach)
- Are any of his friends having similar problems, and are they having any success keeping acne under control? (Risk factors, peer influence for management)
- Is this problem making him feel self-conscious when he wrestles or elsewhere? (Self-esteem, embarrassment, possibility of limiting his sports participation)
- What is the family history of acne? (Risks, perceptions of care and outcomes)

José responds that he is not taking any medications or working. He has not had any other rashes, boils, or changes in his health. He uses a gel to groom his hair sometimes. He has not seen a curandera. Yes, some of his friends also have acne. One has seen a doctor and has some medications that are helping; others are just using over-the-counter treatments as far as he knows. For his wrestling, he wears ear guards that cover part of his cheeks and have a strap under his chin and through his hair but no other special gear. He has been wrestling all summer about twice a week to get ready for the wrestling season, but the coach checks out the team members' skin to be sure they don't have infections. He is embarrassed by the lesions, especially when he dresses for wrestling, but has not considered stopping the sport and doesn't feel depressed because of his appearance.

Physical Examination

Upon physical examination, you find that he has open and closed comedones on his face and forehead, back of the neck, and chest. There are also multiple papules and pustules in all stages of healing (> 40) and his skin is erythematous in the affected regions. There are no nodules, abscesses, or rashes consistent with MRSA, *herpes gladiatorum*, or *tinea corporis*. Height, weight, blood pressure, and the remainder of the physical examination are within normal limits for this Tanner stage 4 male. He does not have gynecomastia, hypertension, enlarged liver, edema, or other signs of anabolic steroid use or endocrine abnormalities.

Making the Diagnosis

This history and physical examination are consistent with a diagnosis of acne. He has papulopustular acne or inflammatory acne (Gupta et al., 2009) with pustules and lesions extending over a wide area but no nodules or cysts.

Comedonal acne has more comedones with little inflammation. Nodular acne or nodulocystic acne has nodules along with the other lesions. Pomade acne would be more pronounced on his forehead (Halder & Nootheti, 2003), steroid-induced acne is more prominent on the trunk, shoulders, and upper arms (Lembo, 2006). A single lesion would be suggestive of another diagnosis such as a MRSA abscess or localized infection.

Staging the severity of the condition is important to select the appropriate management strategy. Acne is sometimes graded as mild if there are less than 15 lesions and mostly comedones. It is considered moderate if there are 15 to 50 papules and pustules and rare cysts. Severe acne is defined as a predominance of nodules and cysts. Acne fulminans is an acute disorder that requires intensive treatment. It is rare but would present with ulcerative, nodular lesions on the face and upper trunk accompanied by fever, leukocytosis, elevated sedimentation rate, and polyarthritis (Paller & Mancini, 2006).

Other diagnoses to consider but that do not fit this picture include folliculitis, perioral dermatitis, rosacea, and seborrheic dermatitis (Roebuck, 2006).

Do you need to do anything to confirm the diagnosis, such as laboratory studies? ▉

No laboratory studies are recommended in general management of acne. Endocrine studies would be needed if an endocrine evaluation was merited based upon the physical findings.

Management

Therapeutic plan: What will you do therapeutically? ▉

The plan is determined by the type and severity of the acne and needs to be customized to improve the patient's adherence to the plan. The goals are to:

- Decrease excess sebum
- Decrease the abnormal keratinization and desquamation in the pilosebaceous follicle
- Decrease the colony count of *P. acnes*
- Decrease inflammation
- Decrease the risks of scarring

Decreasing embarrassment and increasing self-esteem are also important goals.

Treatment Options

You need to understand the various treatment options before you can create an individualized plan for this Hispanic adolescent. "Topical therapy is the standard of care for acne" (Strauss et al., 2007, p. 653).

The mainstay and first treatment of acne is a topical retinoid. Topical retinoids are also a mainstay of maintenance therapy. Their primary mechanism of action is normalization of follicular keratinization and perhaps facilitation of follicular penetration of other agents. These products help prevent microcomedones, the precursor of all the other lesions of acne. Retinoids are drying and somewhat irritating to the skin. Application on alternate nights or just two to three times per week is sometimes needed at the beginning of therapy (Roebuck, 2006). Retinoids should be applied to very dry skin to avoid the irritating effects. Alternative choices are azelaic acid or salicylic acid preparations, but these are less effective agents (Strauss et al., 2007).

Benzoyl peroxide is the next therapeutic agent commonly used for acne management. It serves as an antibacterial, comedolytic agent and oxidizing agent. It is available in a variety of concentrations and vehicles though there is little evidence to evaluate the efficacy of these different formulations (Strauss et al., 2007). Gels, topical cleansers, pads, and creams are all available. Benzoyl peroxide is the most common ingredient in over-the-counter acne products (Institute for Clinical Systems Improvement, 2006).

Topical antibiotics are used for moderate and severe acne conditions. *Propionibacterium acnes* is an anaerobic bacterium present in pilosebaceous follicles. The antibiotics reduce colonization and may possess direct anti-inflammatory effects. A combination of erythromycin or clindamycin and a topical retinoid are more effective than either agent alone. Combining either of these agents with benzoyl peroxide decreases bacterial resistance and enhances efficacy and again, combining the products is more effective than using either product alone (Strauss et al., 2007).

Oral antibiotics are considered the standard of care for moderate and severe acne and treatment-resistant forms of inflammatory acne (Strauss et al., 2007). Doxycycline and minocycline are more effective than tetracycline; minocycline may be more effective than doxycycline. Erythromycin should be used only in those who cannot use the tetracyclines because bacterial resistance is common. Trimethoprim-sulfamethoxazole can be used when the other antibiotics cannot be used. Azithromycin has also been used. There are no studies that support use of ampicillin, amoxicillin, or cephalexin according to the expert panel of the American Academy of Dermatology (Strauss et al.). Because antibiotic resistance is increasing and there are some side effects of antibiotics, they should all be used for as short a time as possible. Vaginal candidiasis is a problem for female patients with all the antibiotics. Doxycycline is associated with photosensitivity. Minocycline may cause pigment deposition in skin, mucous membranes, and teeth. Pigmentation may occur in acne scars, anterior shins, and mucous membranes. Autoimmune hepatitis and serum sickness-like reactions are all rare occurrences with minocycline (Strauss et al.).

Hormonal agents may also be helpful in treatment of acne among women. These decrease androgen levels and thus the production of sebum. Oral contraceptives, spironolactone, and cyproterone acetate are among these types of agents. Oral corticosteroids used in short courses of high dose may be beneficial in patients with highly inflammatory disease but are not considered mainstays of treatment (Strauss et al., 2007).

Oral isotretinoin, a vitamin-A derivative, is approved for treatment of severe acne. It can also be used in less severe cases where either physical or psychological scarring is occurring. It is a potent teratogen and has many other serious adverse effects so it should only be prescribed by physicians knowledgeable in its administration and monitoring. Female patients must participate in the iPLEDGE program (http://www.ipledgeprogram.com). Mood disorders, depression, and suicidal ideation have been reported in addition to other effects summarized in Table 31-1.

The summary of a plan for management of acne of different types and in different levels of severity is found in Table 31-2.

In José's case, it would be appropriate to prescribe a topical retinoid, benzoyl peroxide, and a topical antibiotic. You choose adapalene 0.1% cream because it is effective and has fewer problems with burning and drying than other agents, and 1% clindamycin with 5% benzoyl peroxide (Duac gel), which should be easy for him to use. You prescribe the adapalene for use at night. The Duac can be applied after the adapalene. Use of an oral antibiotic such as doxycycline is also an option, but you choose to begin more conservatively and then see if it should be added to the regimen later.

Educational plan: What will you do to educate him and his mother about acne and its management? ■

Points to make through discussion include:
- Explain the diagnosis and its pathophysiology, chronic nature, and need for maintenance after it is brought under control.
- Explain the use of the various agents you are prescribing: adapalene 0.1% cream, 1% clindamycin with 5% benzoyl peroxide (Duac), and their side effects.
- Reassure them that acne is very treatable but results may not be apparent for 6 to 12 weeks. He will need to be patient until the improvements begin.
- Alert him that an increase in the number of lesions is common as all the developing ones in the skin layers emerge, but this effect will subside as the lesions are eliminated.
- Warn him that some mild irritation and drying may occur at the beginning of treatment, but this response should subside over time.
- Advise him to:
  - Avoid harsh cleansers and wash with mild soap and water morning and night.
  - Use a noncomedogenic sunscreen to minimize sun exposure and photosensitivity and a noncomedogenic moisturizer if needed to combat dryness.
  - Avoid over-the-counter acne products at the same time as the prescription ones are being used.

Table 31-1   Therapeutic Agents Used for Acne

Class	Drug	Dose	Mechanism of Action	Comments
I. Topical Keratolytic or Comedolytic Agents				
Retinoids	Tretinoin (Retin A, Avita)	0.01% to 0.25% gel, 0.25% to 0.1% cream 0.1% microgel	Normalizes follicular keratinization and possibly enhances follicular penetration of other agents. Promotes drainage of comedones and development of new ones.	Topical therapy is considered the standard of care for acne. Topical retinoids are generally applied in the evening to dry skin. Azelaic acid and salicylic acid are alternates.
	Adapalene (Differin)	0.1% gel or cream	Normalizes follicular keratinization and possibly enhances follicular penetration of other agents. Prevents microcomedones.	Less irritating and better tolerated than other topical retinoids (Zaenglein & Thiboutot, 2006).
Benzoyl peroxide	Benzoyl peroxide	Various strengths, cream, gels	Benzoyl peroxide reduces colonization of *P. acnes* and reduces inflammation. Also reduces antimicrobial resistance.	Commercial products are available without prescription or in combination with topical antibiotics. Applying the retinoid medication to the benzoyl peroxide pad and then wiping the face with the combination assures even distribution of both products and enhances compliance.
II. Antibiotics			These drugs penetrate the follicle and sebaceous gland well and decrease colony counts. Suppress *P. acnes* and decrease inflammation.	
A. Topical	Clindamycin	1% solution, lotion, gel, pledget		Evoclin Foam is a foam version that is more acceptable for hair areas. It is odorless, nonstaining, and easier to apply to large

Table 31–1 Therapeutic Agents Used for Acne (Continued)

			areas such as the back and chest (Roebuck, 2006).
	Clindamycin with benzoyl peroxide	1% clindamycin with 5% benzoyl peroxide (Benzaclin or Duac)	*P. acnes* is less resistant to combination products than topical antibiotics or benzoyl peroxide alone.
	Erythromycin	1% to 2% solution, 3% gel or swabs	High rate of antimicrobial resistance.
	Erythromycin with benzoyl peroxide	3% with benzoyl peroxide 5% gel (Benzamycin)	*P. acnes* is less resistant to combination products than topical antibiotics or benzoyl peroxide alone.
		Decrease *P. acnes* colonies and thus reduce inflammation. Used with topical products.	
B. Oral			Considered standard of care for moderate to severe acne and treatment-resistant forms. Because bacterial resistance is increasing, these should not be used in those with less severe acne and the duration should be limited.
	Tetracycline	500 mg to 1,000 mg in 1–4 divided doses	Less effective than doxycycline or minocycline (Strauss et al., 2007). Should be taken on an empty stomach and not before bedtime because ulceration of the esophagus can occur. Photosensitivity is common (Haider & Shaw, 2004).

(continues)

Table 31-1   Therapeutic Agents Used for Acne (Continued)

	Erythromycin	500 mg to 2,000 mg in 1–4 divided doses.	Should only be used in those who cannot use tetracycline (pregnant women or those < 8 years of age) (Strauss et al., 2007).
	Minocycline	50 mg to 200 mg in 1–2 divided doses. Extended release tablets are available.	More effective than tetracycline and doxycycline. Associated with pseudotumor cerebri, blue-gray hyperpigmentation, and drug-induced lupus, so it is a less desirable choice (Haider & Shaw, 2004).
	Doxycycline	50 mg to 200 mg in 1–2 divided doses. Adoxa available in several dosages in a pack similar to contraceptive packaging to help with daily dosing determination.	More effective than tetracycline.
	Trimethoprim with sulfamethoxazole	160 mg TMP/800 mg SMZ PO q12h	Effective where other antibiotics cannot be used.
Systemic Retinoid	Isotretinoin (Acutane)	Decreases sebum production with resulting decrease in *P. acnes* bacteria and inflammation.	Used only for severe nodular acne or moderate acne that has been resistant to all other treatments or in cases of severe psychological distress. Requires cholesterol level,

Table 31-1   Therapeutic Agents Used for Acne (Continued)

				triglyceride level, and liver function tests. Teratogenic. Associated with depression and suicide. Affects skin and mucous membranes, may decrease bone density, alter light sensitivity and vision, and cause GI effects and elevated triglyceride and cholesterol levels (Gupta et al., 2009). Prescribers must follow iPLEDGE. Not for primary care providers.
Other Treatments	Oral contraceptives			May help women who fail conventional acne therapies. Reduces androgen production.
	Spironolactone	50–200 mg daily	Antiandrogenic effects	Sometimes used in adult women if high testosterone levels are felt to be a contributing factor. May decrease sodium and increase potassium levels, so these need to be monitored.
	Intralesional injections	Triamcinolone 2–10 mg/cc	Rarely used to inject large acne cysts	Risk of skin atrophy. Not for primary care providers.
	Tea tree oil			Effective in one study, though onset of action is slower than with other topical treatments (Strauss et al., 2007).

Sources: Gupta, A. K., Cooper, E., Cunliffe, W., Gover, W., Melissa, D. (2009). Oral isotretinoin for acne (protocol). *Cochrane Database of Systematic Reviews, 1,* 1–10; Haider, A., & Shaw, J. C. (2004). Treatment of acne vulgaris. *Journal of the American Medical Association, 202,* 726–735; Roebuck, H. L. (2006). Acne: intervene early. *The Nurse Practitioner, 31,* 25–53; Strauss, J. S., Krowchuk, D. P., Leyden, J. S., Lucky, A. W., Shalita, A. R., Siegfried, E. C., et al. (2007). Guidelines of care for acne vulgaris management. *Journal of the American Academy of Dermatology, 56,* 651–663; Zaenglein, A. L., & Thiboutot, D. M. (2006). Expert committee recommendations for acne management. *Pediatrics, 118,* 1187–1199.

Table 31-2 Outline of Care for Acne			
Acne Type	**Medications**	**Education**	**Comments**
Comedonal	Topical retinoid	Apply to entire affected area. May need to begin with every other night or 2–3 times per week at beginning until skin adapts.	Alternatives for patients intolerant of retinoids may be azelaic acid or salicyclic acid preparations, but these are less effective.
Papulopustular: mild	Topical retinoid plus benzoyl peroxide or a combination product	Benzoyl peroxide can bleach clothing.	
Moderate, nodular	Topical retinoid plus oral antibiotic plus benzoyl peroxide or combination benzoyl peroxide/topical antibiotic product		Oral antibiotics should be prescribed for 3–6 months, tapering and discontinuing as soon as possible to reduce antibiotic resistance. Antiandrogens can be considered for females with hyperandrogenemia.
Severe, nodular	Isotretinoin		Because of several potentially severe side effects, it should be prescribed by a provider experienced with its use and compliant with the iPLEDGE program. Usually primary care providers refer to dermatologists at this level of care.
Maintenance	Topical retinoid +/- benzoyl peroxide or combination benzoyl peroxide/topical antibiotic product		

Source: Adapted from Zaenglein, A. L., & Thiboutot, D. M. (2006). Expert committee recommendations for acne management. *Pediatrics, 118,* 1187–1199.

- Avoid oily pomades and keep his hair off his face.
- Avoid squeezing or manipulating the lesions because this will increase infection in the skin.
- Assure Jose and his mother that most foods are not related to acne.
- Tell him that his acne is not directly related to his wrestling contact with other students, but his ear guard may be a source of some acne lesions on his cheeks. Wrestling, however, can lead to other skin infections and he should watch for any other lesions that are different from the acne ones he currently has.

When do you want to see this patient back again? ■

Generally you want to see new patients beginning acne management in about 6 weeks to assess response to medications and to support the patient as he takes on this new management regimen. You may need to increase the level of care, reduce it, or move to a maintenance program after initial success.

José and his mom seem to understand the regimen as explained and ask appropriate questions. You choose to get a translator for your discussion with the mother so that José is not expected to fulfill that role. You also hand him the prescriptions to give a nonverbal gesture of your trust in him as the primary manager of his condition and his ability to make decisions.

When he returns in 6 weeks, his face and chest have only 15 papules and pustules but there are still many comedones. You congratulate him on his care of his condition and he seems pleased with the progress, although he doesn't like the dryness of his skin and he didn't like the emergence of so many pustules during the first few weeks of the treatment. He does not have more lesions on his cheeks where the ear guards were in place. You elect to continue the treatment for another 6 weeks and then reassess his progress.

Key Points from the Case

1. Guidelines simplify the care of acne. They are based on the severity of the condition.

2. Treatment of acne in a teen requires understanding physiology, activities, cognitive development and experience, and the role of provider as advisor, not director, for care.

3. Activities such as sports or after-school work could influence the development and severity of conditions such as acne and need to be considered in assessment and planning for care.

4. Treatment of acne can be influenced by cultural beliefs and practices as with any healthcare problem. Awareness and openness to other approaches to management is helpful.

REFERENCES

Cohen, B. A. (2005). Disorders of the hair and nails. In B. A. Cohen (Ed.), *Pediatric dermatology* (pp. 201–235). Philadelphia: Elsevier Mosby.

Gollnick, H. (2003). Current concepts of the pathogenesis of acne: implications for drug treatment. *Drugs, 63,* 1579–1596.

Guarnero, P. A. (2005). Mexicans. In J. G. Lipson & S. L. Dibble (Eds.), *Cultural and clinical care* (pp. 330–342). San Francisco: UCSF Nursing Press.

Gupta, A. K., Cooper, E., Cunliffe, W. W, Gover, W., & Melissa, D. (2009). Oral isotretinoin for acne (protocol). *Cochrane Database of Systematic Reviews, 1,* 1–10.

Halder, A., & Nootheti, P. K. (2003). Ethnic skin disorders overview. *Journal of the American Academy of Dermatology, 48,* S143–S148.

Haider, A., & Shaw, J. C. (2004). Treatment of acne vulgaris. *Journal of the American Medical Association, 202,* 726–735.

Howell, L., Kochlar, K., Saywell, R., Zollinger, T., Koehler, J., Mandzuk, C., et al. (2006). Use of herbal remedies by Hispanic patients: do they inform their physicians? *Journal of the American Board of Family Medicine, 19,* 566–578.

Institute for Clinical Systems Improvement. (2006). *Acne management.* Retrieved March 20, 2008, from http://www.icsi.org/acne__for_patients___families__ 17995/acne_management__for_patients___families__2.html

Kerkemeyer, K. (2005). Acne vulgaris. *Plastic Surgical Nursing, 2,* 31–35.

Lembo, R. (2006). Dermatology. In R. M. Kliegman, K. J. Marcdante, H. B. Jensen, & R. E. Behrman (Eds.), *Nelson essentials of pediatrics* (pp. 877–898). Philadelphia: Elsevier Saunders.

Leonard, T., Eady, A., & Leonardi-Bee, J. (2009). Complementary therapies for acne vulgaris (protocol). *Cochrane Database of Systematic Reviews, 1,* 1–14.

Paller, A. S., & Mancini, A. J. (2006). Disorders of the sebaceous and sweat glands. In A. S. Paller & A. J. Mancini (Eds.), *Hurwitz clinical pediatric dermatology* (pp. 185–204). Philadelphia: Elsevier Saunders.

Roebuck, H. L. (2006). Acne: intervene early. *The Nurse Practitioner, 31,* 25–53.

Strauss, J. S., Krowchuk, D. P., Leyden, J. S., Lucky, A. W., Shalita, A. R., Siegfried, E. C., et al. (2007). Guidelines of care for acne vulgaris management. *Journal of the American Academy of Dermatology, 56,* 651–663.

Vandenberg, P., Neumark-Sztainer, D., Cafri, G., & Wall, M. (2007). Steroid use among adolescents. Longitudinal findings from Project EAT. *Pediatrics, 119,* 476–482.

Zaenglein, A. L., & Thiboutot, D. M. (2006). Expert committee recommendations for acne management. *Pediatrics, 118,* 1187–1199.

Chapter 32

The Limping Child

Jan Bazner-Chandler

A child with acute onset of a limp presents a diagnostic problem of some complexity and urgency that requires an efficient and structured sequence of diagnosis and treatment. The etiology can be infection, genetic, developmental disorders, physical injury, neoplastic, hematologic, or vascular. This case study explores the presenting symptoms and signs of this condition and will review the workup and treatment of the underlying causes.

Educational Objectives

1. Define normal gait development as related to developmental age.
2. Apply guidelines for the diagnosis of the child with a limp, taking into consideration the chronological and developmental age of the child.
3. Consider the differential diagnoses of a limp of acute onset.
4. Choose appropriate diagnostic testing and treatment options.
5. Describe desirable outcomes as a function of disease state.
6. Describe treatment, follow-up, and compliance with medical management.

Case Presentation and Discussion

Tyler, a 4-year-old African American male, presents to the clinic with a 2-day history of a limp and now refuses to bear weight. His mother states he felt abnormally warm last night when she put him to bed but she did not take his temperature. Today he has been less active than usual, and his appetite has been poor. He is the youngest of three boys and is usually quite active.

What additional history do you want to collect as the healthcare provider? ■

The healthcare provider must get additional information regarding chief complaint, history of present illness, past medical history, family, and social history in order to make the diagnosis and begin treatment. In this particular case, you will need more information about the following:

- *Characteristics of pain:* Degree of pain using FACES pain tool, pattern (Is there any time of day when the limp is worse? Has the limp or pain interfered with normal activity? Is there any weakness in the extremity?), location, and quality.

- *Activities:* Has there been any trauma, injuries, or potential for child abuse?
- *Recent infections or exposure to infections:* Family and other contacts.
- *Constitutional signs or symptoms:* Weight loss, change in eating or sleep patterns, irritability.
- *Birth, immunization, nutritional, and developmental history:* Any pregnancy, labor, or delivery problems; immunizations to date; details about whether speech and language, personal, social, and fine and gross motor skills are developmentally appropriate for his age based on results of developmental screening.
- *Family medical history:* Stature, cancer, arthritis, inflammatory or sickle cell disease.
- *Socialization:* Day care, babysitter, family members.
- *Medications:* Prescription and over the counter.
- *Environment:* Lead exposure.

History of Present Illness, Family and Social History

Here is what was revealed in the analysis of the symptoms and the family and social history:

> The mother states that Tyler was born full term via a normal spontaneous vaginal delivery. Developmentally he has reached all of his milestones. His immunizations are up-to-date by record review. He has no known allergies. The mother states she took him to the emergency department for a fever, earache, watery eyes, and a cough 1 month ago. He was diagnosed as having an ear infection and a viral upper respiratory infection. His treatment consisted of an antibiotic and cough syrup. He had two doses of acetaminophen for fever after the emergency room visit but none since. Currently there are no immediate family members who are sick with infectious diseases. There was no known trauma. An uncle has the sickle cell trait but Tyler has tested negative for the trait. A grandmother has type 2 diabetes, hypertension, and arthritis.

Physical Examination

What information do you want to collect from the physical examination? ■

It is important to examine the child to identify the anatomic location of the pain. The examiner must determine what body segment is creating the problem. Observation will reveal body habitus such as preference for supine, side lying, or prone position. Immobility or pseudoparalysis is an indicator of pain. Hip flexion and external rotation are positions of relative comfort for a painful hip, as is flexion of the knee. The presence of guarding (resistance to motion with gentle passive movement) can indicate the location of the pain. Range of motion of each body segment should be measured along with circumference and length of each body segment in the lower extremities. Asymmetry of the thighs or legs may suggest a chronic condition. The examiner should obtain and record vital signs, perform a vascular examination, and determine if erythema or edema is present.

The essential features of the examination of the extremities are inspection, palpation, and range of motion testing. It is important to inspect the extremities for evidence of deformity, erythema, swelling, effusion, and asymmetry. Palpate for edema, pulses, and manifestations of tenderness or guarding. Examine each joint for range of motion and note any restrictions. The child should be placed prone if possible, with the knees flexed; rotate the hip in and out to check for asymmetry. Examine the child's shoes for wear patterns and fit. Observe the pattern of walking. In the ambulatory older infant, toddler, or small child, have the child walk back to the caretaker while you observe their gait. In the toddler or small child, the use of distraction can often get the child to cooperate. A child with an inflammation of the hip will keep the hip in a position of flexion, abduction, and external rotation because this position reduces pressure from increased fluid within the joint capsule. In the presence of bacterial infection, any motion is exquisitely painful. The examiner should be aware that developmental dysplasia can cause asymmetric abduction without severe pain. A modified log roll test may help to determine the severity of hip irritation. The child lies supine and the examiner gently rotates the involved limbs from side to side.

Tyler's physical examination reveals the following: temperature 37.6°C (99.7°F), heart rate 124, respiratory rate 36, blood pressure 115/76, and weight 24 kg (52 lbs 12 ozs).

General appearance: The child is lying across his mother's lap, immobile but alert and responsive. His skin shows no erythema or rashes.

Neurological: Deep tendon reflexes on the right are 2+ and not determinable on the left due to pain.

Orthopedic:

- No abnormal curvature of the spine; no hair tufts or dimples are noted.
- When asked to locate his pain, he points to the groin and upper thigh.
- All upper extremity joints have full range of motion with no swelling, erythema, or pain with palpation.
- His right ankle, knee, and hip have unrestricted pain-free motion.
- His left hip is held flexed, abducted, and externally rotated.
- He has guarding and begins to cry and pushes your hand away when you attempt to move the left hip.
- His left knee and ankle are nontender and have no swelling or erythema.
- His leg and thigh measurements are circumferentially equal.
- His leg lengths are equal.

The examiner must also take into account the normal gait of young children. Characteristics of childhood gaits are found in Table 32-1. Because Tyler will not walk, you cannot assess his gait today.

Table 32-1 Gait According to Chronologic Age	
Age	Description of Gait
10–12 months	Cruises while holding onto objects
12–14 months	Walks short distances and stands unaided
17–21 months	Balances on one foot long enough to walk up steps
30–36 months	Balances on one foot for more than a second
36 months	Develops sufficient balance to attain a normal gait pattern

Differential Diagnosis

A limp is defined as any deviation from a normal gait pattern for the child's age. An antalgic limp is caused by pain and is remarkable because the amount of time the patient spends with his or her body supported by the involved extremity is reduced. In contrast, a short leg limp caused by a leg length difference results in a gait in which equal time is spent on both legs. A chronic limp of weeks to months is typically associated with atrophy of the thigh and calf as well. The inability of young children to clearly describe the location and nature of their pain contributes to the diagnostic challenge.

Common causes for antalgic limp are conditions that cause hip pain such as trauma or inflammation. Inflammation, in turn, can be caused by infection, arthritis, neoplasia, and vasculitis. The causes of limp in the pediatric population can be further sorted by age.

For a 4-year-old, the most relevant considerations are:

- Trauma
- Infection
  - Bacterial infection of the hip joint
  - Osteomyelitis of the femur or acetabulum
  - Postviral synovitis (toxic synovitis)
- Developmental
  - Congenital hip dysplasia (CHD)
  - Legg-Calve-Perthes disease (LCPD)
- Autoimmune: juvenile rheumatoid arthritis (JRA), also called juvenile arthritis (JA)
- Hemoglobinopathy: sickle cell disease
- Neoplasia: leukemia or tumor—benign or malignant

Limping is a common clinical problem in childhood. Limping is a gait abnormality due to pain (Fordham et al., 2007). Limping can be the result of a fracture, sprain/strain, or contusion. Overuse syndromes are more common in the school-age child and present as stress fractures, shin splints, Sever's disease, apophysitis of the tibial tubercle (Osgood-Schlatter disease), and chondromalacia patellae. A chronic limp can be the result of developmental hip dysplasia or leg length discrepancy. A history of a limp that appears worse in the morning and gets better with use suggests a rheumatologic process. Night pain, especially if the pain wakes the child from sleep, can be an indicator of a bone tumor. "Growing pains" often present as bilateral leg pain, with pain occurring at night, and no limp, pain, or symptoms during the day. Septic arthritis and transient synovitis both present with decreased motion of the hip. In the African American child with sickle cell disease, the differential diagnosis of osteonecrosis of the femoral head should be considered.

Trauma, resulting in strain, sprain, or fracture, is the most common cause of an acute limp in children. Fractures are more common than sprains and strains in the younger child. Child abuse should be suspected if the injury does not fit the history given, particularly if there is evidence of multiple fractures in different stages of healing or a spiral fracture indicative of a twisting mechanism of injury. Greenstick fractures, which are characterized as incomplete fractures, are seen only in children and are usually the result of a fall. Physeal fractures occur near joints and restrict or impede motion. Overuse syndromes such as Osgood-Schlatter disease (OSD) present as knee pain/limp due to repetitive activities such as running and jumping. OSD is more common in the older school-age child or adolescent (Beach & Ficke, 2007).

Repeated microtrauma with bone collapse following interruption of blood flow to the femoral head is thought to be the cause of Legg-Calve-Perthes disease (LCPD), also known as juvenile avascular necrosis. LCPD is caused by ischemic episode(s) that interrupt the circulation to the capital femoral epiphysis. It accounts for 2% of childhood limps in the 3- to 12-year-old. A positive family history is found in 10% to 20% of cases. Whites are more affected than Asian Americans, and Asian Americans more than African Americans. LCPD typically affects short, active boys with a delay in bone age (Mace, 2006). LCPD is characterized by persistent knee, thigh, or groin pain. The history may include intermittent pain after activity. There may be a painless limp. Physical findings may include atrophy of the quadriceps and thigh with adduction flexion contracture. Children with LCPD can present with an antalgic gait or Trendelenburg gait resulting from pain in the gluteus medius muscle.

Slipped capital femoral epiphyses (SCFE) is a disease frequently seen in adolescents. There is a slightly higher incidence in males and African American children. Incidence is about 1 case per 100,000 people (Adler, 2008). During a period of rapid adolescent growth, the growth plate separates from the femoral neck. A large number of children with this condition are overweight for height. Additional risk factors include malnutrition, endocrine abnormalities, history of chemotherapy, and prior developmental dysplasia of the hip (DDH). Children with SCFE typically have a history that includes hip pain (50%) or knee pain (25%) over several weeks or a minor fall or trauma resulting in inability to bear weight (Adler). Physical findings include loss of complete hip flexion and ability to fully rotate the hip inward. The affected leg may appear shorter.

In an African American child, the possibility of complications of sickle cell disease has to be considered. Osteonecrosis of the femoral head is a common complication in patients with sickle cell disease. Children as young as 5 years of age who present with hip pain during an acute sickle cell crisis have been diagnosed with osteonecrosis of the femoral head (Neumayer et al., 2006). Osteonecrosis of the femoral head occurs in 90% of patients with sickle cell disease, and collapse of the femoral head occurs in 90% of patients within 5 years after the diagnosis of osteonecrosis. The prevalence of the complication peaks during adolescence (Neumayer et al.).

Musculoskeletal tumors, benign and malignant, are another cause for a limp. Malignant tumors, osteosarcoma, Ewing's sarcoma, and rhabdomyosarcoma account for 5% to 10% of malignant neoplasms in children (Junnila & Cartwright, 2006b). Osteosarcoma most often presents in the teenage years during episodes of growth spurts, and presents as pain in the upper arm near the shoulder area or leg pain above or below the knee that awakens the child at night. The child might also have pain at rest. The physical exam may reveal a lump or swelling at the site.

Acute lymphoblastic leukemia (ALL) is the most common malignancy in children; it occurs in 1 to 5 per 10,000 children, with peak incidence in children ages 2 to 5 years. Leukemia can present with nonspecific complaints of fever, bone, or joint pain (Junnila & Cartwright, 2006b). The pain is due to accumulation of blast cells in the bone marrow or joint fluid. The immature blasts crowd out healthy cells in the bone marrow.

Developmental dysplasia of the hip (DDH) can predispose a child to premature degenerative changes and painful arthritis. Hip dysplasia refers to abnormality in size, shape, orientation, or organization of the femoral head. Approximately 1 in 1,000 children is born with a dislocated hip, and 10 in 10,000 may have hip subluxation (Storer & Skaggs, 2006). Intrauterine position, sex, race, and a positive family history are the most important risk factors. A positive Galeazzi sign, inequality in height of knees in a supine position, is caused by hip dislocation or congenital femoral shortening. In the ambulatory child, a positive Trendelenburg sign or limping on the affected side may be a sign of a dislocated hip.

Benign nocturnal limb pains or growing pains present as cramping pains of the thigh, shin, and calf. They affect approximately 35% of children 4–6 years of age (Junnila & Cartwright, 2006b). Pain typically appears in the evening or at night and may awaken the child from sleep. Benign nocturnal limb pain is not associated with a limp (Junnila & Cartwright).

Juvenile rheumatoid arthritis (the most common type of childhood arthritis) can present with a limp. However, in a study by Junnila and Cartwright (2006b), 99% of children with pain as an isolated complaint did not have inflammatory disease. Systemic onset in children younger than 5 years will include a history of febrile episodes and macular or maculopapular rash with only mild joint involvement. Prolonged morning stiffness, swelling, and symptoms of weight loss, fever, and fatigue are suggestive of an inflammatory process such as arthritis and vasculitis (Junnila & Cartwright, 2006a).

In a review of 64 cases with septic arthritis, 33% of the children had been seen by healthcare professionals prior to definitive diagnosis and 33% had been treated previously with antibiotics (Luhmann et al., 2004). Septic arthritis and transient synovitis of the hip can present in a child as both a limp and a painful hip. Accurate diagnosis of septic arthritis is critical because of poor outcomes associated with delay in diagnosis. Septic arthritis of the hip requires surgical drainage and use of intravenous antibiotics.

The most common pathogen in septic arthritis is *Staphylococcus aureus.* Fever, bone pain, swelling, redness, and guarding the affected body part are common. In the infant and younger child, inability to support weight and asymmetric movement of the affected extremity are often early signs. On physical exam, painful swelling and point tenderness over the affected area are cardinal signs of infection/inflammation.

Toxic synovitis (TS) presents similarly to septic arthritis and is most likely a viral synovitis or postviral reactive arthritis that causes inflammation and pain around the hip joint. It most commonly causes a limp with pain. In one prospective study of 243 children under 14 years of age presenting with a limp, the most common diagnosis was transient synovitis (Fordham et al., 2007). The child often has a history of recent upper respiratory infection, pharyngitis, bronchitis, or otitis media. The child with TS is usually afebrile or has a mildly elevated temperature; high fever is rare. The affected hip is usually held flexed, abducted, and externally rotated. The main difference between TS and septic arthritis is that the child with TS does not appear systemically ill. The condition is self-limiting. In review of laboratory studies, white blood cell count (WBC) and erythrocyte sedimentation rate (ESR) may be slightly elevated. Transient synovitis, a self-limiting problem, is treated nonoperatively with oral analgesics and observation.

Making the Diagnosis

To make the correct diagnosis, you need to know the cause of the limp. Certain laboratory and radiographic data will help. In addition, you need to consider the child's age because certain pediatric orthopedic problems occur more often at one age than another.

What laboratory and radiographic data would help you make the diagnosis? ■

The workup for an irritable hip consists of a thorough history and physical examination along with plain radiographs of the hip and laboratory studies including a complete blood count (CBC) with differential, ESR, C-reactive protein (CRP), and blood culture (Luhmann et al., 2004). Anteroposterior and lateral radiographs, ultrasound, and MRI may be needed to differentiate among stress fractures, Legg-Calve-Perthes disease, and osteomyelitis. Anteroposterior and frog lateral views of the hip joint can rule out SCFE, LCPD, bone lesions, or congenital abnormalities. In the nonverbal patient, a screening anteroposterior film from hips to feet may identify any occult fractures. Ultrasound of the hip is useful in identifying fluid in the hip joint.

What imaging or laboratory tests are indicated? ■

In a child in whom the presenting symptoms are inconclusive, radiographic studies, CBC, ESR, and CRP would be indicated. Depending on the results of the blood work, an ultrasound of the hip with needle aspiration would provide the most accurate diagnosis. Delay in treatment of septic arthritis of the hip can lead to destruction of the hip joint, growth plate, and avascular necrosis of the femoral head.

Transient synovitis of the hip can be identified by the healthcare provider based on the history and physical examination. An afebrile, nontoxic-appearing child playing in the examination room and walking with a slight limp of recent onset most likely has transient synovitis and is treated with close monitoring, without need for invasive studies (Caird et al., 2006). Observation of the child for a period of time can help to distinguish between TS and septic arthritis. Children with bacterial infection will rapidly worsen, and children with synovitis will often improve over time. In general, children with septic arthritis appear more acutely ill than those with toxic synovitis (Luhmann et al., 2004). The more difficult patients to diagnose are those that present with a history of recent infection, elevation in temperature, and a painful hip with inability to bear weight.

Is the condition emergent? ■

The most important part of the diagnosis is to ensure that the hip pain is not caused by a bacterial infection of the hip joint. Early, accurate diagnosis of septic arthritis of the hip in children is critical because poor outcomes have been associated with a delay in diagnosis (Kocher, Mandiga, Zurkowski, Barnewold, & Kasser, 2004). Differentiating between septic arthritis and transient synovitis of the hip can be difficult.

Management

Tyler has a history of febrile illness in the past month and treatment with antibiotics for otitis media (OM) and upper respiratory infection (URI). The physical examination is positive for a painful left hip with pain on movement. Given the history and positive physical findings, an anteroposterior and lateral X-ray and laboratory tests including CBC with differential, ESR, and CRP would be indicated. The physiologic response to an early bacterial infection can be variable and can result in serum makers (elevated ESR, WBC, and CRP) of inflammation within the normal range of values (Luhmann et al., 2004). If the laboratory values indicate septic arthritis, an ultrasound with hip aspiration would be indicated.

Medical management differs depending on the diagnosis. In transient synovitis, bed rest, non-weight-bearing activity, and nonsteroidal anti-inflammatory drugs are the standard treatment recommendations. In septic arthritis, the child would need to be managed by an orthopedic surgeon and requires immediate surgical intervention and intravenous antibiotics.

Test Results

After reviewing Tyler's hip X-rays and laboratory values, you make the diagnosis of transient synovitis. The sedimentation rate is 6 mm/hr, C-reactive protein is 0.3 mg/L, and WBC count is 10,000/mm³.

Kocher and associates (2004) developed a clinical prediction algorithm for septic arthritis based on four clinical variables: history of fever, non-weight-bearing, an erythrocyte sedimentation rate of greater than or equal to 40 mm/hr, and serum white blood-cell count greater than 12,000/mm³. When all four variables are present the child has a 99.6% chance of having septic arthritis of the hip (Kocher et al., 2004). C-reactive protein level was added as an important part of the evaluation due to its elevation within 6 to 8 hours after onset of inflammatory process or infection. A C-reactive level of > 2.0 mg/dL is considered positive (Caird et al., 2006). Fever was defined as an oral temperature of 38.5°C (101.3°F) or greater during the week prior to admission (Luhmann et al., 2004).

Plain radiographs of the hip are useful in detecting other causes of hip pain; however, they are not sensitive enough to exclude the diagnosis of septic arthritis (Shah, 2005). An ultrasound of the hip is more sensitive than the plain film in identifying joint effusions of the hip. An ultrasound does not assist in determining the cause and is best used to guide hip aspiration. Diagnostic synovial fluid aspiration remains the gold standard for excluding septic arthritis of the hip (Shah). Specific etiologic agents can be identified through blood, bone, or joint aspirate cultures.

Educational plan: What does the mother need to know about transient synovitis and its management? ■

Transient synovitis is a benign disease, so treatment consists of supportive therapy. The major goal of therapy is to provide comfort and reduce activity until the inflammation subsides (Whitelaw & Schikler, 2008).

The treatment plan for Tyler will be:
- Bed rest or position of comfort for 7–10 days.
- Do not bear weight on affected limb.

- Avoid full unrestricted activity until limp and pain have resolved.
- In a 4-year-old, bed rest for any period of time may be difficult. Position the child on a couch or chair so he or she can observe family activity. Encourage sedentary activities with the help of siblings, such as board games, puzzles, or video games.
- Provide ibuprofen 10 mg/kg per dose given every 6 to 8 hours. The parent may administer it with food or milk to decrease GI upset.
- Return in 24 hours for repeat exam.
- Call if the child has high fever or symptoms worsen.

What medications will provide the best pain relief? ■

Naproxen and ibuprofen are the most frequently prescribed nonsteroidal anti-inflammatory drugs (NSAIDs) used for children. NSAIDs may shorten the duration of symptoms (Whitelaw & Schikler, 2008). In a randomized clinical trial, ibuprofen was found to shorten the duration of symptoms in cases of mild transient synovitis of the hip (Kocher, 2004). In cases of severe transient synovitis, medications such as ibuprofen or acetaminophen may need to be avoided so that symptoms of septic arthritis will not be masked (Kocher). The most important factor in the drug therapy is to make sure the parent/caretaker is giving the medication in the correct dose at the prescribed intervals. NSAIDs should be administered with food to avoid gastrointestinal upset. The parent/caretaker needs to understand that they are giving the medication for the anti-inflammatory effects so the medication needs to be given around the clock, not just when the child has pain or fever.

When do you want to see this child back? ■

Diagnosis of an infected hip is especially difficult in the early phase. The physiologic response to early bacterial infection is quite variable, and serum indicators of inflammation can be within normal range (Luhmann et al., 2004). Follow-up in 12 to 24 hours is crucial to check for changes in the child's condition.

24-Hour Follow-Up

Tyler is seen in the clinic the next morning. According to his mother he has been afebrile and slept through the night. She has given him the prescribed ibuprofen every 6 hours. He is sitting on his mother's lap looking at a picture book. When he is examined he still has some hip irritability and guarding, but is more cooperative than on the previous exam. An appointment is made to return to the clinic in 1 week with instructions to call if the child develops fever or increased pain. The mother is instructed to continue administering the ibuprofen for inflammation until the next visit.

One week later Tyler is seen in the clinic. He is sitting on the floor playing with a truck. His mother states it has been difficult to keep him from running around and playing with his brothers. He has been afebrile. On examination he has no complaints of pain or guarding, with range of motion of the hip. He is able to ambulate without a limp. At this time, you instruct the mother to discontinue the ibuprofen and to let him resume his normal activity. She is to return to the clinic if he becomes febrile or has hip pain.

Tyler's mother asks you if there are any long-term effects that she should watch for.

How will you answer her question? ■

The parent should be informed about the following expected outcomes:
- Transient synovitis requires systematic treatment and typically resolves without complication (Shah, 2005).
- Patients with transient synovitis usually experience marked improvement in 24–48 hours.
- Two thirds to three fourths of patients usually experience complete resolution in 2 weeks.
- The recurrence rate is 4–17%; most recurrences develop within 6 months.
- There is no increased risk for chronic juvenile arthritis.
- There is a slightly increased risk for developing osteoarthritis later in life (Whitelaw & Schikler, 2008).

Key Points from the Case

1. History with an analysis of the presenting symptoms and a physical exam are key to making the proper diagnosis.
2. Review of the causes of acute limping in the child identifies the differential diagnosis that must be considered.
3. Know the key radiographs and laboratory values that are needed to make the correct diagnosis.
4. Management and follow-up care of toxic synovitis are critical points to discuss with the parents.

REFERENCES

Adler, B. (2008). *Slipped capital femoral epiphysis.* Retrieved June 2, 2009, from http://emedicine.medscape.com/article/413810-overview

Beach, C. B., & Ficke, J. (2007). *Limping child.* Retrieved June 2, 2009, from http://emedicine.medscape.com/article/1258835-overview

Caird, M., Flynn, J. M., Leung, L., Millman, J., D'Italia, J., & Dormans, J. (2006). Factors distinguishing septic arthritis from transient synovitis of the hip in children. A prospective study. *Journal of Bone and Joint Surgery, 88*(6), 1251–1257.

Fordham, G., Gunderman, R., Blatt, E. R., Bulas., D., Coley, B. D., Poderbersky, D., et al. (2007). American College of Radiology ACR appropriateness criteria: limping child: ages 0–5 years *American College of Radiology.* Retrieved June 2, 2009, from http://www.guideline.gov/summary/summary.aspx?ss=15&doc_id=11598 &nbr=6011

Junnila, J., & Cartwright, V. (2006a). Chronic musculoskeletal pain in children: part I. Initial evaluation. *American Family Physician, 74*(1), 115–122.

Junnila, J., & Cartwright, V. (2006b). Chronic musculoskeletal pain in children: part II. Rheumatic causes. *American Family Physician, 74*(2), 293–300.

Kocher, M. (2004). Ibuprofen shortened time to symptom resolution in children with transient synovitis of the hip. *Journal of Bone and Joint Surgery, 86*(2), 439.

Kocher, M., Mandiga, R., Zurkowski, D., Barnewold, C., & Kasser, J. (2004). Validation of a clinical prediction rule for the differentiation between septic arthritis and transient synovitis of the hip in children. *Journal of Bone and Joint Surgery, 86*(8), 1629–1635.

Luhmann, S., Jones, A., Schootman, M., Gordon, J. E., Schoenecker, P., & Luhmann, J. (2004). Differentiation between septic arthritis and transient synovitis of the hip in children with clinical predictive algorithms. *Journal of Bone and Joint Surgery, 86*(5), 956–962.

Mace, S. (2006). Legg-Calve-Perthes disease: an update. *Resident and Staff Physician, 52*(7). Retrieved June 2, 2009, from http://www.residentandstaff.com/issues/articles/2006-07_07.asp

Neumayer, L. D., Auilar, C., Earles, A. N., Jergensen, H. E., Haberkern, C. M., Kammes, B., et al. (2006). Physical therapy alone compared with core decompression and physical therapy for femoral head osteonecrosis in sickle cell disease. Results of a multicenter study at a mean of three years after treatment. *Journal of Bone and Joint Surgery, 88*(12), 2573–2582.

Shah, S. S. (2005). Abnormal gait in a child with fever. Diagnosing septic arthritis of the hip. *Pediatric Emergency Care, 21*(5), 336–341.

Storer, S. K., & Skaggs, D. (2006). Developmental dysplasia of the hip. *American Family Physician, 74*(8), 1310–1316.

Whitelaw, C., & Schikler, K. (2008). *Transient synovitis.* Retrieved April 27, 2009, from http://emedicine.medscape.com/article/1007186-overview

Chapter 33

The Late-Preterm Baby Beginning Well-Child Care

Lori J. Silao

Late-preterm infants present a unique situation for the healthcare provider because these infants have higher morbidity and mortality rates than term infants. Thus, they need additional surveillance during their early health supervision visits. The healthcare provider needs to focus on both the infant's gestational age and potential associated problems when examining such patients. In addition, the family must be educated about the need to watch for worrisome signs and symptoms of illness or failure to thrive. Potential problems must first be addressed with parents when their baby is discharged home from the hospital and then continue to be addressed at subsequent health supervision visits.

Educational Objectives
1. Identify potential risk factors and apply management guidelines for the late-preterm infant.
2. Consider the age of the infant's primary caregivers and the impact of their maturity on the management plan developed.
3. Address cultural and socioeconomic factors that may affect the management plan and adherence with the identified plan of care.
4. Identify any infant health problems that may require further evaluation, and make appropriate referrals.

Case Presentation and Discussion

Sandra Jones is a 17-year-old white female who presents to your clinic with her newborn infant boy, Bobby, born at 35 and 4/7 weeks gestation. Sandra and her infant are accompanied by the baby's father who is also 17 years old and in his senior year of high school. They are here for the baby's first visit since being discharged from the hospital 2 days ago. Sandra is concerned that her son does not seem to be eating well and sleeps all the time. Initially, you need to attend to the facts that this is a late preterm infant being cared for by teen parents.

The Late-Preterm Infant

A late-preterm infant is defined as a baby born between 34 and 36 and 6/7 weeks gestation (Engle, Tomashek, & Wallman, 2007). It is known that infants generally gain approximately ½ pound per week during the last 6 weeks of gestation, so an infant born even slightly premature may be at risk for a lower birth weight. Although some late-preterm infants may weigh as much as a term infant, the late-preterm infant is still premature and arrives with his or her own set of potential health risks. Traditionally there have been few studies in this popula-tion (Engle et al., 2007). However, because of the increased number of late-preterm births in recent years and the associated problems these infants experience due to their immature physiologic and metabolic systems, there has been a recent increase in the number of research studies focusing on this cohort of infants. Noteworthy, some interesting early data are beginning to surface regarding in-utero development and postnatal adaptation in this population (Wang, Dorer, Fleming, & Catlin, 2004). Most of the research data point to certain disease processes that seem to be prevalent or place such infants at increased risk for potentially life-threatening situations. Thus, the late-preterm infant must be closely monitored with careful follow-up by the healthcare provider. The most common problems facing this group of infants are discussed in this case study.

Lung Function

Because of the potential for immature pulmonary functioning, the lack of fully mature alveoli units, possible surfactant insufficiency, and delayed intrapul-monary fluid absorption, the late-preterm infant may need oxygen, positive pressure ventilation, and possibly surfactant therapy. Keep in mind that even if a late-preterm infant does not require pulmonary assistance after birth, he or she is still at risk for problems such as apnea that are associated with a poten-tially immature neurologic system. There are very few studies about apnea in this population, but one of the classic studies in this age population suggests that the incidence of apnea in a late-preterm infant is small, reported at 4–7%, compared to 1–2% for a term infant (Ramanathan et al., 2001). Nevertheless, this can be a life-threatening occurrence.

Sepsis

All infants are at risk for sepsis; however, the more preterm the infant is, the higher the risk factor due to the greater immaturity of their immune system. The late preterm infant is most at risk for group B streptococcal (GBS) sepsis; current American Academy of Pediatrics (AAP) recommendations include screening for GBS and sepsis, as well as monitoring the infant in the hospital for 48 hours after birth (AAP, 2004b; Engle et al., 2007).

Hyperbilirubinemia

Jaundice and hyperbilirubinemia occur more commonly in late-preterm infants than in term infants. This is due to a number of factors including the immaturity of the liver in which there are lower levels of the necessary enzymes to synthesize bilirubin, immature gastrointestinal function, and potential feeding difficulties that predispose infants to dehydration, decreased stooling, and subsequent hyperbilirubinemia. The two basic mechanisms that lead to unconjugated hyperbilirubinemia are increased bilirubin production and decreased bilirubin clearance (such as decreased hepatic clearance or increased enterohepatic circulation; Moerschel, Cianciaruso, & Tracy, 2008). Studies investigating the rates of and reasons for readmission to hospitals for the late-preterm infant note that the most common cause of readmissions in this population was hyperbilirubinemia (Engle et al., 2007).

Temperature Regulation and Metabolic Function
Late-preterm infants, like all premature infants, have less body fat present to maintain thermoregulation. Brown-fat accumulation is crucial in the last trimester of pregnancy, and peaks at term. Therefore, the preterm infant does not have this protective insulation and loses heat more rapidly than a term infant does. Cold stress may also lead to hypoglycemia. When combined with the fact that all infants have insufficient metabolic response time when the maternal glucose supply is abruptly cut off, hypoglycemia may be a more persistent problem in the late-preterm infant as opposed to the term infant, who quickly develops the necessary enzymes to combat hypoglycemia.

Immature Gastrointestinal Function and Feeding Problems
As stated previously, the late-preterm infant is at greater risk for gastrointestinal problems than the term infant due to the greater immaturity of his or her gastrointestinal system and slow production of certain enzymes necessary for digestion. In addition, these infants tend to have longer sleep cycles than term infants and must be awakened frequently to eat. They also may not be able to consume the same volume as a term infant, so smaller more frequent feedings become necessary to maintain weight gain and growth and minimize hyperbilirubinemia. These infants may also have issues in coordinating sucking and swallowing that can lead to a delay in successful breastfeeding (Raju, Higgins, Stark, & Leveno, 2006).

Epidemiology

Approximately 13% of all births in the United States result in preterm (less than 37 weeks gestation) deliveries (Davidoff et al., 2006). Interestingly, studies have shown that almost two thirds of all preterm births from the years 1992–2002 were judged to be late-preterm births (Davidoff et al.). Research studies demonstrate that the rise in late-preterm births correlates with the rise in births to women over age 30, the rise in induction rates, multiple births, and the rise in primary and repeat cesarean deliveries (Raju et al., 2006; Trofatter, 2006). Furthermore, various ethnic and sociodemographic subgroups in the United States differ in their rates of premature birth, a factor that is currently being investigated to examine the underlying variables. Factors such as low socioeconomic status, maternal age less than 18 years or advanced maternal age, lack of access to health care, and poor nutritional status all increase the risk of preterm delivery (Polin & Spitzer, 2001).

As reported by Chen and colleagues (2007) in the *International Journal of Epidemiology*, the number of teenage pregnancies in the United States had decreased over 10 years. However, this decline was short lived, with the birth rate for teenagers 15 to 19 rising from 40.5 to 41.9, and then to 42.5 births per 1,000 based on data collected in 2005, 2006, and 2007 respectively (Hamilton, Martin, & Ventura, 2009). Teenage pregnancy continues to be a major social, economical, and healthcare concern in the United States (Chen et al., 2007). Chen and colleagues reviewed multiple studies on teenage pregnancy, and one of the consistently identified adverse outcomes of teenage pregnancy was the increased risk for preterm birth.

In summary, the most common neonatal issues that arise include hyperbilirubinemia, feeding issues, temperature instability, thermoregulation, potential breathing problems, and neonatal sepsis. Thus, prior to the infant's discharge from the hospital, the healthcare provider must be assured that each of these areas of risk is no longer a threat to the infant and that the infant is stable enough to be discharged home. Furthermore, prior to the infant's discharge home, the infant's mother needs careful instructions about feeding and sleep issues, knowledge of signs and symptoms of illness indicating a need to immediately seek care, as well as the date of the first health supervision visit. Close follow-up during the subsequent weeks and the next few months is often necessary so the infant can be carefully evaluated for appropriate growth and development and a healthy progression from the newborn stage to that of the young infant. In addition, if the mother is a teen, her developmental level also needs to be factored into the care plan.

How will you begin your data collection with the information you have just learned? ■

You introduce yourself to Sandra and José, the dad, and ask them how they would like to be addressed (e.g., Sandra and José). You begin by responding that you realize that the first few days and weeks home with a preterm infant are a challenging time for parents and go over the goals for today's visits. You explain that the information you are collecting will provide you with an overview of how things progressed from pregnancy to today's visit. You start by asking Sandra to tell you about how she, the baby, and dad are doing.

Sandra looks tired and says that having the baby early was very scary for her, and motherhood is much more challenging than she thought it would be. She starts to cry and says she is concerned that her son does not seem to be eating as well as he did in the hospital and that he sleeps all the time. You acknowledge her feelings and notice that the father has put his arm around her shoulders as she hugs the baby. Sandra quickly replies, "I'm OK now, I was just upset because I had trouble filling out these forms. We need you to help me and José do them right." She hands you the pregnancy, labor and birth history, and family medical history forms that she completed while waiting to be seen. You decide to go over the forms first to give you some time to dialogue with Sandra and José and to relieve her stress about completing the forms correctly. You will address her obvious stress and emotional needs later during the visit.

What questions will you ask Sandra regarding the pregnancy, labor and delivery, and birth history? ■

Obtaining a complete prenatal and birth history will be a key factor in evaluating subsequent health risk factors for this infant. Starting with the hospital stay, it will be important to find out as much as possible about Bobby's course of hospitalization. You begin with the pregnancy and ask about whether there were any complications other than the prematurity. After birth, was the infant in the neonatal intensive care unit (NICU) or did he remain with the mother or in the newborn nursery? Was he treated with antibiotics and, if so, does she remember their names? Did he have hyperbilirubinemia and/or did he receive treatment; if so, what? Did he have any breathing problems during the hospitalization? What was he fed, how much, and how often, and what was his birth weight?

According to the mother, she and José weren't planning on having Bobby but "things just got out of hand." Bobby was conceived the first time they had sex. She started prenatal care at 5 months gestation and had problems with her blood pressure "going real high" and her feet and hands swelling. She had to see the obstetrician frequently because of her blood pressure and needed to take blood pressure medication, which she is still taking. She went into labor early and delivered Bobby vaginally after a 6-hour labor. He cried right away, and the doctor said he was small but that was expected since he was early. She and the infant stayed in the hospital for 4 days without complications. She can't remember how much he weighed when he went home but "the nurse said he lost a little weight from birth, but that was expected." Bobby is now 6 days old, and this is his first visit to you for follow-up care.

What has been Bobby's course since being discharged home with Mom? ■

The following discussion will help you review common problems seen in the late preterm infant and to determine whether this infant has experienced any of these problems or associated sequelae.

You explain to Sandra that you will check Bobby's weight today and compare it to her discharge papers that she has brought with her. You ask her if she is breastfeeding or bottle feeding, and if bottle feeding, what type of formula she is using; how much does the baby take (or if breastfeeding, how many minutes at the breast and inquire if she switches sides); how often is the infant feeding; how many wet diapers per day and frequency of stooling; how long does the baby sleep; and does the infant have any trouble with breathing, feeding, rashes, or any other concerns she has.

Sandra states that she is trying to breastfeed Bobby, but she isn't very good at it. She states that the nurses told her to feed him every 2–3 hours. She is trying her best but is frustrated that she doesn't seem to have very much milk. She tells you that the baby gets cranky when she tries to put him to breast and that she is so tired now. She tries to switch to both breasts but feels awkward. She says that the nurses told her not to give him anything else but breastmilk, so she hasn't given him a bottle. They did show her how to pump while in the hospital, but she doesn't have a pump at home. Sandra tells you that he seems to have quite a bit of poop, almost every diaper change, so she guesses that there is urine in the diaper as well. She says that Bobby doesn't seem to have any other issues in general, but that he does seem to sleep all the time and she has to wake him up to feed, and then he starts crying because, according to Sandra, he isn't getting very much milk. She is frustrated because she has been told that breastfeeding is best, but José's mother keeps telling her to give the baby a bottle. Before moving on to further discussion, you take this moment to encourage her with the breastfeeding and inform her that you will arrange for a lactation consultant to come to her home to assist her and arrange for her to get a breast pump.

Social and Emotional History

As you begin to obtain a complete history from Sandra regarding her baby, you ask her about home life: her biologic parents, current living arrangements, and future plans for education or a career (both Sandra and José). How are they supporting themselves and the baby (food, shelter, clothing, medical insurance)? What were the issues surrounding the conception and the use of birth control? The possibility of postpartum depression (maternal and paternal) should be assessed using a brief assessment tool such as the Beck Depression Scale (Mancini, Carlson, & Albers, 2007; Whooley, Avins, Miranda, & Browner, 1997).

She reveals that she got pregnant by her Hispanic boyfriend, José, also 17 years of age, and, as a result, Sandra's mother "disowned" her. She is now living with her boyfriend and his family, a large Mexican family. José's mother, father, and four younger siblings are all living in a small three-bedroom house. She and José have no space to themselves. José's parents speak minimal English. Sandra says she feels stressed because she cannot easily communicate with them and has to rely on her boyfriend to translate for her. José's mother tries to help with the baby and has been very helpful with changing diapers and rocking the baby when he cries. She says that she has been happy overall about the pregnancy, although she had no idea about how difficult it was to be a new mom, but that she plans on finishing school because José's mother can help with the baby. She and José have talked about marriage, but are waiting for now. She says she is on WIC and does have Medicaid for insurance.

You use the two-question depression screen that the U.S. Preventive Services Task Force (Gaynes et al., 2005) recommends as a quick screen for adults. The two-question screen is as effective as longer screening tools. The two simple questions to ask are:

During the past month have you been bothered by 1) feeling down, blue, depressed, or hopeless? and 2) feelings of little interest or pleasure in doing things? Sandra answers no to both, and you decide that at this point in time she does not have postpartum depression.

Cultural and Teenage Dynamics

Cultural/socioeconomic factors must always be considered when evaluating patients. The healthcare provider working with ethnically diverse patients must reach out to patients and learn about their cultures, beliefs, and values as well as addressing the dynamics of teenage parenting. Sociodemographic risk factors of teenage pregnancy include poverty, low education level, inadequate prenatal care, and unmarried status (Chen et al., 2007). Thus, one of the most important issues to address in teenage parents is their lack of support as well as the lack of access to resources. Some perceptions of teenage parents include that they lack emotional and mental maturity, lack the ability to provide financial stability due to education interruption or to qualify for particular jobs due to their age, lack preparation for motherhood or fatherhood, and a general feeling that teenagers are unsuitable to be parents because they are still children themselves. This often leads to social abandonment when they become parents and worsens the already turbulent adolescent period (Hanna, 2001).

Cultural diversity can also add to difficulties in teenage parenting. In this particular discussion, the father of the baby is Hispanic, and typically Hispanic households are male-dominated and take great pride in their sons. There may be alternative healthcare practices that affect the care of a newborn and influence when to access traditional medical care. During this past decade great emphasis has been placed on developing family-centered care management strategies. This translates to all aspects of health care, including private physician offices and community clinics. Thus, it is critical to include the family in all decisions regarding care as well as recognizing cultural differences that may affect the delivery of care at home. Explanations should be sensitive to cultural issues and potential barriers to effective communication. Language translators or cultural brokers (individuals who are fluent in the language and sensitive to customs and nuances) may be very helpful. Careful wording of health and social questions is essential as well as explaining the content of the questions and why the healthcare provider needs such information. Identifying cultural beliefs and integrating appropriate management plans is important to the success of the treatment and management plan for the infant and his or her mother. In this case, there may be cultural differences operating between the mother and her Hispanic surrogate family as well as between the mother and the healthcare provider.

What information will be especially important to obtain on this newborn examination? ■

Physical Examination

On physical examination, you find a sleeping male infant who appears comfortable with regular respirations. Vital signs for this age are within normal limits, and auscultation of lungs and heart sounds are also normal. The infant's weight at birth was 5 lbs 5 oz. Current weight is 4 lbs 12 oz (approximately 11% weight loss). This places the infant at approximately the 10th percentile on a premature growth chart for boys, but the current weight loss is the more concerning issue. You notice milia on the infant's nose, and the anterior fontanel is open, of normal size, and flat but not depressed. His skin is slightly jaundiced in color and the mucous membranes are wet. The infant's abdomen is soft and flat with active bowel sounds; the umbilical cord is drying without redness or other abnormalities. The infant's genitalia is Tanner stage 1 with both testicles descended, the penis uncircumcised, and the anus patent. Tone appears to be within normal limits; however, the infant is slightly difficult to awaken but when he does awaken he has a robust cry and is easily soothed.

Making the Diagnosis

The differential diagnoses for assessing a late-preterm infant include carefully evaluating for each of the previously discussed problems that can occur in this population. In this particular case study, the infant's jaundiced skin, slight lethargy, and the poor feeding are red flags that require further evaluation. The healthcare provider should evaluate Bobby for three key potential problems:

1. *Hyperbilirubinemia:* Total and direct bilirbubin levels and the feeding history should provide you with information to distinguish between conjugated versus unconjugated hyperbilirubinemia.

2. *Sepsis:* A complete blood count (CBC) with differential should serve for sepsis screening. Some practitioners may obtain a blood culture at the same time, but usually a CBC is sufficient initially. Infection is also a differential diagnosis for hyperbilirubinemia (Moerschel et al., 2008). The CBC should be similar to a term, healthy infant, which often has an elevated white blood cell (WBC) count for the first 2 weeks of life (up to 30,000 leukocytes), and then decreases to normal adult levels. Of concern would be a low WBC count, a persistently elevated WBC level, or an elevation in the segmental band count on the differential (Polin & Spitzer, 2001).

3. *Dehydration:* Comparison of the infant's current weight compared to birth weight, feeding history including volume and frequency of feedings, as well as the number of wet diapers will help with this assessment. Do a 24-hour recall of feedings, number of wet diapers, and stooling pattern. Normal weight loss for newborns is 5–10% of birth weight for the first week of life. Watch the mother breastfeed her infant to assess proper latch on and sucking by the infant; encourage 10–15 minutes of breastfeeding

on both sides. Approximate the amount of breastmilk the infant is receiving by comparing to how much she pumps in 10–15 minutes. And, of course, make appropriate referrals to lactation consultants as needed.

Do you need to do anything to confirm the diagnosis, such as laboratory studies? ▦

Laboratory studies are needed to confirm the diagnosis, and to monitor the degree of hyperbilirubinemia and the response to treatment. According to the AAP, bilirubin levels should be obtained within the first 24 hours of life, then repeat the test based on identified risk factors from every 4 hours to every 24 hours. When suspecting hyperbilirubinemia, a total serum bilirubin level should be obtained for baseline diagnosis. It is generally accepted that a rise of greater than 5 mg/dL per day of life is concerning. And any level greater than 15 mg/dL requires further investigation and possible intervention (AAP, 2004a). If elevated, but within normal limits for age/gestation, a follow-up level should be obtained the next day. Depending on the severity of hyperbilirubinemia, levels may need to be obtained as frequently as every 4 hours, in which case an infant would need to be hospitalized for the frequent lab draws and management such as phototherapy. Generally, a daily total serum bilirubin level is adequate to monitor the low-risk infant. In addition, a set of electrolytes would be warranted in this infant due to the dehydration. The fractionated bilirubin test is helpful to rule out any other issues that could cause a cholestatic hyperbilirubinemia; however, current guidelines suggest evaluation only if the jaundice persists beyond the normal physiologic period (2 weeks) in newborns. Also, if it had not been obtained in the newborn nursery or neonatal intensive care unit, a direct Coombs test would be necessary to rule out Rh hemolytic disease (Moerschel et al., 2008).

You order the following tests:

- Neonatal bilirubin
- Complete blood count with differential

The indirect bilirubin level comes back at 15 mg/dL on day 6 of life, and the CBC is within normal limits. Fortunately, the mother had a discharge summary from the birth hospital, and the direct Coombs test is negative. With the information that Bobby has had only three wet diapers in the last 24 hours, is not taking adequate amounts of fluids, and has had an excessive weight loss (approximately 11%) within the first few days of life, in combination with the elevated bilirubin level, you decide that this infant's hyperbilirubinemia is exaggerated by poor feeding and mild dehydration with no other signs of sepsis.

Management

How do you plan to treat the hyperbilirubinemia and dehydration? What specifically will you do to bring the bilirubin level to within acceptable range? ▦

The most important therapy to initiate after making the diagnosis will be one that increases bilirubin excretion and includes improved hydration and stooling. Increasing the number of feedings per day will be necessary with possible supplemental breastmilk or formula, usually adding about one additional ounce of formula or breastmilk to each feeding as tolerated. Some infants may even "request" more, and as long as the infant does not have emesis, choking, or overt resistance, he or she can be fed with an ad lib volume. Breastfed infants should continue to be breastfed, optimally 8–12 times per day, 10–15 minutes on each breast. If there is difficulty with breastfeeding, a lactation consult may be initiated. Water or dextrose water supplementation is not recommended (Moerschel et al., 2008). If the mother is still having trouble breastfeeding or her milk production seems low, encourage her to stay hydrated herself and to eat healthy meals. Many new mothers feel that once the baby is born it is a good time to go on a diet, but this is not appropriate for breastfeeding mothers. Also, support her if she chooses not to breastfeed. There is a lot of pressure from society to breastfeed, and many new mothers feel like failures if they are unsuccessful or overwhelmed with the difficulties and frequency of feeding necessary with a poor feeder.

In extreme cases of hyperbilirubinemia or dehydration, hospitalization will be required for intravenous fluid therapy and aggressive monitoring of total serum bilirubin levels. A minimum of daily total serum bilirubin levels is recommended. Home phototherapy could be considered if the infant is close to requiring intensive phototherapy. You will need to order the phototherapy equipment for the mother from a local home healthcare equipment vendor if you decide to use it. The old wives' tale of placing a jaundiced infant near the sunlight still holds true to a certain extent to help assist with mild jaundice. However, issues such as "heat, excessive water loss and dehydration, and unnecessary exposure to ultraviolet light (prevented by window glass) need to be considered" (Polin & Spitzer, 2001, pp. 196–197).

Patient Education

The goals of patient education should be holistic and include addressing the socioeconomic factors/home stresses as well as the infant's medical condition. They are as follows:

1. *Feeding:* The most important thing for this infant's hyperbilirubinemia and mild dehydration is to increase the feedings/intake. The mother is young and is probably lacking support at home in caring for the infant. A lactation consultant should be included if the mother wishes to continue breastfeeding successfully. Sandra should be taught that the infant needs to be fed every 3 hours and to supplement with extra breastmilk or formula as needed due to the hyperbilirubinemia. The mother should contact the healthcare provider if the infant is refusing feedings. Tell her that she

should observe improvement in intake in the next 12 hours. If not, Bobby must be seen immediately for the first morning appointment or taken to the emergency department if he is listless or she is concerned about his general well-being. Instruct the mother to keep a journal to log feeding times, volume and length of feedings, and the number of wet diapers and bowel movements each day.

2. *Jaundice:* Sandra needs to be taught what jaundice/hyperbilirubinemia is and the potential risks of elevated bilirubin levels, such as kernicterus. She should be taught to call the healthcare provider immediately if Bobby shows signs of increased irritability, hypertonia alternating with lethargy, arching, fever, and high-pitched cry (Moerschel et al., 2008).

3. *Infection/thermoregulation:* Instruct the mother that often newborns do not have fevers when they become ill, and may actually have a low temperature. Instruct the mother in how to take the infant's temperature if she has not been taught, good handwashing techniques, and to keep the infant away from ill contacts. Regarding temperature, the Association of Women's Health, Obstetric and Neonatal Nurses (AWHONN) recommends that a good rule of thumb is to dress the infant in one more layer than the mother is wearing (AWHONN, 2007).

4. *Sleeping:* Most infants sleep 18–20 hours per day in the newborn period, and it is not uncommon for infants to sleep through feedings. For newborns, the typical length of sleep between feedings is 2–4 hours, then usually a 30-minute feeding, then back to sleep. Most healthcare providers do not recommend sleeping longer than 4 hours without a feeding, and not exceeding 30 minutes for a feeding. Encourage the mother to wake the infant up for feedings and teach her to always place the infant on his back to sleep.

5. *Referrals:* Due to the mother's young age, it is important to get her the appropriate referrals such as WIC (Women, Infants, and Children) programs, lactation consultants, referral to a teen mom clinic if you have one in your practice setting, and any community organizations (such as the YWCA or YMCA) that help young mothers. Encouraging her to network with other mothers and even other teen mothers is important because her resources may be limited. Web sites such as http://www.youngmommies.com, http://www.teenmotherchoices.org, and http://www.mops.org all offer resources to teenage parents. She should be provided phone numbers for questions and for poison control, and told in case of emergency to call 911. AWHONN has a worksheet for parents on its Web site that helps parents keep information organized for doctor visits (http://www.awhonn.org).

6. *Immunization:* Bobby received his first hepatitis B immunization at birth. You will emphasize Sandra's role in having her son receive all recommended childhood vaccinations on schedule. Tell her that immunization is

the most effective way to avoid vaccine-preventable diseases and to protect her child's health. The AAP and the Centers for Disease Control and Prevention have excellent immunization information for parents. Their Web sites are http://www.aap.org and http://www.cdc.gov, respectively.

You discuss each of these six major areas of patient education with Sandra and provide pamphlets or written information regarding the key points outlined under each patient education point.

When do you want to see Sandra and Bobby back again? ■

You want to see Bobby the next day for a follow-up total serum bilirubin level and to evaluate feedings and stooling. Encourage Sandra to bring her journal with her to the appointment to help quantify this information and include both José and his mother at the appointments, if possible, for additional support to Sandra. Including the grandmother at the appointments and translating information into Spanish for her may improve stress encountered at home from different ideas on how to care for Bobby.

Sandra and her baby return the next day for the follow-up appointment and the total serum bilirubin level is 13 mg/dL. She brings her journal with her with detailed entries on feeding times, volume, and intake/output and has done a good job in increasing the feedings. She quietly tells you that when she left the hospital she did not know she was supposed to wake the baby up to feed and before yesterday's visit had been supplementing formula in between breastfeedings. She also tells you that the lactation consultant is coming over to her house today to help assist with breastfeeding, because she "isn't very good at it," and hopes this will help. You congratulate her on a job well done and encourage her and José to continue doing a great job. You decide to see Bobby again tomorrow to check another bilirubin level and tell Sandra to continue with current management of increased volume intake. At that time you will also expand on your anticipatory guidance discussions, including appropriate car seat positioning and size for a preterm infant, placing Bobby on his back to sleep, and making sure they have a crib that meets current safety standards, among other newborn safety issues.

It will also be important to continue to monitor Sandra's mental health because most mothers do not see their obstetricians for 4–6 weeks postpartum. You encourage José to be at each visit and be involved with activities such as diaper changes, bathing, learning how to give any medications, and participating in feedings as able. You also discuss with José the importance of finishing his high school education and ask him whether he has considered college or vocational school as part of his future plans.

Above all, the healthcare provider must serve as an advocate for these young parents and assist them in not only raising a happy, healthy child, but also continuing their own growth to reach their full potential.

Key Points from the Case

1. Late-preterm infants are more at risk for potentially serious health problems than term infants and require special observations.

2. Hyperbilirubinemia is one of the most common causes of rehospitalization in the late-preterm infant population and needs to be identified early with appropriate management to prevent negative sequelae.

3. Teenage parents often have limited resources and thus need to be supported and encouraged by providing information and teaching from experts such as the nurse practitioner, the physician, physician assistant, and various members of the healthcare team.

4. Appropriate referrals should be made to assist the parents. Finding ways to include the family in planning care and providing education will be key in assuring success at home.

REFERENCES

American Academy of Pediatrics. (2004a). Clinical practice guideline: management of hyperbilirubinemia in the newborn infant 35 or more weeks of gestation. Subcommittee on Hyperbilirubinemia. *Pediatrics, 114*(1), 297–316.

American Academy of Pediatrics. (2004b). Policy statement: hospital stay for healthy term newborns. Committee on Fetus and Newborn. *Pediatrics, 113*(5), 1434–1436.

Association of Women's Health, Obstetric and Neonatal Nurses. (2007). *Late preterm infant initiative.* Retrieved August 7, 2008, from http://www.awhonn.org

Chen, X., Wen, S. W., Fleming, N., Demissie, K., Rhoads, G. G., & Walker, M. (2007). Teenage pregnancy and adverse birth outcomes: a large population based retrospective cohort study. *International Journal of Epidemiology, 36*(2), 368–373.

Davidoff, M. J., Dias, T., Damus, K., Russell, R., Bettegowda, V. R., Dolan, S., et al. (2006). Changes in the gestational age distribution among U.S. singleton births: impact on rates of late preterm birth, 1992–2002. *Seminars in Perinatology, 30*, 8–15.

Engle, W. A., Tomashek, K. M., & Wallman, C. (2007). "Late-preterm" infants: a population at risk. *Pediatrics, 120*(6), 1390–1401.

Gaynes, B. N., Gavin, M., Meltzer-Brody, S., Lohr, K. N., Swinson, T., Gartlehner, G., et al. (2005). *Perinatal depression: prevalence, screening accuracy, and screening outcomes.* Evidence Report/Technology Assessment No. 119. (Prepared by the RTI-University of North Carolina Evidence-Based Practice Center, under Contract No. 290-02-0016. AHRQ Publication No. 05-E006-2.) Rockville, MD: Agency for Healthcare Research and Quality.

Hamilton, B. E., Martin, J. A., & Ventura, S. J. (2009). Births: preliminary data for 2007. *National Vital Statistics Reports, 57*(12), 1–23.

Hanna, B. (2001). Negotiating motherhood: the struggles of teenage mothers. *Journal of Advanced Nursing, 34*(4), 456–464.

Mancini, F., Carlson, C., & Albers, L. (2007). Use of the postpartum depression screening scale in a collaborative practice. *Journal of Midwifery and Women's Health, 52*(5), 420–434.

Moerschel, S. K., Cianciaruso, L. B., & Tracy, L. R. (2008). A practical approach to neonatal jaundice. *American Family Physician, 77*(9), 1255–1263.

Polin, R. A., & Spitzer, A. R. (2001). *Fetal and neonatal secrets.* Philadelphia: Hanley & Belfus.

Raju, T. N. K., Higgins, R. D., Stark, A. R., & Leveno, K. J. (2006). Optimizing care and outcomes for late-preterm (near-term) infants: a summary of the workshop sponsored by the National Institute of Child Health and Human Development. *Pediatrics, 118*(3), 1207–1214.

Ramanathan, R., Corwin, M. J., Hunt, C. E., Lister, G., Tinsley, L. R., Baird, T., et al. (2001). Cardiorespiratory events recorded on home monitors: comparison of healthy infants with those at increased risk for SIDS. *Journal of the American Medical Association, 285*, 2199–2207.

Trofatter, K. F. (2006). *Late preterm birth—AGAIN.* Retrieved August 7, 2008, from http://www.healthline.com

Wang, M. L., Dorer, D. J., Fleming, M. P., & Catlin, E. A. (2004). Clinical outcomes of near-term infants. *Pediatrics, 114*, 1341–1347.

Whooley, M. A., Avins, A. L., Miranda, J., & Browner, W. S. (1997). Case-finding instruments for depression: Two questions are as good as many. *Journal of General Internal Medicine, 12*, 439–445.

Chapter 34

A Child with Short Stature

George Anadiotis

It is not uncommon in medicine to discover a child presenting with one problem that leads to a variety of other concerns and eventually to the underlying etiology. The importance of tying together the physical findings with the history for the patient cannot be overestimated and is essential to achieving a diagnosis and an effective follow-up treatment plan. Identifying the child who is apparently well but short and then moving forward to the issue of a genetic cause with a host of other potential health problems is not an easy step for the healthcare provider, family, and child. However, the outcomes can be very satisfying when the child is on a path towards a more healthy future.

Educational Objectives
1. Identify possible causes of short stature in young girls.
2. Discuss the types of treatment options available.
3. Understand appropriate referral patterns for further treatment.
4. Clarify the role of the primary care provider caring for a child with a genetic condition.

Case Presentation and Discussion

Jane Murphy is a 10-year-old girl who is brought to you by her mother because of concern regarding her height. Upon evaluation, you note that her height is 120 centimeters (48 inches; < fifth percentile) with a weight of 30 kilograms (68.2 pounds; < fifth percentile) and a head circumference of 51 centimeters (20 inches; within normal limits for age 10 years). You talk with Jane's mother about her concerns.

Further discussion with Mrs. Murphy reveals that Jane has occasional visits to a urologist because she was born with a horseshoe kidney, and that she has a heart murmur that was described as innocent. She states that Jane does well in school although she has some social issues including difficulty interacting with other children her age; Jane prefers to play with younger children.

When you ask Jane how she feels regarding her height, she becomes somewhat tearful and tells you that she is the shortest girl in her class and the other girls are growing very rapidly. She often gets teased for being so small. Sometimes when she is out with her friends, other individuals think that she is a younger sister of her friends. At this point,

Jane's mother adds that this has become a more pressing concern for Jane; she has been voicing more frequently how much it bothers her to be small.

Her physical examination reveals a child who appears to be in good health. She has some soft physical findings such as some minimal swelling in her hands and feet, which Mrs. Murphy states has been there since infancy. She has a small chin with a low posterior hairline and posteriorly rotated ears. The rest of her examination does not reveal any health problems. You hear a grade I/VI heart murmur today. You did the head circumference because you were interested in whether she was in proportion or had either macrocephaly or microcephaly. Her head circumference was within normal limits. Head circumference tables are available for older children as well as infants.

What questions are going through your mind at this point? ▧

Within this very brief visit, you should have a variety of questions arising for you as the primary care provider. Questions to consider regarding Jane's findings include:

- How long has Jane been below the fifth percentile on the growth curve?
- Although we know Jane appears to have some social interaction issues, has she ever been assessed for any type of learning disorder?
- Has Jane ever been evaluated by cardiology regarding her murmur?
- Has Jane shown any evidence of starting puberty?
- Has anyone in the family been evaluated for late growth spurts or short stature?
- Have the renal issues been fully evaluated, and can the urologist provide any other information that may be useful?
- Are there any options available for this 10-year-old to increase her growth velocity and final height?

Short Stature

The history and physical examination of this child appear to be consistent with a genetic syndrome, most likely Turner syndrome. The combination of the physical findings such as rotated ears, low posterior hairline, micrognathia, renal abnormalities, and short stature are classic for Turner syndrome. However, there are other genetic causes of short stature that can present somewhat similarly, and they must be ruled out.

The differential of short stature can be quite large. The most common causes are 1) familial short stature in which individuals have normal growth below the fifth percentile with no skeletal delay and normal onset of puberty, and 2) constitutional short stature with normal growth velocity but delayed skeletal maturity. An in-depth family history as well as radiologic studies are necessary to diagnose these types. Other causes include a variety of endocrine abnormalities such as growth hormone deficiency. Chromosomal anomalies such as Turner or Noonan syndrome must also be considered. In this case, the physical features suggest a syndromic cause.

Turner Syndrome

Pathophysiology

Due to the loss of one X chromosome, approximately 50% of individuals with Turner syndrome will show a 45, X karyotype in a phenotypic female. However, this classic chromosomal finding is not the only karyotype that can result in the physical features of Turner syndrome. Mosaicism is fairly common in Turner syndrome. This term indicates the presence of two cell lines in a single individual. Individuals with mosaic cell lines such as 45, X with 46, XX or 46, XY or 47, XXX can all be placed under the Turner syndrome category. Mosaicism with a 46, XX usually results in individuals with a much milder phenotype of Turner features than the classic 45, X individuals.

Clinical Findings

Although Turner syndrome can be diagnosed prenatally or in infancy—especially if a child is born with features such as lymphedema, webbed neck, or cardiac and renal anomalies—many individuals with Turner syndrome are diagnosed later in childhood when they present with short stature but without the other classical physical findings. Common clinical findings are found in Table 34-1. Intelligence in these individuals is normal, but a variety of issues are related to learning disabilities, particularly with mathematics, memory, spatial perception, or visual motor integration as well as issues associated with immaturity, hyperactivity, anxiety, low self-esteem, or even depression (Bondy, 2007; McCauley, Ross, Kushner, & Cutler, 1995; Tyler & Edman, 2004). The psychosocial concerns raised by both Jane and her mother are often the driving factors bringing these children in. They are concerned about being the smallest in the class, especially when other children begin to make fun of them.

As adults, women with Turner syndrome can have health problems such as obesity, and autoimmune issues such as diabetes, hypothyroidism, and inflammatory bowel disease. High-frequency hearing loss occurs in about 25% to 66% of individuals (see Table 34-1).

Epidemiology

Turner syndrome occurs in approximately 1 in 2,000 to 3,000 live female infant births (Frias, Davenport, Committee on Genetics, & Section on Endocrinology, 2003; Nielsen & Wohlert, 1991). It is thought to occur in about 1–2% of all conceptuses; however, the majority of these are spontaneously lost in the first trimester of pregnancy. The retained X chromosome can come from either parent (Tsezou et al., 1999).

Differential Diagnoses

Although Turner syndrome is classically the most common syndrome associated with young women with short stature, it should be noted that Noonan syndrome also presents with similar findings, including poor growth, congenital heart malformations, short stature, renal problems, learning problems, pectus excavatum,

Table 34-1	Common Clinical Findings in Turner Syndrome
Age	**Clinical Findings**
Prenatal	*Increased nuchal translucency
	*Cystic hygromas
	*Coarctation of the aorta and/or left-sided cardiac defects
	*Brachycephaly
	*Renal anomalies
	*Polyhydramnios or oligohydramnios
	*Growth retardation
	*Abnormal alpha fetoprotein, human chorionic gonadotropin, inhibin A, and unconjugated estriol
	Short femurs
Infancy	*Lymphatic effects:* *Edema of hands or feet, *webbed neck
	Cardiovascular: *Left-sided heart anomalies, especially coarctation of aorta (11–40%), bivalve aortic valve (16%), hypoplastic left heart, or elongated aortic arch (50%)
	Skeletal: Broad shield-like chest with inverted or hypoplastic nipples, short fourth metacarpal, short stature, short neck, cubitus valgus, genu valgum, scoliosis (10%), lordosis, growth velocity less than 10th percentile for age (95–100%), developmental dislocated hips (5%)
	Urinary system: Congenital malformations (30–40%)
	Dental: Small mandible, abnormal tooth development and morphology, high arched palate, micrognathia, cleft palate
	Eyes: Epicanthal folds, ptosis, hypertelorism, upward slanting palpebral fissures, Red-green color deficiency (8%), strabismus, or hyperopia (25–30%)
	Ears: Hearing problems, ear malformations, chronic otitis media, low-set ears
	Dermatologic: *Low posterior hairline, nail hypoplasia/hyperconvex uplifted nails, multiple pigmented nevi
	Neurocognitive: Decreased visual-spatial organization, visual-motor skills, social cognition, nonverbal problem-solving, right-left sequencing, nonverbal memory, executive functioning, attention, and self-esteem
Childhood and adolescence	*Unexplained growth failure, declining growth velocity
	Pubertal failure (84%–98%)
	*Amenorrhea with elevated follicle-stimulating hormone (FSH) levels
	Hypertension (25% of girls and higher in adults)

Table 34–1	Common Clinical Findings in Turner Syndrome (Continued)
Adulthood	*Short stature
	Progressive sensorineural hearing loss
	Autoimmune disorders such as inflammatory bowel diseases, juvenile rheumatoid arthritis, Hashimoto's thyroiditis, Graves' disease, myasthenia, or celiac disease (4–6%)
	*Premature ovarian failure
	Glucose intolerance
	Hypothyroidism (24%)
	Liver disease
	Decreased bone density

* indication for screening karyotype

Sources: Data from Bondy, C., for the Turner Syndrome Consensus Study Group. (2007). Care of girls and women with Turner syndrome: a guideline of the Turner syndrome study group. Journal of Clinical Endocrinology and Metabolism, 92(1), 10–25; Doswell, B., Visootsak, V., Brady, A., & Graham, J. M. (2006). Turner syndrome: an update and review for the primary care pediatrician. Clinical Pediatrics, 45, 301–313; Tyler, C ., & Edman, J. C. (2004). Down syndrome, Turner syndrome and Klinefelter syndrome: primary care throughout the lifespan. Primary Care Clinics in Office Practice, 31, 627–648.

impaired blood clotting, webbed neck, low hairline, low-set ears, and scoliosis. This syndrome may occur in males or females. It is caused by genetic mutations of chromosome 12q24.1, including genes PTPN11, KRAS, and RAF1. The karyotype is different from that of Turner syndrome.

Making the Diagnosis

What test will you order to make the diagnosis of Turner syndrome or another chromosomal condition? ▪

Diagnostic Testing

The diagnosis of Turner syndrome is confirmed by obtaining high-resolution chromosome studies.

You discuss the possibility of a genetic cause for Jane's short stature and kidney problem with Jane and her mother. They agree to testing and you send them off for high resolution chromosome studies. The results shows a 45, X karyotype as you suspected. You might choose to call a geneticist and consult with him or her regarding testing at this point or make a referral and then let that person decide what studies are necessary. In this case, you are fairly confident about the diagnosis and a karyotype is a basic genetics test. Other diagnoses might require considerably more studies including metabolic assays and others. In that case, given the expense, it would probably be better to send the child off and let appropriate studies be ordered from there.

Management

How will you begin management of this child with the genetic condition of Turner syndrome? ■

Because genetic conditions do not occur very often in your daily primary care practice, you go online to see if there are guidelines for care of these children prepared by experts from across the country. The National Institutes of Health and the American Academy of Pediatrics are good places to start. Online, you quickly find that guidelines have been developed by the National Institutes of Health, National Institute of Child Health and Human Development, and Turner Syndrome Consensus Study Group (Bondy, 2007). Earlier guidelines were published in 2003 by the American Academy of Pediatrics (Frias et al., 2003). You feel prepared now for the Murphys' return visit.

> Jane and her mother return to the clinic to learn the results of the chromosome studies. You tell them what the syndrome is and explain that the condition was not the fault of either parent. Turner syndrome is caused by a loss of an X chromosome, so the underlying chromosomal defect cannot be repaired. However, there are a variety of treatments that can positively affect the symptoms of the genetic disorder, including help with her short stature.

Management of Turner Syndrome

Your management plan generally follows the national guidelines. Here is the information you learned from your study before seeing the family.

Short Stature

Short stature is one of the most common findings associated with Turner syndrome, affecting almost all of the girls with this diagnosis. The mean final height in untreated women is 143 cm, or only 4' 9" (57 inches). Growth hormone has been approved for the treatment of short stature and is considered the standard of care for a child with Turner syndrome. The best time for it to be started would be when the child's height falls below the fifth percentile. For approximately 50% of girls, that would occur between 2 and 3 years of age. Starting children on growth hormone at an early age is important, because gains of 8 to 10 centimeters (about 3 to 4 inches) have been noted if individuals receive at least 6 years of growth hormone (Bondy, 2007; Tsezou et al., 1999).

Starting Jane on growth hormone at age 10 years will not give her as much additional height as it would had she been started at age 2 or 3 years, but some increase in growth velocity and final height can be anticipated.

Cardiovascular Issues

Jane requires a cardiovascular evaluation, although her murmur sounds innocent. Even if there is no evidence of a murmur, all children with the diagnosis of Turner syndrome should be evaluated by a cardiologist and have an echocardiogram, an ECG, and other studies as necessary. Cardiovascular anomalies are thought to occur in 20% to 40% of affected individuals or more, and many of these congenital heart problems can be repaired through intervention. Hypertension occurs in about 25% of girls and is an important risk factor for dissecting aneurysms, another health problem for Turner syndrome patients (Bondy, 2007).

Endocrinology

An endocrine evaluation is extremely useful because gonadal dysgenesis is common (90%) in Turner syndrome (Doswell et al., 2006). Many girls will require sex hormone replacement in order to begin puberty. It should be noted that a variety of issues are associated with sex hormone replacement. It can be initiated early in some individuals, whereas other individuals who are still working on gaining height may have their estrogen therapy delayed until as late as 15 years of age to allow them to achieve their maximum height potential. Although secondary sexual characteristics can develop in individuals with mosaicism, even those individuals should have their endocrine system evaluated because they may also require estrogen therapy.

In the majority of cases, individuals with Turner syndrome are not able to bear children. It is the responsibility of the primary care provider to discuss reproductive options such as adoption or medically assisted reproduction with individuals who have this diagnosis when they are at an age for comprehension. Occasionally, a rare individual may have sufficient ovarian function to ovulate and may become pregnant; however, there is an increased risk of fetal chromosomal abnormalities or miscarriages in such women so genetic counseling is important. Pregnancy with a donated egg is more commonly achieved (Doswell et al., 2006).

Neurocognitive Issues

Many individuals with Turner syndrome have a specific set of cognitive functioning differences in the areas of decreased visual-spatial organization, social cognition, nonverbal problem-solving, right-left sequencing, executive function, attention, and self-esteem (Bondy, 2007; Doswell et al., 2006; McCauley et al., 1995; Romans, Stefanatus, Roeltgen, Kushner, & Ross, 1998; Ross, Zinn, & McCauley, 2000).

Psychosocial Support

It is important for the primary care provider to assess the psychological support that is available to the child and family. Involvement with local Turner syndrome support groups or the Turner Syndrome Society of the United States (http://www.turnersyndrome.org) is a way of allowing individuals to interact with other families who have similar problems. Literature should be supplied to the family about Turner syndrome, and other resources should be available including therapy resources if they are needed. The American Academy for Pediatrics provides information for medical providers.

Genetics Issues

Genetic conditions, as do other chronic conditions, affect families for many years, influencing decisions about childbearing, health care, social relationships, finances for health insurance, and many other aspects of life. Consultation with a genetics clinic or geneticist can be very helpful in answering a family's questions.

Other Healthcare Needs

A variety of other abnormalities are associated with Turner syndrome, including hearing loss, strabismus, obesity, glucose intolerance, hypertension, thyroid dysfunction, orthopedic issues, and urinary tract abnormalities, among others. Each of these systems needs to be evaluated in a child with Turner syndrome, and appropriate referrals will need to be made (Bondy, 2007; Donaldson, Gault, Tan, & Dunger, 2006; Doswell et al., 2006; Tyler & Edman, 2004).

Given the national guidelines for treatment of girls with Turner syndrome (Bondy, 2007), you talk with the family to describe the plan and rationale for each step. You arrange for her:

- Referrals for care:
  - A pediatric endocrinologist for growth hormone and estrogen therapy to increase her height and then to induce puberty at the appropriate time
  - A pediatric cardiologist for evaluation and monitoring of her cardiac status
  - A pediatric genetics clinic for further discussion of Turner syndrome and its influences on Jane and the family
- Evaluations to assess needs for care:
  - By an audiologist for hearing loss
  - By an ophthalmologist
  - By an orthodontist
  - An educational evaluation by her school's personnel

You also describe the current national guidelines for them and begin the screening and on-going monitoring protocol for Turner syndrome (Bondy, 2007). Thus, you also order T_4 and thyroid stimulating hormone (TSH) tests for thyroid function, celiac screen (TTG-Ab), liver function tests, fasting blood sugar, lipids, CBC, and creatinine and BUN for kidney functioning.

You also give the family the Web site for the Turner Syndrome Society of the United States with the suggestion that meeting other girls who also have Turner syndrome might be very helpful to Jane, and meeting their parents would be helpful to Mr. and Mrs. Murphy.

You consider whether Jane would benefit from some counseling regarding her self-esteem and feelings about being teased due to her size. You decide to wait on this given the number of other evaluations scheduled. Perhaps with more information, the initiation of growth hormone therapy, and meeting some other girls with the condition, Jane will begin to feel better about herself, but you note that this issue needs monitoring both short-term and long-term.

When do you want to see this family back again? ■

You schedule the family to return to the clinic after the evaluations have occurred to review Jane's overall health status and to see how various therapy programs are evolving.

The family returns in 3 months, having been to the endocrinologist, cardiologist, urologist, ophthalmologist, audiologist, genetics clinic, and orthodontist. She also has an educational evaluation scheduled in the next few weeks. The endocrinologist has started her on growth hormone treatment, which has been accepted positively by Jane. The cardiologist identified a bicuspid aortic valve but does not want to do anything at this time to repair it. Her blood pressure is normal. The urologist was surprised to learn that Jane has Turner syndrome and will follow her regularly, but did not find significant urological problems at this time. Her hearing and vision are normal so she will return for annual evaluations. The geneticist provided them with more information about Turner syndrome, its inheritability, and the health issues they need to monitor.

Jane reports that when kids tease her, she tells them that she has Turner syndrome and is hoping that she will grow a bit faster now that she is getting treatment. Her friends are supportive. Her mother and father are beginning to accept the fact that their daughter has a genetic condition with many health issues to face as she matures, but are hopeful that with good care she can avoid significant problems. They have not yet made contact with the Turner Syndrome Society but know when the next meeting in their area is to be held and plan to attend with Jane.

You congratulate them on their progress navigating all the healthcare evaluations and assure them that you will be available at any time and will continue to oversee the various specialties' plans to help Jane. You also alert them that positive mental health and strong self-esteem are important for Jane and suggest that they return any time they see Jane becoming stressed so appropriate mental health interventions can be instituted.

What are some other issues you need to address with the family in the future? ■

You will need to address the following with the Murphys:

- Obesity is a common problem for individuals with Turner syndrome. Jane needs a healthy diet and plenty of exercise. You will monitor her weight carefully as she moves into adolescence.
- Finding a sport that Jane can be successful in, such as dance, gymnastics, or swimming.

- The probability that Jane will not have children or will achieve pregnancy with difficulty.
- The long-term health problems such as diabetes and autoimmune diseases that Jane needs to be monitored for.
- Scoliosis may emerge as an issue when she is growing more rapidly.
- Many girls with Turner syndrome have neurocognitive problems such as visual-spatial deficits, poorer nonverbal memory, problems perceiving social situations appropriately, and attention deficits, which may yet emerge in Jane. They will need to monitor her progress in school and socially because educational help can be provided to keep her functioning at age level if such problems arise.

Not all of these can be addressed at once, but these will need to be priorities for discussion over the next several years.

Key Points from the Case

1. Young females with short stature require a variety of evaluations including a genetic evaluation for the possibility of Turner syndrome.
2. An individual diagnosed with Turner syndrome can have a variety of organs affected, and a thorough work-up is required once a diagnosis is made.
3. Future issues such as growth, reproduction, obesity, diabetes, vision, hearing, cardiovascular system, autoimmune disorders, learning, psychological, and other issues will also need to be monitored by the primary care provider.

REFERENCES

Bondy, C., for the Turner Syndrome Consensus Study Group. (2007). Care of girls and women with Turner syndrome: a guideline of the Turner Syndrome Study Group. *Journal of Clinical Endocrinology and Metabolism, 92*(1), 10–25.

Donaldson, M. D. C., Gault, E. J., Tan, K. W., & Dunger, D. B. (2006). Optimizing management in Turner syndrome: from infancy to adult transfer. *Archives of Diseases in Children, 91*, 513–520.

Doswell, B., Visootsak, V., Brady, A., & Graham, J. M. (2006). Turner syndrome: an update and review for the primary care pediatrician. *Clinical Pediatrics, 45*, 301–313.

Frias, J. L., Davenport, M. L., Committee on Genetics, & Section on Endocrinology. (2003). Health supervision for children with Turner syndrome. *Pediatrics, 111*(3), 692–702.

McCauley, E., Ross, J. L., Kushner, H., & Cutler Jr., G. (1995). Self-esteem and behavior in girls with Turner syndrome. *Journal of Developmental and Behavioral Pediatrics, 16*, 82–88.

Nielsen, J., & Wolhert, M. (1991). Chromosome abnormalities found among 34,910 newborn children: results from a 13-year incidence study in Arhus, Denmark. *Human Genetics, 87,* 81–83.

Romans, S., Stefanatus, G., Roeltgen, D., Kushner, H., & Ross, J. L. (1998). Transition to young adulthood in Ullrich-Turner syndrome: neurodevelopmental changes. *American Journal of Medical Genetics, 79,* 140–147.

Ross, J., Zinn, A., & McCauley, E. (2000). Neurodevelopment and psychosocial aspects of Turner syndrome. *Mental Retardation and Developmental Disabilities Research Reviews, 6,* 135–141.

Tsezou, A., Hadyiathanasiou, C., Gourgiotis, D., Galla, A., Kavazarakis, E., Pasparaki, A., et al. (1999). Molecular genetics of Turner syndrome: correlation to clinical phenotype and response to growth hormone. *Clinical Genetics, 56,* 441–446.

Tyler, C., & Edman, J. C. (2004). Down syndrome, Turner syndrome and Klinefelter syndrome: primary care throughout the lifespan. *Primary Care Clinics in Office Practice, 31,* 627–648.

Index

Note: Entries followed by "b" indicate boxes; "f" figure; "t" tables.

A

AAFP (American Academy of Family Physicians), 346–357
AAP (American Academy of Pediatrics)
  diagnostic criteria of
    AOM, 351–352
    childhood obesity, 90
    OME, 346–357
  recommendations of
    autism screening, 27–28, 35, 39
    bilirubin level testing, 501
    fluid replacement, 397–398
    four-stage overweight approach, 95
    GBS sepsis screening, 494
    genetic condition treatment, 512
    immunization, 504
ABA (Applied Behavior Analysis) program, 37–38
abuse situations, 193–206
  case presentation for, 193–198, 200, 204
  diagnosis of, 193–200
    drawings as indicators, 201
    interviews, 193–199
    physical examinations, 199–200
    risk factors, 193–195
    signs/symptoms reviews, 202–203
  epidemiology/etiology of, 193–195
  fundamental contexts of, 193–195, 205
  management of, 203–204
    abuse consequences, 204
    therapeutic plans, 203–204
  objectives for, 193
  reporting of, 194–200, 203
  resources for, 205–206
Accutane. *See* isotretinoin (Accutane)
ACE (angiotensin-converting enzyme) inhibitors, 280
acne (adolescents), 467–480
  case presentation for, 467–468, 470, 479
  diagnosis of, 469–471
    diagnostic testing, 471
    differential, 469–470
    history-taking, 469–470
    physical examination, 470
  epidemiology/etiology of, 468–469
    cultural/ethnic factors, 469
    pathophysiology, 468
  fundamental contexts of, 467–468, 479
  management of, 471–479
    care plan, 478t
    education plan, 473–474
    follow-up visits, 479
    iPLEDGE program, 473
    medications, 472–473, 474t–478t
    therapeutic plans, 471–473
  objectives for, 467
  resources for, 479–480
ACS (American Cancer Society)
  cervical cancer detection guidelines, 444
  Pap smear recommendations, 428
acute lymphoblastic leukemia. *See* ALL (acute lymphoblastic leukemia)
acute *vs.* chronic diarrhea, 391–392. *See also* diarrhea/vomiting
acyclovir, 463
AD (atopic dermatitis), 455–466
  case presentation for, 455, 457–458, 459, 463–464
  diagnosis of, 456–459
    differential, 459
    history-taking, 459
    physical examination, 456
  epidemiology/etiology of, 456–457
  fundamental contexts of, 455–456
  management of, 459–464
    antibiotics, 462–463
    antivirals, 463
    Atopiclair, 463
    follow-up visits for, 463–464
    medications, 460–463, 461t
    MimyX for, 463
    parental/patient education for, 463–464
    PUVA therapy for, 462
    RAST/SPT, 458
    systemic steroids for, 462

TCIs for, 462
topical corticosteroids for, 460–462,
461t
triggers of, 458–459
objectives for, 455
resources for, 465–466
AD (autism disorder), 28, 30f
adapalene (Differin), 474t–477t
adenovirus, 378, 388
ADHD (attention deficit hyperactivity
disorder), 175–192
case presentation for, 176, 178, 180, 186,
189–190
diagnosis of, 176–181
AAP guidelines, 178–179
comorbidities, 179–180, 179t
Conners' Scales, 180–181
diagnostic testing, 180–181
differential, 179t
DSM-IV-TR criteria, 176–178,
177t–178t
physical examinations, 180
Vanderbilt assessment, 180–181
fundamental contexts of, 175, 191
management of, 182–190
appetite and, 188
cardiac problems and, 187–188
family education, 182
follow-up visits, 189–190
medications, 182–187, 183t–185t
sample approach, 187t
sleep disturbances and, 188–189
objectives for, 175
prognosis for, 190
resources for, 191–192
adolescent-specific concerns
acne, 467–480
birth control, 427–440
depression, 207–220
diagnostic reasoning for, 1–8
fatigue, 59–72
late-preterm infants (adolescent parents),
493–506
LGBT issues, 221–231
PPEs, 133–163
vaginal discharge, 441–454
aeroallergens, 458–459
albuterol, 260
ALL (acute lymphoblastic leukemia),
486–487
Allegra. *See* fexofenadine (Allegra)
alpha-glucosidase inhibitors, 278
Alpha Keri soap, 460
American Academy of Neurology Practice
Parameters, 330

American Academy of Child and Adolescent
Psychiatry, 65
American Academy of Dermatology,
472–473
American Academy of Pediatric Dentistry,
409, 412–413
American Academy of Pediatrics. *See* AAP
(American Academy of Pediatrics)
American Cancer Society. *See* ACS
(American Cancer Society)
American Community Survey, 225
American Diabetes Association, 269–271,
271t, 278
amoxicillin, 353, 355t, 423, 472–473
amoxicillin/clavulanate (Augmentin), 355t
ampicillin, 472–473
anemia (toddlers), 291–320
case presentation for, 291–295, 315–316
diagnosis, 296–309
anemia as symptom, 301–303
anemia phases, 300–302
diagnostic testing, 308–313,
310t–312t
differential, 296
environmental toxins, 296–299,
298t–299t
history-taking, 292–293
hypothyroidism, 306–307, 309
I PREPARE mnemonic, 298–299, 299t
ICD-9 codes, 313t
IDA, 300–303, 300t, 308
lead poisoning, 303–305, 309
leukemia, 305–306
lymphoma, 305–306
pathophysiology, 299–301
physical examinations, 294–296, 295t
systems reviews, 293–295
warfarin toxicity, 306, 308
epidemiology/etiology of, 296
fundamental contexts of, 291, 317
management of, 313–327
care plans, 315–316
follow-up visits, 316–317
medications, 314–315
objectives for, 291
resources for, 317–320
angiotensin-converting enzyme inhibitors.
See ACE (angiotensin-converting
enzyme) inhibitors
antibiotics
oral, 353–354, 353t, 399, 421, 462–463,
472–473
topical, 472
antidepressants, 215–219, 217t
antidepressants, tricyclic, 218
antihistamines, 68, 343t

antihistamines/mast cell stabilizers, 343t
antihistamines/vasoconstrictors, 343t
antipyrine/benzocaine (Auralgan), 356t
antivirals, 463
appendicitis, 395–396
Applied Behavior Analysis program. *See* ABA
    (Applied Behavior Analysis) program
Aquaphor, 460
AS (Asperger syndrome), 28
ASDs (autistic spectrum disorders), 28–40,
    29t, 30f. *See also* language/social delays
    (toddlers)
Atopic dermatitis. *See* AD (atopic dermatitis)
Atopiclair, 463
Attention deficit hyperactivity disorder. *See*
    ADHD (attention deficit hyperactivity
    disorder)
Augmentin. *See* amoxicillin/clavulanate
    (Augmentin)
Auralgan. *See* antipyrine/benzocaine
    (Auralgan)
Autism and Developmental Disabilities
    Monitoring Network, 29
autistic spectrum disorders. *See* ASDs (autistic
    spectrum disorders)
autoimmune hepatitis, 472–473
Aveeno soap, 460
Avita. *See* tretinoin (Retin-A, Avita)
avoidance, healthcare, 223–224
avulsion. *See also* oral trauma
    permanent incisors, 405–414, 409f
    primary incisors, 405–414, 408f
AWHONN (Association of Women's Health,
    Obstetric and Neonatal Nurses), 503
azathioprine, 462
azelastine HCl (Optivar), 343t
azithromycin, 353–354, 353t, 355t, 383–384

B
bacturia, 418–419
barrier method/spermicides, 433
benzocaine/antipyrine (Auralgan), 356t
benzoyl peroxide, 472, 474t–477t
best evidence *vs.* best practice, 1–5, 372–374
Biaxin. *See* clarithromycin (Biaxin)
biguanides, 278
birth control (adolescents), 427–440
    case presentation for, 427–428, 434,
        437–439
    diagnosis of, 428–430
        diagnostic testing, 428
        history-taking, 429–430
        physical examination, 428
    fundamental contexts of, 427, 439
    management of, 430–439
        COC pills, 435b–437b
        contraceptive options, 430–434, 431t

counseling, 437–438
    follow-up visits, 438–439
objectives for, 427
resources for, 439–440
bisexual issues. *See* LGBT (lesbian, gay,
    bisexual, and transgendered) issues
blood glucose diaries, 268t
BMI (body mass index), 89–90
Bogalusa Heart Study, 272–273
Bordetella pertussis, 379t
BRAT (bananas, rice, applesauce, toast) diet,
    399
breastfeeding/slow weight gain (infants),
    103–114
    case presentation for, 103–111
    diagnosis of, 108–109
    first visit, 104–108
        breastfeeding observations, 108
        history-taking, 105–107
        maternal *vs.* infant problems,
            105t–107t
        physical examination, 107
    fundamental contexts of, 103, 111
    management of, 109–111
        AAP recommendations, 104
        follow-up visits, 109–111
        guidelines, 104, 104t, 112t
        Healthy People 2010 goals, 104
        support concerns, 104
    objectives for, 103
    resources for, 113
Bright Futures guidelines, 86–87
bronchiolitis, 380
budesonide, 260
bullous impetigo, 459
bupropion (Wellbutrin), 218
busy/inattentive child, 175–192. *See also*
    ADHD (attention deficit hyperactivity
    disorder)
    case presentation for, 176, 178, 180, 186,
        189–190
    diagnosis of, 176–181
    follow-up visits for, 189–190
    fundamental contexts of, 175, 191
    management of, 182–190
    objectives for, 175
    prognosis for, 190
    resources for, 191–192

C
calicivirus, 388
Campylobacter jejuni, 388
care models, 5
caregiving teams, 5–6
CARS (Childhood Autism Rating Scale), 37
case studies (pediatric primary care)
    for developmental problems, 9–72

fatigue (adolescents), 59–72
    gross motor delays (infants), 11–26
    language/social delays (toddlers),
        27–42
    school failure/refusal problems,
        43–58
    diagnostic reasoning for, 1–8
for diseases, 232–518
    acne (adolescents), 467–480
    anemia (toddlers), 291–320
    birth control (adolescents), 427–440
    cough, 377–386
    fever, 233–250
    headache, 321–335
    high blood sugar/overweight,
        267–290
    itchy rash, 455–466
    limp, 481–492
    oral trauma, 405–416
    recurrent ear infections (toddlers),
        347–358
    red eye (preschoolers), 335–346
    short stature, 507–518
    syncope, 359–376
    urinary urgency/incontinence
        (preschoolers), 417–426
    vaginal discharge (adolescents),
        441–454
    vomiting/diarrhea, 387–404
    well-child care (late-preterm infants),
        493–506
    wheezing, 251–266
for functional/mental health problems,
    73–230
    abuse situations, 193–206
    ADHD, 175–192
    breastfeeding/slow weight gain,
        103–114
    constipation (school-age children),
        115–132
    depression (adolescents), 207–220
    LGBT issues (adolescents), 221–231
    overweight (preschoolers), 85–102
    PPEs (adolescents), 133–163
    sleep patterns (infants), 163–175
    well-child care (infants), 75–84
CBCs (complete blood counts), 382–383,
    487–488, 500–501
CBT (cognitive behavior therapy), 214–215
CDC (Centers for Disease Control and
    Prevention)
    childhood obesity diagnostic criteria of, 90
    fluid replacement guidelines, 397–398
    immunization recommendations, 504
    Youth Behavior Study, 210–212
cefdinir (Omnicef), 353–354, 353t, 355t
cefpodoxime (Vantin), 353–354, 353t, 355t

Ceftin. See cefuroxime (Ceftin)
ceftriaxone (Rocephin), 353–354, 353t, 356t,
    421
cefuroxime (Ceftin), 353–354, 353t, 355t
Celexa. See citalopram (Celexa)
Centers for Disease Control and Prevention.
    See CDC (Centers for Disease Control
    and Prevention)
cephalexin, 421, 472–473
ceramide-based creams, 460
cerebral palsy. See CP (cerebral palsy)
CereVe, 460
cetirizine (Zyrtec), 343t
CHAT (Checklist for Autism in Toddlers), 35
CHD (congenital hip dysplasia), 484–487
Checklist for Autism in Toddlers. See CHAT
    (Checklist for Autism in Toddlers)
child abuse situations, 193–206
    case presentation for, 193–198, 200, 204
    diagnosis of, 193–200
        drawings as indicators, 201
        interviews, 193–199
        physical examinations, 199–200
        risk factors, 193–195
        signs/symptoms reviews, 202–203
    epidemiology/etiology of, 193–195
    fundamental contexts of, 193–195, 205
    management of, 203–204
        abuse consequences and, 204
        therapeutic plans, 203–204
    objectives for, 193
    reporting of, 194–200, 203
    resources for, 205–206
child protective authorities, 194–200, 203
Childhood Autism Rating Scale. See CARS
    (Childhood Autism Rating Scale)
Childhood Depression Inventory, 211–213
Chlamydia trachomatis, 379t, 382–383, 382t
Chlamydophila pneumonia, 378–379, 379t
chronic diarrhea vs. acute diarrhea, 391–392.
    See also diarrhea/vomiting
chronic fatigue vs. fatigue, 59–72. See also
    fatigue (adolescents)
citalopram (Celexa), 215–219, 217t
clarithromycin (Biaxin), 353–354, 353t, 355t
Claritin. See loratadine (Claritin)
clavulanate. See amoxicillin/clavulanate
    (Augmentin)
Cleocin. See clindamycin (Cleocin)
clindamycin (Cleocin), 353–354, 353t, 356t,
    474t–477t
clinical trials and studies
    American Community Survey, 225
    Bogalusa Heart Study, 272–273
    DCCT, 274–275
    ERIC, 274
    Kinsey Institute studies, 225–226

NHANES, 88
SEARCH for Diabetes in Youth Study,
    272–274
TADS, 213
TODAY Study, 277
TRIGR study, 273–274
cluster headache, 322, 324–328. *See also*
    headache
CMV (cytomegalovirus), 235–237
CNDC (chronic nonspecific diarrhea of
    childhood), 391–392
COC (combined oral contraceptive) pills,
    435b–437b
cognitive behavior therapy. *See* CBT
    (cognitive behavior therapy)
combined oral contraceptive pills. *See* COC
    (combined oral contraceptive) pills
complete blood counts. *See* CBCs (complete
    blood counts)
congenital hip dysplasia. *See* CHD (congenital
    hip dysplasia)
Conners' Scales, 180–181
consciousness loss, 359–376
    case presentation for, 360, 366–368, 370,
        372–373
    diagnosis of, 363–373
        ECGs, 370
        emergent evaluations, 370, 371f
        history-taking, 363–367
        imaging studies, 370
        laboratory blood work, 369–370
        physical examinations, 367–368
        red flags, 364–365
    epidemiology/etiology of, 360–361, 361t
        causal factors, 360–361, 361t
        definitions, 360
        recurrent episodes, 363
    fundamental contexts of, 359–360, 374
    management of, 372–373
        best practice evidence, 372–373
        referral *vs.* admission indictors, 372
    objectives for, 359
    resources for, 374–375
constipation (school-age children), 115–132
    case presentation for, 115–116, 119,
        122–123, 126, 128
    encopresis, 115–130
        diagnostic testing for, 120–121
        epidemiology/etiology of, 116–117,
            117–118
        follow-up visits for, 126, 130
        history-taking for, 118–119
        management of, 124t–125t, 126–130,
            129t
        medications for, 124t–125t, 129t
        parental education for, 127–128
        physical examinations for, 120–122

prognosis for, 130
    Rome III criteria for, 117t
    fundamental contexts of, 115–116,
        130–131
    objectives for, 115
    resources for, 131–132
contact dermatitis, 459
contraception (adolescents), 427–440
    case presentation for, 427–428, 434,
        437–439
    diagnosis of, 428–430
        diagnostic testing, 428
        history-taking, 429–430
        physical examination, 428
    fundamental contexts of, 427, 439
    management of, 430–439
        COC pills, 435b–437b
        counseling, 437–438
        follow-up visits, 438–439
        options, 430–434, 431t
    objectives for, 427
    resources for, 439–440
corticosteroids
    inhaled, 260
    oral, 473
    topical, 460–461, 461t
cough, 377–386
    case presentation for, 377–378, 381,
        383–384
    diagnosis of, 378–383
        clinical manifestations, 380
        common pneumonia syndromes, 382t
        diagnostic testing, 382–383
        differential, 380–381
        history-taking, 378–379
        Mycoplasma pneumoniae, 377–385
        physical examination, 381–382
        pneumonia, 378–383
    epidemiology/etiology of, 378–380
        common pathogens, 379t
        pathophysiology, 378–379
    fundamental contexts of, 377–385
    management of, 383–385
        educational plans, 384
        follow-up visits, 384
        hospitalization *vs.* home care, 383
        medications, 383–385
        pathogen transmission, 384–395
        prognosis, 384–395
    objectives for, 377
    resources for, 385
CP (cerebral palsy), 19–20
critical thinking skills, 1–8
    best evidence *vs.* best practice and, 1, 5
    care models and, 5
    caregiving teams and, 5–6
    complicating contexts of, 3–5

comorbidities, 4–5
cultural, 5
developmental, 3
family-centered care, 4
evidenced based care and, 1–2
fundamentals contexts of, 1–2, 6
problem domains and, 2–3
processes for, 5
resources for, 7
crown fracture, 405–414, 410f. *See also* oral
trauma
cultural contexts, 5
cyclosporine, 462
Cymbalta. *See* duloxetine (Cymbalta)
cystic fibrosis, 380
cytomegalovirus. *See* CMV (cytomegalovirus)
cytotoxic diarrhea, 390

D
DCCT (Diabetes Control and Complications
Trial), 274–275
decongestants, 353
delays, language/social, 27–42
ASDs, 28–40, 29t, 30f
AAP screen recommendations for,
27–28, 35, 39
ABA and, 37–38
AD, 28, 30f
AS, 28
CARS and, 37
CHAT and, 35
diagnosis of, 33–35, 34b
diagnostic testing for, 35–37, 36f
DSM-IV-TR criteria for, 30f
epidemiology/etiology of, 29, 31
expected outcomes for, 39
history-taking for, 31–32
M-CHAT and, 35, 36f
management of, 37–39
PDD-NOS, 28
PDDST-II and, 35
physical examinations for, 33
plans, diagnostic, 37
plans, educational, 37–39
plans, intervention, 37–38
TEACCH and, 37–38
case presentation for, 27–28
developmental milestones and, 28, 29t
fundamental contexts of, 27–28, 39
objectives for, 27
resources for, 40–41, 40b
dental trauma, 405–416
case presentations for, 405–406, 411–413
diagnosis of, 405–414
avulsion, permanent incisors,
405–414, 409f

avulsion, primary incisors, 405–414,
408f
crown fracture, permanent incisor
with/without pulp exposure,
405–414, 410f
history-taking, 406
PERRLA mnemonic, 407
physical examination, 406–407
epidemiology/etiology of, 407–411
fundamental contexts of, 405, 414
management of, 411–414
complications, 412–414
prognosis, 411–414
objectives for, 405
resources for, 414–415
Departments, governmental
DHHS. *See* DHHS (Department of Health
and Human Services)
USDA. *See* USDA (United States
Department of Agriculture)
Depo-Provera. *See* medroxyprogesterone
(Depo-Provera)
depression (adolescents), 207–220
case presentation for, 207–208, 218–219
diagnosis of, 211–213
Childhood Depression Inventory,
211–213
diagnostic testing, 212–213
differential, 212–213
physical examinations, 212–213
symptom analyses, 211–212
epidemiology/etiology for, 208–211
biological factors, 209
characteristics, 208
comorbidities, 209
definitions, 208
genetic factors, 209–210
pathophysiology, 208–209
psychosocial factors, 210
theoretical frameworks, 209–210
Youth Behavior Study, 210–212
fundamental contexts of, 207, 219
LGBT issues of, 227–228. *See also* LGBT
(lesbian, gay, bisexual, and
transgendered) issues
management of, 213–219
CBT, 214–215
follow-up visits, 219
medications, 215–219, 217t
patient/family education, 218–219
psychoeducation, 213–214
referrals, 213
serotonin syndrome, 217–218
TADS, 213
thought logs, 215, 216f
objectives for, 207
resources for, 210, 219–220

dermatitis, atopic. *See* AD (atopic dermatitis)
DES (dysfunctional elimination syndrome),
   418
developmental contexts, 3
developmental milestones, 11–18, 13t–15t
   ASDs and, 28, 29t
   fine motor, 29t
   gross motor, 29t
   language, 29t
   social, 29t
developmental problems
   diagnostic reasoning for, 1–8
   fatigue (adolescents), 59–72
   gross motor delays (infants), 11–26
   language/social delays (toddlers), 27–42
   school failure/refusal problems, 43–58
DHHS (Department of Health and Human
      Services)
   adolescent risk-taking data of, 429
   recommendations of
         adolescent exercise, 438
         HPV vaccine, 438–439
diabetes/overweight, 267–290
   case presentation for, 267–269, 275–276,
      283–284
   diagnosis of, 268–276
         ADA criteria, 270–271, 271t
         blood glucose diaries, 268t
         diabetes, 269–284
         differential, 275–276, 275t
         history-taking, 267–268
         obesity, 271–284
         physical examination, 268–269
         prediabetes, 270–271, 271t
   epidemiology/etiology of, 269–275
         Bogalusa Heart Study, 272–273
         DCCT, 274–275
         ERIC, 274
         pathophysiology, 269–271
         SEARCH for Diabetes in Youth Study,
            272–274
         TODAY Study, 277
         TRIGR study, 273–274
         type 1 diabetes, 273–275, 275t
         type 2 diabetes, 269–271, 275t
   fundamental contexts of, 267–268, 284
   management of, 270t, 276–284
         CDC Healthy Weight
            recommendations, 278–279
         comorbidities, 280–281
         depression, 281
         developmental factors, 279–280
         DHHS recommendations, 279
         dyslipidemia, 280–281
         education plans, 282–284
         follow-up visits, 284
         hypertension, 280

         medications, 277–278
         microvascular complications, 281
         NDEP, 270t
         nutritional changes, 278–279
         physical activity changes, 279
         renal disease, 281
         sociocutural factors, 281–282
         therapy goals, 277
         treatment options, 277–278
   objectives for, 267
   resources for, 270t
Diabetic ketoacidosis. *See* DKA (diabetic
      ketoacidosis)
diagnoses. *See* diagnostic case studies
*Diagnostic and Statistical Manual of Mental
      Disorders. See DSM-IV-TR (Diagnostic
      and Statistical Manual of Mental
      Disorders, Fourth Edition, Text
      Revisions)*
diagnostic case studies
   for developmental problems, 9–72
         fatigue (adolescents), 59–72
         gross motor delays (infants), 11–26
         language/social delays (toddlers),
            27–42
         school failure/refusal problems,
            43–58
   diagnostic reasoning for, 1–8
   for diseases, 232–518
         acne (adolescents), 467–480
         anemia (toddlers), 291–320
         birth control (adolescents), 427–440
         cough, 377–386
         fever, 233–250
         headache, 321–335
         high blood sugar/overweight,
            267–290
         itchy rash, 455–466
         limp, 481–492
         oral trauma, 405–416
         recurrent ear infections (toddlers),
            347–358
         red eye (preschoolers), 335–346
         short stature, 507–518
         syncope, 359–376
         urinary urgency/incontinence
            (preschoolers), 417–426
         vaginal discharge (adolescents),
            441–454
         vomiting/diarrhea, 387–404
         well-child care (late-preterm infants),
            493–506
         wheezing, 251–266
   for functional/mental health problems,
      73–230
         abuse situations, 193–206
         ADHD, 175–192

breastfeeding/slow weight gain,
    103–114
constipation (school-age children),
    115–132
depression (adolescents), 207–220
LGBT issues (adolescents), 221–231
overweight (preschoolers), 85–102
PPEs (adolescents), 133–163
sleep patterns (infants), 163–175
well-child care (infants), 75–84
diagnostic reasoning, 1–8
    best evidence *vs.* best practice and, 1, 5
    care models and, 5
    caregiving teams and, 5–6
    complicating contexts of, 3–5
        comorbidities, 4–5
        cultural, 5
        developmental, 3
        family-centered care, 4
    evidenced based care and, 1–2
    fundamental contexts of, 1–2, 6
    problem domains and, 2–3
    processes for, 5
    resources for, 7
diaries, blood glucose, 268t
diarrhea/vomiting, 387–404
    case presentation for, 387–388, 394–395,
        400
    diagnosis of, 392–397
        death risk factors, 391–392
        diagnostic testing, 396–397
        differential, 393t, 395–396
        history-taking, 391–395
        hospitalization risk factors, 391–392
        telephone consultations, 391–395
    epidemiology/etiology of, 388–395
        acute *vs.* chronic diarrhea, 391–392
        causative agents, 388–389
        CNDC, 391–392
        pathophysiology, 389–390
    fundamental contexts of, 387, 400–401
    gastroenteritis, 397–401
    management of, 397–400
        feeding resumption, 397–399
        follow-up visits, 399–400
        hydration/rehydration, 397, 398t
        medications, 399
    objectives for, 387
    resources for, 401–402
Differin. *See* adapalene (Differin)
diphenhydramine, 68
discussion of cases. *See* case studies (pediatric
    primary care)
diseases
    acne (adolescents), 467–480
    anemia (toddlers), 291–320
    birth control (adolescents), 427–440

cough, 377–386
diagnostic reasoning for, 1–8
fever, 233–250
headache, 321–335
high blood sugar/overweight, 267–290
itchy rash, 455–466
limp, 481–492
oral trauma, 405–416
recurrent ear infections (toddlers), 347–358
red eye (preschoolers), 335–346
short stature, 507–518
syncope, 359–376
urinary urgency/incontinence
    (preschoolers), 417–426
vaginal discharge (adolescents), 441–454
vomiting/diarrhea, 387–404
well-child care (late-preterm infants),
    493–506
wheezing, 251–266
DKA (diabetic ketoacidosis), 267–268,
    267–269, 275t
domains, problem, 2–3
Dove soap, 460
doxycycline, 383–384, 472–473, 475t–477t
drawings as abuse indicators, 201
drug therapies. *See* medications
*DSM-IV-TR (Diagnostic and Statistical
    Manual of Mental Disorders, Fourth
    Edition, Text Revisions)*
    AD diagnostic criteria, 30f
    ADHD criteria
        criteria, 176–178, 177t–178t
duloxetine (Cymbalta), 218
dysenteric diarrhea, 390
dysfunctional elimination syndrome. *See* DES
    (dysfunctional elimination syndrome)
dyshidrotic eczema, 459

E
ear infections (toddlers), 347–358
    case presentation for, 347–348, 351,
        354–355
    diagnosis of, 350–356
        AOM, 347–356
        diagnostic testing, 352
        history-taking, 348–351
        OME, 347–356
        physical examination, 351
    epidemiology/etiology of, 348–350
        pathophysiology, 350–351
        risk factors, 349–350
    fundamental contexts of, 347–348, 357
    management of, 352–356
        AAP recommendations, 353–356
        education plans, 354
        follow-up visits, 354–355
        medications, 352–356, 353t, 355t

SNAP, 353
   therapeutic plans, 352–353
objectives for, 347
resources for, 357–358
EBV (Epstein-Barr virus), 235–237
educational objectives. *See* objectives
Effexor. *See* venlafaxine (Effexor)
Elestat. *See* epinastine HCl (Elestat)
Elidel. *See* pimecrolimus (Elidel)
Emadine. *See* emedastine difumarate
   (Emadine)
emedastine difumarate (Emadine), 343t
Emergency contraception, 434
encopresis (school-age children), 115–132
   diagnosis of, 117–122
      diagnostic testing, 120–121
      history-taking, 118–119
      physical examinations, 120–122
      Rome III criteria for, 117t
   epidemiology/etiology of, 116–117,
      117–118
   fundamental contexts of, 115–116, 130–131
   management of, 124t–125t, 126–130, 129t
      follow-up visits, 126, 130
      medications, 124t–125t, 129t
      parental education, 127–128
   objectives for, 115
   prognosis for, 130
   resources for, 131–132
Entamoeba histolytica, 388
environmental toxins, 296–299, 298t–299t
Epiceram, 460
epidemiology/etiology
   of developmental problems
      fatigue (adolescents), 60–61
      gross motor delays (infants), 11–18
      language/social delays (toddlers),
         28–31
   of diseases
      acne (adolescents), 468–469
      AD, 456–457
      anemia (toddlers), 296
      cough, 378–380
      diarrhea/vomiting, 388–395
      fever, 234–239
      headache, 322–324
      late-preterm infants (well-child care),
         494–496
      oral trauma, 407–411
      overweight/high blood sugar,
         269–275
      recurrent ear infections (toddlers),
         348–350
      red eye (preschoolers), 336
      syncope, 360–361, 361t
      urinary urgency/incontinence
         (preschoolers), 418–419

vaginal discharge (adolescents), 446
      wheezing, 252–259
   of functional/mental health problems
      abuse situations, 193–195
      constipation (school-age children),
         116–117, 117–118
      depression (adolescents), 208–211
      overweight (preschoolers), 88–90
      sleep patterns (infants), 163–166
epinastine HCl (Elestat), 343t
EPR-3 (Expert Panel Report 3) guidelines,
   259–260
Epstein-Barr virus. *See* EBV (Epstein-Barr
   virus)
ERIC (Epidemiology of Diabetes Interventions
   and Complications), 274
erythromycin, 353–354, 353t, 383–384,
   472–473, 475t–477t
erythromycin/sulfisoxazole (Pediazole), 356t
Escherichia coli, 388, 418, 420
escitalopram (Lexapro), 217t
estrogen/progesterone, 430–431, 431t
etiology. *See* epidemiology/etiology
Eucerin soap, 460
evidenced-based care case studies
   for developmental problems, 9–72
      fatigue (adolescents), 59–72
      gross motor delays (infants), 11–26
      language/social delays (toddlers),
         27–42
      school failure/refusal problems,
         43–58
   diagnostic reasoning for, 1–8
   for diseases, 232–518
      acne (adolescents), 467–480
      anemia (toddlers), 291–320
      birth control (adolescents), 427–440
      cough, 377–386
      fever, 233–250
      headache, 321–335
      high blood sugar/overweight,
         267–290
      itchy rash, 455–466
      limp, 481–492
      oral trauma, 405–416
      recurrent ear infections (toddlers),
         347–358
      red eye (preschoolers), 335–346
      short stature, 507–518
      syncope, 359–376
      urinary urgency/incontinence
         (preschoolers), 417–426
      vaginal discharge (adolescents),
         441–454
      vomiting/diarrhea, 387–404
      well-child care (late-preterm infants),
         493–506

wheezing, 251–266
for functional/mental health problems,
73–230
abuse situations, 193–206
ADHD, 175–192, 175–193
breastfeeding/slow weight gain,
103–114
constipation (school-age children),
115–132
depression (adolescents), 207–220
LGBT issues (adolescents), 221–231
overweight (preschoolers), 85–102
PPEs (adolescents), 133–163
sleep patterns (infants), 163–175
well-child care (infants), 75–84
Expert Panel Report 3 guidelines. *See* EPR-3
(Expert Panel Report 3) guidelines

F

FACES pain tool, 481–482
family-centered care, 4
fatigue (adolescents), 59–72
case presentation for, 59, 62–63, 67, 69–70
cultural influences on, 60–61
development factors of, 61
diagnosis of, 64–66, 65t
24-hour diet recall, 62, 63t
differential, 64–66
fatigue as symptom, 59–60
history-taking, 61–64, 63t
laboratory tests, 64–65, 65t
epidemiology/etiology of, 60–61
fundamental contexts of, 59, 71
management of, 66–69
follow-up visits, 69–70
medications, 68
patient education, 68–69
sleep hygiene measures, 67, 70t
therapeutic management plans, 67–69
objectives for, 59
prognosis for, 69–70
resources for, 71–72
female athlete triad, 143–144, 157
Ferber method, 169–170
fertility awareness, 433
fever, 233–250
case presentation for, 233–234, 240,
243–244, 247
diagnosis of, 239–242
CMV, 235–237
CMV-caused IM, 238–247
diagnostic error sources, 246–247
diagnostic testing, 240–246,
245t–246t
differential, 233, 239–240, 241t
EBV, 235–237
history-taking, 239–240

HIV, 235–237
IM, 234–237
pharyngitis, 235–247
sensitivity *vs.* specificity, 240–242
toxoplasmosis, 235–236
epidemiology/etiology of, 234–239
common infectious agents, 234–238,
236t–237t
cultural/ethnic factors, 238–239
pathophysiology, 234–238
fundamental contexts of, 233–234, 247
management of, 242–247
educational plans, 243–244
medications, 243
sports participation and, 247
therapeutic plans, 242–243
treatment options, 243
NEEDS mnemonic, 234
objectives for, 233
resources for, 248–249
fexofenadine (Allegra), 343t
fluoxetine (Prozac), 215–219, 217t
fluvoxamine (Luvox), 215–219, 217t
food allergies, 458–459
foreign body aspiration, 380
four-stage overweight approach, 95
functional/mental health problems
abuse situations, 193–206
ADHD, 175–192, 175–193
breastfeeding/slow weight gain, 103–114
constipation (school-age children),
115–132
depression (adolescents), 207–220
diagnostic reasoning for, 1–8
LGBT issues (adolescents), 221–231
overweight (preschoolers), 85–102
PPEs (adolescents), 133–163
sleep patterns (infants), 163–175
well-child care (infants), 75–84
fundamental contexts
of developmental problems
fatigue (adolescents), 59, 71
gross motor delays (infants), 11–12, 25
language/social delays (toddlers),
27–28, 39
of diseases
acne (adolescents), 467–468, 479
AD, 455–456
anemia (toddlers), 291, 317
birth control (adolescents), 427, 439
cough, 377–385
diarrhea/vomiting, 387, 400–401
fever, 233–234, 247
headache, 321–322, 332
late-preterm infants (well-child care),
493, 505
limp, 481–482, 491

oral trauma, 405, 414
overweight/high blood sugar,
    267–268, 284
recurrent ear infections (toddlers),
    347–348, 357
red eye (preschoolers), 334, 335–336
short stature, 507–508, 516
syncope, 359–360, 374
urinary urgency/incontinence
    (preschoolers), 417, 425
vaginal discharge (adolescents),
    441–452
wheezing, 251–252, 264
of functional/mental health problems
    abuse situations, 193–195, 205
    ADHD, 175, 191
    breastfeeding/slow weight gain
        (infants), 103, 111
    constipation (school-age children),
        115–116, 130–131
    depression (adolescents), 207, 219
    LGBT issues, 221–223, 229
    overweight (preschoolers), 85, 98–99
    PPEs, 133, 158–159
    sleep patterns (infants), 163, 172
    well-child care (infants), 75–76, 82
Furadantin elixir, 423

G
gait abnormality, 481–492
    case presentation for, 481–483, 488–491
    diagnosis of, 481–488
        diagnostic testing, 487–488
        differential, 484–487
        gait by chronological age, 484t
        history-taking, 481–482
        physical examination, 482–483
        symptom analyses, 482
        transient synovitis, 489–491
    fundamental contexts of, 481–482, 491
    management of, 488–491
        educational plan, 489–490
        follow-up visits, 490–491
        medications, 490
    objectives for, 481
    resources for, 491–492
gastroenteritis, 387–404
    case presentation for, 387–388, 394–395,
        400
    diagnosis of, 392–397
        death risk factors, 391–392
        diagnostic testing, 396–397
        differential, 393t, 395–396
        history-taking, 391–395
        hospitalization risk factors, 391–392
        telephone consultations, 391–395
    epidemiology/etiology of, 388–395

acute *vs.* chronic diarrhea, 391–392
causative agents, 388–389
CNDC, 391–392
pathophysiology, 389–390
fundamental contexts of, 387, 400–401
management of, 397–400
    feeding resumption, 397–399
    follow-up visits, 399–400
    hydration/rehydration, 397, 398t
    medications, 399
objectives for, 387
resources for, 401–402
gay issues. *See* LGBT (lesbian, gay, bisexual,
    and transgendered) issues
GBS (group b streptococcal) sepsis, 494
Giardia lamblia, 388
goals/objectives. *See* objectives
governmental departments/agencies
    DHHS. *See* DHHS (Department of Health
        and Human Services)
    USDA. *See* USDA (United States
        Department of Agriculture)
gross motor delays (infants), 11–26
    diagnosis of, 19–21
        CP, 19–20
        cultural/ethnic factors, 20–21
        developmental milestones and,
            11–18, 13t–15t
        epidemiology/etiology of, 11–18
    fundamental contexts of, 11–12, 25
    management of, 21–25
        educational plans, 23
        follow-up visits, 23–24
        preventive measures, 24–25
        prognosis, 24
        therapeutic plans, 21–22
        treatment options, 22–232
    objectives for, 11
    resources for, 25–26
group b streptococcal sepsis. *See* GBS (group
    b streptococcal) sepsis

H
Haemophilus influenzae, 349
Hank's balanced salt solution, 409, 412
headache, 321–335
    case presentations for, 321–322, 327–328,
        330–332
    diagnosis of, 324–328
        diagnostic testing, 327–329
        differential, 324, 325t
        history-taking, 324–327, 329t
        physical examinations, 327–328, 329t
    epidemiology/etiology of, 322–324
        cluster headache, 322, 324–328
        IHS classification, 322–324
        migraine, 322–328

pathophysiology, 322–323
social factors, 324
trigeminal autonomic cephalalgias, 322, 324–328
TTHs, 322, 324–328
fundamental contexts of, 321–322, 332
management of, 328–332
American Academy of Neurology Practice Parameters, 330
behavioral, 332t
follow-up visits, 332
medications, 331–332
PedMIDAS tool, 330–332
therapeutic plans, 328–330
objectives for, 321
resources for, 333
healthcare avoidance, 223–224
healthcare case studies
for developmental problems, 9–72
fatigue (adolescents), 59–72
gross motor delays (infants), 11–26
language/social delays (toddlers), 27–42
school failure/refusal problems, 43–58
diagnostic reasoning for, 1–8
for diseases, 232–518
acne (adolescents), 467–480
anemia (toddlers), 291–320
birth control (adolescents), 427–440
cough, 377–386
fever, 233–250
headache, 321–335
high blood sugar/overweight, 267–290
itchy rash, 455–466
limp, 481–492
oral trauma, 405–416
recurrent ear infections (toddlers), 347–358
red eye (preschoolers), 335–346
short stature, 507–518
syncope, 359–376
urinary urgency/incontinence (preschoolers), 417–426
vaginal discharge (adolescents), 441–454
vomiting/diarrhea, 387–404
well-child care (late-preterm infants), 493–506
wheezing, 251–266
for functional/mental health problems, 73–230
abuse situations, 193–206
ADHD, 175–192
breastfeeding/slow weight gain, 103–114

constipation (school-age children), 115–132
depression (adolescents), 207–220
LGBT issues (adolescents), 221–231
overweight (preschoolers), 85–102
PPEs (adolescents), 133–163
sleep patterns (infants), 163–175
well-child care (infants), 75–84
Healthy People 2010 goals, 104
HEAT (Healthy Eating and Activity Together) Initiative, 96
hemoglobin/hematocrit counts. *See* H&H (hemoglobin/hematocrit) counts
hemolytic uremic syndrome. *See* HUS (hemolytic uremic syndrome)
hepatitis
autoimmune, 472–473
hepatitis B immunizations, 503–504
H&H (hemoglobin/hematocrit) counts, 428
high blood sugar/overweight, 267–290
case presentation for, 267–269, 275–276, 283–284
diagnosis of, 268–276
ADA criteria, 270–271, 271t
blood glucose diaries, 268t
diabetes, 269–284
differential, 275–276, 275t
history-taking, 267–268
obesity, 271–284
physical examination, 268–269
prediabetes, 270–271, 271t
epidemiology/etiology of, 269–275
Bogalusa Heart Study, 272–273
DCCT, 274–275
ERIC, 274
pathophysiology, 269–271
SEARCH for Diabetes in Youth Study, 272–274
TODAY Study, 277
TRIGR study, 273–274
type 1 diabetes, 273–275, 275t
type 2 diabetes, 269–271, 275t
fundamental contexts of, 267–268, 284
management of, 270t, 276–284
CDC Healthy Weight recommendations, 278–279
comorbidities, 280–281
depression, 281
developmental factors, 279–280
DHHS recommendations, 279
dyslipidemia, 280–281
education plans, 282–284
follow-up visits, 284
hypertension, 280
medications, 277–278
microvascular complications, 281
NDEP, 270t

nutritional changes, 278–279
physical activity changes, 279
renal disease, 281
sociocutural factors, 281–282
therapy goals, 277
treatment options, 277–278
objectives for, 267
resources for, 270t, 285–290
hip dysplasia, 484–487
HIV (human immunodeficiency virus), 235–237
hormonal agents, 472–473
HPV (human papilloma virus) vaccine, 438–439
human immunodeficiency virus. *See* HIV (human immunodeficiency virus)
human metapneumovirus, 379t
human papilloma virus vaccine. *See* HPV (human papilloma virus) vaccine
HUS (hemolytic uremic syndrome), 395–396
Hylira, 460
hyperactivity. *See* ADHD (attention deficit hyperactivity disorder)
hypnotics, 68
hypothyroidism, 306–307, 309

I

I PREPARE mnemonic, 298–299, 299t
ICD-9 codes, anemia, 313t
IDA (iron deficiency anemia), 300–303, 300t, 308. *See also* anemia (toddlers)
Identifying and Preventing Overweight in Childhood, 96
IHS (International Headache Society) classification, 322–324
IM (infectious mononucleosis), 234–237
immunizations
    AAP recommendations for, 504
    HPV vaccine, 438–439
    for late-preterm infants, 503–504
impetigo, 459
Impruv, 460
inattentive/busy child diagnoses. *See also* ADHD (attention deficit hyperactivity disorder)
    case presentation for, 176, 178, 180, 186, 189–190
    diagnosis of, 176–181
    follow-up visits for, 189–190
    fundamental contexts of, 175, 191
    management of, 182–190
    objectives for, 175
    prognosis for, 190
    resources for, 191–192
infant/newborn-specific concerns
    breastfeeding/slow weight gain, 103–114
    diagnostic reasoning for, 1–8

gross motor delays, 11–26
sleep patterns, 163–175
well-child care
    infants, 75–84
    late-preterm infants, 493–506
infectious mononucleosis. *See* IM (infectious mononucleosis)
influenza, 379t
inhaled corticosteroids, 260. *See also* corticosteroids
insulin, 268t, 277–278
International Headache Society classification. *See* IHS (International Headache Society) classification
intrauterine devices, 433
intussusception, 395–396
iPLEDGE program, 473
iron deficiency anemia. *See* IDA (iron deficiency anemia)
isotretinoin (Accutane), 473, 477t
itchy rash, 455–466
    AD (atopic dermatitis), 455–464
        antibiotics for, 462–463
        antivirals for, 463
        Atopiclair for, 463
        diagnosis of, 456, 459
        differential diagnosis for, 459
        epidemiology/etiology of, 456
        follow-up visits for, 463–464
        history-taking, 459
        management of, 459–464
        medications for, 460–463, 461t
        MimyX for, 463
        parental/patient education for, 463–464
        pathophysiology of, 457
        physical examination, 456, 459
        presentation of, 457–458
        PUVA therapy for, 462
        RAST/SPT, 458
        systemic steroids for, 462
        TCIs for, 462
        topical corticosteroids for, 460–462, 461t
        triggers of, 458–459
    case presentation for, 455, 459, 463–464
    fundamental contexts of, 455–456, 464
    objectives for, 455
    resources for, 465–466

J

JRA (juvenile rheumatoid arthritis), 484–487

K

ketotifen fumarate (Zaditor), 343t
Kinsey Institute studies, 225–226
Klebsiella pneumoniae, 421

L

language/social delays (toddlers), 27–42
  ASDs, 28–40, 29t, 30f
    AAP screen recommendations for,
      27–28, 35, 39
    ABA and, 37–38
    AD, 28, 30f
    AS, 28
    CARS and, 37
    CHAT and, 35
    diagnosis of, 33–37, 34b
    diagnostic testing for, 35–37, 36f
    DSM-IV-TR criteria for, 30f
    epidemiology/etiology of, 28–31
    history-taking for, 31–32
    M-CHAT and, 35, 36f
    management of, 37–39
    PDD-NOS, 28
    PDDST-II and, 35
    physical examinations for, 33
    prognosis for, 39
    TEACCH and, 37–38
  case presentation for, 27–28
  developmental milestones and, 28, 29t
  fundamental contexts of, 27–28, 39
  objectives for, 27
  plans for, 37–39
    diagnostic, 37
    educational, 37–39
    intervention, 37–38
  resources for, 40–41, 40b
late-preterm infants (well-child care),
      493–506. *See also* well-child care
  case presentation for, 493, 496–501, 504
  diagnosis of, 496–501
    cultural/teenage dynamics, 499
    diagnostic testing, 501
    differential, 500–501
    history-taking, 496–499
    physical examination, 500
    social/emotional history, 499–500
  epidemiology/etiology of, 494–496
    common issues, 495–496
    definitions, 494
    hyperbilirubinemia, 494–495
    jaundice, 494–495
    lung function, 494
    metabolic function, 495
    sepsis, 494
    temperature regulation, 495
  fundamental contexts for, 493, 505
  management of, 501–504
    follow-up visits, 504–505
    immunizations, 503–504
    parent education, 502–504
    referrals, 503

  therapeutic plans, 501–502
  objectives for, 493
  resources for, 505–506
law enforcement authorities, 194–200, 203
LCPD (Legg-Calve-Perthes disease), 484–487
lead poisoning, 303–305, 309
Legg-Calve-Perthes disease. *See* LCPD (Legg-
      Calve-Perthes disease)
lesbian issues. *See* LGBT (lesbian, gay,
      bisexual, and transgendered) issues
leukemia, 305–306
leukemia, lymphoblastic, 486–487
levocabastine HCl (Livostin), 343t
Lexapro. *See* escitalopram (Lexapro)
LGBT (lesbian, gay, bisexual, and
      transgendered) issues, 221–231
  adolescent sexual expression, 225–227
    American Community Survey, 225
    epidemiology/etiology of, 225–227
    Kinsey Institute studies, 225–226
  case presentation for, 221, 224–229
  definitions for, 222t
  diagnosis of, 228
  fundamental contexts of, 221–223, 229
  management of, 229
  objectives for, 221
  related health risk factors of, 221, 223–228
    depression, 227–228. *See also*
      depression (adolescents)
    healthcare avoidance, 223–224
    mental health risks, 223
    STDs, 221, 223, 226–228
    suicide risks, 227–228
    violence risks, 223, 227–228
  resources for, 230
limp, 481–492
  case presentation for, 481–483, 488–491
  diagnosis, 481–488
    diagnostic testing, 487–488
    differential, 484–487
    gait by chronological age, 484t
    history-taking, 481–482
    physical examination, 482–483
    symptom analyses, 482
    transient synovitis, 489–491
  fundamental contexts for, 481–482, 491
  management of, 488–491
    educational plan, 489–490
    follow-up visits, 490–491
    medications, 490
  objectives for, 481
  resources for, 491–492
Livostin. *See* levocabastine HCl (Livostin)
loratadine (Claritin), 343t
loss of consciousness, 359–376
  case presentation for, 360, 366–368, 370,
      372–373

diagnosis of, 363–373
    diagnostic testing, 363
    ECGs, 370
    emergent evaluations, 370, 371f
    history-taking, 363–367
    imaging studies, 370
    laboratory blood work, 369–370
    physical examinations, 367–368
    red flags, 364–365
epidemiology/etiology of, 360–361, 361t
    causal factors, 360–361, 361t
    definitions, 360
    recurrent episodes, 363
fundamental contexts of, 359–360, 374
management of, 372–373
    best practice evidence, 372–373
    referral *vs.* admission indictors, 372
objectives for, 359
resources for, 374–375
Luvox. *See* fluvoxamine (Luvox)
lymphoblastic leukemia, 486–487
lymphoma, 305–306

M

M-CHAT (Modified Checklist for Autism in
    Toddlers), 35, 35f
Macrodantin, 423
macrolides, 383–384
management
    of developmental problems
        fatigue (adolescents), 66–69
        gross motor delays (infants), 21–25
        language/social delays (toddlers),
            37–39
    of diseases
        acne (adolescents), 471–479
        AD, 459–464
        anemia (toddlers), 313–327
        birth control (adolescents), 430–439
        cough, 383–385
        diarrhea/vomiting, 397–400
        fever, 242–247
        headache, 328–332
        late-preterm infants (well-child care),
            501–504
        limp, 488–491
        oral trauma, 411–414
        overweight/high blood sugar, 270t,
            276–284
        recurrent ear infections (toddlers),
            352–356
        red eye (preschoolers), 340–344
        short stature, 512–516
        syncope, 372–373
        urinary urgency/incontinence
            (preschoolers), 420–425

vaginal discharge (adolescents),
    449–452
wheezing, 251, 260–264
of functional/mental health problems
    abuse situations, 203–204
    ADHD, 182–190
    breastfeeding/slow weight gain
        (infants), 109–111
    constipation (school-age children),
        124t–125t, 126–130, 129t
    depression (adolescents), 213–219
    LGBT issues, 229
    overweight (preschoolers), 94–95
    PPEs, 152–158, 152t, 154t–155t
    sleep patterns (infants), 168–172
mast cell stabilizers/antihistamines, 343t
medications
    for developmental problems
        fatigue (adolescents), 68
        language/social delays (toddlers),
            37–39
    for diseases
        acne (adolescents), 472–473,
            474t–478t
        AD, 459–464
        anemia (toddlers), 314–315
        asthma, 260
        birth control (adolescents), 430–439
        cough, 383–385
        diarrhea/vomiting, 399
        fever, 243
        headache, 331–332
        limp, 490
        overweight/high blood sugar,
            277–278
        recurrent ear infections (toddlers),
            352–356, 353t, 355t
        red eye (preschoolers), 341–342, 343t
        STIs, 451–452, 452b
        urinary urgency/incontinence
            (preschoolers), 421–422
        vaginal discharge (adolescents),
            451–452, 452b
    drug names/classes
        ACE inhibitors, 280
        acyclovir, 463
        adapalene (Differin), 474t–477t
        albuterol, 260
        alpha-glucosidase inhibitors, 278
        Alpha Keri soap, 460
        amoxicillin, 353, 355t, 423, 472–473
        amoxicillin/clavulanate (Augmentin),
            355t
        ampicillin, 472–473
        antibiotics, oral, 353–354, 353t, 399,
            421, 462–463
        antibiotics, topical, 472

antidepressants, 215–219, 217t
antidepressants, tricyclic, 218
antihistamines, 68, 343t
antihistamines/mast cell stabilizers,
  343t
antihistamines/vasoconstrictors, 343t
antipyrine/benzocaine (Auralgan),
  356t
antivirals, 463
Aquaphor, 460
Atopiclair, 463
Aveeno soap, 460
azathioprine, 462
azelaic acid, 472
azelastine HCl (Optivar), 343t
azithromycin, 353–354, 353t, 355t,
  383–384
benzoyl peroxide, 472, 474t–477t
biguanides, 278
budesonide, 260
bupropion (Wellbutrin), 218
cefdinir (Omnicef), 353–354, 353t,
  355t
cefpodoxime (Vantin), 353–354,
  353t, 355t
ceftriaxone (Rocephin), 353–354,
  353t, 356t, 421
cefuroxime (Ceftin), 353–354, 353t,
  355t
cephalexin, 421, 472–473
ceramide-based creams, 460
CereVe, 460
cetirizine (Zyrtec), 343t
citalopram (Celexa), 215–219, 217t
clarithromycin (Biaxin), 353–354,
  353t, 355t
clindamycin (Cleocin), 353–354,
  353t, 356t, 474t–477t
COC pills, 435b–437b
corticosteroids, inhaled, 260
corticosteroids, oral, 473
corticosteroids, topical, 460–461,
  461t
cyclosporine, 462
decongestants, 353
Dove soap, 460
doxycycline, 383–384, 472–473,
  475t–477t
duloxetine (Cymbalta), 218
diphenhydramine, 68
emedastine difumarate (Emadine),
  343t
Epiceram, 460
epinastine HCl (Elestat), 343t
erythromycin, 353–354, 353t,
  383–384, 472–473, 475t–477t

erythromycin/sulfisoxazole
  (Pediazole), 356t
escitalopram (Lexapro), 217t
estrogen/progesterone, 430–431, 431t
Eucerin soap, 460
fexofenadine (Allegra), 343t
fluoxetine (Prozac), 215–219, 217t
fluvoxamine (Luvox), 215–219, 217t
Furadantin elixir, 423
hormonal agents, 472–473
Hylira, 460
hypnotics, 68
immunizations
  HPV vaccine, 438–439
Impruv, 460
insulin, 268t, 277–278
isotretinoin (Accutane), 473, 477t
ketotifen fumarate (Zaditor), 343t
levocabastine HCl (Livostin), 343t
loratadine (Claritin), 343t
Macrodantin, 423
macrolides, 383–384
medroxyprogesterone (Depo-
  Provera), 431t, 432
meglitinides, 278
melatonin, 68
metformin, 277
MimyX, 463
minocycline, 472–473
mirtazapine (Remeron), 218
mycophenolate mofetil, 462
naphazoline HCl/pheniramine
  (Naphcon A, Opcon-A), 343t
Nouriva Repair, 460
NSAIDs, 490
olopatadine HCl (Patanol, Pataday),
  343t
paroxetine (Paxil), 215–219, 217t
penicillin, 353
pimecrolimus (Elidel), 462
prednisolone, 260
progesterone only contraceptives,
  431t, 432
retinoids, topical, 472, 474t–477t
SABAs, 260
sertraline (Zoloft), 215–219, 217t
SSRIs, 215–219, 217t
Stelatopia, 460
steroids, oral, 260
sulfamethoxazole, 421
sulfonylureas, 278
tacrolimus (Protopic), 462
TCIs, 462
tetracycline, 475t–477t
thiazolidinediones, 278
tretinoin (Retin-A, Avita), 474t–477t
TriCeram, 460

trimethoprim-sulfamethoxazole,
421–423, 475t–477t
Vaseline, 460
venlafaxine (Effexor), 218
zinc, 399
for functional/mental health problems
constipation (school-age children),
124t–125t, 129t
depression (adolescents), 215–219, 217t
overweight/high blood sugar,
277–278
immunizations
for late-preterm infants, 503–504
off-label use of, 68
warfarin, toxicity, 306, 308
medroxyprogesterone (Depo-Provera), 431t,
432
melatonin, 68
mental/functional health problems, 73–230
abuse situations, 193–206
ADHD, 175–192
breastfeeding/slow weight gain, 103–114
constipation (school-age children),
115–132
depression (adolescents), 207–220
diagnostic reasoning for, 1–8
LGBT issues (adolescents), 221–231
overweight (preschoolers), 85–102
PPEs (adolescents), 133–163
sleep patterns (infants), 163–175
well-child care (infants), 75–84
metformin, 277
migraine, 322–328. *See also* headache
milestones, developmental, 11–18, 13t–15t
MimyX, 463
minocycline, 472–473
Mirena intrauterine device, 433
mirtazapine (Remeron), 218
models of care, 5
Modified Checklist for Autism in Toddlers. *See*
M-CHAT (Modified Checklist for Autism
in Toddlers)
mononucleosis. *See* IM (infectious
mononucleosis)
Moraxella catarrhalis, 349
MRSA (methicillin-resistant *Staphylococcus
aureus*), 458, 469–470
Mycobacterium tuberculosis, 379t
mycophenolate mofetil, 462
Mycoplasma pneumoniae, 377–385
case presentation for, 377–378, 381,
383–384
diagnosis of, 378–383
clinical manifestations, 380
common pneumonia syndromes, 382t
diagnostic testing, 382–383
differential, 380–381

history-taking, 378–379
physical examination, 381–382
pneumonia, 378–383
epidemiology/etiology of, 378–380
common pathogens, 379t
pathophysiology, 378–379
fundamental contexts of, 377–385
management of, 383–385
educational plans, 384
follow-up visits, 384
hospitalization *vs.* home care, 383
medications, 383–385
pathogen transmission, 384–395
prognosis, 384–395
objectives of, 377
resources for, 385
MyPyramid, 94–97, 438

N

NAEPP (National Asthma Education and
Prevention Program) guidelines,
259–260, 261t–263t
naphazoline HCl/pheniramine (Naphcon A,
Opcon-A), 343t
Naphcon A. *See* naphazoline HCl/pheniramine
(Naphcon A, Opcon-A)
National Association of Pediatric Nurse
Practitioners, 96
National Center for Health Statistics, 88
National Diabetes Education Program. *See*
NDEP (National Diabetes Education
Program)
National Guideline Clearinghouse, 96
National Health and Nutrition Examination
Survey. *See* NHANES (National Health
and Nutrition Examination Survey)
National Institutes of Health. *See* NIH
(National Institutes of Health)
National Sleep Foundation, 68
Natural family planning, 433
NDEP (National Diabetes Education Program),
270t
NEEDS (Nutrition, Elimination,
Education/Environment,
Development/Daycare, and
Sleep/Sexuality) mnemonic, 234
newborn/infant-specific concerns
breastfeeding/slow weight gain, 103–114
diagnostic reasoning for, 1–8
gross motor delays, 11–26
sleep patterns, 163–175
well-child care
infants, 75–84
late-preterm infants, 493–506
NHANES (National Health and Nutrition
Examination Survey)
overweight data of, 88

NIH (National Institutes of Health), 512
nonsteroidal anti-inflammatory drugs. *See* NSAIDs (nonsteroidal anti-inflammatory drugs)
Noonan syndrome, 508
Norwalk virus, 388
Nouriva Repair, 460
NSAIDs (nonsteroidal anti-inflammatory drugs), 490
nummular dermatitis, 459

O

obesity. *See* overweight (preschoolers)
objectives
  for developmental problems
    fatigue (adolescents), 59
    gross motor delays (infants), 11
    language/social delays (toddlers), 27
  for diseases
    acne (adolescents), 467
    AD, 455
    anemia (toddlers), 291
    birth control (adolescents), 427
    cough, 377
    diarrhea/vomiting, 387
    fever, 233
    headache, 321
    late-preterm infants (well-child care), 493
    limp, 481
    oral trauma, 405
    overweight/high blood sugar, 267
    recurrent ear infections (toddlers), 347
    red eye (preschoolers), 335
    short stature, 507
    syncope, 359
    urinary urgency/incontinence (preschoolers), 417
    vaginal discharge (adolescents), 441
    wheezing, 251
  for functional/mental health problems
    abuse situations, 193
    ADHD, 175
    breastfeeding/slow weight gain (infants), 103
    constipation (school-age children), 115
    depression (adolescents), 207
    LGBT issues, 221
    overweight (preschoolers), 85
    PPEs, 133
    sleep patterns (infants), 163
    well-child care (infants), 75–76
off-label drug use, 68

olopatadine HCl (Patanol, Pataday), 343t
Omnicef. *See* cefdinir (Omnicef)
Opcon-A. *See* naphazoline HCl/pheniramine (Naphcon A, Opcon-A)
Optivar. *See* azelastine HCl (Optivar)
oral antibiotics. *See* antibiotics
oral steroids, 260
oral trauma, 405–416
  case presentations for, 405–406, 411–413
  diagnosis of, 405–414
    avulsion, permanent incisors, 405–414, 409f
    avulsion, primary incisors, 405–414, 408f
    crown fracture, permanent incisor with/without pulp exposure, 405–414, 410f
    history-taking, 406
    PERRLA mnemonic, 407
    physical examination, 406–407
  epidemiology/etiology of, 407–411
  fundamental contexts of, 405, 414
  management of, 411–414
    complications, 412–414
    educational plans, 414
    follow-up visits, 414
    prognosis, 411–414
  objectives for, 405
  resources for, 414–415
oro-motor development, 15–16
osmotic diarrhea, 390
overweight (preschoolers), 85–102
  BMI and, 89–90
  Bright Futures themes and, 85–86, 86–87
    developmental surveillance, 87
    healthy weight, 87–88
    injury prevention, 87
    nutrition, 87–88
    oral health, 87
    physical activity, 87–88
    safety concerns, 87
  case presentation for, 85–88, 90–93, 97–98
  comorbidities of, 90
  diagnosis of, 93
    diagnostic criteria, 90
    history-taking, 90–92
    physical examinations, 92–93
  epidemiology/etiology of, 88–90
  fundamental contexts of, 85, 98–99
  high blood sugar. *See* overweight/high blood sugar
  management of, 94–95
    AAP four-stage approach, 94–95
    follow-up visits, 98
    nutrition guidelines, 94

physical activity guidelines, 94
USDA MyPyramid, 94, 96–97
objectives for, 85
prevention of, 96–98
family motivation for change, 96
parenting skills, 96
therapeutic plans, 96–97
resources for, 99–101
overweight/high blood sugar, 267–290
case presentation for, 267–269, 275–276, 283–284
diagnosis of, 268–276
ADA criteria, 270–271, 271t
blood glucose diaries, 268t
diabetes, 269–284
differential, 275–276, 275t
history-taking, 267–268
obesity, 271–284
physical examination, 268–269
prediabetes, 270–271, 271t
epidemiology/etiology of, 269–275
Bogalusa Heart Study, 272–273
DCCT, 274–275
ERIC, 274
pathophysiology, 269–271
SEARCH for Diabetes in Youth Study, 272–274
TODAY Study, 277
TRIGR study, 273–274
type 1 diabetes, 273–275, 275t
type 2 diabetes, 269–271, 275t
fundamental contexts of, 267–268, 284
management of, 270t, 276–284
CDC Healthy Weight recommendations, 278–279
comorbidities, 280–281
depression, 281
developmental factors, 279–280
DHHS recommendations, 279
dyslipidemia, 280–281
education plans, 282–284
follow-up visits, 284
hypertension, 280
medications, 277–278
microvascular complications, 281
NDEP, 270t
nutritional changes, 278–279
physical activity changes, 279
renal disease, 281
sociocutural factors, 281–282
therapy goals, 277
treatment options, 277–278
objectives for, 267
preschoolers and. *See* overweight
(preschoolers)

resources for, 270t

P

Pap smears, 428
ParaGard intrauterine device, 433
parainfluenza virus, 378, 379t
parasitic agents, 388
parenteral fluids, 399
paroxetine (Paxil), 215–219, 217t
Participation sports examinations. *See* PPEs
(participation sports examinations)
Pataday. *See* olopatadine HCl (Patanol, Pataday)
Patanol. *See* olopatadine HCl (Patanol, Pataday)
pathogens
Bordetella pertussis, 379t
Campylobacter jejuni, 388
Chlamydia trachomatis, 379t, 382–383, 382t
Chlamydophila pneumonia, 378–379, 379t
Entamoeba histolytica, 388
Escherichia coli, 388, 418, 420
Giardia lamblia, 388
Haemophilus influenzae, 349
Klebsiella pneumoniae, 421
Moraxella catarrhalis, 349
Mycoplasma pneumoniae, 377–385
Propionibacterium acnes, 472
Salmonella, 388
Shigella, 388
Staphylococcus aureus, 388, 458, 469–470, 487
Streptococcus pneumoniae, 349, 378–379, 379t, 382–383, 382t
transmission of, 384–395
Paxil. *See* paroxetine (Paxil)
PDD-NOS (pervasive developmental disorder, not otherwise specified), 28
PDDST-II (Pervasive Developmental Disorder Screening Test), 35
pediatric primary care case studies
for developmental problems, 9–72
fatigue (adolescents), 59–72
gross motor delays (infants), 11–26
language/social delays (toddlers), 27–42
school failure/refusal problems, 43–58
diagnostic reasoning for, 1–8
for diseases, 232–518
acne (adolescents), 467–480
anemia (toddlers), 291–320
birth control (adolescents), 427–440
cough, 377–386
fever, 233–250

headache, 321–335
high blood sugar/overweight,
    267–290
itchy rash, 455–466
limp, 481–492
oral trauma, 405–416
recurrent ear infections (toddlers),
    347–358
red eye (preschoolers), 335–346
short stature, 507–518
syncope, 359–376
urinary urgency/incontinence
    (preschoolers), 417–426
vaginal discharge (adolescents),
    441–454
vomiting/diarrhea, 387–404
well-child care (late-preterm infants),
    493–506
wheezing, 251–266
for functional/mental health problems,
    73–230
    abuse situations, 193–206
    ADHD, 175–192
    breastfeeding/slow weight gain,
        103–114
    constipation (school-age children),
        115–132
    depression (adolescents), 207–220
    LGBT issues (adolescents), 221–231
    overweight (preschoolers), 85–102
    PPEs (adolescents), 133–163
    sleep patterns (infants), 163–175
    well-child care (infants), 75–84
Pediazole. *See* erythromycin/sulfisoxazole
    (Pediazole)
PedMIDAS tool, 330–332
penicillin, 353
permanent sterilization, 433–434
PERRLA mnemonic, 407
persistent cough, 377–386
    case presentation for, 377–378, 381,
        383–384
    diagnosis of, 378–383
        clinical manifestations, 380
        common pneumonia syndromes, 382t
        diagnostic testing, 382–383
        differential, 380–381
        history-taking, 378–379
        physical examination, 381–382
        pneumonia, 378–383
    epidemiology/etiology of, 378–380
        common pathogens, 379t
        pathophysiology, 378–379
    fundamental contexts of, 377–385
    management of, 383–385
        educational plans, 384
        follow-up visits, 384

hospitalization *vs.* home care, 383
    medications, 383–385
    pathogen transmission, 384–395
    prognosis, 384–395
Mycoplasma pneumoniae, 377–385
objectives of, 377
resources for, 385
Pervasive Developmental Disorder Screening
    Test. *See* PDDST-II (Pervasive
    Developmental Disorder Screening Test)
pharyngitis, 235–247
pimecrolimus (Elidel), 462
pink eye. *See* red eye (preschoolers)
pityriasis rosea, 459
PMDD (premenstrual dysphoric disorder), 432
pneumonia
    case presentation for, 377–378, 381,
        383–384
    diagnosis of, 378–383
        clinical manifestations, 380
        common pneumonia syndromes, 382t
        diagnostic testing, 382–383
        differential, 380–381
        history-taking, 378–379
        physical examination, 381–382
        pneumonia, 378–383
    epidemiology/etiology of, 378–380
        common pathogens, 379t
        pathophysiology, 378–379
    fundamental contexts of, 377–385
    management of, 383–385
        educational plans, 384
        follow-up visits, 384
        hospitalization *vs.* home care, 383
        medications, 383–385
        pathogen transmission, 384–395
        prognosis, 384–395
    Mycoplasma pneumoniae, 377–385
    objectives of, 377
    resources for, 385
postconcussive syndrome, 142–143
PPEs (participation sports examinations),
    133–163
    case presentation for, 134, 140–142, 145,
        157–158
    clearance, 137t–139t, 158
        condition-based, 137t–139t
        preparticipation permission, 158
    diagnoses and, 151
    follow-up visits for, 158
    forms for, 135f–136f
    fundamental contexts of, 133, 158–159
    history-taking for, 141–142
    management of, 152–158, 152t, 154t–155t
        concussion, 152t
        family planning/lifestyle issues, 158
        female athlete triad, 143–144, 157

fractures, 144–145
general, 153, 154t–156t, 157
medroxyprogesterone (Depo-
Provera), 145
musculoskeletal disorders, 144–145
postconcussive syndrome, 142–143
second-impact syndrome, 158
objectives for, 133
physical examinations for, 145–151
diagnostic testing, 145, 151
features of, 150t
musculoskeletal, 145–149, 146f–149f
readiness factors for, 140–142
resources for, 159–160
risk factor assessments, 134
prediabetes, 270–271, 271t
prednisolone, 260
pregnancy testing, 428
premenstrual dysphoric disorder. *See* PMDD
(premenstrual dysphoric disorder)
preschooler-specific concerns
anemia (toddlers), 291–320
diagnostic reasoning for, 1–8
language/social delays (toddlers), 27–42
overweight, 85–102
red eye, 335–346
urinary urgency/incontinence, 417–426
presentation of cases. *See* case studies
(pediatric primary care)
primary care case studies
for developmental problems, 9–72
fatigue (adolescents), 59–72
gross motor delays (infants), 11–26
language/social delays (toddlers),
27–42
school failure/refusal problems,
43–58
diagnostic reasoning for, 1–8
for diseases, 232–518
acne (adolescents), 467–480
anemia (toddlers), 291–320
birth control (adolescents), 427–440
cough, 377–386
fever, 233–250
headache, 321–335
high blood sugar/overweight,
267–290
itchy rash, 455–466
limp, 481–492
oral trauma, 405–416
recurrent ear infections (toddlers),
347–358
red eye (preschoolers), 335–346
short stature, 507–518
syncope, 359–376
urinary urgency/incontinence
(preschoolers), 417–426

vaginal discharge (adolescents),
441–454
vomiting/diarrhea, 387–404
well-child care (late-preterm infants),
493–506
wheezing, 251–266
for functional/mental health problems,
73–230
abuse situations, 193–206
ADHD, 175–192
breastfeeding/slow weight gain,
103–114
constipation (school-age children),
115–132
depression (adolescents), 207–220
LGBT issues (adolescents), 221–231
overweight (preschoolers), 85–102
PPEs (adolescents), 133–163
sleep patterns (infants), 163–175
well-child care (infants), 75–84
problem domains, 2–3
progesterone/estrogen, 430–431, 431t
Propionibacterium acnes, 472
Protopic. *See* tacrolimus (Protopic)
Prozac. *See* fluoxetine (Prozac)
pseudomembranous colitis, 395–396
psoralen plus ultraviolet A light therapy. *See*
PUVA (psoralen plus ultraviolet A light)
therapy
psoriasis, 459
psychoeducation, 213–214
PUVA (psoralen plus ultraviolet A light)
therapy, 462

R
radioallergosorbent/skin prick testing. *See*
RAST/SPT (radioallergosorbent/skin
prick testing)
rash, itchy, 455–466
AD, 455–464
antibiotics for, 462–463
antivirals for, 463
Atopiclair for, 463
diagnosis of, 456, 459
differential diagnosis for, 459
epidemiology/etiology of, 456
follow-up visits for, 463–464
history-taking, 459
management of, 459–464
medications for, 460–463, 461t
MimyX for, 463
parental/patient education for,
463–464
pathophysiology of, 457
physical examination, 456
presentation of, 457–458
PUVA therapy for, 462

RAST/SPT, 458
systemic steroids for, 462
TCIs for, 462
topical corticosteroids for, 460–462,
    461t
triggers of, 458–459
case presentation for, 455, 459, 463–464
fundamental contexts of, 455–456
objectives for, 455
resources for, 465–466
RAST/SPT (radioallergosorbent/skin prick
    testing), 458
reasoning, diagnostic, 1–8
best evidence *vs.* best practice and, 1, 5
care models and, 5
caregiving teams and, 5–6
complicating contexts of, 3–5
    comorbidities, 4–5
    cultural, 5
    developmental, 3
    family-centered care, 4
evidence-based care and, 1–2
fundamental contexts of, 1–2, 6
problem domains and, 2–3
processes for, 5
resources for, 7
recurrent ear infections (toddlers), 347–358
case presentation for, 347–348, 351,
    354–355
diagnosis of, 350–356
    AOM, 347–356
    diagnostic testing, 352
    history-taking, 348–351
    OME, 347–356
    physical examination, 351
epidemiology/etiology of, 348–350
    pathophysiology, 350–351
    risk factors, 349–350
fundamental contexts of, 347–348, 357
management of, 352–356
    AAP recommendations, 353–356
    education plans, 354
    follow-up visits, 354–355
    medications, 352–356, 353t, 355t
    SNAP, 353
    therapeutic plans, 352–353
objectives for, 347
resources for, 357–358
red eye (preschoolers), 335–346
case presentation for, 335, 338, 344
conjunctivitis, 336–344
    diagnosis of, 338–340
    differential diagnosis of, 339–340
    educational plans for, 344
    epidemiology/etiology of, 336
    history-taking, 336–338, 337t
    management of, 340–344

medications for, 341–342, 343t
    physical examinations, 338
    therapeutic plans, 340–341
fundamental contexts of, 334, 335–336
objectives for, 335
resources for, 345
Remeron. *See* mirtazapine (Remeron)
renal disease, 281
resources
for developmental problems
    fatigue (adolescents), 71–72
    gross motor delays (infants), 25–26
    language/social delays (toddlers),
        40–41, 40b
for diagnostic reasoning, 7
for diseases
    acne (adolescents), 479–480
    AD, 465–466
    anemia (toddlers), 317–320
    birth control (adolescents), 439–440
    cough, 385
    diarrhea/vomiting, 401–402
    fever, 248–249
    headache, 333
    late-preterm infants (well-child care),
        505–506
    limp, 491–492
    oral trauma, 414–415
    overweight/high blood sugar, 270t
    recurrent ear infections (toddlers),
        357–358
    red eye (preschoolers), 345
    short stature, 516–517
    syncope, 374–375
    urinary urgency/incontinence
        (preschoolers), 426
    vaginal discharge (adolescents),
        453–454
    wheezing, 264–266
for functional/mental health problems
    abuse situations, 205–206
    ADHD, 191–192
    breastfeeding/slow weight gain
        (infants), 113
    constipation (school-age children),
        131–132
    depression (adolescents), 210, 219–220
    LGBT issues, 230
    overweight (preschoolers), 99–101
    PPEs, 159–160
    sleep patterns (infants), 172–173
    well-child care (infants), 83
respiratory syncytial virus. *See* RSV
    (respiratory syncytial virus)
Retin-A. *See* tretinoin (Retin-A, Avita)
retinoids, topical, 472, 474t–477t
rhinovirus, 379t

Rocephin. *See* ceftriaxone (Rocephin)
Rome III criteria, 117t
rotavirus, 388
RSV (respiratory syncytial virus), 349, 378–379

S
SABAs (short acting beta$_2$-agonists), 260
safety net antibiotic prescription. *See* SNAP
    (safety net antibiotic prescription)
Salmonella, 388
school-age children-specific concerns
    ADHD, 175–193
    for adolescents. *See* adolescent-specific
        concerns
    constipation, 115–132
    diagnostic reasoning for, 1–8
    PPEs, 133–163
    recurrent ear infections, 347–358
    school failure/refusal problems, 43–58
school failure/refusal problems, 43–58
    case presentation for, 43, 45–46, 49–50, 55
    diagnosis of, 43–46
    fundamental contexts of, 43, 56
    management of, 47–55
    objectives for, 43
    resources for, 56–57
SEARCH for Diabetes in Youth Study,
    272–274
second-impact syndrome, 158
secretory diarrhea, 390
selective serotonin reuptake inhibitors. *See*
    SSRIs (selective serotonin reuptake
    inhibitors)
sensitivity *vs.* specificity, 240–242
separation anxiety, 170–171
sepsis screening, 494
serotonin syndrome, 217–218
sertraline (Zoloft), 215–219, 217t
sexual orientation issues (adolescents),
    221–231
    adolescent sexual expression, 225–227
        American Community Survey (U.S.
            Census Bureau), 225
        epidemiology/etiology of, 225–227
        Kinsey Institute studies, 225–226
    case presentation for, 221, 224–229
    definitions, 222t
    diagnosis of, 228
    fundamental contexts of, 221–223, 229
    management of, 229
    objectives for, 221
    related health risk factors, 221, 223–228
        depression, 227–228. *See also*
            depression (adolescents)
        healthcare avoidance, 223–224
        mental health risks, 223
        STDs, 221, 223, 226–228

    suicide, 227–228
    violence risks, 223
    resources for, 230
sexually transmitted diseases. *See* STDs
    (sexually transmitted diseases)
Shigella, 388
short acting beta$_2$-agonists. *See* SABAs (short
    acting beta$_2$-agonists)
short stature, 507–518
    case presentation for, 507–508, 511–512,
        514–515
    diagnosis of, 507–512
        diagnostic testing, 511
        differential, 508–511, 510t–511t
        epidemiology/etiology, 509
        history-taking, 507–508
        physical examination, 508–509
        Turner syndrome, 509–516,
            510t–511t
    fundamental contexts for, 507–508, 516
    management of, 512–516
        AAP guidelines, 512
        cardiovascular issues, 512–513
        endocrine issues, 513
        follow-up visits, 515–516
        genetic issues, 514
        neurocognitive issues, 513
        NIH guidelines, 512
        psychosocial support, 513–514
        referrals, 514–515
        Turner Syndrome Consensus Study
            Group guidelines, 512
    objectives for, 507
    resources for, 516–517
skin barrier dysfunction, 457
sleep patterns (infants), 163–175
    case presentation for, 163–166, 169–172
    cultural/ethnic aspects of, 167
    diagnosis of, 164–165, 168
        developmental issues, 166
        history-taking, 164
        normal sleep physiology, 165–166
        trained night feeders, 166
        physical examinations, 166–167
    epidemiology/etiology of, 163–166
    fundamental contexts of, 163, 172
    management of, 168–172
        Ferber method, 169–170
        follow-up visits, 171–172
        routine establishment, 170–171
        separation anxiety, 170–171
        therapeutic plans, 168–171, 169b
    objectives for, 163
    resources for, 172–173
SNAP (safety net antibiotic prescription), 353
SNOUT mnemonic, 241t
social/language delays (toddlers), 27–42

ASDs, 28–40, 29t, 30f
    AAP screen recommendations for, 27–28, 35, 39
    ABA and, 37–38
    AD, 28, 30f
    AS, 28
    CARS and, 37
    CHAT and, 35
    diagnosis of, 33–35, 34b
    diagnostic testing for, 35–37, 36f
    DSM-IV-TR criteria for, 30f
    epidemiology/etiology of, 29, 31
    history-taking for, 31–32
    M-CHAT and, 35, 36f
    management of, 37–39
    PDD-NOS, 28
    PDDST-II and, 35
    physical examinations for, 33
    plans, intervention, 37–38
    prognosis for, 39
    TEACCH and, 37–38
  case presentation for, 27–28
  developmental milestones and, 28, 29t
  fundamental contexts of, 27–28, 39
  objectives for, 27
  plans for
    diagnostic, 37
    educational, 37–39
    intervention, 37–38
  resources for, 40–41, 40b
specificity vs., sensitivity, 240–242
spermicides, 433
SPIN mnemonic, 241t
sports examinations (adolescents), 133–163
  case presentation for, 134, 140–142, 145, 157–158
  clearance, 137t–139t, 158
  diagnosis of, 151
  follow-up visits for, 158
  forms for, 135f–136f
  fundamental contexts of, 133, 158–159
  history-taking for, 141–142
  management of, 152–158, 152t, 154t–155t
    concussion, 152t
    family planning/lifestyle issues, 158
    female athlete triad, 143–144, 157
    fractures, 144–145
    general, 153, 154t–156t, 157
    medroxyprogesterone (Depo-Provera), 145
    musculoskeletal disorders, 144–145
    postconcussive syndrome, 142–143
    second-impact syndrome, 158
  objectives for, 133
  physical examinations for, 145–151
    diagnostic testing, 145, 151
    features of, 150t
    musculoskeletal, 145–149, 146f–149f
  readiness factors for, 140–142
  resources for, 159–160
  risk factor assessments, 134
SSRIs (selective serotonin reuptake inhibitors), 215–219, 217t
staged overweight approach, 95
Staphylococcus aureus, 388, 458, 469–470, 487
stature, short, 507–518
  case presentation for, 507–508, 511–512, 514–515
  diagnosis of, 507–512
    diagnostic testing, 511
    differential, 508–511, 510t–511t
    epidemiology/etiology, 509
    history-taking, 507–508
    physical examination, 508–509
    Turner syndrome, 509–516, 510t–511t
  fundamental contexts for, 507–508, 516
  management of, 512–516
    AAP guidelines, 512
    cardiovascular issues, 512–513
    endocrine issues, 513
    follow-up visits, 515–516
    genetic issues, 514
    neurocognitive issues, 513
    NIH guidelines, 512
    psychosocial support, 513–514
    referrals, 514–515
    Turner Syndrome Consensus Study Group guidelines, 512
  objectives for, 507
  resources for, 516–517
STDs (sexually transmitted diseases), 221, 223, 226–228
Stelatopia, 460
steroids
  oral, 260
  systemic, 462
Streptococcus pneumoniae, 349, 378–379, 379t, 382–383, 382t
studies (pediatric primary care)
  for developmental problems, 9–72
    fatigue (adolescents), 59–72
    gross motor delays (infants), 11–26
    language/social delays (toddlers), 27–42
    school failure/refusal problems, 43–58
  diagnostic reasoning for, 1–8
  for diseases, 232–518
    acne (adolescents), 467–480
    anemia (toddlers), 291–320
    birth control (adolescents), 427–440
    cough, 377–386
    fever, 233–250

headache, 321–335
high blood sugar/overweight,
    267–290
itchy rash, 455–466
limp, 481–492
oral trauma, 405–416
recurrent ear infections (toddlers),
    347–358
red eye (preschoolers), 335–346
short stature, 507–518
syncope, 359–376
urinary urgency/incontinence
    (preschoolers), 417–426
vaginal discharge (adolescents),
    441–454
vomiting/diarrhea, 387–404
well-child care (late-preterm infants),
    493–506
wheezing, 251–266
for functional/mental health problems,
    73–230
abuse situations, 193–206
ADHD, 175–192
breastfeeding/slow weight gain
    (infants), 103–114
constipation (school-age children),
    115–132
depression (adolescents), 207–220
LGBT issues (adolescents), 221–231
overweight (preschoolers), 85–102
PPEs (adolescents), 133–163
sleep patterns (infants), 163–175
well-child care (infants), 75–84
suicide risks, 227–228
sulfamethoxazole, 421
sulfonylureas, 278
syncope, 359–376
case presentation for, 360, 366–368, 370,
    372–373
diagnosis of, 363–373
    diagnostic testing, 363, 368–370
    ECGs, 370
    emergent evaluations, 370, 371f
    history-taking, 363–367
    imaging studies, 370
    laboratory blood work, 369–370
    physical examinations, 367–368
    red flags, 364–365
epidemiology/etiology of, 360–361, 361t
    causal factors, 360–361, 360–363,
        361t
    definitions, 360
    recurrent episodes, 363
fundamental contexts of, 359–360, 374
management of, 372–373
    best practice evidence, 372–373
    referral vs. admission indictors, 372

objectives for, 359
resources for, 374–375
systemic steroids, 462

T
T-cell downregulation, 457
tacrolimus (Protopic), 462
TADS (Treatment of Adolescent Depression
    Study), 213
TCIs (total calcineurin inhibitors), 462
TEACCH (Treatment and Education of Autistic
    and Related Communication-
    Handicapped Children) program, 37–38
teams, caregiving, 5–6
teen-specific concerns
    acne, 467–480
    birth control, 427–440
    depression, 207–220
    diagnostic reasoning for, 1–8
    fatigue, 59–72
    late-preterm infants (adolescent parents),
        493–506
    LGBT issues, 221–231
    PPEs, 133–163
    vaginal discharge, 441–454
telephone consultations, 391–395
tension-type headaches. See TTHs (tension-
    type headaches)
tetracycline, 475t–477t
therapeutic management. See management
thiazolidinediones, 278
tinea corporis, 459
TODAY Study, 277
toddler-specific concerns. See also
    preschooler-specific concerns
    anemia, 291–320
    diagnostic reasoning for, 1–8
    language/social delays, 27–42
    recurrent ear infections, 347–358
topical medications
    antibiotics. See antibiotics
    corticosteroids. See corticosteroids
    retinoids, 472, 474t–477t
total calcineurin inhibitors. See TCIs (total
    calcineurin inhibitors)
toxic megacolon, 395–396
toxic synovitis. See TS (toxic synovitis)
toxins, environmental, 296–299, 298t–299t
toxoplasmosis, 235–236
transgendered issues. See LGBT (lesbian, gay,
    bisexual, and transgendered) issues
trauma, oral, 405–416
    case presentations for, 405–406, 411–413
    diagnosis of, 405–414
        avulsion, permanent incisors,
            405–414, 409f

avulsion, primary incisors, 405–414, 408f
    crown fracture, permanent incisor with/without pulp exposure, 405–414, 410f
    history-taking, 406
    PERRLA mnemonic, 407
    physical examination, 406–407
    epidemiology/etiology of, 407–411
    fundamental contexts of, 405, 414
    management of, 411–414
        complications, 412–414
        educational plans, 414
        follow-up visits, 414
        prognosis, 411–414
    objectives for, 405
    resources for, 414–415
Treatment and Education of Autistic and Related Communication-Handicapped Children program. See TEACCH (Treatment and Education of Autistic and Related Communication-Handicapped Children) program
Treatment of Adolescent Depression Study. See TADS (Treatment of Adolescent Depression Study)
tretinoin (Retin-A, Avita), 474t–477t
TriCeram, 460
tricyclic antidepressants, 218
trigeminal autonomic cephalalgias, 322, 324–328. See also headache
TRIGR study, 273–274
trimethoprim-sulfamethoxazole, 421–423, 475t–477t
TS (toxic synovitis), 487
TTHs (tension-type headaches), 322, 324–328. See also headache
tuberculosis, 380
Turner syndrome, 507–518
    case presentation for, 507–508, 511–512, 514–515
    diagnosis of, 507–512
        diagnostic testing, 511
        differential, 508–511, 510t–511t
        epidemiology/etiology, 509
        history-taking, 507–508
        physical examination, 508–509
    fundamental contexts for, 507–508, 516
    management of, 512–516
        AAP guidelines, 512
        cardiovascular issues, 512–513
        endocrine issues, 513
        follow-up visits, 515–516
        genetic issues, 514
        neurocognitive issues, 513
        NIH guidelines, 512
        psychosocial support, 513–514

        referrals, 514–515
        Turner Syndrome Consensus Study Group guidelines, 512
    objectives for, 507
    resources for, 516–517
type 1 diabetes, 273–275, 275t
type 2 diabetes, 269–271, 275t

U
United States departments and agencies
    DHHS. See DHHS (Department of Health and Human Services)
    USDA. See USDA (United States Department of Agriculture)
urinary urgency/incontinence (preschoolers), 417–426
    case presentation for, 417–420, 422, 425
    diagnosis of, 417–430
        diagnostic testing, 419, 421–422
        differential, 420
        history-taking, 417–420
        physical examination, 418
        UTI, 417–425
    epidemiology/etiology of, 418–419
        pathophysiology, 418
        social/economic factors, 419
    fundamental contexts of, 417, 425
    management of, 420–425
        complications, 425
        dysfunction elimination syndrome, 422
        follow-up visits, 424–425
        medications, 421–422
        patient education, 424
        vesicoureteral reflux, 422–424
    objectives for, 417
    resources for, 426
urine human chorionic gonadotropin testing, 428
USDA (United States Department of Agriculture), 94–97, 438
UTI (urinary tract infection), 417–425. See also urinary urgency/incontinence (preschoolers)

V
vaginal discharge (adolescents), 441–454
    case presentation for, 441–444, 446, 448, 451
    diagnosis of, 441–448
        CDC Five Ps, 442–443, 443b
        chlamydia trachomatis, 446–447
        diagnostic testing, 444–448
        gonorrhea, 447
        HIV, 448
        physical examination, 444–446
        sexual history-taking, 441–444, 443b

STD risk factors, 445b
syphilis, 447
epidemiology/etiology of, 446
fundamental contexts of, 441–452
management of, 449–452
contraceptive need, 448–451
counseling, 449–451
follow-up visits, 452
STI medications, 451–452, 452b
objectives for, 441
resources for, 453–454
Vanderbilt assessment, 180–181
Vantin. *See* cefpodoxime (Vantin)
Vaseline, 460
vasoconstrictors/antihistamines, 343t
VCUG (voiding cystourethrogram), 422
venlafaxine (Effexor), 218
vesicoureteral reflux. *See* VUR (vesicoureteral
reflux)
ViaSpan, 409
violence risks, 223, 227–228
voiding cystourethrogram. *See* VCUG (voiding
cystourethrogram)
vomiting/diarrhea, 387–404
case presentation for, 387–388, 394–395,
400
diagnosis of, 392–397
death risk factors, 391–392
diagnostic testing, 396–397
differential, 393t, 395–396
history-taking, 391–395
hospitalization risk factors, 391–392
telephone consultations, 391–395
epidemiology/etiology of, 388–395
acute *vs.* chronic diarrhea, 391–392
causative agents, 388–389
CNDC, 391–392
pathophysiology, 389–390
fundamental contexts of, 387, 400–401
gastroenteritis, 397–401
management of, 397–400
feeding resumption, 397–399
follow-up visits, 399–400
hydration/rehydration, 397, 398t
medications, 399
objectives for, 387
resources for, 401–402
VUR (vesicoureteral reflux), 418, 422–423

W

warfarin toxicity, 306, 308
WBC (white blood cell) counts, 500
weight-related concerns
breastfeeding/slow weight gain (infants),
103–114
high blood sugar/overweight, 267–290
overweight (preschoolers), 85–102

well-child care
infants, 75–84
AAP initial visit recommendations,
75
Bright Futures guidelines for, 79–80
case presentation for, 76–79, 81–82
diagnosis of, 78–82
follow-up visits for, 80–81
fundamental contexts of, 75–76, 82
military family needs and, 81–82
newborn jaundice, 77–82
objectives for, 75–76
resources for, 83
late-preterm infants, 493–506
case presentation for, 493, 496–501,
504
diagnosis of, 496–501
epidemiology/etiology of, 494–496
fundamental contexts for, 493, 505
hyperbilirubinemia, 494–495
immunizations, 503–504
jaundice, 494–495
lung function, 494
management of, 501–504
metabolic function, 495
objectives for, 493
resources for, 505–506
sepsis, 494
temperature regulation, 495
Wellbutrin. *See* bupropion (Wellbutrin)
wheezing, 251–266
case presentation for, 251–252, 259–260,
263
diagnosis of, 252–253, 259–260
diagnostic testing, 259
EPR-3 guidelines, 259–260
history-taking, 252–253
NAEPP (National Asthma Education
and Prevention Program)
guidelines, 259–260, 261t–263t
NHLBI guidelines, 259–260
physical examinations, 252–253, 259
severity classification, 259–260
epidemiology/etiology of, 252–259
AAP tobacco smoke policy statement,
255
asthma, 253–257
Asthma and Allergy Foundation cost
data, 254
causal factors, 257, 257t
CDC data, 253–255
child wheezers, 258–259
infant wheezers, 258
National Center for Health Statistics
data, 254–255
NHANES III data, 254–255
NHIS data, 255

pathophysiology, 255–257, 256f
risk factors, 258–259
fundamental contexts of, 251–252, 264
management of, 251, 260–264
environmental factors control, 260,
263
follow-up visits, 263–264
medications, 260–263
objectives for, 251
resources for, 264–266
white blood cell counts. *See* WBC (white
blood cell) counts
WHO (World Health Organization)
fluid replacement guidelines, 397–398
pneumonia data, 379–380
WIC (Women, Infants, and Children) program,
503
World Health Organization. *See* WHO (World
Health Organization)

Y
Youth Behavior Study, 210–212
youth/young adult-specific concerns
acne, 467–480
birth control, 427–440
depression, 207–220
diagnostic reasoning for, 1–8
fatigue, 59–72
late-preterm infants (adolescent parents),
493–506
LGBT issues, 221–231
PPEs, 133–163
vaginal discharge, 441–454

Z
Zaditor. *See* ketotifen fumarate (Zaditor)
zinc, 399
Zoloft. *See* sertraline (Zoloft)
Zyrtec. *See* cetirizine (Zyrtec)